DEDICATION

To the real heroes of patient education—
those nurses and other health care providers
who are on the front lines educating
and empowering patients and their families.

Authors

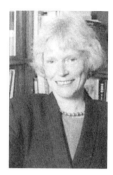

Sally Heller Rankin began her career in social work in the 1960s and became convinced while making home visits that clients needed more than she could offer as a caseworker. She noted their needs for health education at that time and decided to pursue nursing. She received her BSN from California State University, Los Angeles.

After working as a staff nurse at Duke University Medical Center and in inservice education, she obtained her MSN from Duke University where she taught for 2 years. During her years at Duke she began work on the first edition of *Patient Education: Issues, Principles, and Practices.* Returning to California in the early 80s, she taught at Mt. St. Mary's College and the University of Southern California and then moved to the San Francisco area. Sally completed her Ph.D. at the University of California-San Francisco (UCSF) in 1988, and then went on the faculty, receiving her certificate from Sonoma State University as a Family Nurse Practitioner in 1991. Following 5 years at Boston College she returned to UCSF where she is currently an Associate Professor and Director of the Family Nurse Practitioner Program. Her clinical practice areas have included cardiac nursing, diabetes education, and primary care practice in student health. Sally received the Distinguished Alumna award from Duke University School of Nursing, the Carol Lindeman New Investigator Award from the Western Institute of Nursing, and is a fellow in the American Academy of Nursing.

Her work in the area of patient education has been informed by her research interests in the area of chronic illness, especially coronary artery disease and diabetes mellitus, both diseases that take a tremendous toll on the individual and family members. Dr. Rankin completed a study of women recovering from myocardial infarction in 1995, completed a second study of elders recovering from MI in 1998, and is currently the Principal Investigator of an intervention study that attempts to improve health outcomes for unpartnered elders post-MI or bypass graft surgery; these studies have been funded by the National Institute of Nursing Research.

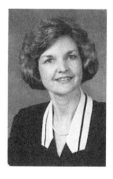

Karen Duffy Stallings began her career as a psychiatric staff nurse at Duke University Medical Center after graduating with her BSN from Boston College. Her master's degree in Adult Education is from the University of North Carolina at Chapel Hill. This formal education was enhanced with rich learning gained from the patients and families to whom she provided care and dedicated nurse colleagues committed to patient empowerment. She worked as a staff nurse and head nurse in a family medicine program, where she participated in the teaching of medical residents and nursing students. It was during this time that she and Sally Rankin began work on the first edition of Patient Education. Karen later served as a hospital staff development coordinator for oncology, orthopedics, and psychiatry, provided continuing education courses for nurses and directed a Refresher Program for inactive RNs who wished to resume their clinical practice.

Her involvement with the North Carolina's AHEC (area health education centers) Program has developed over most of her twenty five years as nurse and has afforded opportunities to teach, consult, and promote interdisciplinary approaches to patient education among the state's health care providers.

Karen's current position is that of Associate Director in the North Carolina AHEC Program Office. She provides leadership and administrative support for initiatives in nursing, mental health, and health promotion which link NC university health science centers and the state's communities in efforts to meet primary health care needs. She oversees a grants program to develop clinical experiences for undergraduate and graduate nursing programs in rural primary care sites. She is also an adjunct instructor for the University of North Carolina at Chapel Hill School of Nursing. In addition to work in her home state, Karen is a national speaker and consultant on the topic of patient education.

Contributors

Ronna E. Krozy received her basic nursing education at Beth Israel Hospital School of Nursing, Boston, MA, her B.S. and M.S. in Community Health Nursing from Boston College, and her Ed.D. in Health Education, with a subspeciality in Sex Education, from Boston University. She has been teaching Community Health Nursing since 1973 and has served as Department Chair. Dr. Krozy has developed numerous community-based programs on health promotion, sexuality, and aging, with particular emphasis on incorporating cultural competence. She created and serves as faculty coordinator for the Por Cristo-BSCON Health Project, teaching community health nursing through an overseas immersion experience in Ecuador.

Barbara E. Hollinger is an Associate Clinical Professor at the University of California, San Franciso in the Department of Family Health Care Nursing. She completed her B.S. in Nursing from California State University, Sacramento and her M.S. in Nursing with a Family Nurse Practitioner (FNP) specialty from California State University, Fresno. Her work experience includes 2½ years working in the Andes in Peru, 10 years as an FNP in a predominantly farm worker clinic in Firebaugh, California, and current practice at the UCSF School of Nursing faculty practice at Valencia Health Services in the Mission District of San Francisco. Her special interest in cross cultural nursing led to her master's thesis "Health Perception for the Hmong" based on an ethnographic study done in Fresno, California and the development of a UCSF course entitled Farm Worker Primary Health.

Ellen M. Robinson received her Ph.D. in Nursing with a concentration in Ethics at Boston College, Chestnut Hill, MA in 1997. Her dissertation, entitled, "Wives Struggle in Living Through Treatment Decisions for Their Husbands with Advanced Alzheimer's Disease," was supported by a National Research Service Award and by a Pre-Doctoral Fellowship through the Department of Veterans' Affairs. Dr. Robinson completed a fellowship in medical ethics at Harvard Medical School, Division of Medical Ethics, in 1998. She is currently a clinical nurse specialist at Massachusetts General Hospital (MGH), where she serves on the hospital's Optimum Care Committee, one of the country's oldest ethics consultation committees dealing with end-of-life treatment issues confronting patients, families, and health care providers. In addition, Dr. Robinson serves leadership position on the Ethics in Clinical Practice Committee, one of MGH's Patient Care Services Collaborative Governance committees.

Marilyn P. Verhey received her baccalaureate degree in Nursing, a master's degree in Psychiatric and Community Mental Health Nursing, her doctorate in Curriculum, Instruction, and Administration from Boston College. She is a professor in the School of Nursing at San Francisco State University, where she teaches community health education program planning and evaluation. Dr. Verhey serves as a Clinical Nurse Specialist for Patient Education at the University of California, San Francisco Medical Center. She was the consultant to the Department of Veterans' Affairs National Interdisciplinary Patient Education Task Group and developed a program of community-based health education services at the Mission High School Health Center. Dr. Verhey also holds a master's degree in Library Science from the University of Illinois and has a strong interest in client access to health information.

Karen S. Zeliff is a medical librarian who received her MLS from the University of North Carolina at Greensboro in 1990. As an Outreach Librarian for the Greensboro Area Health Education Center/Moses Cone Health System her primary responsibility was to train health providers to use the Internet to access information for their clinical practice and professional education. Currently, as Director of Education Technology Services for the AHEC, the primary focus of her work has been to develop Internet-based health information and education resources.

Reviewers

Patricia M. Bufalino, RN, MA, MN, FNP
Associate Professor of Nursing
Riverside Community College
Riverside, California

Fran London, RN, MS
Health Education Specialist
The Emily Center, Phoenix Children's Hospital
Phoenix, Arizona

Sheila Stroman, PhD
Assistant Professor of Nursing
University of Central Arkansas
Conway, Arkansas

Mary Welhaven, RN, PhD
Associate Professor
Winona State University-Rochester Center
Rochester, Minnesota

Shila Wiebe, RN, MSN
Director of Undergraduate Nursing Program
Azusa Pacific University, School of Nursing
Azusa, California

Preface

Seventeen years ago the first edition of *Patient Education: Issues, Principles, and Guidelines* reflected our youthful enthusiasm for an area of health care and nursing practice that was in its infancy. We were certain that patient education was the panacea for frustrated patients and dissatisfied nurses and we naively believed that we could improve health care through the publication of the text. While we continue to believe in patient education as a vehicle for empowering patients and enhancing nursing satisfaction, we have extensively revised earlier editions to reflect the increasing complexity of health care, the growth of nursing as a discipline, and the exponential changes in patient education wrought by such electronic technology as the Internet.

The text is designed to be helpful to students in both generic and advanced practice nursing programs. Additionally, advanced practice nurses will find this edition even more useful than previous editions in terms of dealing with systemwide issues that affect the delivery of patient education. We believe that members of all health care disciplines will find the book valuable, but because the authors are themselves nurses practicing in nursing arenas, the work draws heavily on nursing examples and the science and research of our discipline. Since all health care providers share a central interest in the welfare of patients, readers from other disciplines will appreciate the patient-centered approach.

NEW TO THIS EDITION

Added to the fourth edition are four totally new chapters, as well as others that have been extensively revised.

Chapter 2: Health Promotion: Models and Applications to Patient Education: The growing interest in health promotion and its relationships to patient education is reflected in chapter two, a chapter that is inclusive of such fed-eral publications as the *Guide to Clinical Preventive Services* and Healthy People 2010.

Chapter 3: Integration of Cultural Systems and Beliefs: A concerted effort to include more content on culture and the importance of integrating cultural systems, beliefs and alternative healing practices with patient education strengthens the text and prepares the nurse for practice in an increasingly multicultural society.

Chapter 11: Patient Education Resources on the Internet: The amazing growth of the Internet as a tool for health education is integrated into the text in an innovative chapter on using the Internet to find and evaluate educational resources.

Chapter 14: Community-Based Patient Education Programs: Lastly, a chapter on moving patient education beyond the walls of the hospital describes innovative programs that have been established using indigenous community resources to extend the scope of patient education.

NEW FEATURES

Other new features include a user-friendly layout that utilizes color and icons representative of situations commonly confronted in patient education. Material that is considered especially important to the practicing nurse is featured in boxes that summarize key content areas; for example, the material previously covered in a question and answer "roundtable" format is now presented in easy-to-read boxes. We are hopeful that this new format will enable the busy nurse or student to quickly access helpful ideas. Case studies are liberally employed throughout the text to demonstrate methods of applying teaching-learning principles to real-life situations. Strategies for critical analysis and application to each chapter continue to be important features of this book.

ORGANIZATION

In response to nursing educators' requests, the fourth edition includes more theory-based chapters as well as the application of theoretical principles to clinical practice. Previous editions of the text were organized into three sections; the fourth edition has been reorganized into two sections: principles of contemporary patient education and applications of the principles in nursing practice. We are confident that this reorganization, in concert with other format changes, will make the text more easily accessible to our readers.

Our commitment to patient education has not changed, as we continue to view it as an essential patient empowerment tool, even though our new practice settings have changed since we wrote the first edition of this book. The first author's involvement as a family nurse practitioner in the education of students in primary care has enhanced her appreciation of the need for patient education on health promotion and disease prevention. Additionally, her research on recovery from major cardiac events has underscored the vulnerability of patients who often lack access to the most basic forms of information that would greatly enhance their recovery. The second author's work in the provision of continuing education to health care providers in the state of North Carolina and for numerous organizations throughout the country has increased her awareness of wider system issues that affect the provision of patient education in diverse settings. Her work as project director, writer, and teacher for the video teleconference project "Integrating Patient Education in Your Nursing Practice" involved sharing the stories of nurses in a variety of practice settings throughout the United States who are role models as patient educators. Feeling powerless is perhaps the most devastating aspect of illness for a patient. Patient education can be implemented by the nurse as the most effective means of returning control to the patient. Patient education can reduce feelings of helplessness and enhance the patient's ability to be the chief decision maker in the management of health and illness problems. We view patient education as the *essence* of nursing practice. In today' tumultuous health care climate created by changing mandates for health care reform, the incursion of managed care into domains that were previously solely within the purview of health care providers, the growing presence of uninsured people with little or no access to health care, and the increased acuity of patients, confident and competent nurses are even more important in the delivery of quality patient care and patient education than when this book was first written.

Sally H. Rankin, RN, PhD, FAAN
Karen Duffy Stallings, RN, MEd

Acknowledgments

Our years in nursing education and practice have provided us with a deep appreciation of our profession. The jewel in the crown of nursing practice is without doubt patient education; we are proud to be able to elucidate this jewel for continuing generations of students and practicing nurses. As we speak to audiences on the topic of patient education, we are encouraged by the comments of staff nurses who are working across all health care settings. In particular, we recognize the expertise of nurses who assume leadership roles in managed care, making patient education its centerpiece. We are awed by the dedication of nurses working in acute and primary care settings who struggle to clarify the intricacies of complex medical regimen, and we appreciate the educators who speak to the utility of our textbook.

Our text has been enhanced by the excellent work of our contributing authors: Barbara Hollinger, Ellen Robinson, Ronna Krozy, Karen Zeliff, and Marilyn Verhey. Each has highly developed knowledge in areas that have added immeasurably to the fourth edition. We would also like to express our appreciation to two advanced practice students, Rebecca Johnson and Patricia Dennehy, who while enrolled in the masters program at the University of California, San Francisco, gave generously of their time to assist the authors in gathering material, developing excellent case studies based on their own practice settings, and offering suggestions for improvement. Additionally, GlaxoWellcome, Inc., which sponsored the video production, "Integrating Patient Education in Your Nursing Practice," provided permission for use of material and photos in the fourth edition of our text. We gratefully acknowledge the generous contributions of Donna Mitchell and Horizon Video Productions (Durham, NC) who extracted the photographic images and quotes for our use from their original production. We thank the following nurses, who shared "pearls of wisdom" regarding the importance of patient education in their nursing practice: Avni Cirpilli, Lois Pradka, Janice McCartney, Marilyn McNeely, Frankie Ballard, Carolyn Holloway, Ellen Wheaton, and Nelda Bostick.

We appreciate the guidance offered by nursing editors at Lippincott Williams & Wilkins during the various revisions of this book; in particular, we recognize Carol Loyd, Nicole Walz, and Margaret Zuccarini for their help and encouragement with the fourth edition. Lastly, we gratefully acknowledge the love and support of our families, which is visible to us between the lines of the text. A special note of gratitude goes to Amy Rankin-Williams, Bill and Rob Rankin, and Frank, Sarah, and Emily Stallings.

Contents

Principles of Contemporary Patient Education

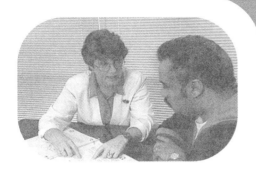

Patient Education in Nursing Practice

LEARNING OBJECTIVES

After reading this chapter, the nurse or student nurse should be able to:

1. Describe patient education as a dimension of nurse caring.

2. Define patient education.

3. Discuss the role of patient education in a reformed health care system.

4. Describe the relationship between patient education and discharge planning.

5. Describe the process of integrating patient education into nursing practice.

> *N*urses become experts in coaching a
> patient through an illness.
>
> (BENNER, 1984)

> *F*eeling powerless is perhaps the most
> devastating aspect of illness for a patient.
> Patient education is the most effective means
> of returning control to the patient by
> reducing feelings of helplessness and
> enhancing the ability to be the chief decision
> maker in the management of one's health and
> illness problems.
>
> (RANKIN & STALLINGS, 1990)

INTRODUCTION

Patient Education as a Dimension of Nurse Caring

> *N*urses clearly see themselves as advocates,
> as persons who stand along side of and
> empower patients and their families to have a
> voice when they are weak and vulnerable.
>
> (BENNER, 1984)

Caring is an integral part of nursing practice. However, studies show that this hidden work may go unrecognized by patients and their families, except when the behaviors and attitudes associated with nurse caring are missed. Caring—which helps to heal, cure, and improve a patient's health—is the essence of nursing. In several studies that describe the process of nurse caring, shared vulnerability between the nurse and the patient, and activities directed toward the welfare of the patient are identified. Nurse caring includes behaviors such as active listening, comforting, getting to know the patient as a person, respecting the patient, touching the patient, providing

information to the patient to help decision-making, recognizing that patients know themselves best, perceiving patient needs, and providing good physical care (Wolf, Giardino, Osborne, & Ambrose, 1994).

Caring includes being a patient advocate, empowering the patient to make informed decisions, and promoting autonomy. Simultaneously, caring includes making the patient feel safe, comforted, and valued (Tanner, Benner, Chesla, & Gordon, 1993). The accuracy and fidelity of clinical and caring knowledge are clarified through scientific knowledge, clinical outcomes, and personal and social understandings as they become available. Thus, clinical reasoning and caring practices are socially embedded (Benner, Tanner, & Chesla, 1996).

Patient education is a dimension of nurse caring when it considers the best interests of the patient and recognizes that the best case manager for a patient is ultimately the patient himself or herself. Nurse caring is a delicate balance of comfort and challenge and a creative ability to maximize resources for the patient's benefit. Research shows that as novice nurses move through the developmental stages of advanced beginner, competent, proficient, and expert practice, patient education becomes an integral part of nurse caring (Benner 1982, 1984; Benner & Wrubel, 1989; Benner & Tanner, 1992, 1996).

We hope that the issues, principles, and practices addressed in this text will help nursing students and novice nurses develop survival skills for teaching. For nurses working toward expert practice, we hope the text will promote a creative integration of patient education with various practice and patient populations. Furthermore, we hope expert nurses will discover validation for their teaching efforts and a call to provide leadership in research, education, and practice arenas. The stereotypical images of a caring nurse, developed early in childhood, can influence the willingness and effectiveness of nurses to become patient teachers.

We are aware, as nurse educators, that much literature is available on patient education. When we first planned this book, we thought strongly that another *how-to* approach to patient education was not needed. Instead, we examined issues that arise in our own practice environments and issues suggested by our colleagues. The first seven chapters present principles of contemporary patient education and address pressing concerns around leadership issues and administrative support for patient education, influencing and understanding patient decisions, effective work with high-risk populations, legal and ethical concerns related to patient education, and motivational theories.

As we designed the remaining chapters, we responded to nurses' questions about applying the principles of patient education. Nursing faculty members also identified specific needs of their students in the implementation of patient education. In summarizing these evaluations, we developed Chapters 8 to 15 to guide nurses from all types of practice settings as they integrate patient education into their nursing practice. We found that nurses wanted realistic approaches that consider the pressures of time, extensive patient care responsibilities, and paperwork overloads. Staff nurses find they must possess teaching skills, astutely define patient learning needs, and know how to involve patients' families. In addition, they want reassurance that patient education can be an integral part of patient care. We have attempted, throughout the text, to offer practical, realistic approaches.

How Does Patient Education Begin?

It was a rainy Saturday. In an upstairs bedroom, four sisters opened a doll hospital. Dolls of various sizes were placed carefully in shoe boxes, and each box was labeled with the patient's name. The patients were all sick, but the specific illness did not matter. The four little nurses scurried busily among the patients, giving baths, administering shots with pins from their mother's sewing basket, and applying scarf bandages and Band-Aids. They reassured their patients they would take care of everything and make them better soon. Eventually, the sisters' mother called the girls to lunch. This completed the recoveries of all the patients. The sisters dressed the dolls, put them back in their usual places, and cleaned up the messy bandages to prevent discovery of their magic treatments.

Years later, the four sisters went off to college. One sister chose to study nursing, and her first day of clinical was, in many ways, as full of adventure as that rainy Saturday. The nursing student walked onto the floors of hospitals with excitement, fear, and a certain reverence. She watched the nurses rush about, answering calls and caring for sick patients. Each nurse was assigned a patient, and the young student reached anxiously for the chart. She hoped for a patient who needed dressing changes, injections, or treatments she had never performed. She hoped she would be able to decipher the doctor's handwriting and understand the medical jargon. Would she have to make an occupied bed? Would there be an intravenous or central venous pressure line?

Many nurses are first attracted to the profession during childhood, perhaps prompted by the desire to help people become healthier and happier and to end their pain. They may view the fields of medicine and nursing as cloaked in mystery and may hope to evoke cures. During nursing school, or early in one's nursing career, a nurse may discover that he or she cannot fix everything or relieve all the pain. Most nurses come to terms with their own strengths and limitations and realize that the effectiveness of one's work is determined more by the ability to influence, rather than by the ability to control people. Also, most nurses learn that the control exercised in the hospital does not necessarily help patients or their families adjust after discharge. Despite well-meaning and knowledgeable advice, patients do not always follow a nurse's directions.

Patients often have many health problems,

are sicker than imagined, and may be discharged from the hospital earlier than a nurse wishes. Nurses must provide care in various settings, including ambulatory care, acute care, home care, and long-term care. Educating patients is part of the care nurses provide in all these settings. Rarely is there enough time to teach patients and families all they need to know, and often patients are too sick to participate. Nurses must be skilled in assessing each patient's needs and in setting priorities to meet the most critical of these needs before the patient's discharge from care (see Chapters 8 and 9). Moreover, patients are influenced by beliefs and values often different from the nurse's. Many patients have limited reading or writing skills; others do not speak English fluently. Nurses must be open, flexible, and creative (see Chapters 3 and 9).

Nurses as Part of a Team

The health care delivery system is driven by economic reality (ie, limited financial resources in the era of managed care) and nursing care must be defined, qualified, and quantified. Nurses must communicate with administrators and patients and must learn to provide effective interventions and quality, cost-effective care through nursing care management systems (see Chapter 13). Thus, nurses do not interact with patients in a vacuum. Rather, nurses are members of a larger team, which includes various health care professionals. Each team member has a special expertise or contribution, and learning to work in harmony with other team members can be more challenging than learning technical skills.

Changing one's view of patients is another challenge. Patients are not just recipients of care; instead, they and their families are at the head of the health care team. By recognizing their right to choose their own futures and by willingly sharing our knowledge with them, a nurse can shift his or her focus to true patient education—a practice based on influence, not control. The nurse also learns to appreciate the roles of the other team members and to find ways to articulate the contributions of each team member in helping patients and their families.

OVERVIEW OF NURSING PRACTICE AND PATIENT EDUCATION

We find that our patients are much more aware of healthcare and what it can offer them. They expect to collaborate, by letting us know how they perceive their needs and asking us what we can do for them. We share the practice of patient and family education.

C.H. (STALLINGS, 1996)

During the past three decades, patient education has become widely recognized as a professional role of nurses. The growth of consumerism and the self-help movement has motivated people to take responsibility for their own health. Simultaneously, this growth and self-help movement has motivated nurses and other health care professionals to implement patient education and to recognize its importance in patient care.

Providing patient education is central to the role of every nurse who provides patient care, regardless of job title or clinical setting. Current models of nursing education should address basic skills needed for contemporary nursing practice: critical thinking, relationship skills, care management skills, primary care skills, and community-focused skills (Balik, 1998).

Changing Environment of Health Care Delivery

When I worked in the hospital, I developed many skills and a broad base of clinical knowledge. In many ways it prepared me well for home health nursing. But I had to learn to be very flexible in my approach.

J.M. (STALLINGS, 1996)

Because of the changing environments of health care delivery, today's nurses practice in various settings, and patient education is integrated in the nursing care delivered in these settings. The expertise nurses develop as patient teachers is carried to new roles and practice settings. Although each setting has unique challenges, the core competencies needed to teach patients are relevant to providing quality care in hospitals, subacute settings, rehabilitation and long-term care facilities, retirement communities, health maintenance organizations, preferred provider organizations, specialized inpatient and outpatient settings (including ambulatory care, urgent care, birthing centers, and day care centers), schools, mental health centers, rural health centers, and home health and hospice agencies. Emerging integrated delivery systems welcome nurses with the following skills:

- Competency to practice in settings with little direct supervision
- Ability to integrate care with other providers across multiple care settings
- Qualitative and quantitative research skills
- Telephone case management
- Use, development, and evaluation of care protocols
- Strong skills in physical assessment and patient teaching for complex and chronically ill populations (Balik, 1998).

Patient care increasingly takes place in the home, where home health care nurses provide skilled, efficient care to patients with complex and chronic illnesses. Under the constraints of managed care (eg, limited number of approved visits, limited time for visits because of heavy caseload), this care must be administered within a short time. Nurses must adapt to the logistical and clinical components of caring for a patient at home and to the patient's resources, needs, and the patient and family's learning capacity. Nurses gain autonomy as they adapt the equipment, procedures, themselves, and their own resources to the situation. Nurses must be creative, innovative, and flexible (Neal, 1999).

The knowledge and skills to provide patient education and the ability to work as a member of an interdisciplinary team are critical factors to a nurse's effectiveness in various practice settings. Nurses describe patient education as a key to enhancing job satisfaction, because it creates greater patient and nurse autonomy. In addition, nurses in advanced practice attribute success in obtaining new employment positions to possessing skills and experience in patient education.

Patient Education in Advanced Practice

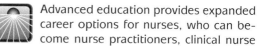 Advanced education provides expanded career options for nurses, who can become nurse practitioners, clinical nurse specialists, and nurse midwives. The roles of advanced practice nurses (APNs) change rapidly with increased authority in primary care settings and more patient management in the inpatient setting. Managed care, which promotes use of the least costly provider to deliver care, explains the growth in career options for APNs. Implementing preventive and health promotion interventions, counseling and patient education expertise, and providing family support to people with chronic illness and disability, are some of the factors that make APNs valued providers (Gilliss & Mundinger, 1998).

The public has been highly satisfied with nurse practitioner care (Office of Technology Assessment, 1986). Double-blind comparisons of physician and nurse practitioner practice indicate that management of uncomplicated, primary care problems has the same, if not better, outcomes for nurse practitioners (Mundinger, 1994). One of the reasons cited for public approbation of the nurse practitioner role is the amount of patient teaching performed by nurse practitioners. One physician explained that he preferred to hire nurse practitioners instead of physician assistants because of the patient education preparation that nurses have in their educational programs. Health education, preventive care, and counseling have become valued by health care consumers and purchasers of health care. Nurses must be part of health care teams for patients to have access to these newly visible services (Mundinger, 1996). ∎

One nurse practitioner describes her collaborative practice with a physician at a large, university medical center: "We work well together and we comanage all of the prenatal patients. The physician sends the client for her first prenatal visit to me, because I will do the physical examination and prenatal workup and all of the necessary teaching related to diet, physical and environmental factors associated with pregnancy, guidelines for management of common problems, and instructions related to subsequent visits. The physician I work with is more interested in the problems and pathology, whereas I'm more interested in the day-to-day management of the prenatal patient.

Certified nurse midwives also bring a nursing background and preparation to advanced clinical practice. Patients frequently state that they chose midwifery services because of excellent patient education and patient empowerment to participate in preventive care, prenatal care, and the delivery experience.

Nursing centers, nurse-managed centers, and community nursing centers have become recognized providers of ambulatory health care. Often affiliated with schools of nursing, they employ a combination of registered nurses (RNs), APNs, and other health professionals. Centers that employ APNs can provide an array of high-quality and cost-effective services. Health education and risk reduction are key components of the care that is provided (Bellack, 1998).

A Tradition of Teaching

> We are in the information age and providing patient and family education is the essence of our practice. As nurses, we have been taught by our discipline and throughout our education the importance of teaching.
>
> **A.C. (STALLINGS, 1996)**

Teaching was recognized as a function of nursing when Florence Nightingale wrote her significant treatises on nursing (Nightingale, 1860). Throughout the history of nursing, nurses have empowered patients to take responsibility for their own health. Some of this power has been returned to nursing, thus increasing the profession's credibility and viability.

In the words of Virginia Henderson, "The unique function of the nurse is to assist the person, sick or well, in the performance of those activities contributing to health or its recovery (or to a peaceful death) that he would perform unaided if he had the necessary strength, will or knowledge. And to do this in such a way as to help him gain independence as rapidly as possible" (Henderson & Nite, 1960). Patient education ensures such individualized care.

Although teaching has always been an integral part of nursing practice, nursing education has not always prepared nurses for the teaching role. In the early part of this century, the National League for Nursing (NLN) voiced concern that nursing education dealt only with disease and not with preparation for teaching (National League for Nursing Education, 1918). The NLN has continued to advocate the importance of educating nurses to teach. In 1993, Redman voiced the concern that, without master's level courses in patient education, graduate nursing education cannot yet commit to prepare nurses for patient education as a specialty (Redman, 1993a; Redman & Braun, 1991).

In 1975, the American Nurses Association (ANA) published a document, *The Professional Nurse and Health Education*. It stated that the professional nurse's responsibility includes "teaching the patient and family relevant facts about specific health-care needs and supporting appropriate modification of behavior." The ANA's Model Nurse Practice Act (1979) defines patient education as a component of the RN's practice. LPNs are responsible for reinforcing what is taught. References to patient education are found in health care agency policies, nursing job descriptions, and the ethics codes of nursing organizations. Furthermore, the courts have consistently upheld the rights of patients to know about their health problems and treatments. Patient education has become a professional expectation and a legal duty of nurses.

Patient Partnership Versus Patient Compliance

Patients have a right to receive appropriate education and to use the knowledge they gain to participate in decision making. However, patients also have a responsibility to participate in their own care decisions and care processes.

(JCAHO, 1996)

A recent nursing graduate shared the following: "I think patient education is an important part of the care patients receive. We should be willing to teach patients what we know and help them to understand what choices they have. Sometimes I feel that it really makes a difference and I can tell that the patient understands. But my experiences are not all positive ones and I end up feeling frustrated and angry. After all, patient education takes time from an already busy schedule of patient care. It requires patience and extra effort to explain procedures and answer questions. I usually have to repeat the information several times or try to explain it in a different way so the patient can understand. After all my effort, some patients still don't take medications or treatments as they should. I end up wondering if they just don't want to be well or if they would have taken the information more seriously if it came from a doctor. Then I ask myself, *What did I do wrong?*"

Physicians express similar feelings of frustration when patient education fails. Although we all recognize that patients have the right and free will to make choices, we also question our own skills in teaching our patients.

We wonder, "Should I have done things differently?"

Many health care professionals describe patient education as giving patients information about their problems and treatments. The quality of patient education is perceived to have a direct correlation with the availability of audiovisual programs and patient education materials and resources, and the informative posters in the physician's office. Patient education programs and materials stress the importance of multiple behavior changes, such as taking medications on an appropriate schedule and with correct dose, changing diet, starting exercise programs, and stopping smoking. Nurses and other health care providers tend to prescribe these changes freely to patients by simply instructing patients what they need to do. The nurse may think his or her job is completed once the instruction is given, and that it becomes the patient's responsibility to make these behavior changes. When patients fail to perform the desired behaviors, the nurse may assume the patient was not given enough information or that the patient failed to assimilate it. The nurse may respond by repeating the information or by providing it in a different form. When the behaviors of patients fail to change, should the nurse assume that patients have not learned the facts impressed on them?

Godfrey Hochbaum (1980) suggests that the temptation to give more (or more forceful) information to emphasize possible dire consequences to patients when they do not exhibit desired behaviors, comes from one's own assumptions that human behavior is shaped by rationality and sufficient motivation. When health professionals examine their own health behaviors and note that they often fail to practice what they preach, the challenge of lifelong behavior change is better appreciated.

The behaviors nurses prescribe for patients involve not a single decision, but many difficult daily decisions that often involve pain, expense, social isolation, a perceived loss of independence, and the difficulty of breaking old habits. Changing a single behavior pattern, such as what one eats, is difficult. Nurses frequently ask patients to change two or more behaviors (eg, diet, exercise regimen, and smoking cessation) simultaneously. The term *compliance* not only oversimplifies the way patients are educated, but also overlooks the needed negotiation, coaching, and integration of health practices in the patient's and family's daily life. Chapter 9 provides strategies for goal setting and for supporting patients in behavior change.

When nurses discuss obstacles in providing patient education, they often identify problems motivating patients to change current behaviors to improve the patient's health status. When asked to elaborate, it becomes evident that nurses see motivation and compliance as closely related. The implication is that a sufficiently motivated patient will comply with the doctor's or nurse's instructions.

Many health professionals have justified their involvement in patient education by asserting that it would increase patient compliance; in other words, it would convince patients to follow instructions. Despite teaching, patients frequently do not make the choices recommended to them by nurses, physicians, and other health care professionals (termed as *noncompliance*).

The term compliance implies that nurses may dictate to the patient what is to be done or changed and that the patient must obey. A nurse may be uncomfortable with the patient's right to choose *not* to follow advice or to change his or her behaviors. The nurse should strive to enlist the patient's partnership—rather than compliance—and view patient education as a process of influencing behavior in ways that are acceptable to the patient. An orientation toward cooperation helps the nurse think about his or her own effectiveness in patient education in a different light. Patient education successes have more to do with the patient's preparation to make informed choices than they do with acts of compliance. In fact, if patient education acknowledges the patient's free will to make choices, it must afford understanding of the importance of his or her values and wishes and the ability to participate in decision-making. Chapter 9 provides an in-depth discussion of the issues surrounding patient decision-making.

Compliance with a medical regimen is an important goal of patient education, but it is not the only goal. A significant process occurs between education and compliance, one in which the client internalizes the teaching and then makes informed choices about applying the teaching to his or her life. Compliance is a product not only of learning about the medical regimen, but also of the patient's lifestyle, a complex group of behaviors including social and family patterns, activities of daily living, and dietary, exercise, and sleep patterns.

The term compliance is so ingrained in discussions of patient education that it is difficult to replace it with another term that reflects mutuality. However, we suggest the terms *concurrence* and *cooperation* as alternatives. These terms suggest choice, mutuality of goals, and a patient-provider relationship based on respect and trust.

Reforming Health Care: A Central Role for Patient Education

General Considerations

An intense debate about health care delivery in the United States will continue on both state and national levels. Questions about how to provide universal access to basic health services and how to finance rising health care costs are central to the debate. Millions of Americans have no health care insurance, and thus appropriate and early medical treatment is often avoided or deferred. Uninsured patients often present for treatment only in the event of acute episodes or exacerbation of chronic illness; thus, costs, complications, disability, and mortality increase.

The hopes for a reformed health care system hold promise of the availability and access to early detection and improved management of chronic health conditions, with lower cost and better outcomes. Nursing views itself as a valuable and visible contributor to managed health care systems of the present and future. The ANA is a voice for nursing in the United States, promoting a changed delivery system and featuring consumer responsibility for self-care, informed decision-making, and choices in the selection of health care providers and services (American Nurses Association, 1991). The ANA believes that improving the health of Americans provides a solid foundation for building a strong nation for the 21st century.

The ANA supports many of the proposals that President Clinton announced in his State of the Union address on January 19, 1999. The president cited proposals to increase access to care for the uninsured, bolster the Medicare program, and provide tax credits for those with long-term health care needs and the family members who care for them (American Nurses Association, 1999). In his 1993 address to the nation, President Clinton emphasized that the following guiding stars would categorize a comprehensive, high-quality, and affordable national health care system for all Americans:

1. **Security**—benefits could not be revoked because of loss of employment or health status.
2. **Simplicity**—less paperwork for providers and a simpler system for consumers.
3. **Savings**—Simplified insurance system and incentives to provide cost-effective care.
4. **Increased choices**—consumers choose their health plans.
5. **Improved quality of health care**
6. **Increased individual responsibility**— patients promote their own health and providers use the system prudently.

The image of a reformed system calls for increasing patient involvement in the health care team and for increasing emphasis on the patient's role in improving health status. Patient education is the vital link for patient empowerment to assume these responsibilities.

Reforms in Education

Although it is difficult to achieve a national consensus on basic health care benefits and on how to finance a comprehensive system, health care reforms are sweeping across traditional settings in which nurses are employed and are influencing nursing education. The downsizing, or right sizing, of hospitals moves nurses into community-based practice. The delivery of patient care continues to move closer to home. In nursing schools, increasing emphasis is placed on preparing students for public, community, and home health settings and for delivering preventive health services in the context of managed care. Nursing school curricula emphasize patient education as an integral part of nursing practice. RNs who pursue bachelor of science in nursing (BSN) degrees gain new knowledge of patient education based in many practice settings.

 In addition, nurses enrolled in nurse practitioner and advanced degree programs should refine patient education skills needed for practice. To meet the public's needs for primary care, the expanded training of medical students for generalist roles is accompanied by an increased amount of training in rural, underserved, and community-based sites. Nursing programs are expanding student exposure to include similar clinical training sites. A growing demand for nurse practitioners, nurse midwives, and physician's assistants is also related to improving the access and cost of primary care services to meet the public's needs. Patient education must be a critical component of graduate nursing education programs that prepare nurses to assume advanced practice roles. ■

Beyond Informed Consent

Nurses who were prepared to practice in the 1970s witnessed the importance of providing for the *informed consent* of the patient. The patient's right to know includes the right to know what illness he or she has, the right to know what diagnostic and therapeutic processes will be used, and the right to know what the prognosis for physical recovery is (Regan, 1975). The patient has a right to refuse treatment and to be informed of the consequences of those actions (American Hospital

Association, 1975, 1992). The nature of this contractual agreement guarantees a patient's right to know what he or she can do to effect physical recovery and includes necessary patient education.

Nursing education and literature about informed consent stressed the importance of providing information on diagnosis, prognosis, and proposed treatments or procedures to all patients. In the summer of 1999, the United States Senate passed patient protective legislation, the Patients' Bill of Rights, which the ANA actively supports. Americans are waiting to see what the United States House of Congress and President Clinton (or the next President) will do with this legislation. Redman notes that until the late 1960s, health care professionals shared with patients information that they perceived to be useful. Information thought to be harmful or upsetting (eg, a grim prognosis, a frightening diagnosis, the adverse effects and financial expenses of treatment) was withheld. Presently, health care providers consider the ethical dilemmas of withholding information, and many providers feel obligated to share information in a complete way (Redman, 1993a, 1997). Chapter 6 provides more discussion of informed consent as a special case of patient education, considering its legal and ethical considerations.

Discharge Planning and Patient Education

By the end of the 1970s, patient teaching witnessed a shifting and an expanding list of priorities. No longer were new nurses educated solely for hospital-based practice. Practice in ambulatory care, long-term care, and home care settings helped nurses gain greater appreciation for the vital link between patient education, discharge planning, and continuity of care. Patients were discharged from hospitals to other settings sicker and quicker.

Discharge planning begins on the day of admission; this is a golden rule taught to all nursing students. Until the past decade, however, the number of days a patient stayed in the hospital was flexible and often could be extended to prepare patients and families to assume self-care. As health care costs continued to increase, hospitals were blamed for inefficiency and the amount of money spent to care for patients. American industry and government agencies pressed for changes in health care reimbursement that would build incentives for efficiency and containment of costs to third-party payers.

Medicare began using a prospective payment system called diagnosis-related groups (DRGs). This major trend in reimbursement became law in 1983. With DRGs, payments were no longer made to hospitals based on the costs of services or on the number of days of care provided to a patient. Instead, a predetermined payment was assigned to each of the DRGs. Each DRG has an assigned mean *length of stay* (ie, the number of days Medicare would pay for services). An *outlier cutoff* (ie, the maximum number of days for which a hospital can bill Medicare) was set. To negotiate payment, the hospital had to prove that the client's condition was complicated. Many health care analysts predicted that major insurance companies would adopt similar prospective-pricing payment systems (Vestal, 1995; Malloy & Hartshorn, 1989). Since then, the health insurance industry has introduced sweeping changes, and new alliances for managed health care evolve daily. Cost and quality are the key components of managed health care.

With the advent of DRGs, discharge planning assumed a new meaning. Financial incentives were tied to the discharge date, because hospitals were reimbursed fixed amounts based on these DRGs. The strategies developed for fiscally managing patient care range from new approaches to preadmission screening to inpatient case management, and from outpatient specialty clinics to high-technology home care. Health care systems emerged, linking providers across a continuum of health care settings. Case management involved ensuring continuity of patient care services, maximizing the quality of care, and minimizing the costs. With the advent of each new approach, patient education has taken center stage.

The primary focus of patient education in the 1980s shifted from provider outcomes to patient and family outcomes. Successful patient education could not be guaranteed based solely on the ability and willingness of health care providers to deliver understandable information about diagnosis, treatment, and prognosis. The American Hospital Association published *Guidelines for Discharge Planning* (AHA, 1984) to help hospitals evaluate and improve their discharge planning functions, stressing that each hospital should develop a system based on its own requirements, resources, and the needs of its patients. Today, discharge planning, in most cases, implies patient education and is viewed as part of routine patient care—an interdisciplinary process to help patients and their families develop and implement a feasible posthospital plan of care. The goals for education of all patients must include learning survival skills, recognizing problems after discharge, and making decisions that contribute to self-care management. Special discharge-planning services are warranted when posthospital needs are expected to be complex. The same guidelines can be applied to other settings. Guidelines and methods for integrating discharge planning and patient education planning are covered in Chapter 8.

Growing Needs of Older Patients and People With Chronic Health Conditions

Virtually everyone with a chronic illness has the same desire—to live as independently and with as much dignity as possible, with minimum pain, disability, and social stigma.

(SCHROEDER, 1993)

 The fastest growing segment of our society is our older population. Health care advances and medical technology have helped these patients to live longer; nevertheless, they continue to have chronic health conditions, physical disabilities, and functional limitations.

Thus, they depend heavily on health care services, particularly nursing care. With increases in the number of older patients and the arrival of prospective payment has come a boom in the home health care industry and rehabilitative programs of long-term care institutions. Many treatments and technologies are now used in the home. More acute care is being provided in the home, and nurses recognize that the discharge of patients from the hospital, sicker and quicker, demands the provision of patient and family teaching and continuity with caretakers in the home. ∎

 Recognizing the growing threats of acquired immunodeficiency syndrome (AIDS) and tuberculosis, nurses employed in public health departments have assumed an active role in new prevention and detection programs for high-risk populations. Patient education for prevention is targeted to the homeless, migrant farm workers, and prison populations. Nurses have augmented their skills in patient education with a new understanding of how culture and poverty can influence patient behavior. ∎

A Gallup poll funded by the Robert Wood Johnson Foundation revealed that although one of seven Americans faces major limitations because of chronic illness, one third of these patients do not seek routine or preventive health care; they receive care only for acute problems. The exacerbation of chronic illness is the only time they may access the health care system. Without patient education and patient involvement in care to prevent acute episodes, health care is costlier and quality of life suffers. Chronic disorders account for much of U.S. expenditures on health care in a health care system geared to cure acute diseases. The number of Americans living with chronic health conditions (eg, diabetes, cancer, emphysema, heart disease, muscular dystrophy, spina bifida, AIDS, chronic mental illness, dementia, disabling injuries, alcoholism, blindness, and disabling arthritis) continues to increase.

Heart disease is a major cause of mortality and morbidity among adults who are older than 65 years of age. Structured educational programs that include exercise and modification of risk factors have been shown to reduce the risk of subsequent coronary events. Nurses can become key to providing leadership in the redesign of cardiac rehabilitation services for older adults (Allen & Redman, 1996).

 The following problems, from which older people and persons with chronic health conditions are especially at risk, are priorities in discharge planning and patient teaching:

Medications.
Nutrition and hydration—healing of wounds and infection require good nutrition. The patient may not be motivated to prepare meals or drink fluids as needed.
Unintentional injury—the patient may fall, which is often related to weakness or side effects of medication.
Mobility and transportation—can the patient get transportation to return for appointments, to pick up medications, to get groceries?
Support services needed at home—is assistance needed with meals, treatments, social services?
When and how to seek appropriate treatment—do the patient and family recognize danger signs that need treatment (eg, pain, medication side effects)? Do they know how to get help? Do they know when to go to the emergency room versus the physician's office? ◼

 Nurses also recognize that the caregivers of older patients need support and possible assistance from community agencies to help them succeed in their caregiving roles. They should be alert and attuned to the language and behaviors related to maintaining control, and should teach caregivers about taking a break, provide information about respite services, and encourage caregivers to talk openly about their caregiving experiences so nurses can help them to find the best solutions to caregiving problems. This is especially important in the home care of patients with Alzheimer's disease and other dementias (Szabo & Strang, 1999). ◼

Disease Management: Pediatric Asthma

Patient education is a large piece of the disease management for pediatric asthma. Unless patients and families accept their responsibility to change behaviors, the goals of disease management cannot be met. In these cases, patient education requires much more from providers than simply providing patients and families information. The education must be tailored to individual needs and circumstances. The Childhood Asthma Initiative, designed for children in the New York City homeless shelter system and launched in 1998, uses an innovative interdisciplinary approach that sequences learning according to readiness and interest of each family (Patient Education Management, 1998). Group sessions and individual counseling are standardized, but patients choose how they are sequenced. This means that one family might begin with instruction on how to fit asthma management into its daily life and another family might begin with managing symptoms of the disease.

Patient education is one of four key components of a disease management program for pediatric asthma. The other three components are:

1. Clinical care, including primary care services
2. Psychosocial services, including stress management and social services
3. Environment, including smoking cessation and harm reduction strategies (eg, dust mite, roach, and rodent control) (Patient Education Management, 1998)

Substance Abuse

 Substance abuse, another priority for nursing involvement in health promotion and disease prevention, is a leading cause of death and disability in the United States. Substance abuse involving tobacco, alcohol, and drugs is the primary cause of preventable illness, injury, and death in the United States. Prevention efforts and early intervention are enhanced by the involvement of school health nurses. Nurses in all settings should know how to counsel patients about smoking and about how to refer patients to smoking cessation programs in the community. School-based prevention programs can be effective in imparting peer-pressure resistance skills, because they recognize that prosmoking messages and availability of tobacco in the community challenge the long-term success of these interventions for adolescent tobacco use prevention. They also recognize that political activism is needed (Altman & Jackson, 1998). ∎

JCAHO Standards

General Considerations

In 1993, new hospital accreditation standards published by the Joint Commission on the Accreditation of Healthcare Organizations (JCAHO) made patient and family education outcomes a high priority and a focus survey area. Meeting this requirement to achieve accreditation placed heightened emphasis on patient education activities within hospitals and in their relationships with other posthospitalization health care providers. The JCAHO standards and scoring guidelines for education of patient and family have brought renewed interest, accountability, and leadership for patient education, which has ultimately benefited both nurses and patients.

Staff nurses committed to patient education have long struggled to gain recognition for the skill, time, and resources needed to succeed. Patient education often competes with high-technology nursing skills for recognition. JCAHO supports and requires accountability for all health care providers to show evidence of patient learning outcomes for accreditation. This provides important reinforcement of nursing's long-standing commitment to teach.

The JCAHO upholds the concept of patient-centered care, with patient and family education viewed as a centerpiece for involving patients as members of the health care team. Patient education also is seen as central to processes for quality management. Health care organizations are expected to show evidence of patient learning outcomes, focus on discharge and continuity of care, and coordinate patient teaching across disciplines. The development of patient-centered care guidelines requires renewed attention to the ways patients and families are educated and to innovative approaches to achieve patient outcomes appropriate to the patient's length of stay. Nurses must turn their attention to what the patient and family can do, rather than to what the nurse has taught. Figure 1-1 illustrates how this educational partnership is evaluated and documented in a Neonatal Intensive Care Unit (NICU).

JCAHO Education Function

The JCAHO identifies the goals of patient education outlined in the *Comprehensive Accreditation Manual for Hospitals*. Patient education improves patient health outcomes by promoting healthy behavior and by involving the patient in care and care decisions. Education supports recovery, a speedy return to function, and enables patients to be involved in decisions about their own care (JCAHO, 1998).

These education standards call for a systematic approach to patient education. Scoring guidelines reflect the expectations that all patients will benefit from appropriate education. The accountability for patient teaching lies within the scope of practice of every nurse. Accountability must also be assumed by nurses in management, staff development, and clinical specialist roles to ensure that staff nurses develop necessary skills as patient educators. Many patient educators have not had formal instruction on teaching, and many do not routinely employ teaching skills known to enhance instructional effectiveness (Boswell, Pichert, Lorenz, Schlundt, Penha, Alexander, Davis, Evangelis, Haushalter, Lindsay, Palm, & Suave, 1996). Novice nurses bring enthusiasm and knowledge about patient education to practice, but they look for coaching and modeling to make patient teaching purposeful (Boswell Pichert, Lorenz, & Schlundt, 1990).

Experienced nurses frequently struggle with implementing outdated protocols that are nurse centered and based on outcomes unrealistic for current lengths of stay. Involvement

LUCILE PACKARD CHILDREN'S HEALTH SERVICES AT UCSF

UCSF Stanford Health Care

UNIT NUMBER	
PT. NAME	
BIRTHDATE	

Instructions: Check box when patient understands the content presented. Date and sign at bottom of form. Document problems/issues with learning on the Pediatric Flowsheet or Progress Notes. Patient/Family signs when form complete.

LOCATION	DATE

1. Health Management

a. I have received the following printed materials:
- ☐ Your guide to breast feeding
- ☐ Breastfeeding your ICN baby
- ☐ Taking your child's temperature
- ☐ Car seat information
- ☐ Positioning your baby
- ☐ 17 ways to cope with a crying baby
- ☐ Going home with baby booklet
- ☐ RSV precautions
- ☐ CPR booklet
- ☐ Bathing your baby

b. I know how to

	demo/info given	date	pt/caregiver demo	date	needs rein-forcement	independent	date	NA
Taken my baby's temperature/NL range	☐		☐		☐	☐		☐
Give my baby a bath	☐		☐		☐	☐		☐
Feed my baby with a bottle	☐		☐		☐	☐		☐
Breastfeed my baby	☐		☐		☐	☐		☐
Use breast pump and store breast milk	☐		☐		☐	☐		☐
Prepare and store formula	☐		☐		☐	☐		☐
Clean bottles and nipples	☐		☐		☐	☐		☐
Mix higher calorie formula	☐		☐		☐	☐		☐
Care for my baby's circumcision	☐		☐		☐	☐		☐
Comfort, burp, and position my baby	☐		☐		☐	☐		☐
Care for my baby's skin and cord	☐		☐		☐	☐		☐
Use a bulb syringe	☐		☐		☐	☐		☐
Care for my baby if she/he has a fever	☐		☐		☐	☐		☐

2. Activity

I have reviewed special activity guidelines with my: ☐ Occupational Therapist ☐ Physical Therapist ☐ Nurse

3. Precautions – I know to call the doctor if my baby:
- ☐ has a fever of 101˚F or 38.6˚C
- ☐ has a fever of 99.5˚F or 37.5˚C that lasts over 4 hours
- ☐ has diarrhea and/or vomiting
- ☐ is so sleepy he/she will not wake up to eat
- ☐ is so fussy that he/she will not sleep or eat
- ☐ is breathing very fast or hard and looks pale or bluish
- ☐ has a cough or runny nose lasting over a few days
- ☐ has not wet his/her diapers at least 6 times a day

4. Medications

I know:
- ☐ which medication my child needs and how to give it
- ☐ my baby's medication schedule
- ☐ medication clock
- ☐ what to do if my child vomits or misses a dose
- ☐ what to do if my child gets a dose by mistake

5. Additional information
- ☐ I have a car seat and know how to use it
- ☐ I have seen the CPR video
- ☐ I have received my follow-up Doctor's appointment
- ☐ taken class (date) _____

6. See additional teaching records: ☐ _____ ☐ _____ ☐ _____

7. Other Special Instructions: _____

_____

_____

☐ Translator used for instructions: _____

Patient/Family Signature _____

Instructor Signature:

Name	Title	Date
Name	Title	Date
Name	Title	Date
Name	Title	Date

FIGURE 1-1. Intensive care nursery teaching record. Reprinted with permission from Bisgaard, R., & Luceti, L.

BOX 1-1. JCAHO's Goals of Patient Education

As outlined in the 1998 (JCAHO) Standards, patient education should:

- Promote interactive communication between patients and providers.
- Improve the patient and family's understanding of the patient's health status, health care options, and consequences of options selected.
- Encourage patient and family participation in decision-making about care.
- Increase patient and family potential to follow the therapeutic health care plan.
- Maximize patient and family care skills.
- Increase patient and family ability to cope with the patient's health status.
- Enhance patient and family role in continuing care.
- Promote a healthy patient lifestyle
- Inform patients about their financial responsibilities for treatment when known.

JCAHO defines family as the person(s) who play a significant role in the patient's life. This includes an individual who may or may not be legally related to the patient (JCAHO, 1998).

based on Benner's four stages of development: advanced beginner, competent, proficient, and expert. The JCAHO standards and scoring guidelines and the role of staff development in promoting patient education are more thoroughly discussed in Chapter 5.

Interdisciplinary Teams

The Pew Health Professions Commission (1998) issued its report *Recreating Health Professional Practice for a New Century,* calling for interdisciplinary competence in all health professionals. Describing this competency as essential for the future, the Commission cited the current integrated health care delivery systems evolving toward acute care and chronic care management by interdisciplinary teams of providers, including nurses, physicians, and allied health. The interdisciplinary model uses resources in a timely, efficient way, avoids error and duplication of services, and elicits the expertise of all professionals in an environment of collaboration and consultation (Pew Health Professions Commissions, 1998).

The Pew Commission noted that medical and professional schools must reassess their curricula to ensure that they apply an interdisciplinary vision. Education should be provided in interdisciplinary settings, students should demonstrate interdisciplinary skills, and students should seek work or study experiences that expose them to interdisciplinary care. Incentives for interdisciplinary management of care are found not only in cost reduction but also on patient satisfaction and empowerment of patients for better management of chronic diseases. Competencies needed within interdisciplinary teams include:

- Providing integrated health services
- Emphasizing health promotion and disease prevention
- Functioning in managed care environments
- Evaluating the quality and cost of health care (Pew Health Professions Commissions, 1995)

of nurse managers and educators is needed to promote patient education in the following ways:

Helping nurses define and evaluate patient learning outcomes
Aiding in the identification of critical learning needs and teaching priorities
Promoting innovative programs that ensure continuity of patient education
Reflecting the value of patient education in the nursing performance appraisal system

Suggestions for continuing education that aids skill acquisition in patient education are

When patient and family education is planned and coordinated based on an interdisciplinary model of care, everyone benefits. Numerous examples offered throughout the text describe nurses who work with other disciplines and the opportunities to provide leadership for the team. The goal is not simply providing more teaching, but also helping to assure that the patient and family are the focus of teaching efforts. Overloading the patient is less likely, outcomes can be measured and tracked, and brainstorming by the larger team leads to innovative approaches to challenging patient teaching situations.

Integrating Patient Education in Nursing Practice Education

How patient education is accomplished varies from setting to setting. In outpatient clinics, nurses have a short time with each patient and must teach throughout the encounter; they must set priorities and rely on educational materials appropriate for the patient. In acute care settings, nurses face shortened lengths of patient stay and thus refine their skills at setting priorities and realistic goals, making referrals, and evaluating a patient's ability to perform survival skills. These nurses also must evaluate the patient's readiness and ability to learn and incorporate patient education literature (Doak, Doak, & Root, 1996). In home care settings, nurses share more high-technology care with the family and coordinating community resources in the patient education role. In long-term care, nurses rely on their skilled assessments to set priorities and to develop meaningful plans of care by valuing the input of patients and families; they use patient education to involve the patient and family in restorative care.

The same process for patient education is used by nurses in all settings and with all types of patients. We hope that students and experienced nurses will find the text helpful by applying the principles of patient education described in the following chapters to daily practice. The principles of patient education also are illustrated by case studies throughout this text to provide practical ex-

amples of how to perform various steps of the process. According to Benner, much can be learned from the wisdom of nurses who are expert teachers and coaches. Teaching and coaching are embedded in nursing care and vary based on demands, resources, and constraints of the situation. Yet, she cautions us that learning from experts requires attention to the context and avoidance of hasty generalizations (Benner, 1984).

The Nursing Process

Nurses provide patient care through the application of the nursing process, a problem-solving method designed to meet client needs in a systematic way. The process has four steps:

1. **Nursing diagnoses.** The nurse gathers information about patient needs and formulates a list of nursing diagnoses. Nursing diagnoses are statements of human responses to actual or potential health problems, which the nurse can legally identify and for which the nurse can intervene (Carpenito, 1999). Many nursing diagnoses relate to patient and family learning needs. The nurse focuses on functional problems and daily management.
2. **Plan for care.** The nurse develops the plan for patient care, outlining priorities and client goals (both short- and long-term). Specific learning objectives are part of the patient care plan.
3. **Implementation.** This step details how the plan will be implemented, outlining specific nursing interventions, including patient teaching targeted to meet client goals.
4. **Evaluation.** Evaluation provides information about how well goals were met. During the process of evaluation, nursing diagnoses are either resolved or referred for continuing care. Thus, implementing the nursing process entails more than a cognitive, four-step procedure.

Clinical Decision-Making and Clinical Judgment

Clinical decision-making based on clinical judgments arises from the expert nurse's grasp of qualitative distinctions in individual cases. The nurse must be attuned to each patient situation, with a sense of what is salient and the confidence to set priorities. Clinical judgment is learned through experience (ie, a combination of hands-on care, mentoring, and continuing education with a case study approach.) Expert nurses learn to notice patients and families in new ways and adapt agency patient education resources to culture, beliefs, context, and environment (Benner, et al., 1992). A faculty member who teaches BSN students shared with us one of the difficulties of teaching patient education skills in the undergraduate program: "Students see only a small proportion of the hospital episode. They are not prepared to teach patients during the long run." This text offers case studies, quotes from practicing nurses, and study questions to promote clinical relevance, reflection, and the development of critical thinking.

 The nurse must recognize significant others, especially the family members, who directly influence the patient. When patient education is incorporated throughout the nursing process, it is a tool to empower clients, enabling them to assume an active role in their care and providing a safer transition on the day of discharge. The client who can recognize symptoms and ask for help, who can cope effectively with the exacerbations of chronic illness, and who can prevent injury, accident, and illness, has an autonomy that will help in negotiating an increasingly complex health care system. ■

Patient education plans are part of the total plan for patient care and are targeted to priorities for each patient. Patient education begins with early screening on admission to determine what is likely to cause trouble for this patient and to anticipate functional problems rather than with a preset teaching plan for all patients with a common medical diagnosis (eg, diabetes). The nurse must realistically consider the anticipated length of stay and determine how much and when to teach the patient. For example, nurses report that they must modify standardized teaching plans for patients with diabetes when a patient's needs vary because of age, complications, experience, presenting problem, and other simultaneous health issues. Thus, patient education cannot be accomplished with a cookbook approach and should not be delegated to inexperienced or unlicensed personnel. Effective patient education requires critical thinking and clinical judgments that allow nurses to plan individualized approaches for patient care.

Patient education is not accomplished by simply tucking a list of instructions or a booklet into the patient's hand or instructing him or her to turn on the television to the patient education channel. Patient education requires a *therapeutic relationship* (ie, providing an individualized response to patient needs rather than to a broad medical diagnosis) and the introduction of whatever resources are available to meet those needs.

CHALLENGES IN PATIENT EDUCATION

Preparing Content for Teaching

How can nursing students anticipate patient and family learning needs and prepare the content needed for patient teaching?

Knowledge of the nursing process itself does not assure that one is fully prepared to deliver patient education. Nurses must know about the health problems faced by their clients and must anticipate the needs the client typically exhibits. To be a capable patient teacher, nurses must assess their own learning needs, their patients's needs, and find resources to meet them.

A community health nurse receives the referral of a new client who was discharged from a nearby medical center with a rare diagnosis. The nurse is unfamiliar with the diagnosis, the prognosis, the functional problems typically affecting the patient, and the learning needs of the patient and family. The nurse goes to the medical center library and finds a recent article from a nursing journal describing the disease, epidemiology, clinical characteristics, medical management, and nursing management. Fortunately, the article also outlines nursing diagnoses applicable to patients with this diagnosis, suggests actions, and reviews infection control guidelines. This prepares the nurse to make an individual assessment of the patient and family and to anticipate their needs and priorities. (Chapter 11 provides valuable guidance for nurses who increasingly turn to the Internet for accurate information resources.)

Cultural Sensitivity

Nurses also understand that cultural factors have a profound effect on patient education. Nursing care and the teaching-learning process must consider the cultural diversity of patients and their families (Leininger, 1994). Patient education for chronic diseases, such as hypertension and diabetes, typically target lifestyle changes (eg, dietary habits and daily activities) that may be associated with cultural patterns and traditions. Nurses recognize the need to learn about religions and cultures and the need to incorporate cultural assessment in the process of patient teaching. To design effective patient teaching interventions, nurses need information about how to work with clients from culturally diverse backgrounds.

Providing culturally relevant nursing care (Andrews & Boyle, 1995) requires that the nurse use transcultural concepts in the application of the nursing process, including identifying cultural needs, understanding the cultural context of patient and family, using culturally sensitive nursing strategies to meet mutual goals, using resources from various cultural subsystems in the community, and learning from and responding to culturally diverse situations. Chapter 3 addresses special challenges involved in teaching patients from a different ethnocultural group. Learning and teaching are indispensable and almost unavoidable parts of the nurse-patient relationship; health care workers must be constantly aware that although they are communicating, either verbally or nonverbally, they are also teaching and patients are learning (Henderson & Nite, 1978).

Nurses as Role Models

We realize how important it is that we should be role models for our patients, to practice what we preach. We don't want to tell our patients "you really shouldn't smoke" while we reek of cigarette odor, or tell them "you really should curb your appetite, eat healthy foods, and exercise regularly," when we are overweight and don't exercise ourselves.

E.W. (STALLINGS, 1996)

How important is it for nurses to "practice what we teach" to be positive role models for our patients?

Many nurses and other health care professionals sacrifice their own health practices because of the multiple demands of families, patients, and work (Mateo, 1999). They may smoke, be overweight, exercise poor nutrition and fitness, experience stress-related symptoms, and invite chronic health issues. Also, nursing faculty members and students face academic pressures, late-night reading and writing, demands of caring for children and older parents, and participation in community and church volunteer activities.

One family nurse practitioner described that she has always prided herself in the holistic care she provides to patients and families. Diet, exercise, and stress management are integral to every patient encounter. She coaches her students to make realistic demands of themselves, because they often must balance jobs and families in addition to studies. She felt dishonest, giving advice she did not follow, because she struggled with a serious weight problem and an associated depression. She finally decided to make a change. She joined a weight loss program, started walking, and lost 50 pounds (Gomez, 1999). She says, "Now, when I counsel patients, I do not feel like I am giving them the company line. I know what it is like to struggle with hunger and emotional eating. I can talk with them about their food choices, talking about their emotions rather than insulting them."

Promoting Teamwork

What can nurses do to promote collegiality with other disciplines on the health care team and to help patients reap the benefits of interdisciplinary teaching?

The importance of interdisciplinary involvement by the total health care team is central to effective patient care. The lack of good communication between disciplines often leads nurses to feel they are not valued as patient teachers. Lack of communication can lead to battles about turf and the inability to collaborate, both one-on-one and in team conferences.

Understanding the contributions that other health care professionals can make to patient teaching increases the effectiveness of patient education and improves attempts to develop collegiality and collaboration of the health care team. We have found that members of other health care professions tend to be as involved as nurses are in patient teaching, particularly those nurses who are recent graduates and those who actively pursue continuing education. However, we have also heard nurses generalize that because one physician opposed their patient education efforts, most physicians, for example, are not supportive of patient education. Such assumptions thwart collaboration and the delivery of patient education.

During the last three decades, the emphasis of nursing education and practice has reflected an expanded focus for interdisciplinary pa-

tient teaching efforts. Furthermore, because of nursing's continuous and visible presence at the patient's side, nurses are in the unique position to provide leadership for patient education and to capitalize on the strengths of each discipline for the patient's ultimate benefit. The need to coordinate teaching efforts is especially critical for patients who are acutely ill and who cannot absorb ambitious teaching activities. Nursing involvement is key to ensuring effective patient education with appropriate learning outcomes to empower rather than to overcome the patient.

Case Management

Case management involves leadership from a nurse or another health professional to oversee the process of providing care, with the goal of improving efficiency, increasing effectiveness of interventions, and containing costs. Critical paths, care maps, and other case management tools incorporate patient and family education consistently across the plan of care. This plan for patient learning involves the input of the health care team and a focus on patient learning outcomes. When nurses assume the role of case manager or care coordinator, they must be especially committed to interdisciplinary planning and team building. Chapter 13 addresses in greater detail how patient education is provided in the context of case management.

Staff Development and Continuing Education

Staff development and continuing education, targeted to helping health care professionals increase skills in patient education, must also address the health care team approach. This is accomplished most effectively when members of the health care team engage in the learning experience together. Chapter 5 explores the role of staff development in patient education and offers suggestions for organizing such continuing education programs.

Nurses gain valuable insights that promote the work of the health care team by talking with other health care professionals who are interested in patient teaching. We have initiated such conversations with physicians, dietitians, physical therapists, pharmacists, and hospital social workers. We asked them to tell us how they see their patient teaching roles and how they perceive the nurse's role. Each suggested ways to increase collaboration. These interviews were also an opportunity to teach other health care professionals about the nurse's involvement in patient education and to generate ideas for new teaching programs. Table 1-1 provides some comments from these interviews.

Although the health care team members we interviewed stressed the importance of protocols and organization (eg, development of critical pathways and teaching protocols), they frequently stated that attitudes and skills of people directly influenced the success of teamwork in patient education. They emphasized the following criteria for successful teamwork:

Communication—verbal and written communication, facilitated by planning meetings, care conferences, telephone consultation, good documentation, and "the willingness to go out of our way to communicate with one another"

Mutual respect among disciplines—including recognizing respective areas of expertise, knowing one's limits, and teaching each other

Desire to work as a team—and recognition of a common goal

SUMMARY

The nursing profession embraces patient education as a central factor in the nursing process and as a dimension of nurse caring. During the past three decades, changing needs and mandates have increased the visibility, involvement, and expertise of nurses as patient teachers. Informed consent, discharge planning, the prevalence of chronic health problems, and patient compliance are issues that require nursing leadership in patient educa-

tion. Mandates from JCAHO, debate about the need to reform health care delivery, the emergence of managed care, and the growth of the nurse practitioner movement are also directly related to patient education.

Every nurse, regardless of title, setting, or specialty, is called on to provide patients and families with an opportunity to learn in their health care encounters. Patient education reduces feelings of helplessness, empowers patients, and promotes continuity of care.

In providing care that is truly patient centered, nurses acknowledge the importance of a health care team approach. Nurses must reflect on their roles and the roles of others, and the respective strengths that each brings to patient care. Patient education is built on the foundations of respecting one another, caring, and communicating, not just among the nurse and patient and family, but also among all members of the health care team.

STRATEGIES FOR CRITICAL ANALYSIS AND APPLICATION

1. Review the nine objectives of patient and family education as stated by JCAHO. Provide examples of how the nurse might meet these objectives when caring for a patient and family.
2. Identify a patient, friend, or family member who has a chronic health problem. Ask this person to describe what knowledge and skills are needed to care for him or her. What resources has this person found helpful for learning to manage care?
3. Look for examples in the media of nurses who are providing innovative patient and family education programs in the community. Consider how the need was assessed and how patients and families were involved in the design of those programs.
4. Interview members of other health care disciplines about their involvement in patient education. Then summarize what you learn and discuss how nurses and other health professionals might promote

TABLE 1-1. Comments on Patient Education From Health Care Professionals

PHYSICIANS	DIETITIANS	PHYSICAL THERAPISTS	PHARMACISTS	HOSPITAL SOCIAL WORKERS
What is your involvement in patient education?				
"I teach patients one-on-one. I try to tell them what they want and need to know in language they understand. I want them to understand and agree with the treatment plan, to know what the goals are, and to participate in decision-making." "I try to incorporate patient education into my interaction with the patient. I think you need to be consciously aware of patient education, and you have to have a good feeling that your patients are understanding and doing what you agree is appropriate. I think we assume more than we should."	"We educate patients about the diets they must follow at home. We try to find out what the patient usually eats and how we need to modify this. Sometimes we discuss the diet with the doctor because what he or she orders is inappropriate. We make the necessary changes and teach the patient."	"We inform patients about their disease, about what to expect, and about any procedures that are done. We teach them about ambulation, functional activities, and safety, especially postsurgically. Physical therapists have a large role in educating patients about rheumatic diseases and how to deal with and prevent flareups. We also teach patients about prostheses and help patients with them."	"The pharmacist is often the first person to see patients when they have problems. When patients ask for advice, the pharmacist must know if a referral to other health care providers is needed. The pharmacist also must teach about how a drug works in the body. If the patient knows the reason for taking the drug, he or she is more likely to take it as prescribed. Many patients know nothing about their medication. They don't know what it is or how to store it. Sometimes they don't even take it, depending on how they feel. This is especially true for hypertensive patients."	"Our biggest role is as a hospital, staff, and community liaison. If patients cannot take care of themselves after leaving the hospital, we talk with the patient, doctor, and family about agencies or resources that can help and coordinate the plans. Many families have problems before they even come into the hospital. We help with these too. We give emotional support and answer questions about things patients are really afraid of. Patients tend to tell things to social workers that they are embarrassed to tell doctors and nurses."
How do you see the nurse's role in patient education?				
"I see it as necessary and important. Nurses have a different perspective from mine. The doctor teaches about diagnosis and prognosis; the nurse teaches daily management. There is combined strength. Patients tend to confide different information to nurses. For example, patients are more open about fear of cancer	"Nurses reinforce what the dietitian tells the patient and emphasize the importance of following the diet plan. Nurses tell us what is going on with the patient, and this helps us to evaluate whether the patient understands the diet plan. Nurses also teach medications, treatments, and basic survival skills. They explain what the doctor has	"The role of the nurse is educating and orienting the patient about the disease and reinforcing the teaching of other health care personnel. Nurses give patients emotional support, teach them about activities of daily living, and give general instructions about medications. Nurses reinforce precautions in transfer and positioning. This is crucial. They can help to motivate the	"All patients have a right to know what medications they take, how much, and why. Nurses can teach this when they administer medications. There are so many new drugs. For nurses to teach patients, we need to collaborate. The nurse can reinforce the teaching done by the team and communicate with other	"The nurses do much patient teaching, especially with surgical patients. They answer questions patients never ask their doctors. I get my best referrals from nurses. There's something about hanging an IV bag, giving a shot, washing hair, giving a bath—patients tell things to nurses at these times. Some nurses are very aware of the situation a patient is going

(table continued on page 24)

TABLE 1-1. Comments on Patient Education From Health Care Professionals (continued)

PHYSICIANS	DIETITIANS	PHYSICAL THERAPISTS	PHARMACISTS	HOSPITAL SOCIAL WORKERS
"with the nurse, and talk with me about stomach pain. Nurses clarify and reinforce what I teach. Nurses teach patients and families, especially in dealing with chronic diseases." "Patient education is often left to the nurse. Yet, nurses often lack confidence in their ability to teach."	"said to the patient after the doctor leaves."	"patient and coordinate pain medications with the treatments."	"team members to meet the patient's learning needs. Nurses have a big job to do, and patients expect a lot of them."	"home to and they involve us when we are better able to handle certain kinds of crises."

What increases your collaboration with the nurse and other members of the health care team in patient education?

PHYSICIANS	DIETITIANS	PHYSICAL THERAPISTS	PHARMACISTS	HOSPITAL SOCIAL WORKERS
"Personal knowledge and trust. Having time to get to know other members of the health care team. Asking the patient who is teaching him. The patient is the center of the team and can help me work with the team. Writing and reading interdisciplinary progress notes is important. One of the most crucial things you do for the patient is document how you educate him." "The most important thing is discussion. There has to be a desire on all parts. People can find the time to do it. Take a half hour to discuss a difficult patient and bring in everyone who is involved in the care. You formulate an approach and cross-educate one another. It optimizes patient care for that particular patient, but it also teaches people how to deal with difficult patients.	"We need planning meetings. We need to know what other people are teaching the patient. The patient should not have to hear things repeatedly, in different ways. Protocols for teaching help. You know what other people are teaching, although you don't always know at what level the patient is understanding." "Documentation! The nurse's assessment of the patient's readiness to learn is especially helpful. For team work, people must go out of their way to communicate with one another."	"We should acknowledge that we have the same goal: getting the patient ready to handle discharge. We should plan teaching together and construct teaching programs where we reinforce teaching and give emotional support from admission to discharge." "Nursing shifts change frequently. Therefore, we often have no consistency and have little interaction. Frequent team meetings and good verbal and written communication would increase collaboration in patient education. This would promote mutual respect among the disciplines, cooperation, and knowing how to use other's expertise in different cases."	"Nurses make valuable assessments about the patient and family and what their supports are like. The nursing assessment should be shared more, especially in the progress notes." "There should be continuing education for health care professionals. Pharmacists could teach nurses about new drugs, making nurses better able to teach patients. Pharmacists should be more open to nurses' questions and should encourage their calls."	"Nurses need to know their limits. The patient needs follow-up after discharge to learn and to reinforce teaching. Social workers can help by making referrals that go beyond discharge, but we have to work together and focus less narrowly on rescuing." "Good notes in the patient record are important. I read all the notes, especially the patient's response to the nurses. Details help me assist the family in planning for discharge, such as whether the patient is incontinent or nonambulatory. Notes from the health care team validate what I see. Patient care rounds are also a good opportunity to collaborate."

teamwork in providing patient education. You might pose the following questions to physicians, dietitians, occupational and physical therapists, pharmacists, dentists, and hospital social workers:

How are you involved in patient education?
How do you see the nurse's role in patient education?
How does your role interface with the nurse's role?
How can members of the health care team increase their collaboration in patient education?

REFERENCES

Allen, J., & Redman, B. (1996). Cardiac rehabilitation in the elderly: improving effectiveness. *Rehabilitation Nursing, 21*(4), 182–195.

Altman, D., & Jackson, C. (1998). Adolescent tobacco use and the social context. In Shumaker, S., Schumacker, S., Schron, E., Ockene, J., & McBee, W., (Eds.), *The Handbook of Health Behavior Change*. New York: Springer Publishing Company.

American Hospital Association. (1975). *A patient's bill of rights*. Chicago: Author.

American Hospital Association. (1984). *Guidelines for discharge planning*. Chicago: Author.

American Hospital Association. (1992). *Update on Patient's Bill of Rights*. Available online: www.aha/resource/pbillofrights.html. Accessed July 14, 1999.

American Nurses Association. (1975). *The professional nurse and health education*. Kansas City, MO: Author.

American Nurses Association. (1991). *Nursing's agenda for health care reform*. Washington, DC: Author.

American Nurses Association. (1999). Press Release. Available online: www.nursingworld.org/pressrel/1999/union.htn. Accessed July 12, 1999.

Andrews, M., & Boyle, J. (1995). *Transcultural concepts in nursing care*. Philadelphia: J. B. Lippincott.

Balik, B. (1998). The impact of managed care and integrated delivery systems on registered nurse education and practice. In O'Neil, E., and Coffman, J. (Eds.), *Strategies for the Future of Nursing*. San Francisco: Jossey-Bass Publishers.

Bellack, J. (1998). Changing roles, responsibilities, and employment patterns of registered nurses in ambulatory care settings. In O'Neil, E., and Coffman, J. (Eds.), *Strategies for the Future of Nursing*. San Francisco: Jossey-Bass Publishers.

Benner, C., Tanner, C., & Chesla, C. (1992). *From beginner to expert: Clinical knowledge in critical care nursing* [Video]. Athens, OH: Fuld Institute for Technology in Nursing Education, 28 Station Street, Athens, OH 45701.

Benner, C., Tanner, C., & Chesla, C. (1996). *Expertise in Nursing Practice: Caring, Clinical Judgement, and Ethics*. New York, NY: Springer Publishing Co.

Benner, P. (1982). From novice to expert. *American Journal of Nursing, 82,* 402–407.

Benner, P. (1984). *From novice to expert*. Menlo Park, CA: Addison-Wesley.

Benner, P., & Wrubel, J. (1989). *The primacy of caring: Stress and coping in health and illness*. Menlo Park, CA: Addison-Wesley.

Boswell, E., Pichert, J., Lorenz, R., Schlundt, D., Penha, M., Alexander, S., Davis, D., Evangelist, J., Haushalter, A., Lindsay, L., Palm, M., & Sauve, D. (1996). Evaluation of a patient teaching skills course disseminated through staff developers. *Patient Education and Counseling, 27,* 247–256.

Boswell, E., Pichert, J., Lorenz, R., & Schlundt, D. (1990). Training health care professionals to enhance their patient teaching skills. *Journal of Nursing Staff Development, 6*(5), 233–239.

Carpenito, L. (1999). *Nursing diagnosis: Application to clinical practice* (6th ed.). Philadelphia: J. B. Lippincott.

Doak, C., Doak, L., & Root, J. (1996). *Teaching patients with low literacy skills* (2nd ed.). Philadelphia: J. B. Lippincott.

Gilliss, C., Mundinger, M. (1998). How is the roles of the advanced practice nurse changing? In O'Neil, E., and Coffman, J. (Eds.), *Strategies for the Future of Nursing*. San Francisco: Jossey-Bass Publishers.

Gomez, D. (1999). Caring for others means caring for ourselves. *The American Nurse,* July/August, *31*(4), 5.

Henderson, V., & Nite, G. (1960). *Principles and practice of nursing*. New York: MacMillan.

Henderson, V., & Nite, G. (1978). *Principles and practice of nursing* (6th ed.). New York: MacMillan.

Hochbaum, G. (1980). Patient counseling versus patient teaching. *Topics in Clinical Nursing, 2* (1), 8.

Jackson, B., Smith, S., Adams, R., Frank, B., & Mateo, M. (1999). Healthy life styles are a challenge for nurses. *Image—The Journal of Nursing Scholarship, 31*(2), 196.

Joint Commission on the Accreditation of Healthcare Organizations. (1993, 1998). Education of the patient: Standards and scoring guidelines. In *1998 comprehensive accreditation manual for hospitals (PF-1–PF-11).* Chicago: Author.

Joint Commission on the Accreditation of Healthcare Organizations. (1996). *Educating Hospital Patients and Their Families: Examples of Compliance.* Oakbrook, IL: Author.

Leininger, M. (1994). *Nursing and anthropology: Two worlds to blend.* Columbus, OH: Greyden Press.

Malloy, C., & Hartshorn, J. (1989). *Acute care nursing in the home.* Philadelphia: J. B. Lippincott.

Mundinger, M. (1994). Advanced-practice nursing—good medicine for physicians? *New England Journal of Medicine, 15*(1), 28–33.

Mundinger, M. (1996). New Alliances: Nursing's Bright Future. *Nursing Administration Quarterly, 20*(3), 50–53.

National League for Nursing Education. (1918). *Standard curriculum for schools of nursing.* Baltimore: Waverly Press.

Neal, L. (1999). Neal theory of home health nursing practice. *Image—The Journal of Nursing Scholarship, 31*(3), 251.

Nightingale, F. (1860/1992). *Notes on nursing: What it is and what it is not.* Philadelphia: J. B. Lippincott.

Office of Technology Assessment. (1986). *Nurse practitioners, physicians assistants, and certified nurse-midwives: A policy analysis.* Washington, DC: U.S. Government Printing Office (Health Technology Case Study #37-OTA-HCS-37).

Patient Education Management. (1998). Patient education is a large piece of the disease management puzzle, *5*(10), 121–123.

Pew Health Professions Commissions. (1995). *Critical Challenges: Revitalizing the Health Professions for the Twenty-First Century.* San Francisco: UCSF Center for the Health Professions.

Pew Health Professions Commissions. (1998). *Recreating Health Professional Practice for a New Century, fourth report.* San Francisco: UCSF Center for the Health Professions.

Rankin, S., & Stallings, K. (1990). *Patient education: Issues, principles, and practices* (2nd ed.). Philadelphia: J. B. Lippincott.

Redman, B. (1993a). Patient education at 25 years; where have we been and where are we going? *Journal of Advanced Nursing, 18,* 725–730.

Redman, B. (1997). *The practice of patient education* (8th ed.). St. Louis: Mosby–Year Book.

Redman, B., & Braun, R. (1991). Courses in patient education in masters programs in nursing. *Journal of Nursing Education, 30,* 42–43.

Regan, W. (1975). The patient's right to know. *Regan Report of Nursing Law, 16,* 1.

Schroeder, S. (1993). Chronic health conditions. *Annual Report 1993.* Princeton, NJ: The Robert Wood Johnson Foundation.

Stallings, K. (1996). *Integrating patient education in your nursing practice* [Video]. Reproduced with permission of Glaxo Wellcome Inc. (Produced by Horizon Video Productions, 4222 Emperor Blvd., Durham, NC 27703.

Szabo, V., & Strang, V. (1999). Experiencing control in caregiving. *Image—The Journal of Nursing Scholarship, 31*(1), 71–75.

Tanner, C., Benner, P., Chesla, C., & Gordon, D. (1993). The phenomenology of knowing the patient. *Image—The Journal of Nursing Scholarship, 25*(3), 273–280.

Vestal, K. (1995). *Nursing management concepts and issues* (2nd ed.). Philadelphia: J. B. Lippincott.

Wolf, Z., Giardino, E., Osborne, P., & Ambrose, M. (1994). Dimensions of nurse caring. *Image—The Journal of Nursing Scholarship, 26*(2), 107–112.

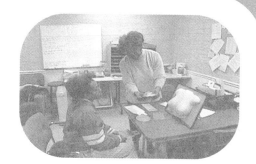

CHAPTER

2

Health Promotion: Models and Applications to Patient Education

LEARNING OBJECTIVES

After reading this chapter, the nurse or student nurse should be able to:

1. Define the terms *health promotion, disease prevention,* and *health maintenance* and give examples of each.

2. Describe the historical transition from a compliance orientation to a health promotion and disease prevention orientation.

3. List five of the six factors used in the Health Belief Model to determine a person's likelihood of complying with health care recommendations.

4. Compare the Health Belief Model with the Health Promotion Model; describe the difference in the definition of health for each model.

5. Recall a community health education dilemma to which the Precede-Proceed Model might be applied.

6. Compare the Care-Seeking Behavior Theory to the Health Promotion Model.

7. List two benefits that would be obtained in using the Self-Regulation Model to guide patient education.

8. Identify the historical origins of *Healthy People 2000* and describe the progress that has been made in achievement of the objectives.

9. Describe a plan for using the *Guide to Clinical Preventive Services* and the *Clinician's Handbook of Preventive Services* in an outpatient family practice setting.

10. List three criteria for prescribing a screening test.

INTRODUCTION

In conjunction with the evolution of highly sophisticated medical and surgical interventions, an appreciation of the importance of promoting healthy lifestyles and reducing risk factors for disease has developed. Health care consumers and providers recognize the importance of promoting healthy lifestyles to prevent the onset of preventable diseases and conditions.

Primary care providers, in particular nurse practitioners, recognize the importance of partnering patient education with health promotion and risk factor reduction to encourage better health outcomes. If patient education were more effectively used to promote health and reduce risk factors, many patient education techniques (discussed in other sections of this book) to intervene with diseases would become unnecessary! ■

This chapter provides important definitions related to health promotion and risk factor reduction, an overview of health belief and health promotion models, and application of cases to the *Guide to Clinical Preventive Services* and *Clinician's Handbook of Preventive Services. Healthy People 2000: Midcourse Review and Revisions* is also examined in terms of how well goals have been achieved and how those that have not been achieved have implications for patient education.

HEALTH PROMOTION, DISEASE PREVENTION, AND HEALTH MAINTENANCE

Definitions

The concepts of health promotion, disease prevention, and health maintenance are interrelated; however, it is important to understand the nuances of each.

Health Promotion

Health promotion includes activities that a person undertakes to enjoy life to the fullest. Generally, health promotion is associated with wellness behaviors rather than with disease prevention. For example, a healthy 32-year-old who walks on a treadmill is performing a health-promoting activity that may prevent disease, but she walks primarily to feel self-actualizing and to enhance her health and well-being.

Other activities and lifestyle decisions that are considered health promoting include deciding not to smoke tobacco, controlling or avoiding ingestion of alcohol, using family planning to promote maternal and child health, seeking psychological counseling to promote mental health, and eating nutritious food for enjoyment and health. Many people can tell a nurse what they do to promote their health; others will be unaware of the concept of health promotion and will focus on disease prevention.

Disease Prevention

Disease prevention is comprised primarily of screening for asymptomatic diseases in children and adults, counseling to prevent diseases and the onset of chronic conditions, and immunizing to prevent diseases. Currently, controversy exists about what screening tests are most essential and what risk factors indicate someone should be screened. The *Guide to Clinical Preventive Services* attempts to answer these questions through a careful review of evidence for and against screening tests. Although there may be overlap between health promotion and disease prevention (and certainly health promotion may aid in disease prevention) the authors generally do not consider disease prevention to reside in the same health-enhancing and self-actualizing arena as health promotion.

Health Maintenance

 Health maintenance involves screening for disease prevention and coun-seling provided by the advanced practice nurse (especially the nurse practitioner). For example, a pediatric or family nurse practitioner performs a Denver Developmental screening test on an eight-month-old infant as a health maintenance activity. If the infant does not meet the appropriate developmental milestones, the nurse practitioner will either continue to monitor the infant (depending on the degree of the developmental delay) or refer the infant and parents for further testing or counseling. Health maintenance is always the first part of the plan when the nurse practitioner charts a SOAP note (Subjective, Objective, Assessment Plan). Making health maintenance a priority helps the nurse practitioner remember that promoting and maintaining health are a crucial part of his or her role. ■

Attention has turned to health promotion and disease prevention. Thus, patient teaching regarding compliance with a medical regimen is still important, but shares the stage with health promotion. Most of the theoretical frameworks of health promotion have evolved from the Health Belief Model.

Understanding Compliance as the Framework for Health Promotion

General Considerations

Before health promotion and health maintenance became well known concepts in the health care lexicon, most health care providers focused on compliance. Health promotion and disease prevention were not common approaches in nursing or other health care arenas in the first half of the 20th century; at that time, health care focused on disease. However, the public has become more knowledgeable about disease prevention and health care providers recognize that preventing major illness is more effective than coping with an established illness. Thus, there has been a burgeoning of health promotion activities. Nevertheless, it is important to understand that the roots of health promotion are in compliance.

Early Approaches to Compliance

Sackett and Haynes (1976) defined compliance as "the extent to which the patient's behavior (in terms of taking medications, following diets or executing other life-style changes) coincides with the clinical prescriptions" (p. 1). They further state that "the presentation of compliance data has clinical relevance only when it is related to the simultaneous achievement of the treatment goals" (p. 3). This definition influenced compliance research and literature in two major ways. First, it indelibly associated the control of illness with compliance to physician-directed regimens (ie, control resulted from complying with the prescribed treatment.) The physician determined the dose and timing of medication, the specific diet to be followed, and the kind of body monitoring to be completed by the patient. Completing these actions as ordered was assumed to lead directly to control of the illness. Compliance was measured by the extent to which the patient accomplished these activities.

Second, the patient's adherence to the prescribed regimen became the focus of the indices of compliance or noncompliance. Noncompliance is defined as "the failure of the patient to fulfill the clinical prescription *as it was intended by the practitioner*" (Hays & DiMatteo, 1981, p. 37). Patient noncompliance with the medical prescription suggested a lack of knowledge, rebellion, or emotional instability (Leventhal, Zimmerman, & Gutmann, 1984; Trostle, 1988).

According to this model, the educator's task involves motivating patients to see the value of treatment plans as a means to attaining health or controlling illness, providing patients with the skills and knowledge needed to manage continuing care without daily professional supervision, and encouraging patients to change behavior patterns to conform with the regimen. The prescriptive, or compliance model was the philosophical basis even in the innovative nurse-managed clinics developed by Allison (1973) and Backscheider (1974), in which Orem's nursing theory of self-care was used to organize the clinic practice. The goal of nursing care was to assist the client in following the prescribed treatment plan; the person's definition of self-care was rarely considered.

Despite prescribed regimens to treat illness and education to inform the patient about the importance of following the medical prescription, the rate of noncompliance is notoriously high. Sackett (1976) reported that compliance with short-term regimens decreases rapidly as the days of treatment increase, and the level of compliance in long-term therapy is approximately 50%. More recent studies of compliance with prescribed drug regimens indicate that compliance continues to be a problem, with 33% of patients never taking their medications (McPhee & Schroeder, 1996).

THE HEALTH BELIEF MODEL

General Considerations

To identify factors that influence compliance or noncompliance with a health care regimen, a group of cognitive and social psychologists began a work group that probed many psychological questions that affect health. Among this group were Bandura, Leventhal, Rosenstock, Becker, and Hochbaum, major contributors to health psychology and, indirectly, to patient education.

The Health Belief Model is a framework that arose from this group. The Health Belief Model was originally developed to predict the likelihood of a person taking recommended preventive health action and to understand a person's motivation and decision-making about seeking health services (Hochbaum, 1958). It has been used recently to explain clinic appointment keeping (Mirotznik, Ginzler, Zagon, & Baptiste, 1998). This model has been adapted for use in predicting compliance with chronic illness regimens (Pham, Fortin, Thibaudeau, 1996).

The Health Belief Model attempts to identify compliers and noncompliers by examining six factors considered important to health care decisions:

1. The patient's perception of the severity of the illness
2. The patient's perception of susceptibility to illness and its consequences
3. Value of the treatment benefits (eg, Does the cost and adverse effects of the treatment outweigh the disease consequences?)
4. Barriers to treatment (eg, degree of social support, expense, regimen complexity, length of treatment, and side effects)
5. Costs of treatment in physical and emotional terms
6. Cues that stimulate taking action toward treatment of illness (eg, illness in family or friends, television or other media coverage, newspaper stories, or health pamphlets)

Demographic variables, such as age, gender, socioeconomic status, and ethnicity, are believed to influence a person's perceptions about the seriousness of health conditions and the need to take action for those conditions (Becker, 1974, 1979; Becker & Janz, 1985; Janz & Becker, 1984; Stout, 1997).

Research Studies

The Health Belief Model has been used in many research studies that cover a wide range of health-related, decision-making situations (Eisen, Zellman, & McAlister, 1992; French, Kurczynski, Weaver, & Pituch, 1992; Galvin, 1992; Laraque, McLean, Brown-Peterside, Ashton, & Diamond, 1997). However, studies using the Health Belief Model have been inconsistent in identifying the differences between those who comply with professional recommendations and those who choose not to comply; similarly, the model has not delivered on its promise to predict those who are likely to engage in health promotion activities.

Studies show various components of the model as effective for prediction, although the model as a whole has not been a consistent predictor of compliance. Janz & Becker (1984) suggest that barriers and costs are the most prominent factors associated with not participating in preventive health practices or maintenance of treatment regimens. However, others have found other variables as more explanatory in terms of supporting the Health Belief Model. For example, Falck and colleagues found that both perceived self-efficacy and susceptibility were the most important factors that explain HIV-risk needle practices among injection drug users, rather than barriers or costs (Falck et al., 1995).

Application of the Health Belief Model

It is possible that the Health Belief Model operates differently in diverse populations with varying conditions. For example, Cerkoney and Hart (1980) found that subjects who perceived their diabetes as serious, and who responded to cues for action, were more compliant with their treatment regimen. The authors state that a positive correlation of $r = 0.50$ ($p < 0.01$) occurred between the subjects' total compliance scores and a composite score of their level of health motivation. This correlation accounted for 25% of the variance in compliance levels of

this sample and could not be used as reliable clinical predictors of compliance. Some of the inconsistency in results is associated with the fact that the components of the model were not operationalized in the same way or applied consistently across studies (Wallston & Wallston, 1984). Additionally, the application of this model to patients with a chronic illness may operate differently than when applied to risk-factor reduction situations.

Although the Health Belief Model acknowledges the importance of a patient's belief in compliance, the assumption is that the variables specified regarding health beliefs are the most significant factors in decision-making about health behaviors. The model also does not offer an explanation of the relationships among the variables or how other aspects of personal experience may affect the way illness treatment is managed or ignored (Conrad, 1985).

THE HEALTH PROMOTION MODEL

General Considerations

Nola Pender, a nurse who began her work in the early 1980s, developed another model that attempts to explain how people arrive at decisions about behaviors toward health promotion (Pender 1982, 1987, 1996). Pender believed that the Health Belief Model focused on an *avoidance orientation* (1982, p. 60) related to seeking preventive care to decrease the probability of negative health and illness outcomes.

Pender theorized that the Health Belief Model did not address positive actions taken to sustain or increase a person's level of health. She maintained that the Health Belief Model was tested on preventive actions requiring the performance of a single act of compliance and was insufficient to explain behavior directed toward health promotion. Pender defined health not as the absence of disease, but as self-actualization. She thought that this definition suggested that health was related to self-initiated behaviors directed toward attaining higher levels of health. From her perspective, defining health as adaptation or stability directed a person's behavior toward health protection or toward avoiding illness and disease.

Health-Promoting Behaviors and Health Protection

Health-promoting behaviors are operationalized for purposes of research as activities that are integrated on an ongoing basis into a person's lifestyle. Health promotion behaviors include exercise, obtaining optimum nutrition, stress management, and the development and maintenance of social support systems. These behaviors are directed toward self-actualization and fulfillment; the behaviors serve to "increase well-being and actualize human health potential" (Pender, 1996, p. 7).

However, *health protection* is described by Pender as the motivation to avoid illness, detect it early, and maintain functioning when ill. Health protection is similar to the concept of health maintenance, a primary focus of the nurse practitioner role. Nurse practitioners and other primary health care providers work to promote health maintenance through the recognition of needed immunizations for adults and children, identification of age-appropriate screening examinations, and clarification of safety issues (eg, seatbelt and child car seat safety, smoking cessation).

The role of the health care professional is to help people overcome barriers to health-promoting activities and support preventive health practices. Assistance by health providers is accomplished by removing genuine barriers (eg, lack of access to care), emphasizing the positive consequences of preferred behaviors, and by reducing the frequency of negative consequences.

Components of the Health Promotion Model

The Health Promotion Model is organized into three categories—individual characteristics

and experiences, behavior-specific cognitions and affect, and behavioral outcome.

The components of the Health Promotion Model are based on many features in the Health Belief Model and on a synthesis of health promotion and wellness literature. In her 1996 text, Pender made major revisions to her original version of the Health Promotion Model (Figure 2-1). Three new variables were added, and the model was revised to highlight individual characteristics and experiences that might influence behavioral outcomes. In addition, the importance of health, the patient's perceived control of health, and cues to action were deleted from the model. Other variables have been repositioned. The new Health Promotion Model is refined and more specific than the old model is.

Individual Characteristics and Experiences

This category includes:

1. **Prior-related behavior**—the habits, skills, and knowledge acquired in the past.
2. **Personal factors** (biological, psychological, multicultural). Personal factors include age, gender, body mass index, self-esteem, perceived health status, and sociocultural variables (eg, race, ethnicity, socioeconomic status, and acculturation).

Behavior-Specific Cognitions and Affect

The behavior-specific cognitions and affect determining health promotion activities are labeled as:

1. **Perceived benefits of action.** (This variable was present in the original model.)
2. **Perceived barriers to action.** (This variable was present in the original model.)
3. **Perceived self-efficacy.** This is the belief people have in their ability to perform behaviors necessary to accomplish the desired action
4. **Activity-related affect.** This new variable

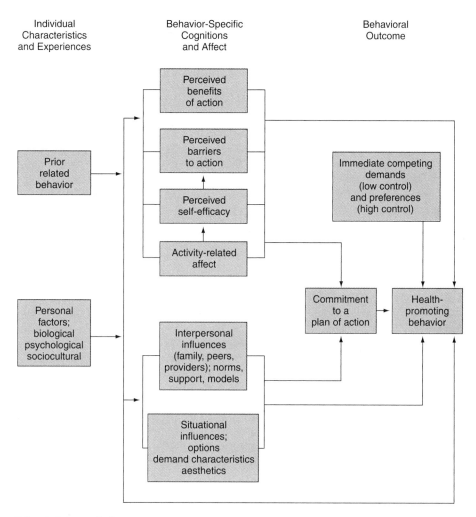

FIGURE 2-1. Pender's Revised Health Promotion Model. From: Pender, *Health promotion in nursing practice* (3rd ed.) © 1987. Reprinted with permission of Prentice-Hall, Inc., Upper Saddle River, NJ.

incorporates the idea that health behaviors can include either negative or positive feeling states or emotional reactions.

5. **Interpersonal influences (family, peers, providers); norms, support, models.** This variable recognizes the importance of other people to influence health-promoting behaviors, social mores, and ways that influence behavior.

6. **Situational influences; options, demand**

characteristics, aesthetics. These are the environmental influences that can modify behavior through the stimulation, safety, and compatibility that they offer.

Behavioral Outcomes

The behavioral outcomes are defined as:

1. **Commitment to a plan of action.** This new variable connotes a person's resolution to

carry out an action and definitive strategies for doing so.

2. **Immediate competing demands and preferences.** This new variable recognizes the rival responsibilities and desires that influence actions.

3. **Health-promoting behavior.** This variable is the end point of desirable health-promoting actions.

Research Studies

Pender and others have reported the results of studies that demonstrated that perceived self-efficacy, benefits, and barriers have been empirically supported as predictors of health-promoting behaviors (Pender, 1996). Demographic variables, such as education, occupation, household size, age, religion, and rural versus urban environment, have also been supported in research related to the Health Promotion Model and generally have a positive relationship with, and are predictive of, health behaviors (Garcia, Pender, Antonakos, & Ronis, 1998; Johnson, Ratner, & Bottorff, 1995; Lusk, Ronis, Kerr, & Atwood, 1994).

Other studies that use the Health Promotion Model to identify health promotion behaviors in middle-aged and older subjects have further confirmed the relationships among various components of the Health Promotion Model and health-promoting behaviors (Walker, Sechrist, & Pender, 1987). Duffy (1988) reported high self-esteem, internal health locus of control (ie, a measure of a person's mastery over his or her health), and good current health related to self-actualization, exercise, and interpersonal support for health promotion activities in middle-aged women. Hawkins and colleagues (1989) found higher self-esteem, internal locus of control, and better health status related to the health promotion activities of regular exercise and sleeping 7 or 8 hours daily. Pender and colleagues (1990) reported that better health status was related to self-actualization, health responsibility, exercise, nutrition, interpersonal support, and stress management. Duffy (1993) reported that subjects who believed that their current health was good, had high self-esteem, and who believed that health was under their own control, more frequently practiced the health promotion activities of self-actualization, nutrition, interpersonal support, stress management, and exercise.

More recently, Bottorff and colleagues have used sophisticated causal modeling techniques to examine the role of cognitive-perceptual factors in health-promoting behavior maintenance in women (Bottorff, Johnson, Ratner, & Hayduk, 1996). Although the cognitive-perceptual factors were an integral part of the model, they contributed little variance to the explanation of specific health-promoting behaviors. This research was based on Pender's earlier version of the Health Promotion Model and highlights some of the difficulties with the earlier version.

Although the authors criticized various portions of the Health Promotion Model in the previous edition of this text (Rankin & Stallings, 1996), Pender's revisions make the model more user-friendly and more likely to explain health outcomes in research and practice settings. Indeed, Pender's willingness to revise and enhance the model is a good example of model respecification, a task that is not frequently assumed by nurse theorists. Her contributions to health promotion have been crucial. Although she does not directly address patient education, her model has many implications for understanding a patient's willingness to undertake health protection and health-promoting activities.

OTHER HEALTH PROMOTION FRAMEWORKS

Three additional health promotion frameworks should be mentioned in this chapter: the Precede-Proceed Model, Care-Seeking Behavior Theory, and the Self-Regulation Model. A fourth model, the Transtheoretical Model of Motivation and Change, is covered in Chapter 4, because it relates more closely to motivation and teaching principles.

The Precede-Proceed Model

Developed by Lawrence Green, a leading public health and health education expert, this model was created for use with people and communities to promote health and, as a desired endpoint, to enhance quality of life (Green, 1980; Green and Kreuter, 1991). The model applies more reasonably to health promotion for aggregates than to individuals, because policy and environmental factors are major components of the framework.

 The model offers a guide to assuring the comprehensiveness of approaches to change through techniques that enable and reinforce change. By involving communities in their own desired changes, the changes are internalized and reinforced rather than created from outside the community. Different from other health promotion models, this model seeks to create change not just through admonitions from health professionals, but through the altering of knowledge, attitudes, and beliefs at a macrosystem level, which alters knowledge at the community or family level (Green, 1999).

A unique feature of the model is that instead of planning interventions to bring about desired outcomes, the nurse starts at the outcome and determines the quality of life of the designated population. The nurse asks, *Why does this group have these health outcomes?* Instead of planning a program to meet the needs of the population, the advanced practice nurse should start with an assessment of the current situation and then try to determine deductively, by working backward, the original cause of the situation. The origin of the problem is referred to as a social diagnosis; it is a type of self-assessment. Once the self-assessment has occurred, an epidemiological diagnosis is made; the epidemiological diagnosis is followed by a behavioral and environmental diagnosis. After the behavioral and environmental diagnoses are made, the educational and organizational structures are considered so that a diagnosis involving these components is made. Last, an administrative and policy diagnosis leads to a plan for health promotion that eventually culminates in methods and strategies to achieve the desired health promoting behaviors. ■

Evaluation is a major part of the iterative process involved in the Precede-Proceed model. The model has been used in programs to decrease child pedestrian injuries (Howat, Jones, Hall, Cross, & Stevenson, 1997) and increase the use of the Glasgow coma scale by emergency department personnel (Macrina, Macrina, Horvath, Gallaspy, & Fine, 1996).

Care-Seeking Behavior Theory

This theory has been developed from Harry Triandis' work related to behavior theory. It was modified by Diane Lauver, a nurse, to represent the reasons that patients seek health care (Lauver, 1992). Lauver posits that psychosocial variables (eg, affect or feelings, expectations and values about outcomes, norms, and habits) influence care-seeking behavior. Preexisting clinical and sociodemographic variables (eg, chest pain, gender) modify the psychosocial variables, but do not directly influence care-seeking behavior. Also, facilitating conditions, such as ease of access to health care and insurance, may influence the psychosocial variables.

Lauver's research primarily has been in the area of women's reproductive health and the decisions women make about care-seeking behavior in the realm of estrogen replacement therapy (Lauver, Settersten, Marten, & Halls, 1999) and mammography (Lauver & Kane, 1999; Lauver, Nabholz, Scott, & Tak, 1997). Her research demonstrates the importance of considering psychosocial variables (eg, anxiety, norms about appropriate actions, and habits) and facilitating conditions (eg, access to health care); these factors appear to influence psychosocial behaviors. The implications are that a nurse would consider the anxiety, mores and norms, habits, and access to care pertaining to a given patient. If the patient represents a particular group for whom preventive action, such as mammography, is feared or not valued—and if this particular patient is also highly anxious, has never participated in preventive screening, and cannot easily access mammography—she is less likely to obtain mammography than is a woman with a different profile.

The care-seeking behavior theory is obviously an outgrowth of the Health Belief Model and the Health Promotion Model. Lauver has reduced the number of variables and simplified the model so that it is easier to test. The emphasis on psychosocial variables seems logical, because most realize that people seek health care based on their own past experiences with illness or health-seeking behavior (habits), their own feelings and beliefs, and the feelings and beliefs expressed by significant others (norms). Pender's most recent Health Promotion Model reflects the importance of psychosocial variables, an example of the cross-fertilization that occurs among nursing theorists.

Self-Regulation Model

Another model that examines decision-making related to health promotion includes the patient's personal meaning of and responses to illness. The self-regulation model was developed from studies that considered the effect of fear-arousing communications on preventive health care actions (Fig. 2-2). For example, in the 1950s, attempts were made to promote polio vaccinations through fear-inducing messages to parents. Studies were conducted using the psychological framework of drive theory that suggested a drive, such as fear (eg, fear of polio), would precede performance of an activity (eg, taking children to be vaccinated). Therefore, fear-arousing information could be used to make people comply with health-related activities (Keller, Ward, & Baumann, 1989; Leventhal & Johnson, 1983; Leventhal, Singer, & Jones, 1985).

Leventhal and colleagues (1985) realized that fear communications initiate problem-solving activities related to the subject's perception of danger. If a patient developed a plan of action to deal with the danger (eg, el-

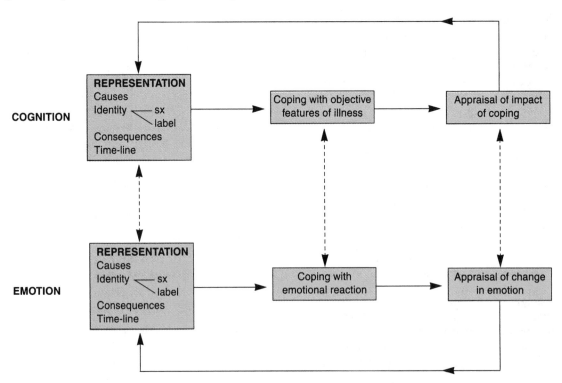

FIGURE 2-2. The Self-Regulation Model. (From: Keller, M. L., Ward, S., & Baumann, L. J. [1989]. Processes of self-care: Monitoring sensations and symptoms. *Advances in Nursing Science, 12*[1], 54–66.) Reprinted with permission.

evated blood sugar), the subject was more likely to take action (eg, eject insulin) to reduce the danger (eg, ketoacidosis). Continuing studies led Leventhal and his colleagues to believe that people generate their own construction or representation of health threats and plan health-related action based on these representations.

Representations of health threats are constructed from accumulated experience and are an integration of knowledge gathered from the media, personal contacts, health professional input, symptoms and body sensations, and past experience with illness. The model views four factors as the key features of a person's construction of health threats:

1. **Identity or identification of concrete symptoms** (eg, a headache means a brain tumor is present)
2. **Cause** (eg, improper food habits or stressful life events)
3. **Time line** or the perception of how long the illness will last (ie, acute or chronic)
4. The patient's perception of the **consequences of the threat**

The action taken will depend on the person's belief that he or she can manage the health threat and the emotional response to the challenge, the person's strategies for dealing with problem situations, and the person's evaluation of whether the action taken is effective (Hamera, Peterson, Young, & Schaumloffel, 1992; Keller et al., 1989; Leventhal, 1982.) Interpretation and synthesis of these factors will influence how a person copes with illness (see Figure 2-2).

Research Studies

Research studies that use the Self-Regulation Model are an expansion of the medical model's conception of compliance as a result of fixed patient characteristics, situational barriers, and inadequate motivation or education. The concepts developed in the Self-Regulation Model suggest that a person's understanding of an illness may be the critical factor in decisions about continuing treatment.

Furthermore, beliefs about illness will de-termine what symptoms people choose to monitor in evaluating health status. The interpretation of symptoms as a health threat will have an impact on a person's actions to correct the problem. For example, if a patient with diabetes interprets lethargy as a normal part of the label "diabetic," he or she may ignore the symptoms of hyperglycemia and fail to adjust diet or medication. The consequences of continuous high blood sugar levels can lead to devastating disabilities with time. Assessing people's representation of illness and connecting the constructions of the illness with self-management choices provides a means of identifying at what point health information may be most helpful to the patient.

In summary, the Self-Regulation Model focuses on the patient's interpretation of the meaning of the illness as a vehicle for understanding why patients comply with health promotion and disease prevention guidelines and medical treatment. However, the model maintains a purely cognitive approach to illness management and does not address health and illness in the context of everyday life. Environmental factors (eg, home and work stresses) are only acknowledged in research as important in the construction of beliefs about the cause of illness. Unrecognized in the model is how modifications in health definitions affect emotions and social activities. Furthermore, this model fails to address how valued social activities (eg, meals with family members) affect emotional adjustment to illness, health definitions, and health practices. The inability to engage in valued social activities may dissuade patients from adhering to the medical regimen.

SUMMARY OF MODELS AND IMPLICATIONS FOR PATIENT EDUCATION

Historical Background of Health Promotion Models

Historically, the Health Belief Model spawned the Self-Regulation Model and later the Health Promotion Model. Rosenstock, Hochbaum, Leventhal, and Kegeles worked together in the Public Health Service in the 1950s and 1960s to ascertain why people failed to seek disease prevention or screening tests for the early detection of asymptomatic disease. In addition to the Health Promotion Model, the influence of the Health Belief Model is obvious when one examines the Care-Seeking Behavior Theory. These models attempt to better discern what characteristics best describe people who would or would not comply with prescribed health promotion and treatment plans. Although they are useful heuristics for trying to explain health promotion behaviors, they are difficult to test in toto and are still more useful as philosophical perspectives to try and understand behavior than they are useful at actually predicting it.

The only model that does not have direct origins in the Health Belief Model is the Precede-Proceed Model. Green has also been engaged in public health research; however, his work generally involves aggregates (ie, groups of people or communities) rather than individuals. Although his model is intuitively appealing, it is probably not as useful to nurses involved either in staff nursing or in primary care, because their focus tends to be more individual and family-oriented, rather than aggregate-based. However, community health nurses trying to work with community aggregates may find the Precede-Proceed Model invaluable.

Models in Context of Patient Education

All of the models discussed are useful for planning patient education oriented toward health promotion.

The Health Belief Model

The Health Belief Model was the first to postulate that a patient's belief in his or her personal susceptibility to, and the severity of a health condition, are important variables influencing the decision to take action to prevent health problems. In terms of patient education, the health care provider should con-sider if the person believes in his or her own personal susceptibility to, and the potential severity of, a health condition. If the health care provider ascertains that the patient has no belief in personal susceptibility to or the severity of a condition, the first step in patient education is to provide information and reality orientation that makes the patient more open to preventive screening and risk factor reduction strategies. Likewise, other variables (eg, benefits, barriers and cost to treatment, and cues to stimulate action) are important to consider when attempting patient education.

The Revised Health Promotion Model

The revised Health Promotion Model makes a unique contribution to patient education through its new focus on commitment to a plan of action and immediate competing demands and preferences. Evaluating the patient's commitment to a plan of action is key to planning an educational intervention. If the health care provider determines a great commitment to promoting healthy lifestyles or to seeking preventive screening, then it is logical to draw up a contract with the patient that specifies what the actions should be and that provides some type of reward. (See Chapter 9 for strategies to develop contracts.) Immediate competing demands and preferences are also important for the nurse or other health care provider to consider before launching patient education. For example, if a young father is worried about losing his job, he is probably less likely to take time off from work to renew a tetanus immunization than would another person whose work situation was more stable.

The Precede-Proceed Model

The Precede-Proceed Model has been used in many different health promotion studies for aggregates or communities with particular needs (eg, communities with high rates of child pedestrian injuries). Its contribution to patient education is generally applicable to certain populations with specified health education needs and includes the "backward" method of assessment; that is, the targeted group participates in determining health-promoting outcomes rather than the nurse or community interventionist, deciding what's best for the population. Nurses and other health care providers working in the area of public health, school health, or with other population aggregates may find that this model provides helpful direction in planning health education.

Care-Seeking Behavior Theory

This theory's primary contribution to patient education is its focus on psychosocial variables that influence care-seeking behavior. Not only do psychosocial variables directly influence care-seeking behavior, but they also are indirectly influenced by preexisting clinical, sociodemographic, and access variables. This theory highlights the necessity to assess psychosocial variables, including feelings and affect, expectations and values, beliefs expressed by significant others (norms), and past experiences with illness (habits). This assessment is critical for determining how to proceed with patient education.

Understanding norms and habits is essential for teaching health-promoting behaviors and for counseling for risk-factor reduction. Patients frequently do not openly express certain norms related to sexual activity or child-rearing (eg, child discipline that includes corporal punishment). The patient's norms may conflict with those of the health care provider, especially if cultural differences between patient and health care provider exist. Therefore, it is important to understand the norms from which different cultural or religious groups operate to help patients engage in health-promoting activities. For example, it is unlikely that counseling will persuade a member of the Jehovah's Witness religious group to use any type of pooled immunoglobulins (eg, those given after exposure to hepatitis A), because Jehovah's Witnesses proscribe against use of blood products. Although attempts should be made to persuade patients to use desirable interventions, religious beliefs must be respected.

Also, a patient's habits are assessed before beginning health-promoting patient education. If a patient had a negative experience with a health screening, he or she may be unlikely to undertake other health screening procedures. For example, a patient who had a negative experience with a sigmoidoscopy is not as likely to agree to a colonoscopy. This example reiterates the importance of conducting a careful patient education assessment before attempting any health promotion patient education.

The Self-Regulation Model

The Self-Regulation Model is useful for trying to understand the cognitive process by which people make decisions regarding health promotion and disease management. This model's contribution to patient education is its focus on the parallel pathways of emotion and cognition. The model denotes that people do not operate solely on cognitive bases, but also process information emotionally. Recognition of the parallel pathways demands that the nurse constantly assess the emotional and cognitive processing. If the emotional pathway is uppermost in priority for the patient, and little cognitive processing occurs, it is unlikely that the patient will undergo health screening or make rational decisions regarding health promotion. Thus the nurse should help the patient use both cognition and emotion to derive health-promoting behavior that is consonant with his or her desired self-actualization.

Summary

In sum, all of the health screening and promotion models presented in this chapter make important contributions to patient education. Pender's Health Promotion model is the only one that focuses on actualizing healthy outcomes, rather than on disease prevention. However, Pender's model intersects health promotion and disease prevention and can be used successfully in either situation to enhance patient education.

HEALTHY PEOPLE 2000 AND 2010

The *Healthy People 2000* document, has been important in guiding the nation toward a health promotion agenda. This document, recently updated to *Healthy People 2010,* focuses on prevention of disability and morbidity. It addresses improvements in the health status of populations most at risk for premature death, disease, and disability, and includes screening interventions to detect asymptomatic diseases before disability, chronicity, or death ensues.

Healthy People 2000 was initiated in 1979 with the publication of *Healthy People: The Surgeon General's Report on Health Promotion and Disease Prevention.* It was revised and amended in 1995 with the publication of *Promoting Health/Preventing Disease: Objectives for the Nation (Midcourse Review and 1995 Revisions).* The publication in 1990 of *Healthy People 2000* was made possible by a consortium of more than 300 organizations, representing all levels of government, professional workers, and people from various sectors of American communities. In 1990, 15 priority areas were established under the headings of preventive services, health protection, and health promotion.

Healthy People 2010 contains 467 objectives in 28 focus (or priority) areas; these focus areas are subsumed under two main goals—to increase quality and years of healthy life and to eliminate health disparities (U.S. Department of Health and Human Services, 2000). New to *Healthy People 2010* is a set of "leading health indicators," which will help people and communities gauge their progress in meeting the objectives. For example, the focus area of tobacco use has two leading indicators: to reduce cigarette smoking by adolescents from 36% to 16% by the year 2010, and to reduce cigarette smoking in adults from 24% to 12% by 2010. These leading indicators give concrete national goals against which communities and the health care providers serving them can measure their own effectiveness.

The vision for *Healthy People 2000* and *Healthy People 2010* moves beyond hospitals and outpatient settings to communities, schools, workplaces, and homes. Thus, the report has major implications for patient education, charging nurses to find methods of implementing health promotion, disease prevention, and health maintenance in practice. Since 1990, progress has been made in the achievement of many of the goals, with 50% proceeding in the right direction, 18% moving in the wrong direction, 3% showing no change from baseline, and the remaining goals having no available data *(Healthy People 2000 Midcourse Review and 1995 Revisions).* Of those objectives that have moved in the wrong direction, special populations, including African American, Hispanic, Asians, Pacific Islanders, American Indians, and Alaskan Natives have been most disadvantaged or less likely to achieve goals. Table 2-1 illustrates the progress on sentinel objectives.

 Related to *Healthy People 2000* is the text *Healthy Children 2000, National Health Promotion and Disease Prevention Objectives Related to Mothers, Infants, Children, Adolescents, and Youth* (1991). Although the objectives are the same as those in the parent text, the objectives have been applied with particular concern to the needs of children and their mothers. The emphasis is on providing community supports to families so that children can develop in optimal situations. Unfortunately, some of the objectives that most affect children's well-being are those that have not been achieved. For example, violent and abusive behavior has increased, rather than decreased. Whether children are the victims of violence or abuse or whether they witness it, the effects are devastating. ∎

GUIDE TO CLINICAL PREVENTIVE SERVICES AND CLINICIAN'S HANDBOOK OF PREVENTIVE SERVICES

Guide to Clinical Preventive Services

The *Guide to Clinical Preventive Services* and *Clinician's Handbook of Preventive Services* are two useful texts developed by the U.S.

TABLE 2-1. Progress in Meeting Objectives

Health Promotion

	RIGHT DIRECTION	WRONG DIRECTION	NO CHANGE/ NO DATA
Physical Activity			
• More people exercising regularly	X		
• Fewer people never exercising			X
Nutrition			
• Fewer people overweight		X	
• Lower fat diets	X		
Tobacco			
• Fewer people smoking cigarettes	X		
• Fewer youth beginning to smoke	X		
Alcohol and other drugs			
• Fewer alcohol-related auto deaths (per 100,000)	X		
• Less ETOH use among youth, (12–17 yrs)	X		
• Less marijuana use among youth, (12–17 yrs)	X		
Family planning			
• Fewer teen pregnancies (per 1,000)		X	
• Fewer unintended pregnancies			X
Mental health and disorders			
• Fewer suicides (per 100,000)	X		
• Fewer reporting stress-related problems	X		
Violent and abusive behavior			
• Fewer homicides (per 100,000)		X	
• Fewer assault injuries (per 100,000)		X	
Educational and community-based programs:			
• More schools with comprehensive school health education			X
• More workplaces with health promotion	X		

Health Protection

	RIGHT DIRECTION	WRONG DIRECTION	NO CHANGE/ NO DATA
Unintentional injuries			
• Fewer unintentional injury deaths (per 100,000)	X		
• More people using auto safety restraints	X		
Occupational safety and health			
• Fewer work-related deaths (per 100,000)	X		
• Fewer work-related injuries (per 100,000)		X	
Environmental health			
• No children with blood lead 25 ug/dL	X		
• More people with clean air in their communities	X		
• More people in radon-tested homes	X		
Food and drug safety			
• Fewer salmonella outbreaks	X		
Oral health			
• Fewer children with dental caries	X		
• Fewer older people without teeth	X		

Preventive Services

	RIGHT DIRECTION	WRONG DIRECTION	NO CHANGE/ NO DATA
Maternal and infant health			
• Fewer low-birth-weight newborns		X	
• More mothers with first trimester care	X		

(table continued on page 42)

TABLE 2-1. Progress in Meeting Objectives (continued)

Health Promotion

	RIGHT DIRECTION	WRONG DIRECTION	NO CHANGE/ NO DATA
Heart disease and stroke			
• Fewer coronary heart disease deaths (per 100,000)	X		
• Fewer stroke deaths (per 100,000)	X		
• Better control of high blood pressure	X		
• Lower cholesterol levels	X		
Cancer			
• Decrease cancer deaths (per 100,000)	X		
• Increase screening for breast cancer (age > 50 yrs)	X		
• Increase screening for cervical cancer (age > 18 yrs)	X		
• Increase fecal occult blood testing (age > 50 yrs)	X		
Diabetes and chronic disabling conditions			
• Fewer people disabled by chronic conditions		X	
• Fewer diabetes-related deaths (per 100,000)			X
HIV infection			
• Slower increase in HIV infection (per 100,000)			X
Sexually transmitted diseases			
• Fewer gonorrhea infections (per 100,000)	X		
• Fewer syphilis infections (per 100,000)	X		
Immunization and infectious disease			
• No measles cases	X		
• Fewer pneumonia and influenza deaths (per 100,000)		X	
• Higher immunization levels (ages 19–35 mos)	X		
Clinical preventive services			
• No financial barrier to recommended preventive services		X	

Preventive Services Task Force, a task force of the Department of Health and Human Services. The first edition of the *Guide to Clinical Preventive Services* was published in 1989, and immediately became an important reference for health care providers concerned about health promotion, health maintenance, and disease prevention.

 Nurse practitioners in particular found this text helpful, and it quickly became required reading; students carry the text to their clinical settings for reference regarding topics as disparate as screening for lead toxicity in infants to counseling to prevent low back pain. Divided into screening, counseling, and immunizations/chemoprophylaxis, the *Guide* provides evidence-based practice guidelines for the wisdom related to various screening, counseling, or immunization practices.

The text is now available in the second edition (1996) and the number of topics evaluated has grown to 70. ∎

Clinician's Handbook of Preventive Services

The *Clinician's Handbook of Preventive Services* is a companion of, and closely related to, the *Guide to Clinical Preventive Services*. The *Clinician's Handbook of Preventive Services* is the cornerstone of the "Put Prevention Into Practice" (PPIP) campaign, which was initiated in 1994 after the U.S. Preventive Services Task Force did its groundbreaking work. The *Clinician's Handbook of Preventive Services*, now in its second edition (1998), provides clinicians with helpful tools for adopting a systematic approach to screening and counseling. Useful features of this book, which are not available in the *Guide to Clinical Preventive Services,* are a resource list for patients, including pamphlets, books, videotapes, and a resource list for providers with supplemental reading on each topic. Any primary care provider would find the patient resource list beneficial for patient teaching efforts.

Clinical Relevance of Health Promotion to Patient Education

Health promotion has become a buzzword for nurses, especially those involved in primary care. Many have jumped on the health promotion bandwagon, especially those of us who have seen the ravages of unhealthy lifestyles. The better educated, affluent consumer demands health promotion from his or her primary care provider and in his or her workplace. Convincing these people that screening and disease prevention is important is usually not a problem; they may request screening tests before the primary care provider suggests them. However, people who cope with many daily problems and limited discretionary income may be less enthusiastic about spending limited funds for taxicabs to clinics, where they can be screened for diseases about which they are unaware and for which they are asymptomatic. If the exigencies of daily life outweigh the promised rewards from obscure screening tests, it is dubious that these people will seek screening tests. Until all Americans can meet their basic survival needs, it is doubtful that screening will be universally accepted.

Health Screening

Screening for health risks is a form of secondary prevention; it is not primary prevention. Screening has been defined as the detection of disease in asymptomatic, apparently healthy people. Screening is the presumptive identification of an unrecognized disease or defect, with tests or examinations that rapidly sort apparently well persons, who probably have a disease, from those who probably do

not. It does not make conceptual or economic sense to screen for all conditions.

The following criteria have been derived for screening that is cost-beneficial:

1. The disease is an important health problem (eg, hypertension) in that many people are susceptible.
2. Accepted therapy is available.
3. Facilities are available for diagnosis and treatment.
4. The disease has an asymptomatic (or latent) phase during which detection and treatment decrease morbidity and mortality.
5. Treatment in the asymptomatic phase yields a therapeutic result.
6. The natural history of the disease is understood.
7. The test(s) for the disease is (are) acceptable and available at a reasonable cost.
8. An agreed-on policy exists regarding whom is to be treated.
9. The cost of case finding and treatment is less than the cost if the disease is discovered when it becomes symptomatic.

Patient education is an important adjunct to screening. If the nurse can help the patient understand why screening is important, the patient is more likely to accept screening. Conversely, it is important that nurses understand why some screening exams are not indicated for particular situations. For example, a healthy 28-year-old male who has had no symptoms of heart disease and does not have a positive family history does not need a resting electrocardiogram, even though he may request one. Therefore, the nurse must understand which forms of disease prevention are most important at which ages and for which populations.

APPLICATION OF RESOURCES: NUTRITION AND WEIGHT

Table 2–1 indicates that a sentinel objective of *Healthy People 2000*—having fewer people overweight—was not achieved at the time of the midcourse review and is an objective in *Healthy People 2010*. Obesity is one of the most significant health problems in westernized countries, and the United States probably has more obese persons than any other country in the world. Approximately 58 million adults in the United States, who are older than 20 years of age, are obese (ie, greater than 20% above desired body weight) (Kuczmarski, Flegal, Campbell, et al., 1994). Obesity is directly and indirectly associated with many diseases (eg, heart disease and diabetes). Obesity frequently begins in childhood with approximately 80% of overweight children becoming overweight adults.

The following case study incorporates information from the *Guide to Clinical Preventive Services* and the *Clinician's Handbook of Preventive Services* to a family that presents to the nurse and nurse practitioner in a midwestern pediatric practice.

C A S E   S T U D Y

THE VAN DAMME FAMILY

HISTORY AND PHYSICAL EXAMINATION
The Van Damme family has been part of the Hollander Family Practice for the past 7 years. The Van Damme's have three children: Anna, 7 years of age; Peter, 5 years of age; and Marta, 9 months of age. Mr. Van Damme is a 28-year-old wheat and dairy farmer and Mrs. Van Damme previously worked as an administrative assistant but now stays home with the children.

Mrs. Van Damme, who has recently discovered that she is pregnant with their fourth child, brings Marta in for her second diptheria-tetanus-pertussis (DTP) injection; Marta had to miss the scheduled 6-month injection because of otitis media. When the nursing staff weighs Marta they note that she weighs 24 pounds and is 27 inches long, placing her above the 100th percentile in weight and just below the

50th percentile in height. Anna weighs 72 pounds (above the 100th percentile for weight). Peter's weight is 35 pounds, which is appropriate for a 5-year-old male. Mrs. Van Damme is 5 feet 6 inches and weighs 164 pounds, which is more than 20% above her desired weight. (Box 2-1 provides a quick, easy method of calculating body weight for adults.)

After the physical examination, the nurse practitioner compliments Mrs. Van Damme on the manner in which she relates to Marta and the two older children. She notes that all three children are progressing well developmentally, and that Marta is almost updated on her immunizations. The nurse practitioner conveys to Mrs. Van Damme that Anna and Marta are overweight and that this is a potential health risk factor. Mrs. Van Damme is surprised to hear that being overweight can be a health risk for children. She notes that everyone in her family has been "solid," but she believes they are all healthy. After further data gathering, the nurse practitioner learns that Mrs. Van Damme's mother and maternal grandmother have the "type of diabetes that old people get." Mr. Van Damme's 58-year-old father recently died from a massive heart attack, which Mrs. Van Damme relates to the downturn in farming profits and the stressors involved in farming.

Plan
The nurse practitioner decides that health maintenance and health promotion are major parts of the plan in the Problem-Oriented Medical Recording that she will enact with the Van Damme family. When the nurse practitioner refers to the *Healthy People 2000 Midcourse Review*, she notes that achievement of the nutrition objective is not being met nationally and that it continues to be an objective in *Healthy People 2010*. More Americans are

(case study continues on page 45)

overweight now than when the objectives were written. A review of the *Guide to Clinical Preventive Services* provides her with helpful patient education and counseling strategies (Box 2-2).

The nurse practitioner reviews Chapter 56 (Counseling to Promote a Healthy Diet) of the *Guide to Clinical Preventive Services.* She learns that reduced intake of dietary fat helps reduce the incidence of coronary artery disease and that intake of dietary fats also may be associated with increased incidence of cancers. Additionally, she notes that increased intake of dietary fiber improves gastrointestinal function; decreasing sodium may help to sodium-dependent cases of hypertension; intake of complex carbohydrates, rather than simple sugars, improves calorie balance and decreases the incidence of dental caries; and that adolescent girls and women generally need more dietary calcium than they usually ingest.

Remembering that Mrs. Van Damme is pregnant, the nurse practitioner reads about the nutritional needs of women, infants, and children. She is particularly impressed by the findings related to breast-feeding (eg, its health benefits and the lower likelihood of adult obesity in breast-fed infants).

Implementation

Armed with this information, the nurse practitioner covers the basics of the food pyramid with Mrs. Van Damme. Based on findings in the *Guide to Clinical Preventive Services* that counseling by dietitians is probably more likely to bring about changes in dietary patterns than counseling by physicians or nurse practitioners, the nurse practitioner refers Mrs. Van Damme to the clinic nutritionist. Finally, the nurse practitioner refers to the *Clinician's Handbook of Preventive Services* and copies down the patient resources dealing with nutrition (Box 2-3).

In the *Guide to Clinical Preventive Services,* Chapter 55 (Counseling to Promote Physical Activity) also provides helpful information related to type 2 diabetes, for which Mrs. Van Damme is at considerable risk based on her family history and her current obesity. The nurse practitioner schedules the Van Damme family for a follow-up visit after the nutritionist appointment. At this time she will cover the guidelines on physical activity and use information from the *Clinician's Handbook of Preventive Services* to make informational materials available to the Van Dammes. The nurse practitioner charts the following SOAP note on Mrs. Van Damme's chart and an appropriate note on Marta's chart.

S: 31-year-old female member of the practice accompanying infant for DPT. Denies concern about her weight or that of her children. Reports positive maternal family history for type 2 diabetes and positive paternal family history (husband's father) for fatal myocardial infarction at age 58. Relates that she is newly pregnant.

O: Height and weight: 5'6" tall, 164 pounds. Pregnancy confirmed with urine test.

A: First trimester pregnancy. Obesity.
Health maintenance:
Appropriate weight loss
Increased physical activity
Diagnostic:
1. Schedule for ultrasound and early pregnancy tests

Patient education:
Refer to nutritionist for dietary counseling for self and children.
Discuss benefits of breast-feeding at the next appointment.
During next appointment discuss benefits of exercise.
Provide patient handouts on weight loss and physical activity for herself and children.

BOX 2-1. Height-Weight Formula for Calculating Adult Body Weight

Female
Allow 100 lbs for first 5' of height and then add 5 lbs for each additional inch above 5'.

Male
Allow 106 lbs for first 5' of height and then add 6 lbs for each additional inch above 5'.

BOX 2-2. Patient Education and Counseling Strategies

1. **Frame the teaching to match the patient's perceptions.** Elicit information about the patient's belief system; match teaching with cultural sensitivity.
2. **Inform patients of the purposes and expected effects of interventions.** Also inform them when to expect these effects. Trace the trajectory of the recovery process and what signifies a recovery or complications.
3. **Suggest small changes rather than large ones.** Patients need to experience success and are more likely to be successful if recommended changes are not overwhelming.
4. **Be specific.** Explain the rationale, demonstrate any needed activities, and write down instructions.
5. **Add new behaviors.** It may be easier to add new behaviors than eliminate old ones. It is usually easier to get patients to add exercise to their daily regimes than to convince them to change their eating patterns.
6. **Link new behaviors to old ones.** If some activities are performed daily, such as brushing one's teeth, it's easier for patients to remember to take medications at the same time they brush their teeth than at other times.
7. **Use the power of the profession.** Health care providers serve as powerful influences in the lives of their patients; it is acceptable and useful to say, "Cigarette smoking is the worst thing that you can do for your health. I would like for you to stop now."
8. **Get explicit commitments from the patient.** Ask patients to describe how they will achieve the recommended health promotion and disease management activities. Obtaining commitments is more likely to result in adherence to the treatment plan.

Both the *Guide to Clinical Preventive Services* and the *Clinician's Handbook of Preventive Services* provide useful health promotion strategies for the Van Damme family. They are essential resources for the nurse practitioner or advanced practice nurse to provide thoughtful patient education that is oriented toward risk factor reduction and health promotion. Additionally, because the objectives for *Healthy People 2000* are constantly being tracked, the advanced practice nurse can easily ascertain the progress that has been made is achieving the various health promotion goals. Although nurses should always individualize treatment plans for each patient, the broad objectives in *Healthy People 2000* offer an overall approach to working with aggregates in achieving healthy lifestyles. They are useful adjuncts to achieving *Healthy People 2000* objectives.

SUMMARY

Chapter 2 provides various frameworks for applying health promotion to patient education. Health promotion was reviewed from its earliest origins in the compliance literature to the more current approach that presumes human beings desire to improve their health status by engaging in healthy lifestyles, undergoing immunizations, and making other various attempts to self-actualize themselves. The

9. **Use a combination of strategies.** Multiple strategies are more likely to result in behavior change than a single strategy. Combinations of group teaching, individual, audio-visual, and printed materials are more likely to bring desired changes than only using printed materials.

10. **Involve office staff.** A team approach facilitates patient education efforts. Some patients may be more attuned to medical assistants or front-office staff in terms of cultural background; thus, their suggestions may be more helpful than those of professional staff. Nurse practitioners and clinical nurse specialists are generally excellent patient educators but at times patients may prefer other professionals.

11. **Refer.** Although health care providers are responsible for patient education for all patients, it may be preferable at times to refer patients for special teaching activities. There are four major referral sources: community groups and agencies, such as diabetes teaching centers at university hospitals; national voluntary health organizations (eg, American Lung Association or the American Cancer Society); instructional references, such as books and videotapes; and other patients who can serve as role models and peer advisors.

12. **Monitor progress through follow-up contact.** Progress can be monitored through telephone calls or office visits. Follow-up should occur frequently so that any problems that arise can be solved, successes can be recognized, and instructions can be reinforced.

Note. From *Guide to Clinical Preventive Services,* 1996.

BOX 2-3. Patient Nutrition Resources

The following books and pamphlets are available from the American Academy of Pediatrics, P.O. Box 927, Elk Grove Village, IL 60009-0927; (800) 433-9016. Internet address: www.aap.org

- The Gift of Love
- Feeding Kids Right Isn't Always Easy
- Tips for Preventing Food Hassles
- Growing Up Healthy: Fat, Cholesterol, and More
- Right from the Start: ABC's of Good Nutrition for Young Children
- What's to Eat? Health Foods for Hungry Children

The following book is directed toward adolescents who participate in athletics, and can be obtained through the American College of Sports Medicine, P.O. Box 1440, Indianapolis, IN 46202-1440; (317) 634-7817.

- Nutrition and Sports Performance: A Guide for High School Athletes Guidelines pertaining to the food pyramid are available from the Cooperative Extension System or by contacting the Superintendent of Documents, U.S. Government Printing Office, Washington, DC 20402; (202) 783-3238. The third citation is available from the Food Marketing Institute, 800 Connecticut Avenue NW, Washington, DC 20006.
- Nutrition and Your Health: Dietary Guidelines for Americans
- The Food Guide Pyramid
- The Food Guide Pyramid: Beyond the Basic 4

Health Belief Model, Pender's Health Promotion Model, Green's Precede-Proceed Model, Lauver's Care-Seeking Behavior Model, and Leventhal's Self-Regulation were reviewed for their applicability to patient education. *Healthy People 2000, A Midcourse Review* was examined in terms of the areas that relate to health promotion. Obesity was used as an example of the one goal that is not currently being met, which has implications for health promotion and patient education. The *Guide to Clinical Preventive Services* and the *Clinician's Handbook of Preventive Services* counseling guidelines for obesity were applied as one approach that uses evidence-based research to provide guidelines for patient education regarding health-promoting lifestyles.

Health promotion is a logical and easy arena in which the nurse can become involved in patient education. Once people understand the reasons for engaging in healthy behaviors, they are frequently amenable to teaching. Motivation toward health promotion, however, remains a problem for patient education; this topic will be covered in Chapter 4.

STRATEGIES FOR CRITICAL ANALYSIS AND APPLICATION

1. Suppose that you are working in an inner city neighborhood in an outpatient clinic that serves primarily new immigrants. These immigrants are struggling to learn English, find jobs, and obtain necessary health care for themselves and their children. Which health promotion model would be most useful in your work with families in this clinic?
2. Apply Pender's Health Promotion Model to the Van Damme family. What are the interpersonal influences (eg, family, peers, providers), norms, and support that might influence Mrs. Van Damme to engage in health promotion behavior? What do you think some of the immediate competing demands might be in Mrs. Van Damme's life that would interfere with health-promoting behavior?

3. Using the *Guide to Clinical Preventive Services* and the *Clinician's Handbook of Preventive Services*, establish a teaching plan related to health promotion and disease prevention for the following situation: Ms. Mahoney is a 55-year-old patient of yours in a family practice. Her most recent fecal occult blood test series that she performed at home was reported by the lab as positive for one of the smears. Ms. Mahoney has resisted having a sigmoidoscopy in the past. What is your recommendation to Ms. Mahoney? Using the patient counseling strategies in Box 2-2, describe your plan for health maintenance and disease prevention.

REFERENCES

Allison, S. D. (1973). A framework for nursing action in a nurse-conducted diabetic management clinic. *Journal of Nursing Administration, 3*(4), 53–60.

Backscheider, J. E. (1974). Self-care requirements, self-care capabilities, and nursing systems in the diabetic nurse management clinic. *American Journal of Public Health, 64*(12), 1138–1146.

Becker, M. H. (1974). The health belief model and sick role behavior. In M. H. Becker (Ed.). *The health belief model and personal behavior.* Thorofare, NJ: Charles B. Slack.

Becker, M. H. (1979). Understanding patient compliance: The contributions of attitudes and other psychosocial factors. In S. J. Cohen (Ed.), *New directions in patient compliance.* Lexington, MA: DC Heath.

Becker, M. H., & Janz, N. K. (1985). The health belief model applied to understanding diabetes regimen compliance. *Diabetes Educator, 11*(1), 41–47.

Bottorff, J. L., Johnson, J. L., Ratner, P. A., & Hayduk, C. A. (1996). The effects of cognitive-perceptual factors on health promotion behavior maintenance. *Nursing Research, 45*(1), 30–36.

Cerkoney, K. A. B., & Hart, L. K. (1980). The relationship between the health belief model and compliance of persons with diabetes mellitus. *Diabetes Care, 3*(5), 594–598.

Conrad, P. (1985). The meaning of medications:

Another look at compliance. *Social Science and Medicine, 20*(1), 29–37.

Duffy, M. E. (1988). Determinants of health promotion in midlife women. *Nursing Research, 37*(6), 358–362.

Duffy, M. E. (1993). Determinants of health-promoting lifestyles in older persons. *Image—The Journal of Nursing Scholarship, 25*(1), 23–28.

Eisen, M., Zellman, G. L., & McAlister, A. L. (1992). A health belief model-social learning theory approach to adolescents' fertility control: Findings from a controlled field trial. *Health Education Quarterly, 19*, 249–262.

Falck, R. S., Siegal, H. A., Wang, J., Carlson, R. G. (1995). Usefulness of the health belief model in predicting HIV needle risk practices among injection users. *AIDS Education and Prevention, 7*(6), 523–533.

French, B. N., Kurczynski, T. W., Weaver, M. T., & Pituch, M. J. (1992). Evaluation of the health belief model and decision making regarding amniocentesis in women of advanced maternal age. *Health Education Quarterly, 19*, 177–186.

Galvin, K. T. (1992). A critical review of the health belief model in relation to cigarette smoking behavior. *Journal of Clinical Nursing, 1*(1), 13–18.

Garcia, A. W., Pender, N. J., Antonakos, C. L., & Ronis, D. L. (1998). Changes in physical activity beliefs and behaviors of boys and girls across the transition to junior high school. *Journal of Adolescent Health, 22*(5), 394–402.

Green, L. W. (1999). What can we generalize from research on patient education and clinical health promotion to physician counseling on diet. *European Journal of Clinical Nutrition, 53*, S9–18.

Green, L. W., & Kreuter, M. W. (1991). *Health promotion planning: An educatinal and environmental approach* (2nd ed). Mountain View, CA: Mayfield.

Green, L.W., et al. (1980). *Health education planning: A diagnostic approach.* Palo Alto, CA: Mayfield.

Hamera, E. K., Peterson, K. A., Young, L. M., and Schaumloffel, M. M. (1992). Symptom monitoring in schizophrenia: Potential for enhancing self-care. *Archives of Psychiatric Nursing, 6*, 324–330.

Hawkins, W. E., Duncan, D. F., & McDermott, R. J. (1989). A health assessment of older Americans: Some multidimensional measures. *Preventive Medicine, 17*(3), 344–356.

Hays, R. D., & DiMatteo, M. R. (1981). Patient compliance assessment. *Journal of Compliance in Health Care, 2*(1), 37–53.

Healthy Children 2000, National Health Promotion and Disease Prevention Objectives related to Mothers, Infants, Children, Adolescents, and Youth. (1991). U.S. Department of Health and Human Services, Public Health Service. Boston: Jones and Bartlett.

U.S. Department of Health and Human Services. (1991). *Healthy People 2000.* Washington, D.C.: Public Health Service, DHHS Pub. Number 91-50212.

Hochbaum, G. M. (1958). *Public participation in medical screening programs: A sociopsychological study.* (Public Health Service Publication No. 572). Washington, DC: U.S. Government Printing Office.

Howat, P., Jones, S., Hall, M., Cross, D., & Stevenson, M. (1997). The PRECEDE-PROCEED model: Application to planning a child pedestrian injury prevention program. *Injury Prevention, 3*(4), 282–287.

Johnson, J. L., Ratner, P. A., & Bottorff, J. L. (1995). Urban-rural differences in the health-promoting behaviours of Albertans. *Canadian Journal of Public Health, 86*(3) 103–108.

Johnson, J. L., Ratner, P. A., Bottorff, J. L., & Hayduck, L. A. (1993). An exploration of Pender's Health Promotion Model using LISREL. *Nursing Research, 42*(3), 132–138.

Kuczmarkski, R. J., Flegal, K. M., Campbell, S. M., Johnson, C. L. (1994). Increasing prevalence of overweight among U.S. adults, The National Health and Nutrition Examination Surveys, 1960–1991. *Journal of the American Medical Association, 272*(3), 205–211.

Laraque, D., McLean, D. E., Brown-Peterside, P., Ashton, D., Diamond, B. (1997). Predictors of reported condom use in central Harlem youth as conceptualized by the health belief model. *Journal of Adolescent Health, 21*(5), 318–327.

Lauver, D. R., Settersten, L., Marten, S., & Halls, J. (1999). Explaining women's intentions and use of hormones with menopause. *Research in Nursing and Health, 22*(4), 309–320.

Lauver, D. R., Kane, J. (1999). A motivational message, external barriers, and mammography utilization. *Cancer Detection and Prevention, 23*(3), 254–264.

Lauver, D., Nabholz, S., Scott, K., & Tak, Y. (1997). Testing theoretical explanations of mammography use. *Nursing Research, 46*(1), 32–39.

Lauver, D. (1992). A theory of care-seeking behavior. *Image—the Journal of Nursing Scholarship, 24*(4), 281–287.

Leventhal, H. (1982). Wrongheaded ideas about illness. *Psychology Today, 16*(1), 48–55, 73.

Leventhal, H., & Johnson, J. E. (1983). Laboratory and field experimentation: Development of a theory of self-regulation. In P. J. Wooldridge, M. H. Schmitt, J. K. Skipper, & R. C. Leonard (Eds.), *Behavioral science and nursing theory*. St. Louis: CV Mosby.

Leventhal, H., Singer, R., & Jones, S. (1985). Effects of fear and specificity of recommendations upon attitudes and behavior. *Journal of Personality and Social Psychology, 2*(1), 20–29.

Leventhal, H., Zimmerman, R., & Gutmann, M. Compliance: A self-regulation perspective. In D. Gentry (Ed.), *Handbook of behavioral medicine*. New York: Guilford Press.

Lusk, S. L., Ronis, D., Kerr, M. J., & Atwood, J. R. (1994). Test of the health promotion model as a causal model of workers' use of hearing protection. *Nursing Research, 43*(3), 151–157.

Macrina, D., Macrina, N., Horvath, C., Gallaspy, J., & Fine, P. R. (1996). An educational intervention to increase use of the Glasgow coma scale by emergency department personnel. *International Journal of Trauma Nursing, 2*(1), 7–12.

McPhee, S. J., & Schroeder, S. A. (1996). General approach to the patient: Health maintenance and disease prevention; and common symptoms. In L. M. Tierney, S. J. McPhee, & M. A. Papadakis (Eds.), *Current Diagnosis and Medical Treatment*. Stamford, CT: Appleton and Lange.

Meyer, D., Leventhal, H., & Gutmann, M. (1985). Common-sense models of illness: The example of hypertension. *Health Psychology, 4*(2), 115–135.

Mirotznik, J., Ginzler, E., Zagon, G., & Baptiste, A. (1998). Using a health belief model to explain clinic appointment-keeping for the management of a chronic disease condition. *Journal of Community Health, 23*(3): 195–210.

Orem, D. E. (1971). *Nursing: Concepts of practice*. New York: McGraw-Hill.

Pender, N. J. (1982). *Health promotion in nursing practice*. East Norwalk, CT: Appleton-Century-Crofts.

Pender, N. J. (1987). *Health promotion in nursing practice* (2nd ed.). East Norwalk, CT: Appleton and Lange.

Pender, N. J. (1990). Expressing health through lifestyle patterns. *Nursing Science Quarterly, 30*(3), 115–122.

Pender, N. J. (1996). *Health promotion in nursing practice* (3rd ed.). Stamford, CT: Appleton and Lange.

Pender, N. J., Walker, S. N., Sechrist, K. R., and Frank-Stromberg, M. Predicting health-promoting life styles in the workplace. *Nursing Research, 39*, 326–332.

Pender, N. J., Walker, S. N., Sechrist, K. R., & Frank-Stromborg, M. (1990). *The Health Promotion Model: Refinement and Validation*. Final Report to the National Center for Nursing Research, National Institutes of Health (Grant#NR01121). Dekalb, IL: Northern University Press.

Pham, D. T., Fortin, F., Thibaudeau, M. F. (1996). The role of the health belief model in amputees' self-evaluation of adherence to diabetes self-care behaviors. *Diabetes Educator, 22*(2), 126–132.

Rankin, S. H., & Stallings, K. D. (1996). Patient Education. Philadelphia: Lippincott-Raven.

Sackett, D. L. (1976). The magnitude of compliance and noncompliance. In D. L. Sackett and R. B. Haynes (Eds.), *Compliance with therapeutic regimens*. Baltimore: The Johns Hopkins University Press.

Sackett, D. L., & Haynes, R. B. (1976). *Compliance with therapeutic regimens*. Baltimore: The Johns Hopkins University Press.

Stout, A. E. (1997). Prenatal care for low-income women and the health belief model: A new beginning. *Journal of Community Health Nursing, 14*(3), 169–180.

Trostle, J. A. (1988). Medical compliance as an ideology. *Social Science and Medicine, 27*, 1299–1308.

U.S. Department of Health and Human Services. (1998). *Clinician's handbook of preventive services*. Washington, D.C.: U.S. Government Printing Office.

U.S. Preventive Services Task Force. (1996). *Guide to clinical preventive services* (2nd ed.). Baltimore: Williams and Wilkins.

U.S. Department of Health and Human Services. (2000). *Healthy People 2010* (Conference Edition, in Two Volumes). Washington, D.C.: .

Walker, S. N., Sechrist, K. R. & Pender, N. J. (1987). The health-promoting lifestyle profile: Development and psychometric characteristics. *Nursing Research, 36*(2), 76–81.

Wallston, B. S., & Wallston, K. A. (1984). Social psychological models of health behavior: An examination and integration. In A. Baum, S. Taylor, & J. E. Singer (Eds.), *Handbook of psychology and health: Vol. IV. Social psychological aspects of psychology*. Hillsdale, NJ: L. Erlbaum Associates.

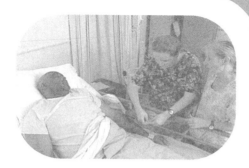

CHAPTER

3

Integration of Cultural Systems and Beliefs

Barbara Hollinger

LEARNING OBJECTIVES

After reading this chapter, the nurse or student nurse should be able to:

1. Apply the Cultural Assessment Framework to better understand the similarities and differences between the mainstream culture and the ethnic or cultural group targeted for patient education

2. Develop a patient teaching plan for a client who is a migrant farm worker.

3. Using the Kleinman Model as part of the assessment, plan a teaching program for a Native American man with diabetes.

4. Plan a culturally-sensitive prenatal teaching plan for a Mexican American adolescent.

5. Assess the acculturation level of various members of a three-generation Vietnamese family.

6. Create a teaching plan for a Hmong toddler with otitis media, using a medical interpreter as a cultural broker.

7. Analyze the stressors facing a hypertensive African American grandmother, who is raising her 2-year-old twin grandsons who have asthma, and identify sources of cultural support that might be available to her.

INTRODUCTION

The Hmong Family: A Case of Cross-Cultural Challenges

Anne Fadiman's 1997 book, *The Spirit Catches You and You Fall Down,* recounts the personal experience of a Hmong family in Merced, California, in the health care system. Lia Lee is 3 months old when she experiences her first seizure. Her American doctors believe she has a disorder caused by damaged cells in the cerebral cortex, transmitting neural impulses simultaneously and chaotically. The Lees think their daughter's condition is caused by a "spirit catching her and making her fall down." The parents' belief is consistent with their belief that soul-stealing spirits are often the cause of illness. The physicians involved are considered the most caring, compassionate, and well trained pediatricians in the area.

This case history spans several years and, despite many changes in medication, several hospitalizations, and the removal of the child from parental custody for several months, the child's seizures are never adequately controlled and she suffers irreversible brain damage. Misunderstandings abound throughout the multiple encounters regarding procedures (eg, spinal taps, blood tests), the lifetime use of medication for a chronic condition, and the roles and responsibilities of the parents and the physicians.

Ethnic Diversity and the Health Care System

The Lee family's story illustrates the complexity of cross-cultural challenges facing all medical professionals in the new millennium. According to the United States Department of the Census, in 1990, 25% of the total U.S. population was comprised of ethnically diverse people. That figure is expected to rise to 33% in year 2000 census, and at current growth rates, should approach 50% by the year 2050. This ethnically diverse population includes an increasing number of foreign-born persons; currently 1 of 13 persons (or 19 million Americans) are foreign-born.

The foreign-born population is not only ethnically diverse, but its attitudes toward its adopted and native countries vary considerably. Some immigrants chose to establish a new life in the United States. Others, such as traumatized refugees fleeing war, ethnic cleansing, or the socioeconomic upheaval after a natural or manmade disaster, may dream of returning to their native country. Some migrant workers have homes and families in their native country and come to the United States to work for a limited time and return home. Even longtime United States residents, whether foreign born or U.S. born, vary tremendously in their level of acculturation. The health professions have begun to acknowledge that the melting pot has become more of an ethnic stew, with each element retaining its own flavor and characteristics.

Because ethnically diverse persons are underrepresented in the health care professions, it can be assumed that other health care providers will increasingly care for persons that are ethnically and culturally different from themselves. Likewise, culturally diverse nurses will care for the full spectrum of patient clientele and also will work cross-culturally.

This chapter presents the Cultural Assessment Framework that is useful for understanding factors that affect patient education in the cross-cultural exchange. Although an in-depth understanding of all ethnocultural groups in the United States is not possible, we hope that nurses will try to explore those cultural groups with whom they regularly interact. In many health care settings, one or two diverse cultural groups form most of the ethnic patient population. All providers are capable of learning a deeper understanding of one or two ethnocultural groups different from their own. Tremendous diversity exists within each cultural group; thus, any framework is only a blueprint; the details of diversity are clarified during individual patient encounters.

Even culturally prepared nurses find themselves teaching patients with cultural backgrounds they are not familiar with. For cases in which a briefer assessment is required, Kleinman's Model is presented. Having a broader idea of the complexity of issues that can influence cross-cultural exchanges can add meaning to a briefer exploration. The clinical relevance of the Cultural Assessment Framework in patient education is presented, along with some factors the nurse should consider when working with special populations within a cultural group (eg, pediatric patients and older people).

In this chapter, *culture* is defined as the sum total of ways of living by a group of human beings (ie, concepts, habits, beliefs, skills, art), which is transmitted from one generation to another. An *ethnic group* is a group of people—racially, linguistically, or historically related—having a common and distinctive culture. Again, as much diversity exists within ethnic groups as exists between them. Hispanics, or Latinos, are often stereotyped as one ethnic group; however, Latinos vary between countries and within the same country, despite sharing Hispanic surnames.

THE CULTURAL ASSESSMENT FRAMEWORK

The framework of Huff and Kline is presented in their book, *Promoting Health in Multicultural Populations*. The framework is designed for use in individual patient encounters and health promotion and disease prevention education activities with small groups or in the community. The Cultural Assessment Framework explores five areas through the following assessment categories (Box 3-1):

1. Culture-specific demographic factors
2. Culture-specific epidemiological and environmental factors

---

BOX 3-1. Cultural Assessment Framework

Factors Pertaining to the Cultural or Ethnic Group

Demographic Factors
- Age profile
- Gender roles
- Social class/Status
- Education/Literacy
- Languages/Dialects
- Religion
- Occupation/Income
- Residence
- Acculturation

Epidemiological and Environmental Factors
- Morbidity rates
- Mortality rates
- Disability rates
- Environmental exposures
- Other environmental risk factors

Group Characteristics
- Cultural/Ethnic identity
- Cosmology
- Time orientation
- Self-Perception
- Community perception
- Social norms, Values, Customs
- Communication patterns

Health Care Beliefs and Practices
- Explanatory models
- Response to illness
- Western health care use
- Health promotion use
- Health behavior practices

Factors Pertaining to the Health Care Provider

Western Health Care Organization and Service Delivery Variables
- Cultural competence/Sensitivity
- Organizational policy and mission
- Facilities and Program preparation
- Evaluation of culturally competent services

Note. From Huff, R. M., & Kline, M. V. (Eds.) (1999). *Promoting health in multicultural populations: A handbook for practitioners.* Thousand Oaks, CA: Sage Publications. Adapted with permission.

3. Cultural characteristics
4. Health care beliefs and practices
5. Western health care organization and service delivery variables

Culture-Specific Demographic Factors

This assessment category evaluates the culture or ethnic group in relation to age, gender, social class or status, education and literacy, language and dialect, religious preferences, occupation and income, patterns of residence, living conditions, and acculturation and assimilation.

Age

Age can affect a given population in terms of demographics or culture. A 1997 National Agricultural Workers Survey of U.S. seasonal agricultural workers indicates that this is a young population (two-thirds of them are younger than 35 years of age). As a cultural factor, age may determine who makes decisions in a family. Age is often a factor in terms of acculturation and language acquisition; younger people are associated with more rapid language acquisition and with faster acculturation.

Gender

In cultural groups, gender is often a factor that affects specific role expectations within a family, decision-making, and client comfort with physical examinations by opposite-gender health care providers.

In the study *Health Perceptions of the Hmong*, which was conducted in Fresno, CA, with Laotian immigrant families (Hollinger, 1984), women were expected to clean the house, cook, wash clothes, garden, do *Pan Dao* (also known as *paj ntaub*, a traditional Hmong textile art), sew, and go to school. One Hmong woman who was interviewed worked outside the home; she described her role primarily in terms of the family. She operated a small gro-

cery store the family owned, but had not been part of the decision to buy the business. The male role was to "support and take care of the family and to help other people" (Hollinger, 1984, pp. 117 and 118) and, in Laos, to be a soldier. The male head of the household made most of the family decisions. Patient teaching related to family planning or even breast-feeding is often much more effective if the family decision-maker is included in the education.

Social Class and Status

The social class and status of an ethnic group is often closely associated with educational level, occupation, and income. English proficiency and greater acculturation are often prerequisites for high educational achievement in the United States. Many professionally trained immigrants experience a decrease in social status and occupation on arrival in this country. It is helpful to know which persons in the ethnic community are held in the highest esteem (eg, clan elders, teachers, or an older grandmother). These people often help a client to make difficult health-related decisions. In every group, some people have great influence among their peers. Making a favorable impression with the cultural broker within the community can greatly affect the entire group's acceptance of a health care provider.

Literacy and Education

Literacy and educational levels are important factors in all aspects of patient education. Among immigrants, rural or urban status in their native country or political upheavals may have affected their educational attainment. Throughout the 1980s and early 1990s, the civil war in El Salvador left many rural Salvadorans in war-conflicted zones with no schools. Those who were literate taught their children what they knew, but rural refugees who fled to the United States often have a much lower educational level than their urban counterparts.

Symbols were designed for teaching low literacy populations; however, they often fail to convey the desired message. A safety study (Domingo, 1992) to determine universal understanding of sketches indicating pain, danger, poison, or death was conducted in California among Mixtec Indian farm workers from Oaxaca, Mexico. The study subjects almost always interpreted the symbols differently from other Mexican farm workers. In Fig. 3-1, which was used in this study, *1c* was meant to indicate pain, yet it brought comments, such as " I don't understand what he has on his back." Drawing *8a*, intended to convey "Danger—no entry for 48 hours," was also confusing. Interpretations included, "Maybe it is dangerous to enter when it is too bright or too dark," and "The intense light from the sun can make you blind."

Language

Language is an important assessment tool. The person's command of the English language is often closely related to his or her level of acculturation. A person's reading and writing proficiency in his or her native language may affect how quickly he or she learns English and is closely related to educational level. A language that is spoken throughout a large geographic area (eg, Spanish) typically has many local dialects; words can have different meanings, depending on the region. Paying close attention to nonverbal cues can help bilingual health care providers understand when they may have used a word or phrase with double meanings to a particular group.

Religious Beliefs

Religious beliefs are crucial to many multicultural groups and often affect health care beliefs. Among the Amish, religion is central to their maintenance of a lifestyle apart from the dominant culture. A recent adolescent study listed church affiliation as a protective factor for youths at high risk. The church has played an integral role in the development and survival of African American communities. Praying for oneself or for others who are experiencing problems is an important spiritual belief.

Occupation and Income

Occupation, income, and place of residence are socioeconomic indicators that may place clients at greater risk for accidents, exposures, or health problems. Many Mexican

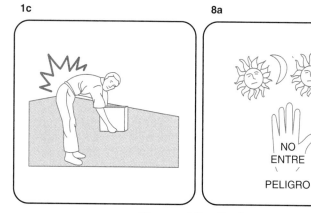

FIGURE 3-1. Pictorial teaching symbols understood differently by Mixtec Indians and Spanish-speaking Mexican American farm workers.

Signs of Confusion

immigrants are employed as seasonal agricultural workers. A 1987 study listed agriculture as the most hazardous occupation, with 49 deaths per 100,000 workers. This statistic surpasses both mining and construction in numbers of fatalities. New immigrants and refugees are more likely to be employed in unskilled, low-wage jobs. Many new immigrants and refugees work as janitors, gardeners, cooks, housekeepers, child-care workers, and home health aides. Low income directly affects residency.

A study was conducted in San Jose, California (Zlolniski & Palerm, 1996) among Mexican immigrants who came to work in the electronics and service industries. Most households spent 40% to 50% of their income on rentals of unsafe, dilapidated, two-bedroom apartments that housed, on average, seven people.

Acculturation is the process of cultural change in people, leading them to adopt elements of one or more cultural groups different from their own. The term is commonly used to indicate the degree to which a person has given up traits of his or her native culture in exchange for elements of the dominant culture. *Assimilation* is defined as cultural and group integration into the political, social, and economic mainstream of the dominant culture. Assimilation is an essential factor in evaluating how to present patient education.

Synthesis: Farm Worker Population

For this chapter, the Cultural Assessment Framework is applied to the U.S. farm worker population. The assessment begins with evaluation of the cultural or ethnic group-specific demographic factors. According to the United States Department of Labor National Agricultural Workers Survey (Mines, Gabbard, & Steirman, 1997), this population is a young population (two-thirds are younger than 35 years of age), male (approximately 80%), and approximately 70% foreign-born. Ninety-four percent of foreign-born farm workers were born in Mexico, with an additional 5%

coming from other Latin countries. Their occupation is comprised of various agricultural tasks. Income for a worker averaged from $5,000 to $7,500 in the survey conducted from 1994 to 1995, with median household incomes between $7,500 and $10,000 annually. Although the majority (60%) of male farm workers are married and although 50% of them have children younger than 18 years of age, many live apart from their families while employed as farm workers. The living pattern showed approximately 50% living with a family member and 50% of all farm workers surveyed living with nonrelatives. Many live in shared living arrangements with five or more people per unit. Most households were in poverty.

Although not addressed in the survey, previous studies have indicated these workers typically have a fifth- or sixth-grade education level. Because 20% of the survey population were in their first year of U.S. farm work and had immediate family in Mexico, it can be assumed that acculturation is low. The language preference is Spanish, but among workers from Oaxaca, Mexico, Mixteco may be the first language, with varying degrees of Spanish fluency. The dominant religion is Roman Catholic, but an increasing number of people adopt Pentecostal, Mormon, or Jehovah's Witness denominations.

Patient Education Implications

For the farm worker population, written, verbal, or video materials must be in Spanish (or Mixteco if available) and geared to a fifth- or sixth-grade reading level. Nurses should reinforce written or symbolic educational materials with verbal explanations and ask for return demonstration of new procedures.

Workers who live in crowded, low-income housing may have inadequate toilet, bathing, refrigeration, and cooking facilities that may further increase health risks. Client education regarding food preparation for patients with diabetes should assess cooking arrangements and food storage availability. Risk reduction for pesticide exposure requires daily bathing and clothing changes. Nurses must assess if workers bathe and wash clothes at home, in the river, or in the local irrigation ditch.

Culture-Specific Epidemiological and Environmental Influences

This second category of the Cultural Assessment Framework has two subcategories:

1. Morbidity, mortality, and disability rates
2. Environmental influences

Despite the difficulty in separating health care access and socioeconomic factors, the morbidity, mortality, and disability subcategory recognizes some specific physical, biologic, and physiologic variations in ethnic and racial groups. For example, a 1988 study of Asian and Pacific Islander Americans in California found that Filipino women older than 50 years of age had a 65% incidence of hypertension; this incidence was higher than that of both African American women (63%) and non-Hispanic white women (47%).

Morbidity and environmental influences are often related. Irish men have the highest death rate from ischemic heart disease in the world, followed by lung cancer. Smoking is believed to account for 26% of premature deaths in Irish men (Purnell & Paulanka, 1998). In this case, the environmental influence of high smoking rates affects the morbidity, mortality, and disability subcategory. Smoking cessation can reduce risk for both ischemic heart disease and cancer.

Environmental racism refers to the tendency for hazardous waste disposal sites to locate in neighborhoods in which people are poor and less politically able to defend their own interests. Environmental racism often occurs in ethnic neighborhoods, increasing the inhabitants' risks for toxic exposures. Inner city environments may expose residents to increased violence, drug dealing, and alcohol abuse.

Synthesis: Farm Worker Population

The second Cultural Assessment Framework category is also applied to the farm worker

population. Among Mexican American migrant workers, infections and communicable and parasitic diseases continue to be major health risks. Tuberculosis rates are increasing among this population; many people acquire the disease after entering the United States. Hepatitis B, amoebic dysentery, shigella, and intestinal parasites are common. A higher incidence of sexually transmitted diseases (eg, syphilis, gonorrhea, chlamydia, and human immunodeficiency virus [HIV]) exists among these workers than in the general population.

Although this population is young, diabetes is a significant risk. Mexican Americans experience five times the incidence of diabetes and an increased risk of diabetes-related complications than does the non-Hispanic white population. Chemical dependency, especially alcoholism, is also increased in Mexican Americans.

Environmental influences consist of physical, biological, and chemical agents. Farm workers are exposed to extremes of hot and cold temperatures, dust, wind, vibration, and noise for those working with farm equipment. Biological exposures include insects, snakes, animals (wild and domestic), and toxic plants. Poison oak is one of the most common dermatological complaints among farm workers. Chemical exposures include fertilizers, cleaning or degreasing compounds, and many classes of pesticides. Farm worker families, including children, also suffer environmental exposures.

 This population is at risk for some of the communicable and parasitic infections. Family is an important cultural value to this population and this can be used in patient education to address some of these issues. For workers who travel without family or relatives, ask how often they hear from family members and ask about how they cope with the isolation and separation. This may be a natural opening for discussing safe sex or alcohol use by focusing on being responsible for the family by not bringing home sexually transmitted diseases or by not mixing drinking with driving. If a patient is thought to have a problem with alcoholism, the nurse might suggest an organization, such as Alcoholics Anonymous, that has Spanish language groups. Some think that the most effective groups for this population are those in which the participants have a similar acculturation level.

The family can also be used when teaching patients about the importance of work safety practices. Many workers dislike wearing cumbersome protective equipment; however, wearing proper equipment might be encouraged by emphasizing to the person how the family depends on the hardworking provider; he should protect himself for the family's sake. ∎

 Patient education regarding child safety must include discussion about the risks of open irrigation canals, the hazards of children riding and playing on tractors and other farm equipment, and the risk of poisoning from chemicals. A coloring book with this information has been developed with bilingual captions and reinforces the message for children. For families that migrate together, older children often help with child care for younger siblings or cousins. Teaching the older children and the parents about safety is another way to prevent accidents. ∎

Cultural Characteristics

The third category of the Cultural Assessment Framework includes general and specific cultural characteristics. These characteristics include how the person or group identifies self, general concepts regarding how natural and supernatural forces interact in the universe, time orientations, communication patterns, social norms, values, and customs. This category also includes the relative priority that the cultural community places on the needs of the person versus the needs of the group.

Among the African American population, age may determine how a person identifies himself or herself. Older people may still use terms, such as Negro or Colored, whereas the 1960s generation may prefer the term Black. African American is the expression more commonly preferred by younger people. African Americans with West Indian heritage may self-identify more with this cultural group.

Views of the Universe

Cultural and ethnic groups view the universe in diverse ways. Some Hmong people believe that those who suffer much in this life may have an easier time in a future life. A *txiv neeb*, or shaman, who was interviewed by the author, thought that this was her third life and that she was blessed with 14 children because of great hardship in her previous life (Hollinger, 1984). Some Mixtec Indians believe that people have spirit animals to assist them in this world. The animal is determined by leaving an infant at a crossroads while the family watches at some distance. The first bird or animal that approaches the child is believed to be that child's spirit animal.

Time Orientation

Time orientation varies among cultures. Among Navajo Indians, the past and present orientation is emphasized, because the Navajo language has no future tense (Purnell & Paulanka, 1998). The European American culture is more future-oriented; investing for later security is encouraged. Many Latin cultures are oriented in the present. For persons in the lower socioeconomic groups, employment is often intermittent. Bringing a child for preventive care (future orientation) and missing a day of work may be seen as jeopardizing a short-term job and illustrates a more present orientation.

Perceptions, Social Norms, Values, and Customs

In the dominant European American culture, self-actualization and competition among peers to achieve are common perceptions. In many cultures, community or family goals take precedence over individual desires. Mixtecs have a strong sense of community and even those who have immigrated to California raise funds to support projects that meet the needs of the home community in Mexico.

Social norms, values, and customs describe accepted and expected behavior among a particular group. Practices regarding birth, marriage, pregnancy, and death are described here. Many East Indians residing in the United States have arranged marriages with women from India. Jewish male infants are circumcised on the eighth day after birth, and the medical procedure is accompanied by a religious ceremony. In Peru and many Latin countries, a cross is placed on the road at the site of a fatal accident.

Communication patterns, including verbal and nonverbal expressions, may vary among cultures. Filipino communication strives to maintain a smooth interpersonal relationship and to avoid confrontation. A hospital director in a San Joaquin Valley community in California had many Filipino employees. An open-door policy was established and the staff was invited to visit him with any concerns or problems that might arise. However, none of the staff members came to the hospital director. When the communication pattern was better understood, employees were encouraged to come together in pairs and each could present the concern of the other; this was a less direct, but more culturally accepted means of communication.

Synthesis: Farm Worker Population

 Cultural characteristics can be applied to the seasonal agricultural worker. Mexican-born farm workers, with family living in Mexico, identify strongly with their Mexican heritage. Many have a fatalistic view of the universe, and health is regarded as a result of good luck, reward for good behavior, or a gift from God not to be taken for granted. These families typically take an active role in caring for a family member who is ill. For example, according to Rehm's 1999 study, when a child suffers from a chronic illness, the family will often make major sacrifices that affect the entire family (eg, relocating to an area perceived to have better health care services). ■

This population has a present-focused time orientation, and its sense of time is more relaxed. Newer immigrants from rural areas may not own a clock or may not know how to tell time. The family is generally considered more important than the individual member. Communication is characterized by *personalismo* or asking about the children or family before discussing the business at hand. Greeting people by name and shaking hands on initial meeting builds an atmosphere of trust. Because education levels are low among this population, television and radio are primary sources of information; written materials may be largely pictorial.

Important cultural values include the importance of family, with children being valued. Men and women have established roles: The man is the head of, and is responsible for the family. The woman cares for the children and is considered the primary purveyor of the culture. Courtesy and respect for adults, elders, teachers, doctors, and authority figures is another important cultural value. Although touching, hugging, and kissing are common forms of expression, this is a modest and private culture in areas of sexuality. Religion is important to most Mexican Americans and most life events are celebrated with a religious ceremony. An isolated client who wears a religious symbol might be encouraged to visit a church with a large Spanish-speaking population.

Patient Education Implications

Emphasizing the importance of responsibility for the family and being a good role model can be a good teaching tactic with Mexican farm worker men. When discussing smoking cessation or second-hand smoke, a good approach might be to discuss how children are most affected by smoking and the role model this behavior creates if the patient smokes. Respect can be shown by acknowledging the physically demanding nature of farm work and the financial insecurity that comes with poorly paid temporary employment. Coming to the clinic for an appointment usually translates into missing a day of work, so caring for as many issues as possible in one visit and trying to accommodate walk-ins on rainy days when clients cannot work are ways of showing respect for the farm worker client.

A study by the Rural Oregon Minority Prenatal Program (Thompson, Curry, & Burton,

1998) among low-income Mexican American women showed that virtually all families had radios and many families subscribed to cable television with a Spanish language channel. Nurses and health care workers should not overlook the opportunities for using the media for health education, especially because many areas only have one or two Spanish-language channels or programs (Fig. 3-2). Public service or health education messages can reach a large proportion of the targeted Spanish speaking population if aired on these stations.

Health Beliefs and Practices

This fourth category encompasses explanatory models of disease and how the culture responds to illness. It also assesses the person's or group's attitude toward Western medicine and preventive medicine. Specific health behavior practices are also examined.

Many non-Western cultures use an explanatory model for the origins of disease. Beliefs regarding disease causality must be consistent with cultural and personal values and behaviors, social training, and often are believed to be linked to an action of a family member,

something happening in the community, or to a supernatural agent. For example, Hollinger was told by family members in Peru that their child has Down syndrome because the mother of the child had spoken ill of her mother-in-law during her pregnancy. A nurse may better understand a culture's specific health behavior practices if he or she understands how culture explains health and illness.

The Hmong View of Illness

The Hmong categorize illness in two ways—illnesses caused by spirits and requiring a spirit healer (eg, a shaman) and illnesses curable by the use of herbs. According to the Hmong, spirit illnesses may be caused by the good shaman spirit, your own body spirits, a spirit from the dead, or an evil spirit. The good spirit of the *txiv neeb* (or shaman) may cause illness by coming to test someone to see if he or she is strong enough to become a shaman. Body spirits could be frightened or stolen away. Illness would result when a few left and death would result when all the spirits left or did not come back. A spirit from the dead could be the spirit of an animal that you mis-

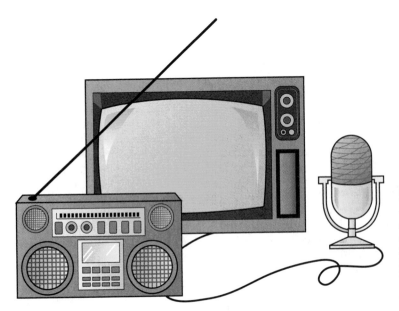

FIGURE 3-2. Local radio and television programs are important venues for disseminating health education information. Many communities have only one or two minority language stations, so public interest programming reaches a wider audience than a similar English-language program.

treated or of a dead person wanting to take you with him or her.

The Hmong's response to illness is consistent with their beliefs. An herbalist would be sought for a nonspirit illness and a shaman for a spirit illness. Because many medicinal herbs available in Laos are not available in the United States, Hmong clients in the study were willing to see Western health care providers for these problems. If a patient saw a medical doctor, did not respond to treatment and became sicker, the family would decide maybe this was a spirit illness. A shaman would be consulted; the shaman would go into a trance state and contact the spirit world. Rituals and ceremonies would be recommended that would placate, bring back, or pay back the offended spirit. Health promotion activities of this population consisted of following customs (eg, observing the postpartum practices), because failure to do so would result in poor health outcomes in the future.

Explanatory Models of Disease: A Peruvian Culture

In the community of Santa Lucia de Pacaraos, Peru, the village's shoe repairman was lame. He used a cane and always carried his right leg at a fixed angle. He believed in and practiced the traditional medicine of this region of Peru and one day recounted how his leg was injured. When he was 9-years-old, he went to the reservoir with two friends. They found some dynamite, and began to play with it. The dynamite exploded and the boy suffered a severe case of *susto* (fright). His fear was so great that his soul left his body. The prescribed treatment required to regain his lost soul consisted of gathering many food items, the national flower *cantuta*, other herbs, and a horse shoe. A ceremony using these items was to be performed three times at midnight, 6:00 AM, and 6:00 PM. The man said he became lame because his family only carried out the ritual twice, thus causing his injury to become permanent. He adamantly be-

lieved that the *susto*, not the dynamite, resulted in his injuries.

Hot and Cold Theory

The hot and cold theory is a belief shared by Mexican Americans and some other Latin cultures. According to this theory, health is maintained when the body maintains proper equilibrium—specifically, a balance between hot and cold elements. Each disease entity is categorized as being caused by hot or cold and must be treated with an opposite remedy to achieve equilibrium of the body. For example, in Peru, rheumatism is a "cold ailment" and is treated with a stinging nettle heated with a small amount of rum and applied to the inflamed joint. Nettles cause a burning sensation when touched and are heated before application; thus, a hot remedy for a cold ailment. An example of using this concept in patient education might be encouraging cold liquids to treat a hot fever.

Synthesis: Farm Worker Population

Among Mexican American farm workers, illness is believed to be caused by the body being out of balance. Cold entering the body may cause an illness and must be treated with a hot element. The definition of what illnesses or treatment remedies are hot or cold varies among regions, but the concept is consistent. A dislocation of a body part or of something in the body may cause illness (eg, as a "fallen fontanel" in infants, or "empacho" in which a ball of food clinging to the stomach wall may cause a bowel obstruction).

Also, certain perceived magical or supernatural causes outside the body (eg, eclipse of the sun) can cause an illness or defect (eg, cleft lip or palate). Last, strong emotional states (eg, fright, rage, jealousy, nervousness) can cause illness. Specific treatments generally correspond to the explanatory model of the illness. For example, a fallen fontanel is treated by holding the infant upside down and pressing up on the palate while someone sucks on the fontanel. Preventing illness is usually done by praying, wearing religious medals, or keeping a small altar of religious relics in the home. Many illnesses are first treated at home by the family with herbs, teas, or medications found in the home or acquired at the local swap meet.

Patient Education Implications

If the client is ill, ask what he or she believes is the cause of the illness. Perhaps medication could be taken with cold water or a hot herbal tea to balance the perceived cause of illness. Mental health issues might be approached by assessing if a strong emotion such as rage, fright, or nervousness may be a contributing factor to the problem. A mental health worker could be presented as a person who can try to help one get his or her life back into balance.

Western Health Care Organization and Service Variables

The fifth and final category of the Cultural Assessment Framework includes the Western health care organization and service variables. This category, which is not included in many assessments, evaluates the cultural competency and sensitivity of the health care provider and the organization that provides services.

Campinha-Bacote and Purnell have established four levels of cultural competency (Fig. 3-3): 1) unconscious incompetence; 2) conscious incompetence; 3) conscious competence; and 4) unconscious competence. The goal is an ongoing process; the caregiver should evaluate at what stage of the continuum he or she is beginning.

Even the most culturally competent provider will experience difficulty providing optimal care if his or her employer has little interest in promoting these services. One should know if the service organization (eg, hospital, long-term care facility, office-based primary care practice) has a policy or mission statement that includes providing culturally competent care. Even the pictures or décor of a waiting area can be tailored to present a comfortable atmosphere to a multiethnic population. Many clinics and hospitals provide regularly sched-

Unconscious Competence
Health care providers are able to automatically provide culturally sensitive care to clients of diverse populations.

Conscious Competence
Caregivers attempt to remedy deficits in knowledge and awareness of the cultural group and begin providing culturally relevant interventions.

Conscious Incompetence
Caregivers have become very aware that cultural differences exist, but lack practical skills in dealing with health needs of diverse populations.

Unconscious Incompetence
Health care providers are unaware that there are differences between themselves and the client.

FIGURE 3-3. Stages of cultural competency.

uled in-service educational programs; this is often an ideal time to promote cultural training. Some clinics sponsor outreach programs to specific ethnic enclaves and use public service radio and television spots to promote healthy and safe lifestyles.

Ideally, a service organization also should have an ongoing evaluation process to measure progress in meeting cultural competency goals. Evaluation should include assessment of management, staff, the facility, and ongoing feedback from the target group.

Synthesis: Farm Worker Population

The fifth category deals with the U.S. health care system's response to the farm worker cultural group. Clinics that target this population should have bilingual signs and educational materials, bilingual and bicultural staff, and professionally trained interpreters (if possible). Ethnic art and posters can provide a welcoming atmosphere.

Because this culture prizes children, a child-friendly waiting area with toys and Spanish or bilingual books presents a family-friendly environment. Some clinics insist that only children with appointments should come with a parent to the clinic, but child care for siblings without appointments can be expensive and difficult to find. Although it may be chaotic to have the whole family present for a visit, it also can be an opportunity to observe general family functioning. Often, evaluating family interactions reveals areas to address in patient education (eg, safety guidance, appropriate discipline, general parenting information). The agency can be instrumental in setting the climate for clinicians to achieve culturally competent care. Clinics can sponsor outreach programs, such as diabetes classes to a migrant camp or participation in cultural fairs. Health care workers and service agencies can learn to effectively use public service announcements on public radio and television.

THE KLEINMAN MODEL

General Considerations

An in-depth cultural assessment is ideal for better understanding the cultural or ethnic groups with whom the nurse has regular contact. When a briefer model is necessary, the Kleinman Model can be used. Arthur Kleinman, a psychiatrist and anthropologist, makes a distinction between illness and disease: *Illness* is the uniquely personal experience that a sick person has of what is happening to him or her. *Disease* is the health care professional's biomedical understanding of the same problem. Thus, people with the same medical diagnosis may experience illness in distinct ways.

Kleinman has developed eight questions to reveal a patient's illness perspective (Box 3-2). The first question—*What do you think has caused your problem?*—may reveal to the nurse some surprising answers. A frustrated clinician, baffled by a confusing clinical presentation, finally asked this question to her patient and was told: "In my country they call this

---

BOX 3-2. Kleinman's Questions

The Kleinman model can be used to assess a patient's own perspective of his or her illness.

1. What do you call the problem?
2. What do you think has caused the problem?
3. Why do you think it started as it did?
4. What do you think the sickness does? How does it work?
5. How severe is the sickness? Will it have a short or a long course?
6. What kind of treatment do you think the patient should receive? What are the most important results you hope he or she receives from the treatment?
7. What are the chief problems the sickness has caused?
8. What do you fear most about the sickness?

Malta Fever" (Brucellosis). Clients from developing countries may be more familiar than the clinician with infectious or tropical diseases common in their country! Typically, the Kleinman questions clarify the patient's explanatory health model and ideas of how this condition would be treated in the client's culture. By asking the patient and the family these questions before initiating patient education, the nurse can receive valuable information to focus patient education.

For example, Rankin, Galbraith, & Johnson (1993) completed a study of Chinese Americans with type II diabetes mellitus. The purpose of the study was to develop an understanding of the meanings Chinese Americans, who have diabetes, attributed to their condition. Question 7 of Kleinman's list—*What are the chief problems the sickness has caused?*—revealed that 33% of the participants felt stigmatized by their families or coworkers because of their diabetes. Many clients or their family members believed that diabetes was contagious. With this information, the nurse can better address these concerns in patient education.

Domains of Influence

Kleinman made another important contribution by recognizing the various domains of influence on a person's beliefs and actions regarding disease and illness. These domains comprise professional, popular, and complementary/alternative areas of influence. The professional domain is the one in which the health care professional operates. The popular domain includes the immediate and extended family and the community. The complementary/alternative domain may include *curanderos,* a Chinese herbalist, a shaman or medicine man, or a wise elder believed to have healing powers. To some ethnic clients, traditional healers are often much more appealing than professional health care providers. They usually are unhurried and make home visits. They know the patient, the family, and understand the culture and language. They offer free or low-cost services, and do not perform invasive physical examinations. They typically do not perform blood or other laboratory tests. They can offer a definite diagnosis without waiting for test results. The nurse educator should not forget the popular and folk areas of influence; in some cases, the nurse may find opportunities to work with complementary/alternative healers.

CULTURAL RELEVANCE

General Principles for Designing and Implementing Culturally Competent Care

Recognizing the need for nursing to take a leadership role in care guidelines for diverse populations, the American Academy of Nursing (AAN) convened an Expert Panel on Culturally Competent Nursing Care to present a set of recommendations to the AAN for consideration, adoption, and action (Box 3-3). The consequences of implementing the recommendations are far-reaching, increasing the knowl-

edge base for providing culturally competent care and widening institutional support at all levels for this increasingly important area. As a result of these recommendations, the need for culturally competent patient education will be routinely considered. With the expanded and available knowledge base, providers can better furnish patient education in an informed, skilled, and culturally sensitive way.

In reviewing the nursing and related literature, the panel also presented some general principles for the design and implementation of culturally competent care. Some of the principles have been included in previous parts of this chapter. These principles include the need to include situation, cultural specificity, norms, values, and communication and time patterns of the cultural group as the foundations for the model.

A cultural group must be empowered to design and support its own solutions to its health care needs. In many cases, patient education or projects are designed for a cultural group without considering what this community has identified as its most urgent priorities. Often the problems of the group are highlighted without considering the strengths and resources within the community. A few years ago in Fresno, California, several homeless women who lived on the streets were attacked and killed. Female patients at Holy Cross Clinic, a homeless clinic in the area, confided to the family nurse practitioner that their time of greatest fear was between 12:00 AM and 6:00 AM. The homeless women would try to stay awake every night during those hours. The nurse practitioner helped the women form a "buddy system." To be a "buddy," the woman had to be drug and alcohol free so she could be responsible for her "buddy." In addition to being an incentive to stay drug free and to increasing security by not being alone, the women could sleep in alternating shifts. The clinic nurse was instrumental in helping the women resolve the problem they identified by relying on each other.

Cultural Brokering

The AAN also presented several conceptual models that use the recommended general principles. For example, *cultural brokering* is

> **BOX 3-3.** Overview of the Recommendations of the American Academy of Nursing Expert Panel for Culturally Competent Care*
>
> The Academy explicitly commits to high quality, culturally competent care that is equitable and accessible.
>
> The Academy will foster research, develop, and maintain expertise and a knowledge base that will:
>
> - examine theories, frameworks and methods
> - be interdisciplinary
> - reflect heterogeneous health care practices
> - identify effective health care delivery models
> - identify how organizations are supportive and successful in fostering increased expertise in this area
> - identify how organizations attract and retain minority, stigmatized, and disenfranchised students, faculty, and clinicians.
>
> The Academy will promote changes in the U.S. health care system, reflecting effective delivery models.
>
> The Academy will collaborate with other organizations in establishing ways to teach health care professionals to provide culturally competent care.
>
> The Academy will collaborate with racial/ethnic nursing organizations to develop models of recruitment, education, and retention of nurses from racial/ethnic minority groups.
>
> In collaboration with other organizations, the Academy will develop a document fostering the inclusion of diversity content in curricula, continuing education, state board examinations, etc.
>
> *Culturally competent care pertains to that of racial/ethnic/stigmatized/disenfranchised populations.

a recommended principle. This concept is based on the use of a middleman to connect diverse subcultures. In relation to health care, brokering is between the patient and the Western health care system. Many view the nurse as the ideal person for this role. In some cases, the nurse may be too representative of the health care system and may also be in need of a middle person. A medical interpreter, in settings where available, can fill this role.

A nurse also may consider forming trusting relationships with cultural insiders who may fill the role of a "cultural guide." Even informed, culturally competent nurses have experiences in which they sense something went wrong with a particular patient encounter. Recounting the situation to a cultural guide can provide insights that are helpful for future encounters. A cultural broker might be another health professional of the culture, a community spokesperson, or a respected elder.

Patient Negotiation

Patient negotiation is helpful when a nurse reaches an impasse with the client about some aspect of patient education. The first step is to listen to the patient's perception of the issues and then try to present the situation from the Western medical perspective. After clearly identifying the areas of conflict, the nurse should select from the list those areas which are nonnegotiable to have the desired patient outcome. Clients often will go to extraordinary lengths to please the provider if they sense negotiation is occurring from a sense of mutual respect. The following example that occurred in an Andean community in Peru illustrates this concept:

> A 2-year-old girl sustained second degree burns over most of her right foot. The physician and nurse visited the family, who lived in a sturdy adobe home with a dirt floor. The burn was dressed

with a Silvadene ointment and bandaged. The next day, the clinicians saw that the child's bandage had been removed and the wound left open to the air. The clinicians reapplied the ointment and bandage and explained their concern about infection and the need to keep the wound clean.

The clinicians came back on the third day and found the bandage off again. Eventually, a better understanding of the mother's concerns led to compromises. From the mother's perspective, health would be restored when a proper balance between hot and cold elements was accomplished. Burns are caused by heat. The ointment was felt to be cool. However, the bandage kept heat in, adding heat to a "heat condition," further disrupting the delicate balance. The mother was happy to use the cream and, despite a busy schedule, chose to carry her daughter everywhere for the time needed to heal, but *without* the bandage. The foot healed well.

In this case, it was important to identify the patient's concept of what caused the condition and how the therapeutic agents were viewed, to negotiate a balance for healing.

Nurses should look for opportunities to encourage minority clients to identify their own health care problems and assist with solutions that use the strengths and resources within the community. By using principles of cultural brokering and negotiating compromises with patients, nurses can work with ethnically diverse clients with respectful open communication.

Acculturation and Assimilation

Acculturation is an important consideration factor when planning patient education. Planning postoperative teaching for a third-generation Japanese American would be different from teaching the same content to a recent Cambodian immigrant. Researchers have described various levels of acculturation. The least acculturated immigrants maintain most of their traditional language and belief systems. The most acculturated immigrants have adopted English, forgotten his or her native language, and accepted the values and belief system of the dominant culture. A bicultural person can operate comfortably in both the traditional and dominant cultural settings. Locke (1992) identifies a fourth marginal level that describes the person who seems to lack any real contact with norms and values from either culture.

Many factors affect acculturation. Among immigrants, the reason for leaving the native country and the attitude toward the departure should be considered. Immigrants making a considered choice to enter the United States in hopes of improved economic opportunities or a better future for their children, will generally acculturate willingly. Persons fleeing natural disasters or war zones are often suffering from post traumatic stress disorder. Some have been tortured. Many hope to return to the country of origin when the crises resolve. Dealing with personal trauma may be a barrier to acculturation. Some persons enter the United States to work for a limited period and have no intention of residing here permanently. Farm workers with material and family ties in Mexico do not perceive the need to acculturate.

Country of birth and age on entry into the United States affect a person's level of acculturation. Those immigrating at a young age and obtaining some education in American schools usually acquire language and social skills more rapidly than their seniors. Each succeeding generation is usually more acculturated than the one before.

Language acquisition is often viewed as the dominant factor in acculturation, but many variables have an impact on language skills. People who join family members or settle into ethnic enclaves have an immediate support group on arrival. Old-timers can significantly buffer the initial culture shock for newcomers. Many newcomers attend English as a Second Language (ESL) classes, but if the newcomer's social group consists primarily of the cultural group, little opportunity exists to practice English outside of the classroom. Women who work within the home or immigrants who work with family or relatives can continue to use their native language. Even if spoken English is learned, reading and writing skills often lag far behind. One argument for bilingual ballots was based on the difficulties new citizens have in deciphering complex "ballot English" and in exercising the right to vote.

Ethnic pride is also a factor in acculturation. Native Americans were here long before European Americans and see no reason to adopt some of the cultural values of the dominant society that are disrespectful of maintaining harmony with nature. Some groups have been more successful in encouraging a bicultural accommodation. A study by Rumbaut (1996) of successful East Indian high school students found much family support for maximal school performance because this would ensure success in a career or business. Most of the these teenagers' social lives, however, remained within the ethnic community.

Complete acculturation need not be a specific goal for clients, but in planning patient education, the nurse must understand where on the acculturation scale the client resides.

Patient Education for Families With Children

Many cross-cultural health care encounters involve young immigrant children or refugee families. There are many things to consider when dealing with patient education issues with these families.

 Pediatric medical problems are common and often can be avoided. Most areas of the world use the metric rather than the English scale for measuring liquids and body temperature. Clients are often unfamiliar with pounds, teaspoons, and Fahrenheit measurements. Many families do not own measuring spoons or cups, because they prepare recipes by adding a handful of or a pinch of an ingredient. Asking a parent to give a teaspoon of medication to a small child may

be interpreted to mean a baby-sized spoon of medication. It is safer to always supply a syringe or measuring cup and indicate the exact amount to be given with each dose.

Many pediatric medications come in liquid form and require refrigeration. Homeless and farm worker families often do not own or have access to refrigerators. Some antibiotics must be kept cold and some (eg, Septra) are stable even in hot conditions (Box 3-4).

Breast-feeding may be abandoned after arriving in the United States. In a 1984 study of the Hmong, Hollinger found that the 26 children born to families before migration were all breast-fed, whereas all of the six infants born in the United States were bottle fed. Reasons for this behavioral change were unclear, but seem to be related to the need to work and go to school. Because many immigrant mothers feel the need to work and help support the family, this may be a common theme. Addressing how some American women manage to combine work and breast-feeding may encourage more immigrant women to continue their traditional practices. Because breast-feeding is not

---

BOX 3-4. Some Common Pediatric Antibiotics and Refrigeration Requirements

Pediazole
Stable up to 1 mo without refrigeration

Septra
Stable up to 1 mo without refrigeration

Amoxicillin
Stable 14 days without refrigeration

Ceclor
Stable 4 days without refrigeration

Ampicillin
Requires refrigeration

Augmentin
Requires refrigeration

commonly seen in public settings, immigrant women may believe that breast-feeding is not commonly done in the United States.

Skin assessment of dark-skinned children can be confusing for clinicians without prior experience. Mongolian spots (dark-bluish areas over the lower back and buttocks) are normal and are present in most Asian, Hispanic, and African American infants. Several common Vietnamese health care practices leave bruises on the skin and should not be mistaken for child abuse. With coining, hot oil is spread over the back, chest, or shoulders and then rubbed with a coin, leaving ecchymotic stripes. Another practice, *cupping*, involves heating small cups and placing the open side on the skin. As it cools, a suction is created that contracts the skin, leaving bruises. Both practices are used to balance the hot or cold element believed to have caused the illness. Rashes in African American children must be palpated for heat, edema, tightness, or induration. Jaundice is best noted in the sclera of the eyes or palms and soles of the hands and feet.

Young children may work in fields or factories in the United States. This is especially true of farm worker children who may work alongside their parents in the fields, because they cannot afford a caretaker at home and because the parents' low wages can be augmented by the children's efforts. Children may be exposed to pesticide residue or drift, or pesticide-contaminated water. Migrant housing is often located adjacent to the fields, so exposures may continue day and night. According to Wilk (1993), children have a disproportionate share of agricultural and workplace fatalities and disabling injuries. Accident prevention should be an ongoing patient education issue for rural families in which farm equipment, grain bins, chemicals, and open irrigation canals are a continual hazard. ∎

Nurses and all health care providers must listen carefully to their clients' concerns about a "cultural illness":

Caida de mollera, or fallen fontanel syndrome, is an example of a Mexican American belief that illness can be caused by physical displacement of a body part. Although considered a culture-bound illness, a study by Trotter (1987) suggests that this condition should be considered more carefully by health care providers. Eighty women who had treated *caida de mollera* in their households in the previous 12 months were asked to list the symptoms that led them to suspect this problem. In order of frequency, the most common symptoms were diarrhea, excessive crying, fever, decreased appetite, restlessness and irritability, watery eyes, inability to nurse, and vomiting. Three case histories based on clusters of symptoms were presented to a panel of physicians. All the physicians agreed that the patients could have been suffering from severe dehydration or a general systemic infection and should have been seen by a health care provider. The women related that they are often reluctant to mention this illness, because providers do not believe in this condition and dismiss their concerns. In this case, failure to take these mothers' concerns seriously could have resulted in great harm to their children.

Patient Education for Families With Adolescents

Among immigrant and refugee families, adolescence is often a time of intergenerational conflict. As teenagers strive to fit in with their peers in the United States, they may question the values of their country of origin. Young people usually acculturate faster than the older generation, which may disrupt the family roles. Conflicts may revolve around acceptable dating behavior or early marriage expectations. Some young Hmong women have marriages arranged at an early age.

Adolescents may balance school with working expectations. Families may have different expectations for daughters than for sons. It is especially important to do a HEADSS assessment—(ie, assess for information about **H**ome, **E**ducation, **A**lcohol and other drugs, **D**epression, **S**ex, and **S**uicide). These teenagers are often overwhelmed young people.

Patient Education for Women

Despite the various social statuses a woman has in different cultures, the time devoted to patient education of women affects not only the female client but the entire family. In many cultures, women are considered the chief source of cultural knowledge and the primary teacher of that culture to the next generation. Women can be wonderful teachers of their beliefs to nurses if providers ask questions in a friendly manner about a cultural symbol you notice on a family member.

In many cultures, the wife, mother, or grandmother is the primary caretaker when a family member becomes ill, and therefore this person must be included in health care instructions. Usually women prepare food throughout the world, and this role usually continues after immigration to the United States. By necessity, teaching about nutrition should always include women if a required special diet is different from the family's usual meals.

In planning patient education for a woman, the first factor to consider is the woman's role within her culture. An 80-year-old great grandmother esteemed for her wisdom and family stories may come to appointments accompanied by extended family with whom she lives. She is in a different situation than an elder living in an extended care facility with infrequent family encounters, despite her children living nearby.

In some cultures, early marriage is expected and a 20-year-old who is not pregnant after five years of marriage may cause great concern for her family. Other immigrant families encourage young women to postpone childbearing, so they can focus on their education and learn skills to contribute to the family. Understanding the role of the woman in her ethnic community can highlight important patient education areas.

Pregnancy, Birth, and the Postpartum Period

Beliefs regarding pregnancy, birth, and the expected behavior during the postpartum period vary among cultures and ethnic groups. Beliefs about food cravings, appropriate weight gain, the postpartum diet, and when to resume sexual activity are important to understand when teaching childbearing patients. For example, Hmong women follow a limited diet, primarily consisting of chicken and rice; they avoid anything cold, and they avoid hard work for one month after the birth. All food and liquids must be hot or warm, and no cold water should be used for bathing. These diet and bathing practices can be accommodated in the hospital, and beliefs about work should be kept in mind when teaching about resumption of activities.

Family Planning

Family planning is another area in which cross-cultural sensitivity is especially important. Limiting family size has been viewed by many minority populations as an attempt to limit the size of their particular population. Refugee populations, who have lost large numbers of their populace to war, may feel a need to replace those killed in the war. Persons migrating from countries with a large infant mortality rate may expect to have larger families to ensure the survival of a few healthy children.

Family spacing (rather than family planning) that emphasizes the improved health of the mother and infant is one possible approach. For recent immigrant groups that are striving to improve their economic status in the United States, the cost of raising and educating children in this country may be an incentive for spacing births.

Cultural factors also may play an important role in the choice of a family planning method. For example, some groups think it improper to touch one's genitals, and methods that require insertion (eg, diaphragm) are less acceptable than other methods (eg, oral contraceptives, Depo-Provera injections).

Cancer Screening

Breast cancer screening is underused by many ethnic populations. African American women suffer a higher mortality rate for breast cancer than Anglo American women (34.8 per 100,000 versus 31.0 per 100,000). This difference in mortality rate is largely attributed to late diagnosis. A 1996 study (Goldsmith & Sisneros) found that 61% of Hispanic farm worker women older than 50 years of age never had a mammogram. Nurses must look for creative ways to teach women about mammography and clinical and self-breast exams.

In one ethnographic study (Chavez, Hubbell, McMullen, Martinez, & Mishra, 1995), knowledge and attitudes about breast cancer risk factors were evaluated. The groups interviewed for the study included Mexican immigrant women, Salvadoran immigrant women, Chicana (United States born) women, Anglo American women, and American physicians. Both the Salvadoran and Mexican immigrant women in the study believed the greatest risk factor for breast cancer was excessive physical use and abuse of the breasts (eg, trauma, excessive fondling, and rough handling during breast-feeding). This information is helpful when teaching breast self-exam techniques. These women also believed the second greatest risk factor included various lifestyle behaviors, such as using drugs and drinking alcohol. Although these behaviors place women at risk for other health problems, these behaviors have not been associated with breast cancer.

An innovative mammogram program was designed to reach African American women 50 years of age and older. This program was developed by Deirdra Forte while she was a student at University of California at Los Angeles (UCLA). Her research showed that older African American women do not visit physicians regularly and are referred less frequently than other groups for mammography. Recognizing that older women congregate and exchange information in beauty salons in ethnic neighborhoods, Ms. Forte recruited beauticians and salons that serve 25 to 50 women on any given Saturday. A culturally sensitive video featuring African American celebrities was shown, and literature designed for this population was distributed. A mobile mammography unit was set up to visit salons on alternating Saturdays to provide on-site screening. This program is a great example of health education targeted for a specific population that uses a regular communication channel normally used by the target group.

Pap smears are another preventive health care practice underused by many ethnic, especially immigrant, women. Data from the National Health Interview Survey indicate that women who speak predominately Spanish are the group least likely to have had a Pap smear in the previous 3 years. Another 1996 study by Goldsmith and Sisneros revealed that 28% of farm worker women had never had a Pap smear.

A project developed to address this population recognized that Tupperware parties are popular with this group, and the project used a similar format to set up educational "Pap parties." A hostess would invite a group of approximately 10 friends into her home; the gathering was sometimes organized around a mother-daughter or husband-wife theme. Education was presented regarding cancer; specific information regarding the cervix, breast, and reproductive organs; self- and clinical breast exams; mammograms; pelvic exams; the Pap smear; and the need for screening and early detection. Women were given information on how to access the health care system, such as making an appointment and transportation issues. Women who attended a "Pap party" were given a modest personal hygiene or health gift and vouchers to receive a second gift were given to those who had a Pap smear. Similar presentations were given at other areas where people congregate, such as laundromats and at health fairs and other public events. The program was successful; more than 2,200 people were contacted through the different outreach methods and more than 300 women visited a clinic for a Pap smear.

Domestic Violence

Domestic violence is an area of concern across every ethnic and socioeconomic group. Among many immigrant groups, additional issues include fear of authorities for undocumented women, inability to speak English, and the vulnerability and isolation because the women's family and support group are in her country of origin. Shelters for battered women may be seen as places that help women leave their husbands and break up the family rather than as centers that help victimized women.

Nurses must educate clients that no person deserves to be mistreated by a domestic partner. However, because women's rights are often perceived differently in diverse cultures, it is often helpful to learn what women of the ethnic group in question have done to address this issue. Women are much more likely to feel empowered if they see other women overcoming the same cultural barriers they have encountered. One such group is called *Lideres Campesinas,* Women Farm Worker Leaders. This group has programs regarding domestic violence and sexual assault, HIV, acquired immune deficiency syndrome (AIDS), a pesticides and work sanitation program, and an economic development program. Fifteen groups currently provide education, often through humorous skits within the community and support groups for women. Many of these groups may have culturally specific videos or literature that nurses can use to teach diverse patient populations.

Patient Education for Senior Citizens

Patient education with older adults among diverse populations carries rewards and challenges. Younger nurses caring for post-World War II immigrants may have the opportunity to hear first-person accounts of how the war both disrupted and mobilized people from throughout the world. The perspectives of Japanese interned in the United States will differ from personal histories of Eastern European Jews who fled Nazi Germany or Filipinos who supported the United States effort and are still waiting to be recognized and compensated for their contributions. Newer immigrants are often less fluent in English, have suffered a tremendous disruption in their expected role within the ethnic community,

and may or may not have legal status in the United States.

Assessment

Planning patient education for seniors involves certain factors. First, the nurse must determine the person's length of stay in the United States, legal status, and general level of acculturation. A client's legal status can have a significant impact on his or her willingness to venture outside of an ethnic enclave or to participate in any program or intervention that might make him or her more visible to the Immigration and Naturalization Service (INS).

Another assessment area is the older man or woman's role in the culture or country of origin and how this role may have changed since immigrating to the United States. Respect for elders is an important cultural value in many cultures and one that is often disrupted because seniors must rely on children or even grandchildren to translate, assist with transportation, and make sense of the new culture.

Nurses must also evaluate the losses the older adult has experienced in his or her life. All seniors should be assessed for depression, especially those who have lost family, suffered physical injury, and lost prestigious employment, status, and country of origin. Inability to sleep or problems with recurrent nightmares may be clues to underlying depression. The ability to absorb the health education needed for coping with a current chronic health condition may be compromised if mental health issues are not dealt with first.

Also, one must evaluate the health care role the older adult plays in the family. In many cultures, grandmothers are the primary care providers in the extended family when someone is ill or has just given birth. It is important to know if alternative health beliefs, medicines, or herbs are being used and if they support or interfere with the desired treatment the nurse wishes to propose. Trying to understand the grandmother's perspective and including her in patient teaching can result in a more harmonious and cooperative relationship.

Death and Dying

Practices around death and dying are often culturally defined. Some ethnic groups believe that a seriously ill person must always have hope and should never be told the status of a terminal illness. The Hmong believe that if a person is told her or she is dying, the medical person essentially condemns him or her to death by encouraging the spirit that takes one's soul away to come closer. According to Fadiman (1997), it would be a great insult for a Hmong to say to one's aged grandparent, "After you are dead," but would express one's death by, "when your children are 120 years old." In some cultures, assessing a client's feelings about heroic measures can be done by presenting a third-person scenario such as, "What would you want done for an ill person who had a medical condition that the doctors had no more treatments that could make the person better?" When issues arise about what to tell the patient regarding a long-term prognosis for a chronic or terminal condition, it is best to discuss with the family what they want shared, and who should be the person to share that information.

Parenting Grandchildren

Many older adults in the 1990s parent grandchildren (or great grandchildren) when the grandchildren's own parents cannot provide care. This issue is common in many minority, especially African American, communities (Kelly et al., 1997). Among immigrant families, seniors may provide child care while the parents work or attend school, but the extended family lives in the same household. Because many senior citizens have chronic health conditions, nurses must assess what psychosocial stressors they may have that may affect their health condition. One 1993 study by Minkler and Roe indicated that 37% of grandmothers reported a decrease in physical and psychological health after becoming primary care givers for their grandchildren.

Intergenerational parenting often keeps an at-risk family intact in a stable and caring environment. Unfortunately, the older caregiver may be placed in a precarious financial situation at a time when he or she faces a fixed income after retirement. Often, informal kinship placement families are not eligible for the same financial aid as are foster care families. Because the most common reason for out-of-home placement for grandchildren is parental abuse or neglect, secondary to substance abuse, children often exhibit special emotional needs and problems at the time of removal from parental custody. Some parenting seniors feel cut off from peers because they lack the time to participate in social activities that might alleviate some of their stress. Nurses working with these families can help the grandparents identify resources that might provide support, enabling them to better meet the needs of the children, and improve their health.

Sometimes respite services can be arranged through ethnic social or religious organizations. Many communities now have support groups available for senior citizens. One source for locating grandparent services can be found through the American Association of Retired Persons (AARP), which has a Grandparent Information Center. Their telephone number is (202) 434-2296.

Working With Interpreters

In many situations, nurses and other health care professionals do not speak the language of the non-English-speaking client. In these cases, the provider will need to use the services of an interpreter. An interpreter is a person fluent in two or more languages, who has been professionally trained to translate oral communication. In many clinics and hospitals, untrained staff, family members, or only partially bilingual persons are asked to interpret complex medical procedures, obtain informed consents, or explain culturally sensitive emotional information. Although professional interpreters are not always available, they should be used whenever possible.

When less-prepared translators are used, look for nonverbal cues from the client or request a return demonstration to be sure the correct message has been conveyed. When medical assistants or nurses are asked to translate, it means they will not perform their other responsibilities during this time. This can lead to resentment from coworkers, who must pick up additional work, or disgruntled patients who must wait longer for services. Many agencies do not list interpreting as part of the job description and do not compensate workers for these skills. Many bilingual persons competent to translate ordinary conversation may be concerned with liability issues when asked to translate informed consent documents or complex medical procedures. Nurses also should be aware that in small communities or small ethnic enclaves, confidentiality may be an issue.

Family members often are asked to serve as translators in medical settings. Because children often learn English more rapidly than their elders, they often are placed in this role. This scenario can cause many problems. In many parts of the world, authority rests with the senior members of the family. In much of rural culture, men have authority over women, and younger Hispanic adults defer to older adults. Having children serve as interpreters places them in a position of control and disrupts the social order. Children are sometimes requested to translate emotional information inappropriate for their age. L. Haffner (1992), an interpreter at Stanford Medical Center, recounts trying to calm a 7-year-old girl who had been requested to tell her pregnant, traumatized mother that she was carrying a stillborn. Women are often reluctant to discuss concerns regarding gynecologic or family planning issues when children (especially sons) are translators. Even when a professional interpreter is used, some clients will hesitate to divulge information regarding sexual or other sensitive issues to an interpreter of the opposite sex. Other issues may arise when more acculturated adults translate for parents. Sometimes they feel reluctant to directly translate information regarding traditional health beliefs or practices, thinking the Western health care provider might react negatively to such information.

Language barriers can arise even when proper translation has occurred, because clients may understand instructions more literally then intended. Although this can occur in English-to-English exchanges, it seems to be more common in cross-cultural situations. A call from a Hispanic client to the Firebaugh Health Center, a clinic in the Central San Joaquin Valley of California, illustrates this. The client had been taking her antibiotic for 3 days and was so hungry she didn't feel she could complete a full 7 days of medication on an empty stomach. She had taken only liquids since beginning the medication; this type of compliance could have serious medical complications for some clients.

Maximizing the Use of an Interpreter

There are several ways to maximize a patient encounter that includes a medical interpreter. The nurse should face and interact directly with the client rather than with the interpreter. This places the clinician in a better position to observe any nonverbal communication with the client. Use short, clear sentences and pause after two to three sentences to allow for translation. The interpreter is more likely to leave out information if too much material is covered between phrases.

Before seeing the client, have a preconference with the translator. After reviewing the chart and deciding on the goals of the client encounter, share the goals and any particular concerns you might have with the interpreter. If you are teaching about diabetes, the interpreter may serve as a cultural broker. Perhaps some cultural-belief information regarding this disease can be shared before the interview. Always try to allow time for the client to ask you questions. When teaching a new procedure, such as insulin administration, allow time for a return demonstration. Having the client recount what he or she understood of the discussion can help clear up any misunderstandings. Finally, to maintain an amicable working relationship with the medical interpreter, respect his or her time. Interpreters often are needed in many areas at once. Jotting down notes to make sure that all pertinent information is covered is much more efficient than having to recall the interpreter later for an essential item overlooked.

SUMMARY

Nurses often are presented with cross-cultural patient education situations. The nurse who works on an ongoing basis with a particular ethnic population is encouraged to acquire an in-depth understanding of that cultural group by exploring the five levels of the Cultural Assessment Framework. During patient education encounters, factors such as specific demographic data, specific risk factors, and the groups' world view and health care beliefs can be incorporated into the teaching and teaching methodology. For cross-cultural patient encounters with an unfamiliar group in which an in-depth exploration is not possible, the Kleinman Model also is proposed as a shorter assessment tool.

The recommendations of the AAN Expert Panel on Culturally Competent Care reinforce the importance of cross-cultural information to nursing and that it must be an essential element of patient care. Cultural brokering and patient-provider negotiation are important elements of culturally competent patient care. The levels of acculturation and assimilation of individuals and families also are major factors to consider in planning patient education.

STRATEGIES FOR CRITICAL ANALYSIS AND APPLICATION

1. Interview a farm worker family. Determine who in the family works and what types of work each member does. Gather information about sanitation in the fields; determine any work-related, chronic or acute health problems that exist, and problems the family has in getting health care. Determine culturally specific illnesses and learn who provides health care for the family (professional, popular, or folk). Plan an educational program designed to reduce the family's risk for injury, pesticide exposure, and overuse syndrome based on the information gathered.

2. Spend an evening watching a commercial non-English television station. Make a list of the commercial products advertised and for what ages they are targeted. Evaluate food or health products listed for health benefit or deficit, such as fat, salt, or sugar content for food, and toy safety. How might this information aid you in patient education for this population?

3. Read more about the principles of yin and yang and plan a diabetes teaching plan for Mr. Chin, a 65-year-old immigrant from China. Base the teaching plan on the concepts of balance between the yin and yang elements.

4. Read the first four chapters of Anne Fadiman's book *The Spirit Catches You and You Fall Down*. Imagine you are a floor nurse caring for Lia, the client in the book. How could you teach this family to give Lia her medication for the seizure disorder consistently?

REFERENCES

American Academy of Nursing Expert Panel On Culturally Competent Nursing Care. (1992). AAN Expert Panel Report: Culturally Competent Health Care. *Nursing Outlook, 40*(6), 227–283.

Campinha-Bacote, J. (1998). *The process of cultural competence in the delivery of healthcare services: A culturally competent model of care.* Cincinnati, OH: Transcultural C.A.R.E. Associates.

Chaves, L. R., Hubbell, F. A., McMullen, J. M., Martinez, R. G., & Mishra, S. I. (1995). Understanding knowledge and attitudes about breast cancer. *Archives of Family Medicine, 4*, 145–152.

Domingo, I. N. (1992). *Drawing from experience: Farm workers evaluation of illustrations used in print safety materials.*

Fadiman, A. (1997). *The spirit catches you and you fall down.* New York: Farrar, Straus & Giroux.

Goldsmith, D. & Sisneros, G. (1996). Cancer Prevention Strategies Among California Farmworkers: Preliminary Findings. *The Journal of Rural Health, 12*(4), 343–348.

Haffner, L. (1992). Translation is not enough. Interpreting in a medical setting. *Western Journal of Medicine, 157*(3), 255–259.

Hollinger, B. (1984). *Health perceptions of the Hmong: An ethnography study.* A thesis submitted in partial fulfillment of the requirements for the degree of Master of Science in the Department of Nursing, California State University-Fresno.

Huff, R. M., & Kline, M. V. (Eds.) (1999). *Promoting health in multicultural populations: A handbook for practitioners.* Thousand Oaks, CA: Sage Publications.

Kelley, S., Yorker, B., & Whitley, D. (1997). To grandmother's house we go and stay: Children raised in intergenerational families. *Journal of Gerontological Nursing, 23*(9), 12–19.

Locke, D. (1992). *Increasing multicultural understanding: A comprehensive model.* Thousand Oaks, CA: Sage Publications.

Mines, R., Gabbard, S., & Steirman, A. (1997). *A profile of US Farm Workers: The National Agricultural Workers Survey, 1-32.* U.S. Department of Labor.

Purnell, L. & Paulanka, B. (1998) *Transcultural health care: A culturally competent approach.* Philadelphia: F.A. Davis Company.

Rankin, S. H., Galbraith, M.E., & Johnson, S. (1993). Reliability and validity data for a Chinese translation of the Center for Epidemiologic Studies Depression (CES-D). *Psychological Reports, 73,* 1291–1298.

Rehm, R. (1999). Religious faith in mexican-american families dealing with chronic childhood illness. *Image—The Journal of American Scholarship, 31*(1), 33–8.

Rumbaut, R. (1996). The new californians: Assessing the educational progress of children of immigrants. *CPS Brief, 8*(3), 1–12.

Thompson, M., Curry, M. & Burton, D. (1998). The effects of nursing case management on the utilization of prenatal care by Mexican-Americans in rural Oregon. *Public Health Nursing 15* (2), 82–90.

Trotter, R. (1987). Caida de mollera: A newborn and early infancy health risk. *Migrant Health Newsline Clinical Supplements, 1985–1987,* 30–31.

Wilk, W. (1993). Health hazards to children in agriculture. *American Journal of Industrial Medicine, 24*(3), 283–290.

Zlolniski, C. & Palerm, J. (1996). Working but poor: Mexican immigrant workers in a low-income barrio in San Jose. *CPS Brief, 8*(9), 7–15.

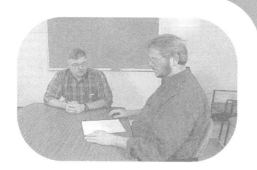

Educational Theories for
Teaching and Motivating Patients

LEARNING OBJECTIVES

After reading this chapter, the nurse or student nurse should be able to:

1. Distinguish between *compliance* and *cooperation* as desirable outcomes for patient education.

2. Define three components of empowerment and apply them to a patient education situation.

3. Compare and contrast the developmental models, self-efficacy theory, and stress and coping theory as useful bases of patient education.

4. Describe Prochaska's stages of change and apply them to smoking cessation.

5. Describe the sequence of events in learning and recount examples of the events as applied to patient education.

INTRODUCTION

Many chapters in this book examine patient education issues from the perspective of health care providers. The authors focus on issues that arise, based on system constraints to effective patient teaching, and contextual and environmental influences that condition the learning situation. This chapter considers the issues the patient faces as a result of various factors, including attitudes, beliefs, and motivational influences. Other influencing factors include teaching and learning theories and their impact on individual patient learning. Additionally, developmental models are discussed to show unique approaches to understanding patients within their biophysical, psychosocial, historical, and environmental contexts.

Factors, such as individual empowerment and motivation, cause each patient to affect the health care system in a unique way and influence the person's decision-making as a consumer of health care services. For example, patients who are highly motivated to learn healthy behaviors, reinforce patient education efforts. This chapter discusses situations in which the patient's values are in conflict with those of the health care provider and in which patient education does not result in the behavioral changes suggested by the provider. In our examination of teaching and learning, the authors consider the steps involved in learning. Effective patient education includes the contextual and developmental status of individuals; therefore, lifespan development and an ecological systems approach to development are presented to focus on the patient's individual situation. Finally, both classic and contemporary learning theories are presented, so that nurses can understand the theoretical underpinnings of patient education. Empowerment has been an important underlying component of our approach to patient education; it is further developed using the work of Paulo Freire.

PATIENT EDUCATION: A PROCESS OF INFLUENCING BEHAVIOR

General Considerations

Patient education was defined by Scott Simonds, Chair of the 1979 National Task Force on Training Family Physicians in Patient Education as:

> *Patient education is the process of influencing behavior, producing changes in knowledge, attitudes, and skills required to maintain and improve health. The process may begin with the imparting of information, but it also includes interpretation and integration of information to bring about attitudinal or behavioral changes that benefit a person's health status.*

This definition seems particularly applicable to the focus of this chapter. Patient education is a holistic process that attempts to change a patient's behavior to benefit his or her health status. The process of patient education begins with assessment of the patient's needs and concerns; then the patient educator sets goals with the patient for desired outcomes. Although patient education includes the imparting of information, the skilled patient educator assists the patient to interpret and integrate the information. Patient education ends with an evaluation of the patient's learning, its usefulness, and the ease with which he or she has integrated it into self-care practices. Patient teaching refers to only one component of the patient education process—the actual imparting of information to the patient.

Patient education is a process that occurs during time, requiring an ongoing assessment of the patient's knowledge, attitudes, and skills. The patient's readiness or motivation to change behaviors—and the obstacles the patient faces to make a behavioral change—are important consideration factors during assessment. (Chapter 8 offers an in-depth discussion of assessment for patient education.)

Most practitioners involved in patient education recognize the impact of the family on the patient's behavior. A close, supportive family unit may facilitate the integration of new health behaviors; a family that faces conflict or that lacks understanding often poses barriers to behavioral change. Strong religious, ethnic, or cultural beliefs may also prevent or influence desired change. The potency of sociocultural belief systems in influencing patient education is discussed in Chapter 3. A Patient and Family Education Assessment Guide, introduced in Chapter 8, provides guidance in examining factors that may promote or impede the process of patient education. The practitioner can then offer the patient and the family assistance in overcoming obstacles to behavioral change.

Compliance Orientation

Compliance and Noncompliance

The authors asked physicians and nurses to share what they consider to be obstacles in their experiences with patient education. All of them identified problems with either motivating patients or with achieving patient compliance. When asked to elaborate, they saw these two issues as closely related. The implication was that a sufficiently motivated patient would comply with the doctor's or the nurse's instructions.

Many of us have justified our involvement in patient education by asserting that it would increase patient compliance (ie, convince patients to follow our suggestions). As research in health education expands, it becomes apparent that, despite teaching, patients frequently do not make the choices recommended to them by nurses, physicians, and other health professionals. This situation is often termed *noncompliance*.

The authors are uneasy with the term *compliance*. It implies that health care professionals dictate to the patient what is to be done or changed, and that the patient is to follow instructions (ie, to obey). Further soul-searching makes us realize that our discomfort stems from the patient's right to choose not to follow our advice, even though we know what is best for him or her. It is natural for health professionals to want patients to choose the recommended course of action; however, what we really should strive to enlist is their partnership or cooperation. We want them to choose what we suggest.

Cooperation

An orientation toward cooperation, rather than compliance, can help a nurse examine his or her own effectiveness in patient education in a different light. Perhaps patient education successes have more to do with a patient's preparation to make informed choices than with compliance? If, in fact, patient education acknowledges the patient's free will to make choices, it must afford understanding of the importance of his or her values, wishes, and ability to participate in decision-making.

Student nurses, acute care and ambulatory nurses, and advanced practice nurses all have experiences with uncooperative patients. These experiences teach a nurse that effective patient education requires an understanding of the factors (eg, values, beliefs, attitudes, current life stresses, religion, previous experiences with the health care system, and life goals) that influence patient decision-making. These experiences also illustrate that patient education involves not just teaching and learning, but also behavioral changes. Patient education providers may begin with giving information and demonstrating skills. However, if the patient is not included in deciding how learning will be applied, and the goals of patient education are not mutually agreed on between the teacher and the learner, then behavioral changes usually will not occur.

Although health professionals tend to view

cooperation with a medical regimen as a single choice, the patient's cooperation with a regimen involves many choices every day. For example, choosing to follow an appropriate diabetes-oriented diet requires constant decisions (often inconvenient and anguishing) throughout each day. The health care professional may expect the patient to do this every day for the rest of his or her life, despite no guarantee that he or she will be free of neuropathy, retinopathy, nephropathy, or other complications. The health professional can offer the patient guidance and support, but health professionals must also be willing to respect the patient's right to make choices that conflict with ours.

However, we reserve the right to keep trying. Despite poor cooperation, a nurse can remain hopeful that the patient will be more open to patient education messages during future encounters. The nurse must also respect the patient's right to change his or her mind. The patient may choose to take the course of action suggested or disregard the actions if he or she judges that the cost or hardship outweighs the benefit. For example, a terminally ill patient may initially decide to take the treatment, but later decide to discontinue chemotherapy because the costly and uncomfortable side effects outweigh the benefits.

THE AGENDA OF EDUCATION

Health care providers bring their own agenda, or purpose, for the health education endeavor to the educational setting. These agendas may vary. Chandler's (1992) characterization of the point of education has four major purposes. (Although this characterization was meant to be applied to primary and secondary school students, it also pertains to the agenda of various health care professionals who provide patient education.) The four purposes are:

1. Prepare students for assumption of adult roles.
2. Provide students with an orientation to improve society.

3. Maintain appreciation of the dominant culture and the status quo.
4. Provide knowledge that liberates people.

The corollary of these purposes to patient education are illustrated in Table 4-1

The first purpose has been a motivating force behind patient education. The second and third purposes also reflect dominant school and patient education purposes. Providing liberating knowledge so that patients can control their own care is part of the empowerment movement, which has generated a great deal of interest but is difficult to institute and perpetuate, particularly at the community level (Israel, Checkoway, Schulz, & Zimmerman, 1994).

Empowerment in Patient Education

The term *empowerment* was introduced in the 1970s with the work of Brazilian educator, Paulo Freire. Freire advocates a participatory educational process, in which people can name their own problems and solutions, and through this process, transform themselves and their communities (Beeker, Guenther-Grey, & Raj, 1998; Freire, 1970; Wallerstein & Bernstein, 1994). Freire purports that education is never neutral, and is always enmeshed in the values of educators. Additionally, people will act on the issues about which they have strong feelings; their identification of issues may coincide with those of the teacher or health care provider.

 The participatory educational process opposes some of the purposes of student and patient education outlined in Table 4-1. When empowerment is applied to an aggregate, such as community empowerment, expectations are that people will listen to each other, compare and contrast central issues in their lives, and together construct new strategies for change (Travers, 1997; Wallerstein & Bernstein, 1994). Community empowerment has been undertaken recently in such attempts as a Hong Kong community-based empowerment program for families

TABLE 4-1. The Purpose of Education

PURPOSE OF STUDENT EDUCATION	EDUCATIONAL PROPONENT	PATIENT EDUCATION COROLLARY
Prepare students for adult role positions	Bobbitt (1924), Finney (1928)	Prepare patients for compliant orderly, obedient positions.
Provide students with an orientation to improve society	Kandal (1941), Kliebard (1987)	Improve patient/health care provider relationships.
Maintain the status quo and reproduce the culture	Broudy (1982)	Maintain the status quo with health care providers dominant.
Provide knowledge that liberates people	Anyon (1980), Freire (1970)	Provide liberating knowledge so that patients control their own care.

Adapted from: Chandler, S. (1992). Learning for what purpose? Questions when viewing classroom learning from a sociocultural curriculum perspective. In H. H. Marshall (Ed.), *Redefining student learning: Roots of educational change* (p. 33). Norwood, NJ: Ablex Publishing.

with a survivor of brain injury (Man, 1999) and a program of parent and family support groups to diminish violent behavior in African-American adolescents at risk. Other well known and successful examples of community empowerment programs include the San Francisco Homeless Prenatal Program (Ovrebo, Ryan, Jackson, & Hutchinson, 1994), the Boston Healthy Start Initiative (Plough & Olafson, 1994), and the Adolescent Social Action Program in New Mexico to decrease alcohol and substance abuse (Wallerstein & Sanchez-Merki, 1994). Although community empowerment is a worthy ideal, its exploration is beyond the scope of this chapter. However, individual empowerment is a strategy to achieve better patient education outcomes. ∎

Individual (Psychological) Empowerment

Individual or psychological empowerment concerns the patient's ability to have control over his or her own life. Israel and colleagues (1994) view individual empowerment as similar to other theoretical constructs, such as self efficacy and self esteem. All three constructs emphasize the development of a sense of mastery, control, and competence. Additionally, empowerment includes the establishment of crit-

ical thinking and analytical skills, which allow the patient to better understand the resources and competencies needed to achieve desired outcomes.

When applied to patient education, the health care professional must provide a framework for creative thinking; assist the patient in raising questions, such as *Why?, How?* and *Who?;* and establish an environment in which genuine dialogue can occur. Lastly, the health care professional encourages the chosen actions and evaluates the results with the patient. Table 4-2 illustrates a model for individual empowerment in patient education situations involving a patient with hypertension.

Although the strategies suggested in Table 4-2 may not be considered desirable by many health care professionals, a significant percentage of hypertensive patients never comply with their medication regimen because of the pharmacologic consequences. Therefore, an empowerment approach is at least as likely to achieve a reduction in blood pressure as the more traditional patient education approach.

Malcolm Knowles, the proponent of *andragogy* (ie, adult learning) attempts to empower adults through the principles he imparts. His important work is covered in Chapter 9.

TABLE 4-2. Components of Empowerment as Applied to Patient Education With a Hypertensive Patient

COMPONENT OF EMPOWERMENT	APPLICATION TO PATIENT EDUCATION
Sufficient knowledge to make rational, informed decisions	Nurse ascertains patient's explanatory model about hypertension (see Chap. 4). Nurse gives patient all information necessary to make informed decision about management of hypertension, including nonpharmacologic (diet, exercise, herbs) and pharmacologic (side effects of medications). Patient is informed of possible complications if high blood pressure is not controlled. Nurse encourages patient to read about hypertension, to talk with friends and relatives.
Sufficient control and resources to implement decisions	Nurse gives patient access to clinic materials on management of hypertension and suggestions for other nonmedical reading. Nurse informs patient of costs of various treatment options. Nurse meets with patient when patient is ready to discuss treatment options and asks patient for decision regarding treatment.
Sufficient experience to evaluate the effectiveness of their decisions	Nurse supports patient in desire to use nonpharmacologic approach. Nurse teaches patient how to monitor his or her own blood pressure at home and asks for a call with weekly readings for 6 weeks. When blood pressure does not respond to nonpharmacologic approach, nurse suggests other nonpharmacologic therapies, such as biofeedback. Nurse continues to monitor patient's blood pressure by telephone and continues to support patient in attempt to achieve blood pressure control without drugs.

Adapted from: "Empowerment: An idea whose time has come in diabetes education," by Funnell, M. M., Anderson, R. M., Arnold, M. S., Barr, P. A., Donnelly, M., Johnson, P. D., Moon, D., & White, N. H. (1991). *Diabetes Educator, 17,* 37–41.

PATIENT DECISION-MAKING: A REVIEW OF THE LITERATURE

A review of patient education literature reveals many of the variables that influence a patient's choices to not follow the recommendations of health professionals. Lack of cooperation is common among patients of all economic and educational backgrounds. Rationalization and denial are recurrent problems encountered in patient education and are often seen in the management of chronic illness. The nature of chronic illness, with its remissions and exacerbations, influences patient attitudes toward adherence and patient teaching; nonadherence in these cases is estimated at 30% to 60% (Cameron & Gregor, 1987). Others report even higher rates of noncompliance with prescribed drug regimens, estimating that up to 50% of all patients fail to achieve full compliance, and as many as 33% never take their prescribed medications (Schroeder & McPhee, 1996).

Anxiety, depression, and anger influence a patient's understanding and, eventually, his choices (Berg, Alt, Himmel, & Judd, 1985; Devine, 1992). In addition, religion, socioeconomic status, ethnicity, family problems, and family experiences influence the patient's course of action (Kloeblen, 1999; Tripp-Reimer & Afifi, 1989). Additional variables, such as the patient's knowledge about the disease and previous contact with the disease, are identified as modifying factors in the patient's consumption of health care services.

Other patient issues that affect patient education include the patient's coping style and locus of control. Lazarus, a cognitive psychologist working in the area of stress and coping, has recognized two primary types of coping: emotion-focused and problem-focused coping (Lazarus, 1999; Lazarus, 1991; Lazarus & Folkman, 1984). Emotion-focused coping in situations of patient education usually includes attempts to appraise the threat involved in an illness. Generally, the efforts involved at appraising and controlling the threat preclude effective patient teaching. For example, if a patient has recently experienced a myocardial infarction (MI) and uses defense mechanisms (eg, denial) as a form of emotion-focused coping, it is unlikely that effective patient teaching can be accomplished. However, if rational, action-oriented coping (problem-focused coping) is used, then the patient will be more open to disease management and necessary lifestyle changes.

Patient education requires the health professional to be open and to desire to discover the variables that influence the patient's choices. Working through, rather than around, patient issues helps nurses intervene most effectively and address the barriers that prevent patients from cooperating. Patient education requires a skilled approach in assessing patient issues and problems and in setting goals with patients. Chapters 8 and 9 help strengthen this approach through use of the nursing process.

MODELS AND THEORIES AS THE RESEARCH AND PRACTICE FOUNDATION OF PATIENT EDUCATION

Various theories and models have been used as the conceptual basis of patient education practice and research. Although Lindeman (1988) and Smith (1989) argue for a singular model that would unify patient education practice and research, others have noted the complexity of the topic and contend pragmatically that different models of patient and health education are needed, depending on the environment, the patient's needs, and many other factors (Haynes, McKibbon, Kanani, Brouwers, & Oliver, 1999; Redman, 1993). We agree with the latter group, and assert that the theories used in research and practice should be chosen carefully to match all situational contingencies. Most patient education research in the past has been atheoretical; this is characteristic of research in many disciplines, especially those that are recent arrivals on the research scene. The following section presents

useful theoretical approaches for patient education.

The Health Belief Model

The Health Belief Model has been the most frequently used theoretical basis for research that examines the efficacy of patient education. The traditional Health Belief Model, also discussed in Chapter 2, was constructed in the 1950s by a group of social psychologists at the United States Public Health Service to predict health behaviors. Built on earlier work of Kurt Lewin, an influential social psychologist, it provides a tool for understanding the patient's perception of the disease and his or her decision-making process in the consumption of health care services. The application of this model in research is often for compliance prediction, and it is also useful for gaining a better understanding of the patient's motivation for seeking and obtaining services.

The Health Promotion Model developed by Pender is discussed in depth in Chapter 2 as is another model pertinent to patient education, the Self-Regulation Model. The foundation for both of these models is the Health Belief Model.

Other Models of Individual Health Behavior

The two theories of *self-efficacy* and *stress and coping* are generally characterized as interpersonal theories of health behavior, whereas the Health Belief Model is characterized as a model of individual health behavior. Interpersonal models of health behavior offer promise for health care providers, because we can become one of the sources of change in our patients' lives according to this formulation.

Self-Efficacy Theory

Social learning theory, also called self-efficacy theory, is a promising theoretical basis for patient education. This theory accounts not only for learner characteristics but also gives direction to the teacher for managing the physical and social environment in which learning occurs (Bandura, 1997; 1977).

Self confidence, also referred to as self-efficacy expectancies to perform certain behaviors, is derived from four discrete sources of information (Bandura, 1982). People with high self-efficacy expectancies (ie, the belief that one can achieve what one sets out to do) are generally healthier, more effective, and more successful than those who have low expectancies (Bandura, 1997). The four discrete sources of information include personal mastery, vicarious experiences, verbal persuasion, and physiologic feedback (Box 4-1).

Personal mastery is the most important of the four sources of information and refers to the patient's perceived confidence that he or she actually performs the desired behavior. An example of personal mastery is the patient newly diagnosed with diabetes, who can perform home blood glucose monitoring successfully. If the patient had experienced many unsuccessful attempts to draw blood and read the glucometer, the sense of personal mastery, or self-efficacy, would be diminished and learning would become more difficult.

The *vicarious experiences* that patients gain from observing role models (eg, other patients, health professionals, family members) are es-

---

BOX 4-1. Clinical Application of Self-Efficacy Theory: Breast-feeding

Personal Mastery

The first-time mother learning to breast-feed her newborn is a good example of the need to develop personal mastery. If the new mother has a difficult time getting her newborn to successfully "latch on," she may begin to feel diminished as a mother. Teaching this new mother may become more difficult for the nurse, because each time she attempts to breast-feed, she may become more stressed and tense. Her newborn, sensing her tension, may become more resistant to feeding at the breast, further diminishing the mother's sense of personal mastery.

Vicarious Experiences

Vicarious experiences may help the first-time mother who is learning how to breast-feed. For example, if the mother watched her own mother successfully breast-feed, she had a significant role model available to her. Likewise, watching friends breast-feed, and viewing educational videos of different women who are breastfeeding provides vicarious experiences and gives the first-time mother an opportunity to develop self confidence.

Verbal Persuasion

Verbal persuasion from lactation consultants is an important source of information for the first-time mother. Lactation consultants can assist with breast-feeding through telephone or in person consultation and encouragement. Breast-feeding groups (eg, La Leche League) also provide an important source of verbal persuasion. The sources of verbal persuasion are important to first-time mothers because they provide answers to questions and, more importantly, provide encouragement, support, and alternate methods of successful breast-feeding.

Physiologic Feedback

Physiologic feedback, as a form of information leading to self confidence, is provided by the infant's weight gains. The first-time mother usually discovers that her infant has gained weight during the second follow-up visit to the pediatric nurse practitioner or physician. This weight gain, a form of physiologic feedback, reinforces the first-time mother's confidence in her abilities to successfully breast-feed her baby.

pecially important for the new learner. For example, a patient with a new ostomy frequently learns better and more quickly how to manage an ostomy if he or she is taught by another person who has also had an ostomy and can role model successful management. Vicarious experiences are more predictive of effective patient education if the role model has similar characteristics to the learner, including age, gender, and ability.

Verbal persuasion reinforces the patient's competence in enacting new behaviors. In a study of recovery from cardiac surgery, patients and their spouses were coached on the telephone by nurses for 8 weeks after hospital discharge regarding various aspects of risk factor reduction (Gortner & Jenkins, 1990). Additionally, the cardiac patients were verbally encouraged to walk and get other forms of exercise as their condition permitted. The encouragement and verbal persuasion were reinforced by the weekly telephone calls. Likewise, elders can serve as peer advisors to other elders when they have both experienced an acute MI (Whittemore, Rankin, Callahan, Leder, & Carroll, 2000). The peer advisors were found to have intervened in situations that involved congestive heart failure, management of physical energy demands, recurrent angina, depression, and obtaining visiting nurse services. They helped older participants by problem solving, and by sharing the common experiences of recovery from an MI.

Physiologic feedback refers to the necessary physical cues patients receive that the behavior they have undertaken is either appropriate or inappropriate, or that alternative actions should be sought. For example, a study of post-MI patients used treadmill testing as a form of physiologic feedback (Ewart, Taylor, Reese & DeBusk, 1983). In a unique attempt to ameliorate the fears of the patients' wives and as a form of enhancing vicarious experiences, the wives were also given the opportunity to use the treadmill; this experience gave them the opportunity to reinforce desired behavior through vicarious experience and their own physiologic feedback (Taylor, Bandura, Ewart, Miller, & DeBusk, 1985).

The use of social learning theory as a theoretical framework to guide patient education research and practice offers a more coherent approach to patient education. Measurement of a patient's confidence, or sense of perceived self-efficacy, usually involves measures that present a singular situation (eg, climbing steps and then asking how confident the person is that he or she can climb three steps, one flight of steps, two flights of steps, and so on). The patient is then asked how confident on a scale of not at all confident (0%) to completely confident (100%) he or she feels in climbing steps. In a study of cardiac patients, experimental study patients who had been coached reported greater self-efficacy in terms of walking and lifting than did the control, or uncoached, group (Gortner, Gilliss, Shinn, Sparacino, Rankin, Leavitt, Price, & Hudes, 1988).

Self-efficacy theory has contributed to the theoretical basis of patient education by specifying mechanisms that enhance learning and by increasing motivation. It has been criticized for its generality and lack of methodologic refinement. In terms of deriving interventions for practice, however, the four discrete sources of information that can result in desired behavior change provide a useful heuristic for designing programs. Table 4-3 suggests different patient education interventions for the various sources of efficacy information with application to a 9-year-old child, newly diagnosed with diabetes, who must learn how to administer insulin.

The following theories are useful in understanding patient responses to threatening situations involving illness. They are also considered interpersonal theories of health behavior.

Stress, Coping, and Social Support

Stress, coping, and social support theories comprise a group of theoretical perspectives derived by various social scientists. The authors have found the cognitive appraisal approach of Lazarus and the sociologic approach of Pearlin as two of the most useful in their own practice. Both of these approaches include social support as an important modifier of stress.

TABLE 4-3. Sources of Efficacy Expectations and Related Patient Education Activity Performance for Newly Diagnosed Children With Type I Diabetes Who Must Learn Insulin Injection

SOURCES OF EFFICACY EXPECTATIONS	RELATED PATIENT EDUCATION ACTIVITY PERFORMANCE
Performance accomplishments	1. Participant modeling; successful injection of insulin by fearful, newly diagnosed, child with diabetes
	2. Performance desensitization: loss of fear of self-injections
	3. Performance exposure: continued successful practice of insulin injection
Vicarious experience	1. Live modeling: demonstration by another child with diabetes of insulin injection procedures
	2. Symbolic modeling: successful insulin demonstration by an age- and gender-matched child with diabetes
Verbal persuasion	1. Suggestion: informing the child on insulin injection techniques and methods to decrease anxiety surrounding it
	2. Exhortation: persuasive coaching by parents and nurse to perform successful insulin injection
	3. Self-instruction: child uses doll to learn insulin injection with persuasion from nurse
Physiologic/emotional arousal	1. Attribution: modification of the threat of injection by attributing the fear to something, or someone, else
	2. Relaxation, biofeedback: modifying threat by deep-breathing exercises before injection

Adapted from: Bandura, A. (1977), "Self-efficacy theory: Toward a unifying theory of behavior change." *Psychological Review, 84,* 191–215.

Historically, stress research was given impetus by the work of two physiologists, Cannon (1939) and Selye (1936, 1952, 1982). Selye generated a tradition, still prominent today in the work of Lazarus and Folkman (1984, 1991, 1999) and others, that posits that the response of the organism is more important than the nature of the stimulus provoking the response. This approach to stress is different from that of epidemiologists and sociologists who are more concerned with the source of stress (ie, the stressors). The authors believe that both perspectives are important to understanding the patient during patient education.

The cognitive appraisal approach assists the health care provider in understanding that the patient's response to a stimulus (eg, stressor) is unique and that the evaluation of the stimulus is influenced by factors within the person and from the stimulus itself. Psychological stress is thus the relationship between the person and the environment that is appraised as exceeding the available personal resources (Lazarus & Folkman, 1984; 1999). Cognitive appraisal is an evaluation of the sit-

uation and includes primary appraisal: *Am I in trouble? Does this situation threaten me?;* and secondary appraisal: *What can I do about it?* A simplified illustration of the stress response according to Lazarus and colleagues is depicted in Fig. 4-1.

Lazarus and his colleagues posit that coping is an ongoing process. Coping does not occur in stages; it is constantly being reworked. Coping comprises cognitive and behavioral efforts to manage specific demands that are appraised by the patient as straining or exceeding personal resources. Lazarus identifies the following coping resources as being available:

Health and energy
Positive beliefs
Problem-solving skills
Social skills
Social support
Material resources

The health care provider usually helps the patient in terms of developing problem-focused coping, because this type of coping is most appropriate when something can be done

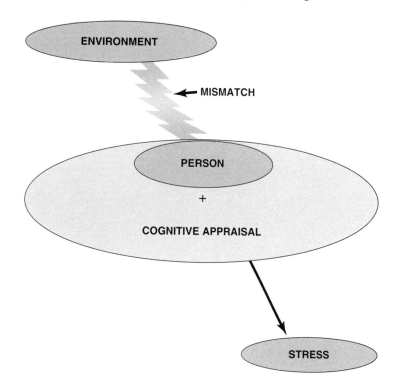

FIGURE 4-1. Depiction of the person–environment mismatch that generates stress.

about the situation. The nurse will offer information to enhance problem-solving and will mobilize socially supportive resources by helping the family understand how it can be most supportive during periods of stress. By referring the patient and family to a hospital social worker or to a case manager, the nurse mobilizes material resources. Table 4-4 illustrates, using the example of a 36-year-old woman with breast cancer, how a nurse might intervene to enhance coping resources with a combination of patient education and other nursing interventions.

The sociologic view of stress is illustrated in Fig. 4-2. This framework postulates that the sources and mediators of stress are located within the social environment of people (Pearlin, Lieberman, Menaghan, & Mullan, 1981; Pearlin & Skaff, 1996). Sources of stress are those stressors in the biologic or social environment that lead to the experience of stress. Stressors consist of life events and persistent life strains that can be physiologic or psychosocial in origin (Pearlin & Schooler, 1978; Pearlin & Skaff, 1996). In the case of a woman with an acute MI, stressors may consist of physiologic risk factors (eg, diabetes mellitus, hypertension) and problems of a psychosocial origin (eg, overeating, smoking, inactivity). Stress mediators are those social resources that help the patient adjust and adapt to the stressors.

Social support is a primary stress mediator and a resource in protecting well-being (Pearlin & Skaff, 1996). Thus, for the woman with an acute MI, stress mediators may include a supportive spouse and family. Mastery is a global sense of control that has repeatedly contributed to well-being. Mastery regulates the impact of stressors and may be elevated or lowered by exposure to stressor conditions (Skaff, Pearlin, & Mullan, 1995). Stress assumes various physiologic and psychosocial manifestations. After an acute MI, stress may be manifested by depression, anxiety, arrhythmias, and pain.

TABLE 4-4. Patient Education and Nursing Interventions to Enhance Coping Resources in a 36-year-old Woman With Breast Cancer

TYPE OF RESOURCE	EXAMPLE OF RESOURCE	NURSING ACTION
Physical resources	Health and energy	Teach importance of diet to maintain strength and decrease cachectic effects.
Psychological resources	1. Positive beliefs	1. Reinforce positive attitudes related to treatment and cure; decrease negative attitudes.
	2. Problem-solving	2. Assist patient in finding solutions to problems within her purview to solve; limit scope of problem-solving to those problems in which the patient can realistically intervene.
Social resources	1. Social skills	1. Refer to American Cancer Society "I Can Cope" groups, Reach to Recovery; reinforce previously developed social skills.
	2. Social support	2. Mobilize family and friends as support. If family and friends are not supportive, refer for counseling if the patient concurs.
Material resources	Money, goods, and services	Refer to hospital social services, discharge planning, and other community agency if the patient concurs. Give information about available services

Adpated from: Lazarus, R. S., & Folkman, S. (1984). *Stress, appraisal, and coping.* New York: Springer.

Adaptation is the dynamic process of adjusting to stress. Although not part of Pearlin's original stress model, it is consistent with his work and with a nursing perspective to view adaptation as the logical outcome of the stress process. Adaptation includes the patient's adjustment to the MI and ongoing coronary artery disease, her perceived quality of life, her assessment of her general health, and her cardiac functional capacity. The nurse who uses a sociologic view of stress in his or her practice of patient education will give more attention to enhancing social resources and decreasing stressors in the social environment than will the nurse who uses a cognitive appraisal view of stress. Both the psychological and sociologic approaches to viewing the stress process are useful for patient education.

DEVELOPMENTAL FRAMEWORKS: THE BASES FOR PATIENT EDUCATION

Developmental frameworks, such as those of Erikson, Piaget, and Duvall, are frequently included in nursing education programs because they offer a theoretical basis to undergird nursing assessment and interventions. Nurses and other health care professionals use the concepts of Erikson's developmental theory when they prepare the young adult for surgery related to repair of a congenital heart anomaly, remembering that the primary task at this developmental stage is to engender intimacy versus despair. They teach a 6-year-old child to administer insulin, recalling Piaget's stage referred to as preoperational development (see Chapter 5). Likewise, the nurse who prepares a family for the birth of a second child recalls that the tasks of the family with preschool children concern integration of the new family member and ways to cope with sibling jealousy. Although these developmental frameworks are useful, they are limited because they do not consider the multiple determinants that influence individual and family development. Therefore, the following two sections discuss two useful theories, Bronfenbrenner's Ecological Systems Theory and Lifespan Development Theory, for understanding the dynamic nature of development and its influence on patient education.

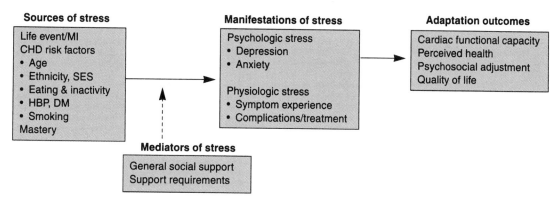

Sources of stress

Life event/MI
CHD risk factors
• Age
• Ethnicity, SES
• Eating & inactivity
• HBP, DM
• Smoking
Mastery

Manifestations of stress

Psychologic stress
• Depression
• Anxiety

Physiologic stress
• Symptom experience
• Complications/treatment

Adaptation outcomes

Cardiac functional capacity
Perceived health
Psychosocial adjustment
Quality of life

Mediators of stress

General social support
Support requirements

FIGURE 4-2. The stress process applied to women with acute myocardial infarctions. CHD, coronary heart disease; DM, diabetes mellitus; HBP, high blood pressure; MI, myocardial infarction; SES, socioeconomic status. Adapted with permission from Pearlin, L. I., Lieberman, M. A., Menaghan, E. G., and Mullan, J. T. (1981). The stress process. *Journal of Health and Social Behavior, 22*, p. 337–356).

Ecological Systems Theory

General Considerations

The 1979 publication of *Ecology of Human Development* by Urie Bronfenbrenner, a child developmental psychologist, highlighted the importance of considering the context of individual development. Bronfenbrenner argues that understanding the developing person without also understanding the ecological niches that govern favorable or unfavorable maturation is impossible. An ecological niche is formed by the intersection of a combination of personal attributes and demographic characteristics (Bronfenbrenner, 1989). Not only is the concept of ecological niche important to understanding development, but it also influences the process of patient education.

 An ecological niche for an adolescent, newly diagnosed with diabetes, might consist of a family that is White, urban, upper middle class, with two parents who both work, three children, and the children attending a private school. The ecological niche for this adolescent may be favorable to patient education and to learning necessary self-care management skills. Contrast this ecological niche and its influence on patient education with an adolescent with diabetes, who is a high school dropout, and lives with a single, unemployed parent, and who has six siblings in a rural, southern U.S. household.

Bronfenbrenner contends that the patient is an actor in this process of development, which is influenced by the environmental context and the reciprocity of the organism. Therefore, in the example above, one cannot assume until more information is available that the second adolescent is incapable of developing diabetes self management skills, although at first glance his or her ecological niche appears less favorable.

Bronfenbrenner's Ecological Framework: Interactive Systems

Other important concepts key to understanding Bronfenbrenner's ecological systems theory include four levels of nested concentric structures that form a model for interactive systems that influence, and are influenced by, the developing person (Fig. 4-3). These interactive systems are microsystems, mesosystems, exosystems, and macrosystems.

Microsystems are the patterns of activities, roles, interpersonal relationships, and material characteristics with which the developing person interacts (Bronfenbrenner, 1979; Bronfenbrenner & Crouter, 1983; Spencer, Dupree, & Hartmann, 1997). Important microsystems with which the

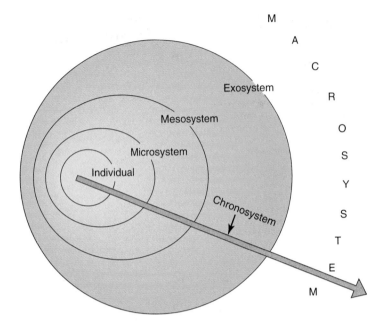

FIGURE 4-3. Bronfenbrenner's ecological framework.

child interacts are the family, peer group, and school. Microsystems are the most basic level of system influencing development. Regarding patient education and its intersection with microsystems, the health care professional who works with a child should consider the quality of family, peer, and school life and how these might influence the child's ability to accept patient teaching.

Mesosystems are interrelated microsystems, such as the interrelationships that occur between a child's family and the school (Bronfenbrenner, 1979). These interrelationships have an impact on the development of the child. Mesosystems have implications for patient education. For example, a child may be enrolled in a school that creates a private environment for children to monitor their blood glucose levels if the family wishes to conceal the child's diabetes. When the family and school have limited understanding of each other or if they interact negatively, the child will not have the environmental supports to maintain the self-care activities taught by the health care professional.

Exosystems are environments and conditions external to the child that indirectly affect the child's development. Examples of exo-systems are parental occupational environments and parental friendships (Bronfenbrenner, 1986). Exosystems are sys-

tems the child infrequently enters, but they are structures that can have major effects on the child's maturation. Exosystems have implications for patient education. For example, parental friendships may affect the manner in which health teaching is interpreted by parents. Parents who are encouraged by their friends to send their child to diabetes camp may open new avenues of patient education for the child who has never been exposed to other children with diabetes. The hospital and health care community are also examples of important exosystems. Schmidt (1990) found that hospitalized children did not have the same levels of fear or postoperative behavior problems as had been reported in an earlier study by Visintainer and Wolfer (1975). This was interpreted as a result of greater parental involvement in the exosystem (ie, the hospital) and more knowledge on the part of children and parents about this influential exosystem. Implications for patient education include enhancing knowledge of parents and children through the schools and the media (especially television) regarding hospitalization so that hospitals as an exosystem are more amenable to children's needs when hospitalized.

Macrosystems are the broadest and most indirect system influences on the child. Macro-systems include the impact of culture, subculture, and embedded belief patterns on the developing child. Macrosystems affect the child through their relationships to the micro-, meso-, and exosystems.

Chronosystems include the dimension of time and were added by Bronfenbrenner in 1986 to expand the theory so that the effects of change, and continuities, on the developing person could be better understood (Bronfenbrenner, 1986). Chronosystems are typically conceived as life transitions. The chronosystem is an important thrust that intersects the other systems (see Figure 4-3).

The importance of understanding chronosystems as related to patient education and children entails a constant attendance to the transitions that children and adolescents encounter during the first 20 years of life. For example, the 12-year-old youth who is diagnosed with insulin-dependent diabetes mellitus (IDDM) is most likely entering the tumultuous years associated with adolescence; peer relationships and being part of the crowd are more important than euglycemia. However, a 3-year-old child diagnosed with IDDM is still within a parentally controlled orbit in which peer relationships are secondary to the family sphere. Thus, the life transitions, or chronosystem effects, encountered by the 12-year-old can be postulated as making adjustment to diabetes more difficult than for a 3-year-old child.

A poignant example of the power of the chronosystem and life transitions was seen when one of the authors facilitated a support group for parents with a child who has diabetes. One mother told the story of her 12-year-old son who had been relatively compliant in terms of insulin injections, diet, and self blood glucose monitoring (SBGM). She related that as he began spending more time after school in the company of friends, she began noticing candy wrappers in his pants pockets. At first he denied he had been eating candy and then he showed her his SBGM log book that he had completed, indicating his blood glucose levels were within acceptable guidelines. Finally, after an upper respiratory infection, he was hospitalized in diabetic ketoacidosis. When he began SBGM again, the nurse noted that he was incorrectly

performing the process so that he fooled his blood glucose monitor, resulting in false low readings. When confronted with his SBGM technique, he readily admitted what he had done but told his parents it was more important to him that he be part of the gang than to have acceptable blood glucose readings. Nurses and other health care providers should realize that chronosystem influences are frequently more significant than long-term health outcomes to patients. Understanding patients from the perspective of life transitions can add greater clarity and direction to patient teaching.

In summary, Bronfenbrenner's Ecological Systems Theory can be a means of sensitizing the health care professional who works with children and adolescents to the various dimensions that influence development not commonly considered in traditional approaches. Although the theory is encumbered by the jargon used by Bronfenbrenner, the importance of considering people in the broadest context of development is an important contribution from Bronfenbrenner's work. ∎

Lifespan Development Frameworks

General Considerations

Lifespan Development Frameworks, also referred to as Life-Course Perspective, evolved in the 1960s and 1970s. It was developed by lifespan developmental psychologists and life-course perspective sociologists. Their research looked at the interrelated effects of age, cohort experience, and nonnormative life events on development.

Unlike Bronfenbrenner, who added the concept of chronosystem almost as an afterthought, the lifespan developmental psychologists had long been involved in longitudinal studies of various U.S. cohorts. Their work also was influenced by the stage developmentalists, such as Erikson and Duvall. However, like Bronfenbrenner, they realized that there was more to development than simply an orderly progression through stages.

Although Ecological Systems Theory is a useful device for considering the many influences on development and their influence on patient education, it pertains primarily to children and adolescents. Lifespan Developmental Frameworks, however, are applicable to people across the life span and add a particularly salient dimension to the work of health care professionals with older patients.

Components of the Lifespan Developmental Framework

The Lifespan Developmental Framework as outlined by various social scientists (Baltes, Reese, & Lipsitt, 1980; Featherman, 1981; Schaie, 1986) is a useful conceptual approach for considering the dynamic, integrated aspects of human functioning (Fig. 4-4). A basic assumption of this model is that biologic, environmental, and behavioral determinants, in conjunction with specified developmental influences, shape the life span of individuals and families. Important developmental influences that should be considered by health care professionals appraising the effects of adult development on patient education include:

Normative age-graded factors (ie, biologic and environmental variables that exhibit a high correlation with chronological age)

Normative history-graded factors (ie, the historical events that influence particular birth cohorts)

Nonnormative factors (ie, life events that occur asynchronously with the life course or that are not experienced by the population at large

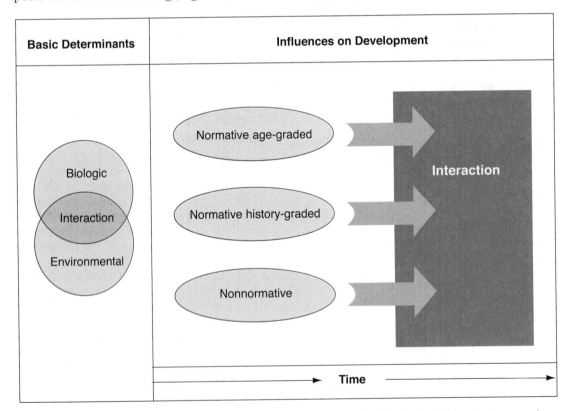

FIGURE 4-4. Determinants and influences on lifespan development: a methodological and theoretical approach. From Life-span Developmental Psychology by Baltes, P. D., Reese, H. W., and Lipsitt, L. P. Used with permission, from the *Annual Review of Psychology*, Volume 31 ©1980 by Annual Reviews www.AnnualReviews.org.

Normative age-graded factors overlap with the psychological and cognitive stages outlined by developmental theorists, such as Erikson and Piaget; they also coincide with normative physical development. Although normative age-graded factors are frequently taken for granted when planning patient education, the importance of considering the effects of age on patient education is illustrated in the case of women with coronary heart disease (CHD). Women are usually older than men when they experience an acute MI, which has implications for recovery and rehabilitation from MI and also may be related to their greater incidence of death from MI (Dittrich, Gilpin, Nicod, Cali, Henning, & Ross, 1988; Vaccarino, 1999). Older women are likely to have preexisting comorbidities that may limit participation in cardiac rehabilitation programs and exercise regimens. For example, limited mobility as a result of osteoarthritis and rheumatoid arthritis, peripheral vascular disease, and orthopedic impairments are comorbid conditions that may impinge on the ability of older women to participate in cardiac rehabilitation programs. Thus, any attempts to effectively educate the older woman post-MI must contemplate preexisting comorbidities and plan methods of exercise that consider them.

Clinical Relevance

Normative Age-Graded Factors

A meta-analysis of diabetes patient education research, examining the effectiveness of diabetes patient teaching interventions found that across 73 studies, normative age-graded factors were especially important (Brown, 1992). Brown's meta-analysis revealed that diabetes teaching interventions were less effective for older patients; for patients older than 55 years, glycosylated hemoglobin levels were only minimally improved by teaching interventions. Brown surmises that older patients with diabetes may need more individualized instruction than younger patients. Also, Brown surmises that instead of mixing diabetes management regimen (ie, insulin versus oral hypoglycemic versus diet) across group

parti-cipants, it might be better to segregate by diabetes type and regimen.

Normative History Graded Factors

 Continuing with the example of older women and acute MI, important normative history graded influences can be identified as attitudes toward promotion, restoration, and maintenance of health. Health promotion, restoration, and maintenance activities relating to CHD include cessation of cigarette smoking, implementation of a proper diet, and regular exercise. Cigarette smoking has been identified as the most prominent risk factor for heart disease in women (Castelli, 1988; Corrao, Becker, Ockene, & Hamilton, 1990). ■ Smoking appears to have synergistic effects, because it increases the risk for heart disease and MI if used in conjunction with oral contraceptives and if hyperlipidemia is present (Corrao et al., 1990; Murdaugh, 1990). The cohort of women who presently experience CHD and MI were naive to the harmful impact of tobacco on the cardiovascular system when they began smoking and thus did not have the benefit of the information available to younger women who currently make decisions regarding smoking. Patient education strategies must be oriented toward improving the quality of life in one's remaining years rather than toward preventing the onset of coronary artery and other vascular diseases.

Other prominent health promotion and restoration activities related to CHD include dietary intake and exercise. Similar to information on the harmful effects of smoking, dietary information was not available to older women when they were young and establishing health promotion activities. Today's cohort of older women (ie, older than age 65) with CHD and MI may have amended their current eating patterns, but previous behaviors may have already established irreversible atherosclerosis. The use of exercise to establish adequate cardiovascular health has health promotive and health restorative functions. However, the cohort of women who are experiencing CHD and MI currently were less likely to engage in health promotive vigorous exercise when they were younger than is found in their more youthful counterparts. Additionally, only a small percentage of women who experience MI are likely to engage in structured cardiac rehabilitative exercise for health restoration (Thomas, Miller, Lamendola, Berra, Hedback, Durstine, & Haskell, 1996). Therefore, health care professionals who seek to provide cardiac rehabilitation and its attendant patient education to older women must consider these history graded factors and amend cardiac rehabilitation programs so that they appeal to older women and are based on their own life experience.

Health maintenance history graded effects include the belief by most women that they were not at risk for CHD and MI because it was considered a male disease. These beliefs, which also have been prominent in the health care community, have resulted in less attention given to the clinical symptoms with which women present with CHD and MI; thus, fewer diagnostic procedures and laboratory tests have been performed that may have assisted in earlier identification of CHD. The patient education implications for these health maintenance history graded effects include the fact that women across the life span need education informing them of their risk for CHD and the symptoms that may indicate angina or MI.

Nonnormative Factors

Nonnormative factors (ie, events that occur unexpectedly during the life span) often offer the greatest challenge to the health care professional who conducts patient education. These factors include the onset of acute or chronic illnesses at times seemingly asynchronous with usual occurrence. For example, most women are unprepared for the diagnosis of MI at the age of 40 years; indeed, 40-year-old men are equally unprepared. Unexpected and severe illnesses are generally unexpected in young children and thus challenge the health care professional who must educate the parents and help the family cope. The family that has an 18-month-old child diagnosed with IDDM, and that faces the challenge of managing the child's illness, is faced with a nonnormative event of monumental proportions. The parents will probably require additional teaching time and additional support in managing potential future losses. During the assessment process, a nurse should recognize nonnormative factors as conceivably requiring more time and greater resources for patient education.

Implications of the Lifespan Framework for Patient Education

At times, health care professionals do not consider the multiple factors that influence a patient's receptivity to patient teaching. If the patient is assessed in the context of the multiple constraints of lifespan development, nurses can better individualize patient education. Examples using the lifespan approach were cited above for older women with CHD. At different ages, people approach learning from distinct vantage points. Remembering that patients are products of the historical eras in which they matured helps nurses shape appropriate patient education for different birth cohorts.

For example, women born during the Baby Boom Era (1946 to 1964) have willingly embraced physical exercise in many different forms. Their mothers, on the other hand, were less likely to exercise to the point of maximal cardiovascular capacity. The female Baby Boomers who have MIs will probably be open to cardiac rehabilitation, whereas their mothers are less likely to become involved. Attitudinal differences toward sexuality, reproductive health, and raising children are major cohort effects found in these two generations of women. These are only a few disparities in these two generations; the health care provider must constantly consider history graded factors, or cohort effects, when planning patient education. Lastly, nonnormative factors challenge the nurse to further individualize patient education efforts so that the patient's own particular experience is viewed from an appropriate perspective.

The next section of this chapter reviews the process of teaching and learning. The theories presented up to this point have been primarily macroanalytical theories of patient and health education. That is, they are useful to understand the broader aspects of patient education. The actual learning process includes microanalytical theories that pertain to particular ideas about how information is actually learned and

processed. This section of the chapter also includes a discussion of motivation.

THE PROCESS OF TEACHING AND LEARNING

Definition of Learning

Learning has been defined as a process involving interaction with the external environment (Gagne & Driscoll, 1988) and as a change
in behavior resulting from reinforced practice
(Huckabay, 1980). The definition by Huckabay, a noted nurse educator, seems especially
pertinent to the learning that must occur
in patient teaching situations involving psychomotor skills. (Chapter 10 provides an in-
depth discussion of psychomotor learning.)
For this chapter's purpose, the authors define
psychomotor learning as pertaining to learning of skills and performance. Learning that
requires a change in feelings or belief (*affective learning*) and learning that requires thinking (*cognitive learning*) may be more difficult
to promote and measure.

Sequence of Events in Learning

Learning and remembering are generally
thought of as orderly sequences of events that
occur in all learners (Fig. 4-5). Gagne and
other educational psychologists (Bigge & Shermis, 1999; Gagne & Driscoll, 1988; Huckabay,
1980; Lewis, Rankin, & Kellogg, 1985) delin-
eate the sequence of learning and remembering as one that occurs in eight phases:

- Motivation
- Apprehending
- Acquisition
- Retention
- Recall
- Generalization
- Performance
- Feedback

Motivation

Motivation can be either intrinsic or extrinsic.
Intrinsic motivation factors (eg, the patient's

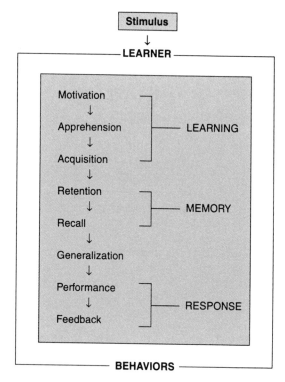

FIGURE 4-5. Sequence of steps involved in learning.

anxiety level, success in past educational settings, and openness to learning) are internally
integrated into the client's personality and
modus operandi. Extrinsic motivation factors
include the learning environment, the pleasure of acquiring new knowledge, and the
type of interaction in the learning process.
Extrinsic motivation factors are the only motivation factors that patient educators can
control. If nurses establish a climate of mutual
trust and safety, the learning environment can
be a positive motivator. Likewise, by injecting
fun and some levity into the learning situation, nurses can make the pleasure of learning
become a positive force.

The type of interaction in the learning
process is another extrinsic motivating factor
that the educator can control. Transactional
analysis provides a vocabulary useful to describing the desired interaction. If our interaction with the learner is structured so that the
adult learner is programmed as the child in an
adult-child or parent-child situation, the inter-

action will have negative motivational effects on the learner. The adult learner will profit most from an adult-adult type of interaction. An example of an adult-adult type of interaction would be that of group learn-ing experiences for ostomy patients, in which one patient would share with the group his or her experiences in coping with the ostomy. Another example of an adult-adult type of interaction includes the patient educator who encourages the client to set his own agenda for learning the management of heart disease. Adult-adult interactions require the client to take responsibility for his or her own learning.

Because motivation also has social and task mastery components, nurses can use these components to enhance a patient's motivation to learn. For example, adolescents have a strong need to belong (affiliative needs). These affiliative needs, and related self-esteem and social approval needs, can be used to enhance internal motivating forces when adolescents learn how to cease smoking or how to manage contraception. The use of peers who role model desired behaviors is an exceptionally strong motivator for adolescents.

The nurse can help the client to recognize the gap between what his or her situation is and what he or she wants it to be. For example, a young couple with whom the authors worked recognized that they did not want to use corporal punishment with their 3-year-old daughter, but they did not know how else to achieve necessary obedience. Once the authors helped the couple recognize the gap, they eagerly asked for and then applied other discipline techniques. Once patients have recognized the gap, they can be effectively motivated with the use of written contracts. (The formulation of contracts is covered in Chapter 9.) If motivational techniques do not seem to work, the nurse should consider reviewing the assessment and then reassessing the patient if necessary. Perhaps something has changed in the patient's own situation and previous motivators are no longer effective. For example, a low-to-moderate level of anxiety is an intrinsic motivator and may be used effectively to motivate the patient with coronary artery disease to learn about necessary diet, medication, and lifestyle changes. However, if this patient has a successful coronary artery bypass graft operation, he or she may think he or she is cured and out of danger; therefore, anxiety may no longer be an effective motivator. The nurse must now reassess the patient and determine other motivators.

Additional questions about motivation exist (eg, *How much responsibility to learn does the patient have?*). When all factors are considered, the patient must ultimately decide whether he or she is going to accept the nurse's attempt to teach, even if acceptance is selective or if all teaching is ignored. Nurses and health care professionals are not responsible for a patient's behavior. They do their best to enhance the learning situation and to use extrinsic motivation factors, but motivation is essentially an inner drive. If a patient does not have this inner drive and sense of personal responsibility, nurses and other health professionals can do little to foster these motivators. Ideally, nurses should teach patients to be their own advocates and to expect patient education services on an inpatient and outpatient basis. Many patients will respond to this approach; various manuscripts have been written detailing the approach that patients should take when dealing with the medical world (Kleinman, 1988; Lewis-Fernandez & Kleinman, 1995; Cousins, 1979; Illich, 1976). However, nurses must recognize the few patients who refuse to take responsibility for their own learning; once a nurse has made every attempt to provide patient education, the nurse must finally release a sense of responsibility for these patients.

Apprehending

During the apprehending phase of learning, learners are exposed to a stimulus, which is then absorbed and processed in a manner that requires discriminative abilities. Patients who are mildly or moderately anxious are often good subjects for patient teaching because they attend to the stimulus with greater care than those who are not anxious. For example, most coronary artery bypass graft surgery patients and their family members are moderately anxious the day before surgery. Their discriminative abilities are heightened, and patient teaching can be extremely effective.

Acquisition

The acquisition phase of learning includes the changes that occur in the central nervous system (CNS) and undergird and concretize the new material. If the learner has a CNS dysfunction, the new material may not be acquired. The patient with a cerebrovascular accident is an obvious example. This patient may apprehend new information, but because of CNS damage, he or she may not perform the desired behavior.

Retention

Retention is the fourth phase of learning. During this phase, the material that was previously apprehended is stored as memories. Age may be an intervening factor in terms of retention, because older people have more problems with short-term memory than with long-term memory.

Recall

Recall is retrieval. During recall, the learner can retrieve his or her new abilities for an external observer or teacher. For example, when parents of an infant with respiratory problems are asked to demonstrate endotracheal suctioning, they recall the basics of sterile suctioning technique, then they organize the procedure systematically and perform the skill safely and correctly.

Generalization

Generalization, the sixth phase in the learning process, is sometimes referred to as the transfer of learning (Bigge, 1992). During generalization, the patient can retrieve something he has learned and apply it within a different situation or context. For example, the parent who has learned the principles of sterile technique in the context of sterile suctioning should be able to apply these techniques to other situations that require sterile techniques.

Performance and Feedback

Performance and feedback are the seventh and eighth phases of learning. Performance is the observable behavior and thus a demon-stration that a change has occurred. Performance is relatively easy to observe in situations of psychomotor learning. However, in situations of affective and cognitive learning, performance is more difficult to observe and frequently must be obtained through verbal methods.

Feedback is the last phase of learning and occurs through reinforcement. Feedback in situations of psychomotor learning is automatic because successful performance of the newly learned information serves as feedback. In situations of affective or cognitive learning, however, feedback is frequently a function of the instructor who encourages the learner by saying "Good," or "That's correct."

Nurses must frequently educate children or adults with learning disabilities; their learning styles may be different and different approaches may be needed. Box 4-2 suggests approaches to match teaching with particular patient disabilities.

Clinical Relevance: Patient Advocacy and Promotion of Change

Anyone who has ever tried to stop smoking, lose weight, or exercise regularly knows how difficult it is to change old behaviors. It may seem at times that patients truly cannot be motivated to change their behaviors. If an empowerment viewpoint is espoused, nurses can recognize that there are times when, given all available information, and after engaging in a fully participatory encounter, patients will still choose not to embrace healthy behaviors.

Gadow's Existential Advocacy

Gadow's work on existential advocacy, which is presented in Chapter 6, further elaborates this view of motivation. Her work demonstrates how the nurse should be a partner with the patient, meet the patient where he or she is, and assist in whatever manner possible in coming to a decision about assuming certain behaviors (Gadow, 1983). Gadow conceptualizes that the patient is on a continuum that stretches between consumerism and paternalism. There-

---

BOX 4-2. Meeting the Needs of Children and Adults With Learning Disabilities

Points to remember

1. **Children with learning disorders** (eg, attention deficit disorder, dyslexia) may learn better using sensory systems—auditory, visual, or tactile—that are different from those used by the patient educator. Also, their learning abilities may be affected by problems affecting memory, language, and motor and integrative process problems.

2. **Auditory learners** are thought to have visual perceptual disabilities (eg, dyslexia). These children and adults learn best through auditory modes; therefore, the nurse should not rely on written teaching materials, but instead use auditory materials, such as tapes, records, and verbal instruction.

3. **Visual learners** often have an auditory perceptual disability. These learners usually have difficulties distinguishing subtle differences in sounds and may have problems picking up cues that they are being spoken to, especially when others are in the same room. These learners do well with films, written materials, and charts. Group instruction may be confusing to these learners.

4. **Tactile learners** are children with learning disabilities that are most amenable to learning that includes hands-on, tactile experience. If they do not have other sensory learning disabilities, they may be good candidates for group games and learning experiences that involve movement.

5. **Integrative process disabilities** usually involve the inability to sequence visual, auditory, or tactile input correctly. Children with these learning disabilities may read words backward, may not correctly process words, or may hear words or sentences improperly, or may not understand the meaning. The most effective learning strategies involve simple instructions with the opportunity for immediate return demonstration.

6. **Short- or long-term memory disabilities** are manifested as the inability to remember information presented recently or in the past. These disabilities often accompany other learning disabilities, adding to the problems involved in achieving effective patient education. Adults or children with memory disabilities need the opportunity for short and frequent teaching sessions.

7. **Language disabilities** are manifested as the inability to answer when some type of response is demanded. The most important response of the nurse educator is to provide sufficient time for the individual to organize his or her thoughts so that a coherent answer can be given. These learners are not good candidates for learning activities that require quick verbal responses (eg, spelling bees).

8. **Motor disabilities** can be exhibited in two different ways—gross and fine motor disabilities. Fine motor disabilities are evident in children or adults who cannot write or draw but possibly can use a computer or paint. Gross motor disabilities frequently result in clumsiness and poor performance in sports activities.

---

fore, the nurse who takes a consumerist view presents the patient with all of the treatment options, with little regard for the patient's personal values and beliefs. Unlike the empowerment approach, the consumerist approach does not allow for reflection and listening. At the other end of the continuum is a paternalistic position, in which the nurse tells the patient what to do and makes decisions for him or her, a position that most nurses eschew.

Prochaska's Stages of Change

One of the most appealing aspects of Prochaska's work is that his stages of change have been applied successfully to some of the most hazardous and unhealthy behaviors, with moderate success. The Transtheoretical Model of Behavior Change is an attempt to explain why some people do not modify risky behaviors, despite adequate information. It has been used to study behaviors most resistant to change, including addictive behaviors, diet and weight control, smoking cessation, sexual behavior related to HIV infection, and other life-endangering behaviors (DiClemente & Prochaska, 1998).

Prochaska and colleagues propose that the stages of change are a "developmental sequence of motivational readiness" that include precontemplation, contemplation, preparation, action, and maintenance (Prochaska, Redding, Harlow, Rossi, & Velicer, 1994, p. 473) [Table 4-5]. Prochaska and colleagues note that the stages of change are not necessarily linear and that people may revert to previous risk-taking behaviors. They suggest that interventions to motivate people must be tailored for each stage. The theory is complex and includes the concept of self-efficacy, which was discussed earlier in the chapter. We refer the interested reader to James Prochaska's 15 years' of publications on change and motivation.

Theories of Learning

Before 1950, comprehensive theories of learning were proposed that asserted an explanation for all types of learning. However, as educational psychologists learned more about the nature of learning, it became clear that single theories could not explain the entire realm of teaching and learning. Therefore, theories emerged that attempted to explain certain

TABLE 4-5. Prochaska's Transtheoretical Model of Motivation and Change as Applied to Weight Loss

STAGE OF CHANGE	PERIOD OF TIME ASSOCIATED WITH STAGE AND CHARACTERISTICS OF STAGE	INTERVENTION
Precontemplation	• 6 mos • Little intent to change • Resistant to change • Defensiveness regarding obesity	Consciousness raising—providing information about health risks related to obesity. Increase awareness of various approaches to weight loss.
Contemplation	• Time in this stage is variable but has been reported from 6 mos to yrs • More serious about changing behavior • Ambivalent about the costs and benefits of changing behavior	Self-reevaluation—thoughtful attention to one's self and problems may provide an opportunity for health care professionals to influence decisions about healthy eating.
Preparation	• Variable period of time • Preliminary healthy behavior attempts, such as brief attempts to eat less	Self-liberation—belief in one's ability and commitment to change. Health care provider can reinforce belief in self through provision of support.
Action	• Usually lasts up to 6 mos • Periods of weight loss interspersed with recidivism and relapse	Helping relationships—need for open, caring, honest relationships can be fulfilled by health care provider.
Maintenance	• Begins 6 mos after successful behavior change in the action stage; may last for years if behavior change was successful • Relapse may occur but is less common than during the action stage	Counterconditioning—substitution of positive behaviors for negative ones. Health care provider can assist with planning meals, suggesting alternative rewards to food. Stimulus control—through restructuring of the environmental access to food can be controlled.

Adapted from: Prochaska, J. O., Redding, C. A., Harlow, L. L., Rossi, J. S., & Velicer, W. F. (1994). The transtheoretical model of change and HIV: prevention: A review. *Health Education Quarterly, 21*, 471–476.

facets of teaching and learning (eg, concept learning, problem solving, skill mastery).

Tables 4-6 and 4-7 present various theories on teaching and learning. The first three theories (mental discipline, natural unfoldment, and apperception) belong to the pre-1950s generation of theoretical precepts that pertain to the process of teaching and learning. They also had their earliest proponents before the 20th century (see Table 4-6). The theories in Table 4-7 have emanated from the various schools of educational psychology that evolved during the 20th century.

Generally, most writers agree that there are individual and interpersonal learning theories. The individual learning theories include the conditioning-behavioristic family, the cognitive-Gestalt-information processing family, and mastery learning. Interpersonal learning theory includes social learning theory. Also included in the interpersonal learning theory group, although not included on the table but discussed earlier in this chapter, are stress and coping theories and developmental theories.

Although learning theories help explain approaches to patient teaching and learning, nurses should remember different theories are used at different times, depending on the situation. An eclectic approach probably serves patients best. The attempt to apply the theories to various patient education situations is more an effort to give concrete illustrations of the theories than an effort to imply that such situations should always be guided by these theories.

The following case study demonstrates the application of behavioristic, cognitive-Gestalt, and social learning theory principles.

CASE STUDY

DIABETES MELLITUS

HISTORY
Claire Patterson is a 25-year-old white woman with IDDM; onset was at age 16. She is 5′, 4″ tall and weighs 125 lb. (4.4 lb. above desired weight). She attended a comprehensive diabetes education program 5 years ago and subsequently controlled her blood glucose levels with multidose insulin therapy. Her glycosylated hemoglobin level recently dropped from 13% to 7%, a desired level.

After marriage and relocation to Los Angeles, she changed physicians and insulin therapy. Her new physician prescribed 28 U of Lente (insulin zinc suspension USP) and 8 U of regular human insulin. She began having seizures in the middle of the night and was hospitalized several times during the month of October. In December, she returned to the comprehensive diabetes teaching program to gain better blood glucose control.

Family Setting
Claire Patterson lived at home with her parents before her marriage. Her mother, a registered nurse, was a primary participant in her daughter's diabetes management. Claire feels that she can openly express her feelings and concerns to her parents. Her mother hesitates between allowing her daughter to be more independent in managing her diabetes and taking control of diabetes management for her daughter because, she says, it "breaks my heart" to see her having convulsions. Claire requested that her mother accompany her to another week-long session at the diabetes teaching center.

Claire's husband is in military service out of state, and portions of the program were audiotaped for his benefit because he could not attend. Both Claire and her husband are motivated to get the diabetes under control so that they can have children.

Identified Problems
Contradicting attitudes about diabetes control resulted from Claire's insulin reactions. The family recognized that long-term complications frequently resulted from high blood glucose levels, but they believed that high blood glucose levels were safer

(case study continues on page 104)

LEARNING THEORY AND KEY PERSONS	ATTRIBUTES OF THE TEACHING/LEARNING PROCESS	NATURE OF LEARNING	APPLICATION TO PATIENT EDUCATION
Mental Discipline			
Plato, Aristotle—early developers M. J. Adler, R. M. Hutchings—contemporary proponents	Teacher trains intrinsic mental power. Learner maintains strict discipline to strengthen mental faculty of attention, memory, will, and perseverance. Rote memory, repetitive drill. Teacher centered with active learners.	Discipline mind and memorization of factual material.	Helpful when teaching exchange diet and basic pathophysiology. Should be used with oral drills.
Natural Unfoldment			
F. Froebel, J.J. Rousseau—early developers P. Goodman, J. Holt, & A. H. Maslow—contemporary proponents	Learner discovers that which nature or a creator has put within him. Teacher waits until learner expresses desire to learn before attempting to teach him or her. Promotes intuitive awareness of self. Learner's feelings are authority for truth. Student centered with active learners.	Self-directed active unfolding of knowledge with intuitive awareness expressed.	Applicable to clients interested in self-care, prenatal clients, well-child care.
Apperception			
J. F. Herbart, E. B. Titchener—original proponents	New ideas are associated with ideas that already exist in the learner's mind. Teacher explains and learner grasps generalizations, relationships, rules, or principles. Teacher centered with passive learners.	Recognition, explanation, or use of understandings, insights, principles, relationships, concepts, theories, or laws.	Applicable to clients who have previous knowledge or experience on which to build (ie, previous surgical experiences, knowledge of medications).

Adapted from: Bigge, M. L., (1976, 1982). Learning theories for teachers, (3rd and 4th ed.), New York: Harper & Row.

TABLE 4-7. Important Twentieth Century Teaching and Learning Theories and Their Application to Patient Education

LEARNING THEORY AND KEY PERSONS	ATTRIBUTES OF THE TEACHING/LEARNING PROCESS	NATURE OF LEARNING	APPLICATION TO PATIENT EDUCATION
Individual Learning Theories			
Conditioning—Behavioristic			
C. L. Hull, E. L. Thorndike— early developers	Involves conditioning or behavior modification. Formation of stimulus-response linkages or response-stimulus reinforcements.	Increased probability of desired response	Useful for reinforcing desired behaviors in children.
E. R. Guthrie, B. F. Skinner, R. Gagne—later proponents	Teacher centered with passive learners.		
Cognitive-Gestalt Information Processing (IP)			
M. Montessori, J. Dewey, K. Lewin, G. W. Allport, E. C. Tolman—early developers	Gains or changes insights, outlooks, or thought patterns. Reorganizes perceptual or cognitive fields. Purposive involvement, problem-solving and problem-raising.	Purposefully acquired insights, principles, relationships, concepts, generalizations, rules, theories, or laws with enhanced scientific outlook and instrumental thinking. Diagnostic reasoning	Applicable to affective learning (ie, working with parents on childrearing issues). Useful when working with groups with common problems (ie, parents of handicapped children, myocardial infarction spouse groups).
J. S. Bruner, M. L. Bigge, M. Deutsch, S. Koch, Newell and Simon, W. Kohler—later proponents	Teacher-student centered with cooperative and interactive inquiry. Information processing model consists of short- & long-term memory. Long-term memory is banked and can be retrieved later for use by short-term memory.		IP is useful for building and connecting information.

Mastery-Learning

B. Bloom, J. Block	Breaks down complex units of instruction into smaller learning units that build on each other. Strives for many (90%) learners, able to achieve or master tasks. Encourages self development.	Increased self esteem from learning results in changed perception of self and external world	Helpful when the information to be taught requires mastery of many skills (ie, patients with diabetes who are insulin-dependent).

Interpersonal Learning Theories
Social Learning

A. Bandura, W. Mischel	Process of learning is influenced by four sources of information: personal mastery, vicarious experiences, verbal persuasion, and physiologic feedback. Learner centered. Teachers can be family members or other learners.	Increased belief that one is capable of performing desired behavior and that the performance will lead to expected outcome	Enhancement of self confidence and self-efficacy can lead to desired health behavior changes and maintenance of desired behavior.

Note. From Bigge, M. C., & Shermis, S. S. (1982, 1992). *Learning theories for teachers* (3rd and 5th eds.) New York: Harper Collins; Bandura, A. (1982). Self-efficacy mechanism in human agency. *American Psychologist, 37,* 122; Glanz, K. Lewis, F. M. & Rimer, B. K. (Eds.). (1990). *Health behavior and health education: Theory, research, and practice.* San Francisco: Jossey-Bass. Adapted with permission.

than the threat of short-term hypoglycemic reactions. Additionally, their experiences with normal, or euglycemic, blood glucose levels led them to believe they were the antecedents of low blood glucose levels.

Goals and Recommended Interventions: Appropriate Teaching and Learning Theories

First, Claire and her family implement an insulin regimen better suited for euglycemia. This goal presumed an understanding of multiple dose, split-mix insulin therapy. The type of learning is cognitive-Gestalt, in which the process of gaining or changing insights is critical. A reorganization of the family's cognitive field and problem-solving abilities is required, one of the attributes of this type of teaching and learning theory. Additionally, insights, concepts, and principles are needed to enhance the Pattersons' scientific thinking because the previous type of learning related to insulin resulted from a stimulus-response or behavioristic-conditioning learning process. In other words, the stimulus of hypoglycemia and convulsions resulted in a response that reinforced high blood glucose levels to diminish the undesired stimulus.

The recommended interventions teach Claire and her mother about her insulin requirements and the need to split the doses into four different injections, so that early morning high blood glucose levels can be accommodated and finer blood glucose control can be maintained. Claire's understanding about the link between high blood glucose levels and diet are reinforced by performing her own glucose monitoring, logging the results at different times during the day, and associating these levels with her food intake. The nurse instructors use a student/teacher-centered, individualized learning situation for Claire, so that she can understand the necessary relationships among diet, insulin, and exercise and then make decisions about adjusting them to maintain euglycemia.

Second, Claire demonstrates the ability to manage her diabetes independently by telephoning the nurse instructors 2 weeks after attendance at the course to report blood glucose levels and insulin dosages. This goal presumes that Claire has learned the principles of insulin, diet, and exercise and their effects on blood glucose levels as outlined in the first goal. An appropriate type of teaching and learning theory for this type of learning situation is social learning.

The recommended interventions include enhancing Claire's perceived self-efficacy or self confidence that she can manage her diabetes without her mother's intercession. The four discrete sources of information leading to perceived self-efficacy include personal mastery, vicarious experiences, verbal persuasion, and physiologic feedback (Bandura, 1982; Strecher, DeVellis, Becker, & Rosenstock, 1986). Claire develops personal mastery through her ability to interpret her blood glucose levels, based on her intake of food during the past 48 hours. Vicarious experiences are an important aspect of teaching and learning theory as applied in the diabetes teaching program. Claire's observation of one of the staff nurses in the program is paramount to her learning. This nurse had diabetes and yet maintained perfect metabolic control during her pregnancy. The nurse who shared this experience contributed to Claire's self confidence. Additionally, the sharing of experiences by other patients who had managed to artfully wrest regulation from family members is an important vicarious learning experience for Claire. An additional recommendation made to Claire by the center staff is that she attend a support group sponsored by the American Diabetes Association in Los Angeles.

SUMMARY

Accepting the patient's prerogative to make a decision contrary to the suggestions offered by the physician and nurse is often difficult. A broader understanding of the patient's choice can be gained from the applications of the Health Belief Model, models of stress and coping, social learning theory, and developmental theories. Learning why these issues arise and how to deal with patient decisions helps the nurse remain committed to patient education. The ultimate role of the health professional is to encourage patients to make informed choices about health, rather than to guarantee compliance or obedience. Principles of empowerment theory are offered as a strategy to enable patients to advocate for their own health education needs.

Understanding the theory related to teaching and learning helps the health professional understand the relationship between knowledge and action. Simply knowing or understanding is insufficient to bring about change in a patient's life; action must follow understanding. The nurse who understands the principles of teaching and learning can better help the client achieve desired health behaviors.

STRATEGIES FOR CRITICAL ANALYSIS AND APPLICATION

1. Using the concept of individual or psychological empowerment, design a program to increase adolescents' ability to withstand peer pressure to smoke.
2. Using Bandura's principles of personal mastery, vicarious experiences, verbal persuasion, and physiologic feedback, design a program to encourage men who are at risk to participate in prostate cancer screening. Which of these principles is the most difficult to incorporate in such a screening program?
3. Which stress and coping model would be most useful in understanding the teaching needs of a second generation, unemployed, Chinese American with NIDDM? Why? In what type of situation would the other stress and coping model be most useful?
4. Using a lifespan developmental perspective, develop an individualized cardiac rehabilitation program for a 75-year-old woman 2 weeks after an acute MI. What are the cohort influences that may mitigate against her participation in cardiac rehabilitation at the YMCA?

REFERENCES

Baltes, P. B., Reese, H. W., & Lipsitt, L. P. (1980). Lifespan developmental psychology. *Annual Review of Psychology, 31,* 65–110.

Bandura, A. (1977). *Social learning theory.* Englewood Cliffs, NJ: Prentice Hall.

Bandura, A. (1982). Self-efficacy mechanism in human agency. *American Psychologist, 37*(2), 122–147.

Bandura, A. (1997). *Self-Efficacy: The exercise of control.* New York: W. H. Freeman.

Beeker, C., Guenther-Grey, C., & Raj, A. (1998). Community empowerment paradigm drift and the primary prevention of HIV/AIDS. *Social Science and Medicine, 46*(7), 831–842.

Berg, C. E., Alt, K. J., Himmel, J. K., & Judd, B. J. (1985). The effects of patient education on patient cognition and disease-related anxiety. *Patient Education and Counseling, 7*(4), 389–394

Bigge, M. L. (1976). *Learning theories for teachers* (3rd ed.). New York: Harper & Row.

Bigge, M. L., & Shermis, S. S. (1992). *Learning theories for teachers* (4th ed.). New York: Harper Collins.

Bigge, M. L., & Shermis, S. S. (1999). *Learning theories for teachers* (5th ed.). New York: Harper Collins.

Bronefenbrenner, U. (1979). *The ecology of human development.* Cambridge, MA: Harvard University Press.

Bronefenbrenner, U. (1986). Ecology of the family as a context for human development: Research perspectives. *Developmental Psychology, 22,* 723–742.

Bronefenbrenner, U. (1989). Ecological systems theory. *Annals of Child Development, 6,* 187–249.

Bronefenbrenner, U., & Crouter, A. C. (1983). The evolution of environmental models in developmental research. In W. Kessen (Ed.), *History, theory, and methods.* Handbook of child psychology. (4th ed., pp. 357–414). New York: John Wiley & Sons.

Brown, S. A. (1992). Meta-analysis of diabetes patient education research: Variations in intervention effects across studies. *Research in Nursing and Health, 15,* 409–419.

Cannon, W. B. (1939). *The wisdom of the body.* New York: Norton.

Castelli, W. P. (1988). Cardiovascular disease in women. *American Journal of Obstetrics and Gynecology, 158,* 1553–1560.

Chandler, S. (1992). Learning for what purpose? Questions when viewing classroom learning from a sociocultural curriculum perspective. In

H. H. Marshall (Ed.), *Redefining student learning: Roots of educational change* (pp. 33–58). Norwood, NJ: Ablex Publishing.

Corrao, J. M., Becker, R. C., Ockene, I. S., & Hamilton, G. A. (1990). Coronary heart disease risk factors in women. *Cardiology, 77* (Suppl.), 8–24.

Cousins, N. (1979). *Anatomy of an illness.* New York: WW Norton.

Devine, E. C. (1992). Effects of psychoeducational care for adult surgical patients: A meta-analysis of 191 studies. *Patient Education and Counseling, 19*(2), 129–142.

DiClemente, C. C., & Prochaska, J. O. (1998). Toward a comprehensive transtheoretical model of change: Stages of change and addictive behaviors. In W. R. Miller, & N. Heather. (Eds.). *Treating addictive behaviors* (2nd ed.), pp 3–24. New York: Plenum Press.

Dittrich, H., Gilpin, E., Nicod, P., Cali, G., Henning, H., & Ross, J. (1988). Acute myocardial infarction in women: Influence of gender on mortality and prognostic variables. *American Journal of Cardiology, 62*(1), 1–7.

Ewart, C. K., Taylor, C. B., Reese, L. B., & DeBusk, R. F. (1983). The effects of early post-infarction exercise testing on self-perception and subsequently physical activity. *American Journal of Cardiology, 51*(4), 1076–1080.

Featherman, D. L. (1981). The *life-span perspective in social science research.* Paper commissioned by the Social Science Research Council for the National Science Foundation. New York: Social Science Research Council.

Finney, R. L. (1928). *A sociological philosophy of education.* New York: Macmillan.

Funnell, M. M., Anderson, R. M., Arnold, M. S., Barr, P. A., Donnelly, M., Johnson, P. D., Moon, D., & White, N. H. (1991). Empowerment: An idea whose time has come in diabetes education. *Diabetes Educator, 17,* 37–41.

Gadow, S. (1983). Existential advocacy: Philosophical foundation of nursing. In C. P. Murphy & H. Hunter (Eds.), *Ethical problems in the nurse-patient relationship* (pp. 40–60). Newton, MA: Allyn & Bacon.

Gagne, R. M., & Driscoll, M. P. (1988). *Essentials of learning for instruction* (2nd ed.). Englewood Cliffs, NJ: Prentice Hall.

Gortner, S. R., Gilliss, C. L., Shinn, J. A., Sparacino, P. A., Rankin, S., Leavitt, M., Price, M., & Hudes, M. (1988). Improving recovery following cardiac surgery: a randomized clinical trial. *Journal of Advanced Nursing, 13*(5), 649–661.

Gortner, S. R., & Jenkins, L. S. (1990). Self-efficacy and activity level following cardiac surgery. *Journal of Advanced Nursing, 15*(10), 1132–1138.

Haynes, R. B., McKibbon, K. A., Kanani, R., Brouwers, M. C., & Oliver, T. (1999). Interventions to help patients to follow prescriptions for medications. *The Cochrane Library (Oxford),* issue 2, pp. 20.

Huckabay, L. (1980). *Conditions of learning and instruction in nursing.* St. Louis: C. V. Mosby.

Illich, I. (1979). *Medical nemesis: The expropriation of health.* New York: Pantheon.

Israel, B. A., Checkoway, B., Schulz, A., & Zimmerman, M. (1994). Health education and community empowerment: Conceptualizing and measuring perceptions of individual, organizational, and community control. *Health Education Quarterly, 21*(2), 149–170.

Kleinman, A. (1988). *The illness narratives: Suffering, healing and the human condition.* New York: Basic Books.

Kloeblen, A. S. (1999). Folate knowledge, intake from fortified grain products, and periconceptional supplementation patterns of a sample of low-income pregnant women according to the Health Belief Model. *Journal of the American Dietetic Association, 99*(1), 33–38.

Knowles, M. (1970). *The modern practice of adult education.* New York: Association Press.

Lazarus, R. S. (1991). *Emotion and adaptation.* New York: Oxford University Press.

Lazarus, R. S. (1999). *Stress and emotion: A new synthesis.* New York: Springer.

Lazarus, R. S., & Folkman, S. (1984). *Stress, appraisal, and coping.* New York: Springer.

Lewis, J., Rankin, S., & Kellogg, J. (1985). Health teaching; module 1. *Foundations of health teaching* (pp. 37–51). Long Beach, CA: Statewide Nursing Program, the Consortium of the California State University.

Lewis-Fernandez, R., & Kleinman, A. (1995). Cultural psychiatry. Theoretical, clinical and research issues. *Psychiatric Clinics of North America, 18,* 433–438.

Lindeman, C. A. (1988). Patient education. *Annual Review of Nursing Research, 6,* 29–60.

Man, D. (1999). Community-based empowerment programme for families with a brain injured survivor: An outcome study. *Brain Injury, 13*(6), 433–445.

Murdaugh, C. Coronary heart disease in women. *Journal of Cardiovasular Nursing, 4,* 35–50.

National Task Force on Training Family Physicians in Patient Education. (1979). *Patient education: A handbook for teachers.* Kansas City, MO: The Society of Teachers of Family Medicine.

Ovrebo, B., Ryan, M., Jackson, K., & Hutchinson, K. (1994). The homeless prenatal program: A model for empowering homeless pregnant women. *Health Education Quarterly, 21*(2), 187–198.

Pearlin, L. I., Lieberman, M. A., Menaghan, E. G., & Mullan, J. T. (1981). The stress process. *Journal of Health and Social Behavior, 22*(4), 337–356.

Pearlin, L. I., & Schooler, C. (1978). The structure of coping. *Journal of Health and Social Behavior, 19*(1), 2–21.

Pearlin, L. I., & Skaff, M. M. (1996). Stress and the life course: a paradigmatic alliance. *The Gerontologist, 36*(2), 239–247.

Plough, A., & Olafson, F. (1994). Implementing the Boston Healthy Start Initiative: A case study of community empowerment and public health. *Health Education Quarterly, 21*(2), 221–234.

Prochaska, J. O., Redding, C. A., Harlow, L. L., Rossi, J. S., & Velicer, W. F. (1994). The transtheoretical model of change and HIV prevention: A review. *Health Education Quarterly, 21*(2), 471–486.

Redman, B. K. (1993). Patient education at 25 years; Where we have been and where we are going. *Journal of Advanced Nursing, 18*(5), 725–730.

Schaie, K. W. (1986). Beyond calendar definitions of age, time, and cohort: The general developmental model revisited. *Developmental Review, 6*, 252–277.

Schmidt, C. K. (1990). Pre-operative preparation: Effects on immediate pre-operative behavior, postoperative behavior and recovery in children having same-day surgery. *Maternal-Child Nursing Journal, 19*, 321–330.

Schroeder, S. A., & McPhee, S. J. (1996). General approach to the patient. In L. M. Tierney, S. J. McPhee, M. A. Papadakis, & S. A. Schroeder (Eds.), *Current medical diagnosis and treatment* (pp. 1–20). Norwalk, CT: Prentice-Hall.

Selye, H. A. (1936). A syndrome produced by diverse nocuous agents. *Nature, 138*(1), 32.

Selye, H. A. (1952). *The story of the adaptation syndrome.* Montreal: Acta.

Selye, H. A. (1982). History and present status of the stress concept. In L. Goldberger & S. Breznitz (Eds.), *Handbook of stress: Theoretical and clinical aspects.* New York: Free Press.

Skaff, M. M., Pearlin, L. I., & Mullan, J. T. (1996). Transitions in the caregiving career: Effects on sense of mastery. *Psychology and Aging, 11*(2), 247–257.

Smith, C. E. (1989). Overview of patient education. *Nursing Clinics of North America, 24,* 583–587.

Spencer, M. B., Dupree, D., & Hartmann, T. (1997). A phenomenological variant of ecological systems theory (PVEST): A self-organization perspective in context. *Development and Psychopathology, 9*(4), 817–833.

Strecher, V. J., DeVellis, B. M., Becker, M. H., & Rosenstock, I. M. (1986). The role of self-efficacy in achieving health behavior change. *Health Education Quarterly, 13*(1), 73–92.

Taylor, C. B., Bandura, A., Ewart, C. K., Miller, N. H., & DeBusk, R. I. (1985). Exercise testing to enhance wives' confidence in their husbands' cardiac capability after clinically uncomplicated acute myocardial infarction. *American Journal of Cardiology, 55*(3), 635–638.

Thomas, R. J., Miller, N. H., Lamendola, C., Berra, K., Hedbäck, B., Durstine, J. L., & Haskell, W. (1996). National survey on gender differences in cardiac rehabilitation programs. Patient characteristics and enrollment patterns. *Journal of Cardiopulmonary Rehabilitation, 16*(6), 402–412.

Travers, K. D. (1997). Reducing inequities through participatory research and community empowerment. *Health Education and Behavior, 24*(3), 344–356.

Tripp-Reimer, T., & Afifi, L. A. (1989). Cross-cultural perspectives on patient teaching. *Nursing Clinics of North America, 24,* 613–619.

Vaccarino, V., Berkman, L. F., Mendes DeLeon, C. F. Seeman, T. F., Horwitz, R. I., & Krumholz, H. M. (1997). Functional disability before myocardial infarction in the elderly as a determinant of infarction severity and postinfarction mortality. *Archives of Internal Medicine, 157,* 2196–2004.

Visintainer, M. A., & Wolfer, J. A. (1975). Psychological preparation for surgical pediatric patients: The effects on children's and parent's stress responses and adjustment. *Pediatrics, 56,* 561–568.

Wallerstein, N., & Bernstein, E. (1994). Introduction to community empowerment, participatory education, and health. *Health Education Quarterly, 21*(3), 141–148.

Wallerstein, N., & Sanchez-Merki, V. (1995). Freirian praxis in health education: Research results from an adolescent prevention program. *Health Education Research, 9,* 105–118.

Whittemore, R. Q., Rankin, S. H., Callahan, C.D., Leder, M. C. & Carroll, D. L. (2000). I pointed out there is a tomorrow: The peer advisor experience providing special support; *Qualitative Health Research, 10*(1), 260–276.

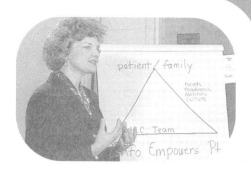

Staff Development in Patient Education: Meeting JCAHO Standards and Beyond

LEARNING OBJECTIVES

After reading this chapter, the nurse or student nurse should be able to:

1. Discuss three roles for staff development in planning organizational approaches to patient education.

2. Outline four JCAHO standards for patient and family education and corresponding teaching targets.

3. Describe continuing education interventions that prepare staff to fulfill JCAHO standards for patient and family education.

4. Identify four barriers perceived by staff nurses in the provision of patient education.

5. Provide examples of educational and institutional support to promote patient education expertise for nurses identified in Benner's four stages of skill acquisition.

6. Provide examples of age-specific approaches for pediatric and geriatric patient education.

INTRODUCTION

JCAHO Focus on Patient Education: Implications for Staff Development

In 1993, the Joint Commission on the Accreditation of Healthcare Organizations (JCAHO) made patient education outcomes a special focus in survey visits. To achieve JCAHO accreditation, health care organizations must show evidence that all patients receive teaching and that health care providers can demonstrate patient learning. In addition to individualized teaching, JCAHO requires an organization-wide patient and family education focus and evidence of the direct impact of education on the patient and family. JCAHO standards require an interdisciplinary approach that includes the patient and family as a part of the health care team. The JCAHO surveys merged hospitals and hospital systems as a single entity, requiring integration of patient education resources and programs. (JCAHO, 1998).

The JCAHO standards place renewed emphasis on the need for all nurses to provide patient education as part of quality care. Many education directors and staff development specialists have been challenged to develop their staff, through continuing education, to be skilled teachers and to demonstrate patient learning outcomes. Staff development specialists facilitate the work of multiple disciplines in combining the contributions that each makes in providing patient teaching; they have also been instrumental in helping merged organizations integrate education programs and design policies on what should be taught to health professionals to spread patient education across the continuum of care. The responsibility to educate patients and families has broad implications for all individuals who hold leadership and management positions in a health care organization (Box 5-1).

This chapter reviews JCAHO Standards and Scoring Guidelines for Patient and Family Education and examines ways that staff development can provide support and leadership in

---

BOX 5-1. Management Responsibility for Patient Education

- Incorporate patient education in the mission and strategic priorities of the organization
- Assure an environment that rewards patient education efforts and outcomes
- Provide an organizational infrastructure to oversee, deliver, and support patient education
- Incorporate patient and staff education into policies, procedures, and protocols
- Ensure that performance improvement efforts address patient education
- Provide critical resources (eg, staff, materials) for patient education

Note. From *Educating Hospital Patients and Their Families,* by (Joint Commission on the Accreditation of Healthcare Organizations), 1996, Oakbrook Terrace, IL. Adapted with permission.

---

achieving successful JCAHO accreditation surveys. Key elements of individual and organization-wide teaching are reviewed and the value of leadership in staff development to promote patient education within an organization is addressed. A workshop plan for nurses and other staff is provided; the workshop addresses patient-centered approaches to patient education, including learning objectives, agenda, content outline, and teaching methodologies. The workshop plan illustrates how Chapters 8 through 12 of the text can be incorporated in a continuing education program.

This chapter also examines how nurses develop clinical expertise in patient teaching, specifically by addressing the work of Benner and her colleagues (Benner 1984; Benner & Tanner, 1987; Benner, Tanner, & Chesla, 1992). This discussion will help the reader discover answers to pressing issues and questions posed by staff development and continuing education professionals. Finally, this chapter provides suggestions for motivating and develop-

---

BOX 5-2. Staff Development Issues

- Motivate staff nurses to teach
- Best use of clinical nurse specialists and patient education specialists
- Promote recognition and charting of patient learning outcomes
- Streamline outdated teaching protocols
- Promote health care team approach
- Determine staff education and training needs

---

ing staff competencies as patient teachers and tailoring patient education with age-specific approaches (Box 5-2).

Need for Innovation

As Director of Educational Services, one of my responsibilities is to bring the staff nurses to an understanding and an appreciation for what the patients' needs are today and how they have changed over the generations we have been in practice. Patient education is a 360-degree event. The process goes on and on. Today's nurse must interact with other members of other disciplines, not just in the hospital, but in the physician's office, the home care agency, wellness settings, rehabilitation, and long term care.

C.H. (Stallings, 1996)

A pressing need exists for innovation in how patients are taught to participate in their care. Rapidly changing models of health care delivery are characterized by short hospital stays and care provided across multiple settings. Most patient education programs developed during the past decade are outdated, be-

cause the current length of hospital stays do not accommodate ambitious learning activities. In fact, teaching programs often become outdated within one year of their creation. Continuing education and coaching, which helps staff revise teaching to focus on survival skills and patient outcomes, is often neglected. Staff becomes frustrated trying to teach too much material in too short a time; many do not know how to streamline teaching. To accommodate patients' need to learn how to manage their care in a limited time, hospitals must refine existing patient education programs and devise teaching interventions that reach homes and outpatient clinics. A strong component of patient education has become a necessity in all clinical services (Wasson & Anderson, 1994). Patient education has become an integral component of case management efforts (Cesta & Falter, 1999). Critical pathways and existing programs must be revised to coincide with carefully tracked outcomes. (Chapter 13 provides guidance in dealing with patient education issues as they relate to case management.)

Depending on one's educational preparation and clinical experience, health care professionals may prioritize aspects of patient education differently. For example, nurses who graduated in the 1970s were taught that patient education always begins with an anatomy and physiology lesson and that informed consent is a primary aim. In the 1980s, basic nursing education stressed discharge planning for high-risk patients but offered less emphasis on individualized teaching for low-risk patients. Nurses educated in the 1990s (and nurses who became case managers) have a heightened awareness of the need to streamline teaching in favor of survival skills. They also developed visible roles in health promotion and disease prevention, rather than restricting to acute illness episodes. These nurses may encounter resistance to redesigning teaching programs with less anatomy and more problem-solving skills from their colleagues who were taught to teach patients only for informed consent.

In every practice setting, various approaches to patient education exist. This variety often causes disagreements among health care professionals on what the priorities for patient teaching are and on how to provide teaching interventions. Many nurses attempt to follow patient education programs and standards based on drastically different lengths of hospital stay. Some nurses practiced at a time when all patient teaching for specific health problems (eg, diabetes, cardiac, prenatal) was delegated to a patient education specialist. These nurses may not accept that their role includes teaching and may have no formal teaching training. In addition, few health care professionals have been offered continuing education opportunities aimed at developing interdisciplinary approaches. Continuing education provides an avenue for uniting practitioners with different perspectives and centralizing efforts to provide innovative new approaches to patient education.

MEETING JCAHO STANDARDS AND BEYOND: PRINCIPLES AND STRATEGIES FOR STAFF DEVELOPMENT

The Challenges for Staff Development

Staff development is defined as employer-sponsored, professional development activities aimed at expanding and improving the competencies of health care professionals (Kelly, 1992). Staff development can help to bridge the gaps between education and practice (Box 5-3). It improves the competencies of health care professionals to provide patient teaching in a rapidly changing health care delivery system. Powerful staff development activities may include:

1. Providing leadership, oversight, or coordination of organization-wide approaches to patient education
2. Providing formal, ongoing, and immediate training about JCAHO Standards and Scoring Guidelines for Patient and Family Education
3. Teaching managers, supervisors, staff

> ## BOX 5-3. Staff Development Roles
>
> - Formal, ongoing training related to work responsibilities (eg, JCAHO standards)
> - Socialization into work setting to increase competence and excellence (eg, coaching, feedback, mentoring staff)
> - Improving group performance to achieve quality and excellence (eg, making sure patient education programs are visible and valued)

nurses, and other providers how to meet JCAHO standards and show evidence of patient learning
4. Helping the organization develop specialized patient education programs and interventions that are realistic for the patient's length of stay, interdisciplinary in their approach, and focused on patient survival skills
5. Identifying barriers that nurses and other providers perceive in the delivery of patient education and designing strategies in partnership with management to break down the barriers
6. Raising awareness of the need for new, innovative approaches to patient education based on patient needs, as opposed to the provider's determination for achieving compliance. These new models for patient teaching span both inpatient and outpatient settings and involve patients in prioritizing learning needs along a continuum of care. They focus on health promotion, risk factor reduction, and disease management.

Organizations cannot afford for staff development to stand on the sidelines of patient education efforts. In the context of JCAHO standards, this chapter outlines the developmental needs of an organization and its staff relative to patient education, and offers suggestions for staff development interventions.

JCAHO Standards
for Patient Education

The Joint Commission on the Accreditation of Healthcare Organizations supports the notion of patient-centered care with patient education as the centerpiece for involving patients as important members of the health care team. Nurses can bring this concept to life by providing patients with information in the right place at the right time.

The stimulus for innovation in patient education resulted from the 1993 JCAHO standards and focus surveys that addressed patient teaching and discharge planning. These standards prompted administrators to review organization-wide approaches and individual patient experiences and to ask, *What is wrong with our patient education programs?* Organizations were forced to acknowledge the priority of educating patients, examine the ways education is delivered, and consider how resources are allocated to patient and family education. In every department, administrators asked, *How do we currently teach patients?* and *Where do we document it?*. The organization's patient education services often lacked structure, function, goals, objectives, and most important, the tracking of outcomes. As members of the management team, staff development professionals must interpret an overall approach and ensure that quality patient education services are provided.

Table 5-1 outlines the JCAHO 1998 standards of goals, objectives, and applications of a patient education program in an organization. This table is useful for teaching managers and staff about JCAHO's expectations for patient and family outcomes. Evaluation of patient education must provide evidence that the organization assesses the need for

TABLE 5-1. Organizational Approach to Patient Education

Goal of patient and family education:	Organizational approach: impact areas
1. To improve patient health outcomes by promoting recovery, speeding return to function, promoting healthy behavior, and appropriately involving the patient in his or her care decisions.	1. Organization's focus on education 2. Direct impact of education on the patient and family 3. Evaluation of the program of patient and family education relative to goal achievement

Education should:	Practical applications
• Facilitate patient's (family's) understanding of patient's health status, health care options, and consequences of options selected • Encourage patient (family) participation in the decision-making process about health care options • Increase patient's (family's) potential to follow the therapeutic health care plan • Maximize patient (family) care skills • Increase patient's (family's) ability to cope with the patient's health status/prognosis/outcome • Enhance patient's (family's) role in continuing care • Promote a healthy patient lifestyle	1. Assess organization-wide patient and family education programs and activities. 2. Organization establishes goals of patient and family education program. 3. Organization allocates resources for patient and family education. 4. Determine specific educational needs of patient and family. 5. Prioritize and sequence educational needs. 6. Present information to patient/family and determine appropriate follow-up. 7. Evaluate if needs met. 8. Compare patient and family activities to organizational goals for quality improvement.

Note. From 1998 *Comprehensive Accreditation Manual for Hospitals,* by Joint Commission on the Accreditation of Healthcare Organizations, Chicago: Author. Adapted with permission.

focused programs and allocates resources to accomplish them. An organization's most important resource is staff nurses who have the skills, interest, and time to teach patients. The JCAHO education standards address that a systematic approach to patient education should be demonstrated throughout the organization, but JCAHO does not describe specific structures or personnel titles. An organization is encouraged to focus on its current processes and on how continuity of care is best accomplished (Box 5-4).

JCAHO standards address patient-focused care, including organizational approaches and individualized patient and family activities. Comparing patient and family activities to the organization's goals is a key component of quality performance (JCAHO, 1998). Table 5-2 lists the four standards that relate to specific educational needs of patients and families, which are defined with targets—or outcomes—for patient-centered interventions.

Implementing an Organization-Wide Approach

The *implementation process* is key to successful patient education outcomes. We provide an example of an orderly process for implementing patient education and discuss the issues confronted during implementation.

The organization must assign responsibility for overseeing or directing the implementation of patient education (eg, to a patient education coordinator or to a director of a department). This individual is referred to as the coordinator, although responsibility for patient education activities is shared throughout an organization and across disciplines. We are familiar with many staff development directors who have been assigned responsibilities as co-ordinators of the organization-wide approach.

Although we have instituted individual patient education programs to meet the needs of particular client groups, we do not recommend this single-shot approach to implementing patient education at the organization level. A single-shot approach tends to be hurried and crisis motivated; staff efforts are typically directed toward the most obvious needy group. Instead, we suggest a JCAHO-validated approach (ie, conducting a systematic patient education needs assessment).

Conducting a Needs Assessment for the Organization

A needs assessment is the cornerstone for planning and implementing patient education. A needs assessment allows long-range planning and direction, so that continuity of program planning is ensured, regardless of leadership or personnel changes.

The American Hospital Association's *Institutional Assessment Guide* (AHA, 1979) continues to provide valuable guidance for hospitals that implement a comprehensive patient education program. The guide also can be modified for use in assessing educational needs in many settings across the continuum of care. Divided into 10 areas, the guide recommends the types of questions that should be asked about each area and lists suggested sources of data (Box 5-5).

Appointing a Steering Committee

The role of the interdisciplinary Patient Education Committee is two-fold. In the short term, we are looking at whether we're actually meeting Joint Commission standards, and if we are not, how can we put new programs and services in place or retire those [that] are no longer as effective as they need to be. Secondly, we act as a resource for reviewing teaching programs and tools and act as a central repository.

C.H. (STALLINGS, 1996)

BOX 5-4. Continuity of Care

- Interdisciplinary coordination
- Interunit and interservice coordination
- Interagency coordination
- Focus on discharge and patient safety

TABLE 5-2. 1998 JCAHO Standards for Patient and Family Education

STANDARD	TARGETS	EVIDENCE
Standard PF.1 Patient/family receive education specific to patient's assessed needs, abilities, and readiness to learn.	• Survival skills for safe discharge • Safe and effective use of medications • Medical equipment • Potential drug-food interactions, modified diets • Community resources • How to obtain further treatment • Ongoing health care needs, hygiene and grooming	Policies/procedures, progress notes, flowsheets, referral/consultation notes, interviews with staff and patients, written information given to patients and families • Patient assessment considers physical and cognitive limitations, language barriers, cultural and religious practices, emotional barriers, motivation to learn, and financial implications of care choices. • Information understandable to patient • Teaching is culturally appropriate • Academic needs met, if appropriate
Standard PF.2 Patient education is interactive.	• Patient/family understanding of current health problem/reason for admission • Patient informed consent • Patient/family understanding of treatment plan and the role they will play in it • Priorities for individual learning needs, sequencing with patient readiness	• Patient learning needs identified • Educational plan implemented with patient feedback • Priorities for education identified for each patient
Standard PF.3 Any discharge instructions given to the patient/family are provided to the organization responsible for patient's continuing care.	• Written discharge instructions, understandable to patient, include lifestyle changes • Continuing care needs/provider identified • Instructions provided to continuing care providers	• Discharge planning involves patient/family • Discharge instructions clear: who is to do what
Standard PF.4 The organization plans and supports the provision and coordination of patient/family education activities and resources.	• Learning environment • Staff competency to teach • Processes and procedures to identify and respond to learning needs • Collaborative/interdisciplinary educational resources and services • Performance improvement process	• Patient education activities and resources provided • Resources provided based on patient needs • Health care team involvement • Education is continuous, safe, timely, efficient, caring, and respectful

Note. From Joint Commission on the Accreditation of Healthcare Organizations, *Comprehensive Accreditation Manual for Hospitals,* 1988. Chicago: Author.

A patient education steering committee should be appointed early in the implementation process. The steering committee acts in an advisory fashion and should include physicians, nurses, members of other health care disciplines, administrators, and others who have an active interest in patient education. A patient education coordinator, hospital education director, or clinical specialist is usually responsible for initiating the committee and should judiciously gather recommendations for committee members. Appointment of physicians should be made by the medical staff, although the coordinator can attempt to have physicians appointed who are known proponents of patient education. Nurses at the decision-making level should be appointed to the steering committee with the input of the

BOX 5-5. Areas of Institutional Review

1. **Hospital philosophy, goals, and policies**
   What is the philosophy of the hospital and what are the goals for patient care? Do these goals require the implementation of patient education? The sources of information include documents that can be obtained from administrators or the board of trustees.

2. **Organization of the hospital staff**
   What types of staff members are employed?

3. **Patient care support staff**
   Who is responsible for orientation of all new hospital patient care staff? Data pertaining to this question can be obtained by contacting department heads or by sending them a questionnaire.

4. **Characteristics of the patient population**
   What are the most common diagnoses, diagnosis-related groups (DRGs), and surgical procedures for the various hospital units? Answers to this question can be procured from the admitting office and its computerized data banks and from medical records. Interviews of various nursing and medical personnel also may be helpful. What are the high risk or high volume diagnoses, patient groups, or product lines that are commonly identified by staff in various departments? For example, because of discharge of newly delivered prenatal patients less than 48 hours after admission, this population may be targeted as high risk.

5. **Patient admission**
   What information is made available to patients *before* admission to inpatient services, short-stay surgery, or outpatient services? Answers to this question should be obtained from various sources. Interviews can be conducted or questionnaires can be sent to admitting and short-stay surgery and outpatient services. Additionally, the public relations department, admitting staff physicians, and community referral agencies should be contacted.

6. **Patient care process**
   How are patient care goals determined and revised? Do the medical, nursing, dietary, and other staff groups use a team planning method to assist in determining goals? Are patients included in the goal planning process? Answers to these questions can be acquired by interviewing head nurses and other unit managers involved in patient care services. Consider mailing questionnaires to patients who have been recently discharged.

7. **Staff perceptions of current and needed patient education programs**
   What patient education programs or activities are currently implemented? Are they conducted on each shift? What resources, in terms of audiovisual, printed, and other media, are being used in these efforts? Interview or send questionnaires to head nurses, appropriate department heads, and supervisors who may be involved with patient teaching.

8. **Adequacy of existing patient education programs for specific populations**
   Are there written goals and objectives for each patient education activity and are they evaluated after the patient completes the activity? Answers to these questions should be obtained for all programs or for activities presently being conducted in the institution. Sources of information include extensive interviews with the staff responsible for the programs, review of written program materials, and participation in a program.

9. **Patient education resources within the hospital**
What types of media are available within the hospital for patient teaching? What types of appropriations have been made for the purchase of audiovisual media, closed circuit television, and software? Where are patient education materials located, catalogued, and reviewed? Does staff use the materials? Are materials up-to-date? The questions can be answered by contacting department managers and hospital administrators and by talking with staff on the units. Chapter 10 in this text offers information about the many types of educational media that can be used to enhance patient learning and how they can be developed and evaluated.

10. **Patient education resources in the community**
Which community patient care agencies provide follow-up care on discharge from the hospital? How do they interpret their role in patient education? Is there a feedback mechanism between the community agency and the hospital? Answers to these questions can be obtained by contacting the community agencies that have been identified by staff as being involved in follow-up care. The discharge planning nurse or social worker should also be contacted. The needs assessment does not have to be conducted in a vacuum; other patient education activities take place while the needs assessment data is gathered.

nursing service coordinator. The historical involvement of other health professionals (eg, dietitians, pharmacists, and physical therapists) makes their membership valued in many institutions. Include other health professionals along the continuum of care, because their cooperation can enhance patient education programs.

After the assessment is complete, the patient coordinator will have a data base to aid the advisory committee in organizing and directing the organization's efforts. While the needs assessment is conducted and the advisory committee is appointed, the committee coordinator should review the literature to learn about *what* types of programs have worked, *why* they have been successful, and *where* they have been implemented. A great deal of information can be gathered from the successes and mistakes of others, and it is limiting to ignore the ever-increasing quantity of material about diverse patient education programs. This also is a propitious time to contact people involved with patient education efforts in other community and inpatient settings. These individuals can share ideas about the needs of the community and help prevent duplication of efforts.

Establishing Goals and Priorities

The perspective of "front-line" staff is critical to the development of realistic, effective, and creative patient education programs. Staff nurses should be asked [for] their assessment of patient education needs and challenges and their suggestions for areas needing improvement.

K.S.

Once the patient education needs assessment is complete, the goals and priorities for program development must be set. The advisory committee should wisely target the patient education programs for implementation (Box 5-6). When attempting to forge new alliances in patient education programs that

BOX 5-6. Staff Questionnaire Regarding Patient Education

This questionnaire asks for your assessment of patient education needs and challenges. It is part of an organization-wide effort to strengthen patient education programs and resources. The perspective of front-line staff is critical to the development of realistic, effective, and creative strategies for patient education.

Please answer all of the questions from your own experiences in your department, service, or unit. If a question does not apply to you, please write N/A. Feel free to add any thoughts, feelings, or opinions to your answers. Whenever possible, please offer suggestions for areas that need improvement.

1. Are you satisfied with the quality of education that your patients receive?
2. Do you think that patient education resources are adequate to prepare patients for discharge from your service?
3. For what **percentage of patients** on your service are interdisciplinary teaching plans (or critical paths) used for patient education?
4. Are current teaching plans realistic based on the average length of patient stay or the number of home visits?
5. Please list the three most frequent patient diagnoses on your service.
6. Please identify three learning outcomes, or survival skills, which are essential for patients with the diagnoses listed in question 5.

7. What is one thing you have done during the past year to improve the patient education that is provided on your service? Feel free to list more than one, if you wish.
8. How would you rate interdisciplinary communication regarding patient education on your service?
   Excellent   Good   Fair   Poor
9. How would you rate the documentation of patient learning outcomes on your service?
   Excellent   Good   Fair   Poor
10. What opportunities are needed for staff to gain additional skills in patient education? Please list specific topics, issues, or needs.
11. Do you think that providing good patient education is valued and recognized by your supervisor?   Yes   No
12. What problem or challenge most frequently prevents patients and families from receiving needed education? Feel free to mention more than one.

_____
_____
_____
_____

Thank you for taking the time to complete this questionnaire. If you have any other ideas or concerns that are not addressed in the questions, you are encouraged to offer additional comments below and on the back of the page.

involve multiple disciplines and care settings, it may be helpful to focus the coordinator's attention and the organization's resources on one or two major start-up programs at a time.

Creating Task Forces for Specific Programs

Nurses have learned the value of involving patients in the design of new patient education programs, often [using] focus groups to gain consumer input and keep the programs patient and family centered. When we ask patients for their input, we must be ready to respond.

K.S. (STALLINGS, 1996)

After priorities and goals are determined, a task force should be appointed to establish a specific patient education program. For example, if the highest priority is to establish or institute a new education program for patients with chronic obstructive pulmonary disease (COPD), then the task force committee should include health professionals in all departments that care for COPD patients. It is essential that a physician is a member of this committee, because approval must be gained from the medical staff to implement the teaching program. One should recognize, however, that including physicians on these task forces does not always guarantee wide medical staff approval. It also is essential that providers who care for patients in the community (eg, physician's office, home health) are included in planning the program, so that it will promote continuity of care.

Evaluating the Program

Evaluation of patient education programs presents some of the most difficult problems encountered in the entire patient teaching venture. (Chapter 12 provides a lengthy discussion of the many aspects and issues associated with the evaluation of patient learning.) We believe that evaluation design is an integral part of program planning. Including a design for evaluation in any proposal for funding will make health care administrators more likely to approve the program. Evaluation frequently occurs after a patient education program has been well established. This type of evaluation procedure should augment a formative evaluation procedure that aids refinement of the educational interventions during a pilot phase.

 Many different outcomes exist, and it is impossible, if not inappropriate, to evaluate all of them. Many nurses and physicians view the outcome of patient education in terms of desired patient compliance. Although compliance is desirable, many other positive outcomes of patient education exist. Therefore, a major issue in evaluation is deciding which outcome should be evaluated and whether this outcome indicates that the program is beneficial. ∎

 The desired outcome must be related to the type of intervention. For example, the desired outcome of educating a group of 13-year-olds on the relationship of cigarette smoking to cardiovascular disease and lung cancer is prevention of smoking. The desired effect of such education with a group of the teenagers' smoking parents, however, is cessation of smoking.

As more research is conducted on the relationship of knowledge acquisition to behavioral change, it becomes clear that acquisition of knowledge does not always guarantee the desired behavioral change. When we apply this concept to our group of cigarette-smoking patients, we may decide that a more realistic immediate outcome is simply knowledge about the effects of smoking. Perhaps later a behavioral change (cessation of smoking) will occur; this may or may not be related to the knowledge acquisition. The effects of peer pressure, family environment, and access to tobacco products for minors are powerful influences (Altman & Jackson, 1998).

Regardless, an argument can be made for improving and increasing the patient's knowledge and understanding of his or her health status, even if it does not lead to improved adherence to and cooperation with the medical regimen. Increasing the patient's understanding of his or her health can be interpreted as part of the patient's legal right to know. A patient deserves the information even if he or she does not choose to act on it. ∎

The following outcomes are defined as important by JCAHO (see Table 2-1) (Iacono & Campbell, 1997; JCAHO, 1996, 1998):

- Patient participation in decision-making about health care options
- The increased potential to follow the health care plan
- The development of self-care skills
- Increased patient and family coping
- Enhanced participation in continuing care
- Healthy lifestyle

Evaluating the costs of patient education is imperative. Hospital administrators must calculate staff time, materials, and education equipment as part of the cost of care. In many cases, well-planned and executed patient education can be shown to decrease length of stay and costs of hospitalization. Documentation of this can be used to justify the professional staff time needed to accomplish teaching before discharge. This information also can be used to determine the efficacy of specialized outpatient teaching programs versus inpatient teaching. It is helpful to consider *which* outcomes to measure for *whom,* and *what* should be done with the findings.

Staffing for Patient Education

*T*he registered nurse cannot delegate patient education to unlicensed personnel or nursing staff [members] who are not prepared to conduct a thorough assessment of learning needs. This is critical thinking that nurses are educated to provide as a piece of patient education.

C.H. (STALLINGS, 1996)

The types of staffing needed for patient education is a thorny issue and must be confronted. It requires more registered nurse (RN) hours to accomplish high-quality patient education. Most licensed practical nurses (LPNs) have not been taught the fundamentals of patient teaching during their formal educational programs and are not prepared to assume this role without additional training and supervision. An organization heavily staffed with LPNs and aides cannot deliver as much high-quality patient education as a larger or more professionally staffed institution can.

We have found that LPNs involved in prenatal education in an outpatient setting were willing and enthusiastic about attending classes but were unprepared and unable to lead patient discussions or to teach or lecture components of the class. LPNs can frequently reinforce patient education performed initially by RNs, but they should not be delegated the primary teaching responsibility. The debate about the appropriateness of delegating patient teaching to multiskilled workers or other unlicensed (less expensive) staff is often encountered by staff development professionals.

Patient teaching is not a procedure, but a process that involves assessment, critical thinking, negotiation, and knowledge about the topic being taught. Professional staff nursing time is required to accomplish patient education. The amount of staff time needed for patient education varies with the number of disease processes covered, and the sophistication and experience of the nurses and other personnel (eg, dietitians). Patient teaching protocols (or care maps) and the amount of preparation the staff has in teaching/learning theory also influence the amount of staff time required to accomplish teaching. Documenting the number of hours required for patient education can be combined with documenting patient response to education; this information eventually helps in evaluating the overall effectiveness of the patient education program. Can nurses allocate time for patient teaching during short hospital stays? How well are nurses prepared to implement standardized teaching plans and individualize them based on patient needs and length of stay?

It is important to assess whether the staff who provide patient teaching has received formal preparation in the use of standardized teaching plans, what teaching resources are provided in the organization, and where staff gets assistance with teaching for difficult patient situations. In short, one hospital discovered in its organizational assessment that the success of its programs hinged on staff development. Most nurses indicated that they had received no formal training to develop teaching plans (Goldrick, Jablonski, & Wolf, 1994).

Political and Financial Issues

Political and financial issues are often encountered in the planning of organizational approaches to patient education. For example, if those who control a budget are opposed to a patient education effort, implementing a program may be more difficult. Our experience is that if healthcare administrators and key physicians believe in the efficacy of patient education, then implementation is fairly straightforward; however, if these individuals think that patient education is not cost-beneficial, patient education programs may be extremely difficult to initiate, especially in light of budget shortfalls and competing demands for scarce resources.

Promoting patient education as a strategy to reduce the high cost of health care through prevention, as a purveyor of better patient services, and as a way of securing more consumer participation is helpful. In some communities with many medical facilities, patient education has been used as an advertising come-on. Programs that have sought the interest of the middle-class, well educated client (eg, programs on cholesterol reduction, stress abatement, parenting, and women's health issues) have been especially popular. Efforts to address health education issues related to social problems (eg, homelessness, teen pregnancy, AIDS, substance abuse) have been largely ignored by both proprietary and nonprofit hospitals, because they address uninsured and underinsured populations.

With rising health care costs, decisions about the expenditure of increasingly tight funds must be made. The public, urged on in many cases by health professionals, is demanding greater technocracy and more lifesaving assistance devices, which cause the costs of health care to skyrocket. To nurses, physicians, and other health care professionals who have been committed to patient education and who have been actively promoting it in their organizations, the JCAHO standards and focus surveys for patient and family education provide important support and ammunition for the effort. The mandates and priorities of JCAHO have required new attention to assessing the learning needs of patients and families and evidence of effective responses to these needs.

JCAHO Standards and Scoring Guidelines

*W*hen Joint Commission [JCAHO] surveyors address the patient education function, they look for adherence to the standards. They look for evidence that the nurse identified priorities for teaching and planned individualized care for patients. They look for evidence of the patient and family's response to care. Does the medical record indicate how the patient responded to teaching, what he [or she] understood? It is important to the Joint Commission that this be reflected in the patient record. We must show that we provided teaching to all patients related to survival skills for safe discharge and strategies to enhance continuity of care.

K.S. (STALLINGS, 1996)

Just as staff nurses must find a way to teach complex information to patients in practical, usable ways, so must staff development present JCAHO standards to staff nurses and members of other disciplines. A theme seen throughout the JCAHO scoring guidelines applies to all four standards; patient education outcomes should be evident in 90% to 100% of patients' records. To score well in a survey, the organization strives to demonstrate that patient education is an integral part of care for every patient, not just patients who receive a specialized teaching protocol.

Hospitalization is a learning experience for every patient and family. Patient outcomes include evidence of the patient's response to teaching. (Chapters 8 through 12 offer examples of the range of needs, interventions, and outcomes that can be documented.) JCAHO surveyors look for evidence that information is understandable and usable to the patient, including considerations of non-English

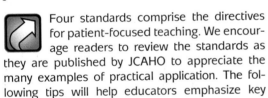

BOX 5-7. JCAHO Focus

- Adherence to standards
- Evidence of priorities, individualized care
- Evidence of patient/family response
- Information understandable, usable to patient
- 91%–100% patients taught
- Continuity of care

speaking patients, patients with low literacy skills, and patients with sight, hearing, and processing difficulties. Educational needs and opportunities should be viewed along the continuum of care and opportunities to incorporate health promotion for patients and families should be identified (JCAHO, 1998).

Evidence of individual patient and family learning include organizational policies and procedures, patient progress notes, flow sheets, referral and consultation notes, interviews with staff, written information provided to the patient and family, and interviews with staff and patients (Box 5-7).

Four standards comprise the directives for patient-focused teaching. We encourage readers to review the standards as they are published by JCAHO to appreciate the many examples of practical application. The following tips will help educators emphasize key points with staff. ∎

JCAHO Standard PF.1

The patient and family receive individualized education specific to their assessed needs, abilities, readiness, and length of stay. The patient and family are educated to increase their knowledge of their diagnosis, treatment options, and skills needed to participate in their recovery and rehabilitation. The assessment considers cultural and religious practices, emotional barriers, physical and cognitive limitations, language barriers, growth and development of the patient, financial implications of are, and patient and family motivation.

Teaching Targets

The patient and family should understand the current health problem or the reason for admission. This sounds obvious, but many patients do not know why they are hospitalized or cannot express it in their own words. Understanding the purpose of the hospitalization, and acknowledging the episode or symptoms that precipitated it, are important lessons in managing chronic illness.

To address health promotion goals, the nurse should consider the following question: *What brought this patient to this place at this time, and could the acute episode have been prevented?* An answer to this question also contributes to the formulation of a teaching plan. The patient and family should be taught about the proposed treatment plan and the role they would play in it. Before a final drug, diet, or exercise regimen is prescribed, teaching should include the expectation the patient will participate actively in his or her recovery in these three areas. Patients should receive an overview of the survival skills needed for discharge and explore their individual learning needs. Teaching priorities are based on survival and safety issues, and patient assessment is key. (Chapters 8 and 9 discuss the process of assessing critical learning needs.) The targets indicate priority areas that must be addressed if they apply to the patient (eg, medications, medical equipment, food/drug interactions, diets, rehabilitation skills, community resources, and ongoing health care needs). Patients must be informed about how to obtain further treatment, including possible emergency treatment and follow-up appointments. ∎

Evidence

All patients receive instruction. In addition, teaching priorities are noted based on the reason for admission, length of stay, and individual safety needs. Many nurses have described the interaction initiated by a JCAHO surveyor with patients. Patients are asked why they are in the hospital, what staff is doing to help them prepare for discharge, and what things the patients expect they will need to do to participate in their own care.

JCAHO Standard PF.2

Patient education is interactive.

Teaching Targets
The process of patient education is interdisciplinary, organized, and should not overwhelm the patient. Health care team involvement strengthens, streamlines, and individualizes care to address the patient's functional problems. Patient teaching focuses on each patient's functional problems; it is not dictated by medical diagnosis. Nurses and other team members focus their teaching on answering the question, *How does this diagnosis affect this patient?* The patient and family are also asked to contribute to this assessment, are actively involved in setting goals for their learning, and indicate preferences for the teaching methods to be used.

Evidence
Patient assessment should include the patient's current understanding of the health problem, statements in the patient's own words that reflect an understanding of the health problem and willingness to participate (ie, readiness), and prior knowledge, beliefs, or values that influence care. Documentation includes quotes from the patient and family about their needs and progress.

JCAHO Standard PF.3

Discharge instructions are given to the patient and the organization responsible for continuing care.

Teaching Targets
Patients receive written instructions that they can understand. (See Chapter 10 for information on preparing one-page discharge instructions that promote patient understanding.) Discharge planning clearly involves the patient and family, and instructions promote safe and continuing care.

Evidence
Documentation reflects discharge and patient preparation. A copy of discharge instructions is in the patient record and has been forwarded to appropriate parties. Instructions are readable, usable, and understandable. A JCAHO surveyor might ask a patient what kinds of written information have been provided and to explain what other instructions he or she has been given about care.

JCAHO Standard PF.4

The organization plans and supports coordinated learning activities and resources based on the patient and family needs.

Teaching Targets
The organizational assessment described earlier in this chapter has resulted in the provision, coordination, and evaluation of quality learning interventions that are based on specific needs. They may include classes, community resources, videos, reading materials, presentations, and various other formats. The staff is provided with education to become skilled patient educators.

Evidence
The patient's attendance at classes and participation in individual teaching sessions and the use of closed circuit television provide documentation. (Chapter 12 provides examples of documentation.) Select learning activities based on individual priority needs and length of stay. Nursing staff and other team members should acknowledge that they might not meet all the learning needs of the patient; instead, the focus is to teach less and reinforce more. The organization-wide needs assessment, resulting programs including standardized approaches, and educational resources used to promote learning, are also documented. Well-prepared staff is the most critical resource for providing patient education.

Preparing for Patient-Centered Care: Profile of a Teaching Program for Nurses and Other Staff

With JCAHO standards to address and with staff representing a diversity of interests and

TABLE 5-3. Workshop: Patient-Centered Approaches to Patient Education

OBJECTIVES	CONTENT	TIME	METHODOLOGY
I. List three goals of patient education.	I. JCAHO Standards and Scoring Guidelines	8:40–9:40 AM	Lecture, discussion, handout
II. Identify four levels of patient learning outcomes.	II. Four levels of evaluation	9:40–10:00 AM	Lecture
III. Describe how the Health Belief Model can be used to understand and influence patient behavior.	III. A. Cooperation vs. compliance B. Barriers to cooperation C. Patient motivation D. Application of model E. Patient decisions	10:15–11:00 AM	Lecture, group exercise, dyads, discussion, handouts
IV. List five concerns of hospitalized patients.	IV. A. Pain B. Cure C. Scarring/deformity D. Burden on others E. Dying	11:00–11:30 AM	Discussion, handouts
V. List four questions a nurse can ask to determine priorities for patient teaching.	V. A. Safe discharge B. Complications/readmission C. Past experience D. Equipment used at home	12:45–2:00 PM	Lecture, case studies, discussion
VI. Discuss guidelines to improve the effectiveness and safety of videotapes and written discharge instructions.	VI. A. Content B. Format C. Organization D. Emergency plan E. Follow-up	2:15–3:30 PM	Lecture, discussion video preview/evaluation
Wrap-up/ Evaluation	Review Objectives I–VI	3:30–4:00 PM	Q & A, discussion

teaching experiences, a formal teaching program can be effective in centralizing organizational values and approaches for patient education. The authors have found that full-day workshops best meet this need, with content and learning activities carefully planned to promote teamwork and critical thinking. Table 5-3 outlines a workshop developed by one of the authors (Stallings, 1996) for interdisciplinary audiences.

Goals of a Workshop

Workshop participants should include staff nurses, educators, nurse managers, and interested members of other disciplines. Participants are instructed that regardless of setting, three universal goals of patient education always exist:

- Developing survival skills
- Recognizing problems
- Making decisions

Addressing these three critical items in a workshop promotes learning retention in the staff. The workshop begins with a simple set of concepts, which are reinforced throughout the day. Participants may come to a workshop feeling overwhelmed at the prospect of teaching sick patients in limited time. The workshop is intended to empower staff members, giving them permission to teach smarter instead of faster and harder. The three universal goals are applied to the four JCAHO standards, demonstrating how the goals are a template for accreditation. Using small group discussions and case study analysis, participants examine how the JCAHO might survey for outcomes and try to develop examples of learning outcomes that could be accomplished in various settings, from intensive to long-term care. Participants review hot buttons (key compliance challenges) common to the JCAHO survey and how they are addressed in their practice area (Box 5-8).

Principles to Application

In workshops, methods to streamline documentation and provide a snapshot of the patient's involvement in learning are discussed. The way patient education is currently provided by the participants is explored, often exposing issues over discipline turf battles and lack of coordination, which adversely affect patient-centered approaches. The focus of the workshop shifts to the process of patient education from a patient's perspective. The issue of compliance is highlighted as workshop participants are asked to answer a survey about their own health behaviors (eg, smoking, seat belt use, diet, exercise, and medication use). Participants, in analyzing why they often do not practice what they preach to patients, identify the challenges of motivating patients to change their behaviors. The wisdom of expecting three or four simultaneous lifelong behavior changes is questioned. The steps of the Health Belief Model are reviewed, with strategies for addressing barriers and influencing patient decisions to-

ward healthy lifestyles. Patient concerns are also discussed. Recommendations are offered to sequence patient education, based on the priority concerns of patients. Priority for education about pain and pain management is discussed.

Critical needs for patient teaching are identified, based on the content of Chapters 8 through 12. Principles for streamlining teaching are introduced and applied to case studies. This part of a workshop often evokes lively discussion and differing opinions, based on the practice and education backgrounds of the participants. With the use of case studies, practice and feedback are provided to identify no more than three or four critical learning objectives for each patient, finding ways to teach and observe performance as an integral part of care, and document based on what the patient accomplished or demonstrated.

Because of the importance placed on media for patient learning, the workshop concludes with a lecture and critique of patient education handouts and videos. These teaching tools must reflect the same targeted, streamlined approach based on length of stay, and the effectiveness of these tools must be evaluated. The information presented to participants is derived from Chapter 10 of this book. Examples of short, effective instructions are provided. The importance and challenges of creating a single, one-page, interdisciplinary set of

---

BOX 5-8. Hot Buttons: Key Compliance Challenges in JCAHO Surveys

- Teaching about potential food and/or drug interactions
- Culturally relevant strategies and resources
- Age-appropriate teaching (especially for older patients, children, adolescents)
- Assessment of readiness to learn; emotional, physical, cognitive, and language barriers to learning
- Teaching about personal hygiene for

patients who can no longer follow normal routine
- Teaching about medications patient will manage at home
- Diet teaching for patients who are on a new or modified diet
- Proof of teaching through documentation
- Policy on how teaching is to be accomplished across the continuum of care

discharge instructions is emphasized. As video and computer-assisted instruction become more sophisticated and affordable, they will allow practical application for patient education in both homes and hospitals. Continuing education offerings must prepare staff to use these technologies wisely and to evaluate their effectiveness (Redman, 1993; Wasson & Anderson, 1994). Throughout the workshop, participants are asked to describe barriers in their work setting that may prevent them from effectively providing patient education. As staff development practitioners know, learners often identify administrative and educational issues. Educators must carry the messages between staff and management to help address the barriers.

Confronting Barriers to Patient Teaching

These workshops (that the authors have conducted) identified four recurring themes as barriers that limit staff nurses' abilities to teach patients effectively: time restrictions, need for teaching skills, haphazard teaching efforts, and lack of notice or reward. When these barriers are addressed with ongoing training and management support, patient education and staff satisfaction can be significantly enhanced (Boswell, Pichert, Lorenz, & Schlundt, 1990; London, 1999).

Barrier 1: Time Restrictions
Teaching is often reported as time consuming, unrealistic, and competitive with other facets of work. Nurses often perceive patient education as an activity separate from routine care and formal in design. Because of this perception (which often arises in settings that have used a patient educator or clinical nurse specialist), staff nurses benefit from coaching and example to incorporate teaching into every patient encounter. Outdated protocols or teaching plans also make teaching in today's environment impossible.

Staff development must assess the work setting and determine how to destroy barriers. Can patient education experts be used for coaching staff? Do teaching plans need to be streamlined and accompanied by new teaching materials? Finally, do demands of paperwork, staffing, and supervision legitimately prevent staff from the patient contact required for teaching?

Barrier 2: The Need for Teaching Skills
Nurses state they lack the skills needed for teaching. Specifically, they ask for modeling and coaching from experienced teachers, such as clinical nurse specialists and patient educators. Many nurses have told us that they have little confidence in their teaching and would like to observe expert teachers. This request goes beyond a class in which the expert shares tips for teaching. A preceptor model of observation, demonstration, and coaching can potentially create much greater productivity from the expert teachers as they develop a staff of confident teachers and become resources for difficult teaching situations. Many nurses lack skills for group teaching, even though they are skilled at individual and family teaching.

Barrier 3: Haphazard Teaching Efforts
Nurses often identify patient teaching efforts as haphazard and not directed to discharge priorities. Patient teaching materials are not readily available or are outdated; many teaching programs are outdated. For example, one postpartum nursing unit had a flow sheet designed to streamline documentation of patient teaching with a check-off format. However, it contained more than 40 learning objectives that staff felt responsible for teaching. Because most patient stays were less than 72 hours, teaching was not feasible and the staff felt frustrated. When Stallings met with the nurses to discuss how to streamline teaching, she discovered that some items on the flow sheet were repetitive and some were best taught after discharge. The remaining items were divided into four topical areas with four key learning objectives related to feeding, hygiene and rest of mother, managing the baby's schedule and the mother's needs, and trouble signs that needed immediate attention. The staff felt confident focusing teaching and assessing patient outcomes on only four areas. To

accompany the streamlined teaching plan, a new discharge instruction sheet was developed, following the same format.

In many cases, interdisciplinary approaches to patient education depend on leadership from staff development and an honest appraisal of sacred cows (ie, well-established programs that are no longer realistic, but ones that people insist should be conducted because of past success or politics) that exist in the institution. If teaching plans are unrealistic, new documentation forms will create more work instead of streamlined work. Staff development personnel may need to advocate for revised teaching plans.

Barrier 4: Patient Education is Neither Noticed Nor Rewarded

Nurses state that patient education is neither noticed nor rewarded. They believe that more recognition should be given to involvement in patient education and it should be evaluated in the performance appraisal system. Patient education is creative work, requiring astute assessment and energetic involvement with the patient and family to make every moment count. If the staff perceives that rewards and recognition are based on the number of patients cared for, the number of committees served on, or the ability to troubleshoot technical equipment, it is not likely to place priority on patient education activities.

Patient education is often invisible in management's eyes because it is frequently undocumented, unmonitored, and underappreciated for the skill and experience it demands. Patient education efforts should be described, monitored, and marketed so that nurses receive credit for their work and strive to increase the amount of teaching that is provided (Goldrick et al., 1994). Staff development's role includes improving documentation and visibility of teaching efforts, promoting accountability of all staff through performance reviews, and sponsoring special events that recognize patient education efforts. An annual "Patient Education Week" that includes displays, guest speakers, special awards to individuals and units, and recognition of patient education outcomes and commitment by top administrators can also provide a needed boost for staff.

Promoting Skill Acquisition in Patient Education

Patient and family teaching must be focused on survival skills. What three or four critical behaviors are needed [by patients/families], what problems must they [patients/families] be able to recognize, and how should they [patients/families] get help to handle these? Staff nurses must be teachers and coaches. The practice of novice nurses can be best supported with realistic teaching plans, critical paths, and teaching tools. Overly ambitious teaching plans will frustrate staff and overwhelm patients, empowering neither.

K.S. (STALLINGS, 1996)

Nurses know that the anatomy and physiology lesson is not what keeps patients safe when they go home. Psychomotor skills and problem-solving are what patients need. Nurses must help patients to integrate these behaviors in their daily lives so, first, they'll remember how to do them, and second, that they will be skilled enough do them right.

K.S. (STALLINGS, 1996)

Despite intensive educational efforts to teach, coach, and standardize approaches for patient education, staff development professionals recognize that nurses have different developmental needs in the process of becoming expert teachers. Patricia Benner (Benner et al., 1992) has convincingly explained that nurses live in different clinical worlds.

The clinical judgment and intuition needed to streamline teaching, provide culturally sensitive care, and engage with patients and families, requires that nurses move from a theoretical, abstract base to a concrete world. Developing judgment and intuition occurs as the nurse learns through experience and reflection. Only by passing these developmental milestones can nurses eventually arrive at the expert stage of practice. The expert nurse can grasp the whole situation, set priorities, and confidently individualize patient care.

Applying Benner's work, the strategies that most effectively promote development of expertise in patient education can be incorporated in staff development efforts. Staff development can be targeted to different clinical worlds and can build teamwork to accomplish patient education (Fig. 5-1).

Figure 5-1 is based on Benner's description of the process of skill acquisition. One cornerstone of this process is the nurse's ability to translate theoretical knowledge into nursing's art and know-how, and to be guided by principles rather than explicit directions. The nurse also becomes able to use intuition, recognizing what is salient in an individual situation. The nurse can detect subtle cues. Clinical knowledge enables the nurse to attend to the patient's situation and needs as a whole, with teaching the patient and family as an integral part of care. Rather than feeling overwhelmed, expert nurses feel confident and powerful in complex situations and adapt care based on individual patient priorities. Clinical judg-

ment is embedded in practice (Benner et al., 1992).

What is required for a novice nurse to successfully progress to expert practice? Benner describes the developmental steps associated with *advanced beginner* (generally the first 2 years of practice), *competent, proficient,* and *expert.* By understanding each stage, the capacity of the nurse to accomplish patient education is better appreciated. This understanding also helps staff developers design effective coaching and preceptor interventions to support a nurse's development of expertise in patient education. Benner's work helps educators carefully choose preceptors who best match the needs of their learners. Although many organizations traditionally assign preceptor responsibilities to their expert nurses, Benner leads one to question this wisdom and to consider using the expertise of nurses at all stages of development to support one another in practice.

Table 5-4 applies Benner's work to identify both the interests and educational needs of nurses at each stage of development.

Advanced Beginner Stage

The advanced beginner nurse must master technical skills and learn to organize nursing care. Attuned to rules and procedures, the nurse is dependent on the availability of a preceptor to provide teaching and coaching in each situation. The nurse does not feel fully re-

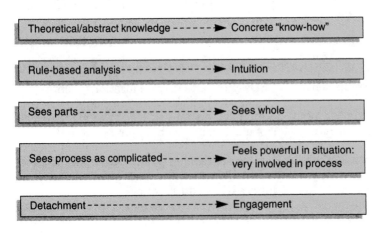

FIGURE 5-1. Patient education science and art: a process of skill acquisition. The *arrows* refer to the process of skill acquisition as a nurse moves from beginner to expert. (Adapted with permission from Benner, P., Tanner, C., & Chesla, C. (1992). *From Beginner to expert: Clinical knowledge in critical care nursing* [video]. Athens, OH: Fuld Institute for Technology in Nursing Education.

TABLE 5-4. Promoting Skill Acquisition in Patient Education

BENNER'S STAGES	DEVELOPMENTAL FOCUS	EDUCATIONAL/INSTITUTIONAL SUPPORT FOR:
Advanced beginner	• Develops technical mastery and organization. • Needs other staff to delegate up. • Manages situations by rules, procedures. • Learns by situation. • Does not feel fully responsible.	• Awareness of agency standards, resources, programs for patient education • Skills for integrating patient and family in patient's care • How to teach skills • Developing explanations to share with family • How-to of documentation
Competent	• Sees relationships among aspects of a situation; pattern analysis. • Desires to limit unexpected. • Deliberately plans and sets goals. • Notices patient/family in new ways; personalizes care. • Feels whole burden of health care team.	• Family assessment • Group teaching skills • Home visits • Negotiating learning contracts • Case study analysis, exemplars • Leading/participating in health care team processes and critical path design
Proficient	• Recognizes patterns. • Sees changing relevance. • Increasingly senses what is salient. • Is attuned to situation; not detached.	• Documentation that supports individualized care • Clinical career ladder based on exemplars that illustrate critical thinking • Permission to break the rules • Support for complex patient situations
Expert	• Develops clinical grasp of whole situation. • Is at home in rapidly changing situations. • Attends to context and environment. • Makes decisions based on qualitative distinctions/what it means for *this* patient.	• Roles in case management • Teacher for competent-proficient • Facilitates patient care rounds • Designs product line models

Note. Adapted with permission from Benner, P., Tanner, C., Chesla, C., (1992). *From Beginner to Expert: Clinical Knowledge in Critical Care Nursing,* [Video], Athens, OH: Fuld Institute for Technology in Nursing Education.

sponsible and is often overwhelmed with the simultaneous demands of a clinical situation.

Staff development efforts for advanced beginners are often best fulfilled by unit-based preceptors. They focus on awareness of agency standards, resources, standardized teaching programs, and critical paths; ways to integrate patient and family teaching into all aspects of care; how-to aspects of teaching individual patients; developing explanations of diagnoses and procedures to share with families; and documenting the outcomes of learning.

Competent Stage
Nurses in the competent stage of practice begin to see patterns and recognize relationships among the various aspects of a situation; they have experienced similar situations and have learned from them. The nurse no longer views

the patient and family as adding to the demands of providing care, but begins to interact with them and personalize care. Desiring to limit the unexpected, the nurse in this stage engages in deliberate planning and goal setting and feels responsible for all aspects of the patient's care.

Staff development efforts to support the competent nurse may include classes or workshops in family assessment, group teaching skills, learning contracts, and case study analysis. The nurse may be interested in and may benefit from making home visits, leading health care team conferences, and serving on committees to design new critical paths. Competent nurses should be engaged as preceptors for beginners, because they can remember how they learned and can still appreciate the needs of novice and advanced beginner nurses.

Proficient Stage

Nurses in the proficient stage recognize patterns. They can see differences in patients and the need to individualize teaching. They confidently streamline teaching, redefine priorities, and break the rules in ways that benefit the patient. Proficient nurses have an increased sense of what is salient in a situation and can teach in ways that are culturally sensitive. They detect subtle cues (eg, patient stress, pain, family dynamics, denial, depression) and are attuned to the situation.

Staff development efforts for these nurses should focus on achieving documentation that supports and reflects individualized care. Clinical career ladders, based on exemplars that illustrate critical thinking, help proficient nurses demonstrate their significant contributions and development of clinical judgment. Although proficient nurses may still need support and resources for complex patient situations, they are skilled at coaching and precepting other nurses in most patient education situations and should be involved as teachers and mentors. Proficient nurses should define patient education successes based on the patient's learning and right to choose rather than on compliance; the failure to define patient education in this manner may result in disillusionment and detachment, rather than in engagement of nursing practice. The nurses must be encouraged to respect intuition. The nurse, in truly listening to the patient and family, may decide to put aside the teaching checklist.

Expert Stage

> *M anagers and administrators must provide expert nurses the freedom to develop innovative new programs that may not look anything like the programs of the past, but [may] help us to achieve health outcomes by working in concert with the community.*
>
> **(RIBISL & HUMPHREYS, 1998; LABONTE, 1994)**

Expert nurses demonstrate an excellent clinical grasp of the whole situation (ie, the patient, the family, the environment) and are comfortable in rapidly changing situations. They attend to context and environment and can make the qualitative distinctions that are crucial in complex situations. Expert nurses can provide valuable coaching for competent and proficient nurses; however, they are not the best choice to precept beginners because they are developmentally distant from the issues beginners experience.

Although beginners strive to learn and follow the rules, experts have learned the conditions under which to safely bend or break rules to meet patient needs. Expert nurses are suited to roles, such as case manager and clinical specialist, in which they must handle complex situations. They also are valuable resources for facilitating patient care rounds and assisting in the development of multiservice product line models for patient education.

 The expert nurse practitioner performs many functions as a primary care physician does (eg, health maintenance examinations, management of common acute conditions and some chronic conditions). However, the nurse practitioner is an expert in patient teaching and counseling. Studies indicate overwhelming satisfaction with nurse practitioners and patients are particularly pleased with the health education they provide. (Mundinger, 1994) ■

CLINICAL APPLICATIONS

Motivating Staff

How can we motivate staff to become involved in patient education?

In workshops, nurses and other health professionals frequently complain that they cannot improve their patient education skills because of heavy patient loads and difficulty scheduling time away from the patient care area to attend workshops. Other offerings have been proven to be an effective means of imparting teaching and learning principles and securing interest in patient education without spending a day away from the patient care area. Self directed learning packages, computer-assisted instruction, computerized inventory of teaching materials and checklists, an inhouse newsletter with teaching tips, and opportunities for staff to team with experienced educators for peer review of their teaching, are effective strategies for staff development.

Continuing Education, Seminars, and Classes

The opportunity for acute care staff to make home visits with a seasoned home care nurse has also been proven helpful in honing discharge teaching skills. The bonus of giving continuing education units may be influential, especially to nurses who work in states with mandatory continuing education requirements. We have offered many brief seminars to nurses as a means of teaching cultural assessment, goal setting, and documentation strategies and have found them to be successful. We typically used case studies and role-play in these seminars to enhance the learning process. Sometimes participants are asked to develop their own teaching programs, and to apply the content learned in the seminar.

The actual disease process or health promotion content that must be conveyed to patients is another problematic aspect. Many nurses say that they do not know what to teach. Most nurses usually have the pertinent information, but anxiety can be decreased by helping the staff to organize and review the information that patients need. Frequently, staff members become so enthusiastic about teaching after attending these classes that they recognize other areas of need and develop teaching protocols with little assistance from the patient educator. Seminars and classes satisfy both intrinsic and extrinsic motivational factors for the staff. Negative intrinsic factors, such as anxiety about lack of knowledge, are modified; positive extrinsic factors, such as gaining continuing education units, are resolved.

Patient Education-Oriented Nursing Rounds

Nursing rounds oriented toward patient education can be an effective motivating force. In

these cases, nurses or other health professionals should be asked to prepare information about a patient with whom they are familiar. This material may be related to assessment of the client's education needs, goal setting, the process of teaching skills, or any patient education task. Nursing rounds are an excellent means of learning from others and of expanding one's repertoire of patient education behaviors.

Reward and Incentive Programs

Reward and incentive programs for staff who provide patient education can be a strong motivator. Sometimes the reward is the ability to move from night or evening shifts to day shifts. Another possibility is for a staff nurse who has developed special skills to advance a clinical career ladder. Rewards and incentives show other staff members that patient education activities are valued in their institution.

Peer and Colleague Support

Peer support is an important motivating factor for the staff. Staff members who can convene on a formal or informal basis to discuss their problems and their successes in patient education can add an impetus to the widespread adoption of patient education efforts. The nursing profession suffers from a lack of internal validation. Too often we think we are the only ones on the battle lines, and we refuse to allow ourselves to ask for support when we need it. Greater team efforts and support within nursing would improve patient education efforts and would act as a motivator to inexperienced nurses who look for guidance.

The benefits that accrue from increased physician-nurse collegiality motivate staff. Nurses who know that physicians approve of their patient education efforts will experience confirmation and validation as motivators. Because collegiality is a two-way proposition, nurses also must validate the patient education efforts of physicians. Collegiality as a motivator can, and should, extend to other health care team members. Another extrinsic motivator is a nurse's better sense of his or her own professional identity in these collegial relationships.

Teaching the Older Patient

JCAHO mandates age-specific approaches. As the population we serve ages, the need for teaching older patients increases. Because staff education is conducted to address this patient group, what are some of the special aspects and needs related to teaching the older patient and his or her family that should be addressed?

Although many health professionals recognize that the differences among older patients and middle-aged adult patients call for modified patient teaching, they mistakenly approach the older patient as if he or she is a child. Although some common qualities among the two age groups exist, a health professional who takes this approach displays a lack of sensitivity and insults the patient.

As people grow old, their cognitive efficiency declines. Older people have been found to have increasing difficulty understanding complex sentences, to be less proficient in drawing inferences, to demonstrate problems with perceptual motor tasks, and to have more difficulty in determining the point of a story (Eliopoulos, 1997). Institutionalized older persons do even more poorly on tests of cognitive ability than do their counterparts living in the community. When teaching older patients, the following points should be remembered:

- Present information at a much slower rate than usual.
- Speak in a low tone of voice; older persons hear low tones better than high-pitched sounds.
- Allow plenty of time for the assimilation and integration of conceptual material; emphasize concrete rather than abstract material.
- Reduce environmental distracters.
- Keep in mind that any or all of the following causes may be related to the older client's reduced capacity to learn: cerebral changes, psychosocial issues, and changes in self concept with probable loss of self esteem.
- Be aware that group experiences can

improve the older client's problem-solving ability.
- Remember that older clients are cautious and do not make changes easily.

Nurses must take more time teaching older patients, and educational material should be delivered in small increments, so that the material can be integrated. Increased compliance to medications can be enhanced with a reminder calendar.

Older patients take 80% or less or 120% or more of essential medications than is prescribed (Hawe & Higgins, 1990) This finding supports the need for continued teaching emphasis on the importance of taking prescribed drugs in the recommended dosages.

Active participation of a spouse or family member can facilitate and reinforce teaching of older patients regarding medication and other prescribed treatments (Murdaugh, 1998). Health professionals should be aware of the causes of an older individual's reduced capacity to learn, so that they can intervene and perhaps change these modifiable causes (eg, psychosocial losses, low self esteem). Other modifiable causes include problems related to multiple medications or medications that are incorrectly used. Additionally, physiologic causes, pertaining to reduced ability to learn, include conditions such as hypoglycemia secondary to diabetes mellitus, and hypoxia secondary to congestive heart failure.

 Many skills involving social interaction can be successfully taught in a group setting (eg, helping older patients to acquire assertiveness skills to secure better housing or more neighborhood police protection). In deference to the cautiousness and reluctance to make changes that older people may display, the health professional should avoid making changes in the medical regimen, whenever possible, and should attempt to maintain a constant environment and schedule for the older patient. ∎

 Many older learners prefer to learn alone, and if this is the case, provide them with teaching materials. However, be certain to return to discuss the contents and to help them problem solve. Older patients may have difficulty following recommendations because of misunderstanding, physical limitations, or financial barriers, so they need to be assessed well (London, 1999). ∎

Teaching Children

How is the teaching of children and adolescents different from the teaching of adults? What principles should we prepare staff to apply in teaching these patients and their families?

Children are not small adults. Teaching them demands ingenuity and a different approach. An adolescent's learning needs vary from those of children and from those of adults, and, therefore, are discussed separately.

Teaching and learning principles, when applied to children, should always consider the growth, development, and cognitive levels of the child. Table 5-5 is based on Piaget's well-known work regarding the development of perceptual and cognitive processes from infancy through adolescence (Piaget & Garcia, 1974). We purposely chose Piaget instead of Erikson, because of the belief that understanding the cognitive processes is of equal importance to understanding the developmental processes for pediatric patient education. Table 5-5 outlines the cognitive and perceptual stages of development and suggests an approach to pediatric patient teaching.

Before embarking on pediatric patient education, remember that children have shorter attention spans, have greater need for support and nurturance, and learn more easily through active participation than do adults. Therefore, material must be presented in abbreviated format during a short time. Staff members must remember to consistently and persistently show affection and to offer praise to young clients during education sessions. By actively involving children in the learning process, we help them to more readily assimilate the information.

An old adage states that the child's play is his work. In this play, he integrates new and unfamiliar information. Play, therefore, becomes a primary vehicle through which he learns about his disease or acute problem, about what will happen, and about how to take care of himself to the best of his ability. Play therapy should also be used to help the child to integrate and understand the painful or frightening experience he has undergone. Follow-up to surgery and procedures is just as important as preparation for these events because most children have many unresolved feelings and questions that need expression.

The following case study illustrates the appropriate teaching for a 10-year-old boy with newly diagnosed idiopathic recurrent seizures.

CASE STUDY

A CHILD WITH NEWLY DIAGNOSED IDIOPATHIC SEIZURES

HISTORY

Eric experiences his first generalized, tonic-clonic (grand mal) seizure during recess at elementary school. He is hospitalized immediately for observation and a diagnostic workup.

Patient Education

Eric's primary nurse initiates patient education. Remembering that Eric's stage of cognitive development had been characterized by Piaget as *concrete operational thought,* she begins by teaching him the basic pathophysiology of seizure activity (Piaget & Garcia, 1974). Eric does not have abstract thought processes, but he understands the simple drawings the nurse provides of the brain and her explanation that the seizures were caused by too much electrical activity in the brain.

The nurse does not stress the term electrical activity; instead, she compares the problem in his brain to "an electric toy train that goes so fast that it runs off the track." She completes her analogy by saying that the medication he was going to take every day would act on his brain as if it were "slowing down the speed of the electric train." Eric's nurse remains aware that at

(case study continues on page 134)

this stage of development in the child's language skills, he may not always manage to indicate whether he has fully comprehended her explanation. Thus, she uses much repetition and asks Eric many questions.

Children from ages 7 years to 12 years generally can handle many of the aspects of their medical regimen. Eric is made responsible for administering his own medication at the prescribed times. He begins preparing and taking the medication himself while he is still hospitalized.

Children of Eric's age are more socially involved with their peers than are younger children, and it is important not to disrupt their attempts to join groups and participate in team sports. Eric is told that he can ride his bike as long as he wears his bike helmet and is accompanied by another child or an adult. He is also informed that he can continue swimming as long as someone is with him.

Finally, Eric is taught to begin to recognize the signs of his aura. The nurse defines an aura as the peculiar sensations Eric would grow to know as a warning sign of a seizure. After determining that Eric has previously experienced nausea and vomiting with the flu, she tells him that an aura is the special warning that takes place before a convulsion, just as there was a certain warning that occurred before vomiting. Eric is told that when he began to recognize his aura, which might be a smell, sound, color, or sensation, he should try to lie down immediately.

The teaching includes both of Eric's parents, so they can reinforce the information imparted to Eric and offer support to him during the teaching sessions. The nurse presents the material to Eric during three half-hour sessions, so that he has an adequate amount of time to assimilate the information and to ask questions. She also spends time with Eric's parents alone, giving them more detailed information and answering their questions.

Discharge

Eric is discharged from the hospital; he and his parents are encouraged to call the nurse, the pediatric nurse practitioner, or the pediatrician if they have questions or if they experience any problems. They also are assisted by the hospital librarian, who provided articles and Internet resources.

Teaching Adolescents

Adolescents have a different cognitive style from that of the school-age child. Piaget asserts that at the age of 12 years, children develop *formal operational thought* (Piaget & Garcia, 1974). During adolescence, the ability to think abstractly becomes well developed. Cognitive processes are of an adult type, and the adolescent develops the ability to reason deductively. Therefore, when considering the cognitive style to use during patient teaching, be aware that the adolescent can be taught in a fashion similar to the way an adult is taught.

The aspect of the adolescent's development that clearly differentiates him from the adult, however, is his social development and the importance of his peer group. Knowledge of the adolescent's psychosocial task—identity versus role confusion, as defined by Erik Erikson—is of primary importance to the health care provider who works with the adolescent in a patient education setting (Erikson, 1993). The nurse must remember that because the adolescent develops his identity in relation to his peers and in opposition to his parents, teaching should be performed without the parents present.

 Use of support groups for families with children with type I diabetes has been found to be an effective strategy in dealing with younger (11 years to 14 years of age) adolescents. One author, Rankin, facilitated a family support group for 3 years, in which parents and children attended on a monthly basis. Although parents and children were frequently separated

TABLE 5-5. Cognitive States and Approaches to Patient Education With Children

COGNITIVE STAGE	APPROACH TO TEACHING
Ages Birth to 2 yrs—Sensorimotor Development	
Begins as completely undifferentiated from environment. Eventually learns to repeat actions that have effect on objects. Has rudimentary ability to make associations.	Orient all teaching to parents. Make infants feel as secure as possible with familiar objects in home environment. Give older infants an opportunity to manipulate objects in their environments; especially if long hospitalization is expected.
Ages 2–7 yrs—Preoperational Development	
Has cognitive processes that are literal and concrete.	Be aware of explanations that the child may interpret literally (eg, "The doctor is going to make your heart like new" may be interpreted as "He is going to give me a new heart"); allow child to manipulate safe equipment, such as stethoscopes, tongue blades, reflex hammers; use simple drawings of external anatomy because children have limited knowledge of organs' functions.
Lacks ability to generalize.	Comparisons to other children are not helpful, nor is it meaningful to compare one diagnostic test or procedure to another.
Egocentrism predominates.	Belief that he causes events to happen may result in guilty thoughts that he caused his own pain, hospitalization, and so forth; reassure child that no one is to blame for his pain or other problems.
Has animistic thinking (thinks that all objects possess life or human characteristics of their own).	Anthropomorphize and name equipment that is especially frightening.
Ages 7–12 yrs—Concrete Operational Thought Development	
Has concrete, but more realistic, objective, cognitive processes.	Use drawings and models; children at this age have vague understandings of internal body processes; use needle play and dolls to explain surgical techniques and facilitate learning.
Is able to compare objects and experiences because of increased ability to classify along many dimensions.	Relate his care to other children's experiences so he can learn from them; compare procedures to one another to diminish anxiety.
Views world more objectively and is able to understand another's position.	Use films and group activities to add to repertoire of useful behaviors and to establish role models.
Has knowledge of cause and effect that has progressed to deductive logical reasoning.	Use child's interest in science to explain what has happened and what will happen to him; explain medications simply and straightforwardly (eg, "This medicine [insulin] unlocks the door to your body's cells just as a key unlocks the door to your house. By unlocking the door to the cell, the insulin can deliver the food and energy in your blood to the cell."(

Note. From (1980) *Emotional care of hospitalized children* (pp 38–50), Petrillo, M., & Sanger, S. Philadelphia: J. B. Lippincott and Kolb, L. C. *Modern Clinical Psychiatry* (9th ed, pp 90–91), 1977, Philadelphia: W. B. Saunders. Adapted with permission.

for different activities, many parents stated that the opportunity for their children to be in contact with other adolescents who have diabetes was a singular experience occurring only during the meetings.

On occasion, parents and children met when there were topics of interest to both. For example, representatives from local diabetes summer camps attended the meetings to orient parents and children to camp possibilities. The most popular joint speaker, however, was a young man with diabetes, who had not been well controlled metabolically during adolescence and who, at the age of 23 years, was experiencing complications related to retinopathy. This speaker served a twofold purpose: First, he allowed children and adolescents an opportunity to see a young adult who had participated successfully in all types of sports and was determined to live as fully as possible, thus modeling a realistic role to adolescents. Second, the speaker's retinopathy that had resulted from a period of multiple hyperglycemic episodes allowed the parents to understand that parental control would probably be inadequate to protect their children from the excesses of adolescence. ■

Frequently, we assume that adolescents have more knowledge about their own anatomy and physiology than they do. This applies to functions of body organs and to sexuality. Illustrations are helpful with this age group, although they can be more sophisticated than those used with the school-age population.

Honesty with adolescents is crucial. If a change in body image is expected as a result of surgery or during the course of a disease, the adolescent must be adequately prepared; body image is of paramount importance to this age group. Because of the desire to be one of the gang and to look like everyone else, the adolescent who faces a change in appearance will need help from health care professionals in camouflaging the change.

Developmental readiness for learning should not be equated with biologic growth or maturation. When teaching adolescents, it is important to explain the illness and ensure an understanding about why they need to follow particular health care regimens. Nurses can empower teens who face chronic illness and disabilities by fostering self esteem, promoting independence through self-care and decision-making, encouraging socialization with peers (those with and without similar disabilities), advocating for verbal communication, and promoting coping and stress management skills (Ferri & Veroneau, 1998; Muscari, 1998a, Muscari, 1998b).

 Don't miss the opportunity with adolescents for health promotion teaching. Epidemiological data related to chronic illnesses clearly show that the following six types of behaviors are the leading causes of morbidity and mortality in our country, and patterns are established during youth: (Orlandi & Dalton, 1998)

1. Behaviors contributing to injury (intentional and unintentional), such as reckless driving
2. Tobacco use
3. Alcohol and other drug use
4. Sexual behaviors that contribute to unwanted pregnancy and STDs (including HIV)
5. Unhealthy dietary patterns
6. Physical inactivity ■

When school-age children and adolescents are hospitalized for extended periods, JCAHO requires that, to assist them in keeping up with their school work, the hospital has a plan to serve as a liaison between student, parents, and school district (Iacono & Campbell, 1997).

SUMMARY

We still have nurses who practice unhappily in their organizations because they teach patients in a way that does not work. Therefore, the patients are not successful, and the nurses are not successful, and the organization as a whole will suffer. There is a great need for staff development. If we could gather all of the expert nurses who feel very powerful about the way they are teaching, and pair them up with other nurses in a mentoring relationship, I think that we would come a long way in improving the welfare of patients and the job satisfaction of nurses.

Nurses have always put the safety of our patients first. And this will continue into the future. The core competencies we bring to the healthcare arena to help our patients take responsibility for health behaviors and achieve better health outcomes will be a key to our success in our individual careers and as a profession.

K.S. (STALLINGS, 1996)

Staff development practitioners are poised to make important contributions to patient teaching efforts (providing leadership to assess needs, developing educationally sound programs, and advocating for needed resources). The work of staff development includes interpreting JCAHO standards, promoting patient-centered approaches, streamlining or replacing outdated programs, and forging alliances that are multidisciplinary and multisetting.

The role of staff development goes beyond helping the organization achieve a successful JCAHO survey. All continuing education programs must address implications for patient education. Workshops that expose staff to innovative approaches and skills for patient education should be offered and should address realistic strategies for teaching and documenting. As staff development professionals identify barriers encountered in the provision of patient teaching, they must address those issues honestly. Unit-based teaching and coaching should be provided to individual nurses to build the acquisition of skills and expertise in patient education. The strengths of nurses as coaches and teachers of others is

perhaps our greatest resource for improving patient education outcomes.

Staff development can help the organization to tailor its patient education programs to a growing population that is culturally diverse and growing older.

Finally, staff development can increase the visibility of patient education efforts in the organization. This can be accomplished by sponsoring special events and recognition, bringing in national experts as guest speakers, and promoting patient education activities as integral to clinical ladders and performance review systems.

STRATEGIES FOR CRITICAL ANALYSIS

1. How can the respective strengths of nurses in each of Benner's four stages contribute to the development of a new patient education program for prenatal clients?
2. Describe two strategies that could be used by a staff development coordinator to increase administrative support for patient education efforts.
3. Describe an age-specific approach for teaching a newly diagnosed 8-year-old girl about how to manage diabetes.
4. Describe an age-specific approach for teaching a newly diagnosed 14-year-old girl about how to manage her diabetes.
5. The input of front-line staff is key to quality improvement efforts in patient education. Interview five staff nurses, using the questions in Box 5-6. (Staff Questionnaire). Based on the interviews, what patient education and staff education needs should be addressed? Describe strategies for meeting these needs.

REFERENCES

American Hospital Association. (1979). *Implementing patient education in the hospital.* Chicago: Author.

Altman, D., & Jackson, C. (1998). Adolescent tobacco use and the social context. In Shumaker, S, Schron, E., Ockene, J., & McBee, W. (Eds.).

The Handbook of Health Behavior Change. New York: Springer.

Benner, P. (1984). *From novice to expert: Excellence and power in clinical nursing practice.* Menlo Park, CA: Addison-Wesley.

Benner, P., & Tanner, C. (1987). Clinical judgment: how expert nurses use intuition. *American Journal of Nursing, 87*(1), 23–31.

Benner, P., Tanner, C., & Chesla, C. (1992). *From beginner to expert: Clinical knowledge in critical care nursing* [Video]. Athens, OH: Fuld Institute for Technology in Nursing Education, 28 Station Street, Athens, OH 45701.

Boswell, E., Pichert, J., Lorenz, R., & Schlundt, D. (1990). Training health care professionals to enhance their patient teaching skills. *Journal of Nursing Staff Development, 6*(5), 233–239.

Cesta, T., & Falter, E. (1999). Case management; Its value for staff nurses. *American Journal of Nursing, 993*(5), 48–51.

Eliopoulos, C. (1997). *Gerontological Nursing.* Philadelphia: Lippincott-Raven.

Erikson, E. (1993). *Childhood and Society.* New York: W. W. Norton.

Ferri, R., & Veroneau, P. (1998). Initiating a dialogue with the adolescent patient. *The American Nurse, 30*(6).

Goldrick, T., Jablonski, R., & Wolf, Z. (1994). Needs assessment for a patient education program in a nursing department. *Journal of Nursing Staff Development, 10*(3), 123–130.

Hawe, P., & Higgins, G. (1990). Can medication education improve the drug compliance of the elderly? Evaluation of an in-hospital program. *Patient Education and Counseling, 16,* 151–160.

Iacono, J., & Campbell, A. (1997). *Patient and Family Education: The compliance guide to the JCAHO Standards.* Marblehead, MA: Opus Communications.

Joint Commission on the Accreditation of Healthcare Organizations. (1996). *Educating Hospital Patients and Their Families: Examples of Compliance.* Oakbrook, IL: Author.

Joint Commission on the Accreditation of Healthcare Organizations. (1998). *Comprehensive accreditation manual for hospitals.* Chicago: Author.

Kelly, K. (1992). *Nursing staff development: Current competence and future focus.* Philadelphia: J. B. Lippincott.

Kolb, L. C. (1977). *Modern Clinical Psychiatry* (9th ed.). Philadelphia: W. B. Saunders.

Labonte, R. (1994). Health promotion and empowerment: Reflections on professional practice. *Health Education Quarterly, 21,* 253–268.

London, F. (1999). *No Time to Teach.* Philadelphia: Lippincott, Williams, & Wilkins.

Mundinger, M. (1994). Sounding board. Advanced practice nursing—Good medicine for physicians? *New England Journal of Medicine, 303*(3), 211–213.

Murdaugh, C. (1998). Problems with adherence in the elderly. In Shumaker, S, Schron, E., Ockene, J., & McBee, W. (Eds). *The Handbook of Health Behavior Change.* New York: Springer.

Muscari, M. (1998a). Coping with chronic illness. *American Journal of Nursing, 983*(9), 20–22.

Muscari, M. (1998b). Rebels with a cause: When adolescents won't follow medical advice. *American Journal of Nursing 98*(9), 26–35.

Orlandi, M., & Dalton, L. (1998). Lifestyle interventions for the young. In Shumaker, S, Schron, E., Ockene, J., & McBee, W. (Eds). *The Handbook of Health Behavior Change.* New York: Springer.

Petrillo, M., & Sanger, S. (1980). *Emotional care of hospitalized children.* Philadelphia: J. B. Lippincott.

Piaget, J., & Garcia, M. (1974). *Understanding Causality* (D. Miles & M. Miles, Trans.). New York: W. W. Norton.

Redman, B. (1993). Patient education at 25 years: where we have been and where we are going. *Journal of Advanced Nursing, 18,*(8) 727–728.

Ribisl, K., & Humphreys, K. (1998). Collaboration between professionals and mediating structures in the community: toward a "third way" in health promotion. In Shumaker, S, Schron, E., Ockene, J., McBee, W. (Eds). *The Handbook of Health Behavior Change.* New York: Springer.

Stallings, K. (1996). *Integrating patient education in your nursing practice* [Video]. Reproduced with permission of GlaxoWellcome, Inc. Produced by Horizon Video Productions, 4222 Emperor Boulevard, Durham, NC 27703.

Wasson, D., & Anderson, M. (1994). Hospital-patient education: Current status and future trends. *Journal of Nursing Staff Development, 10*(3),147–151.

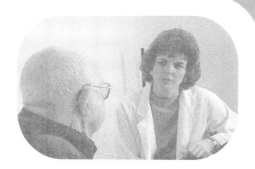

Informed Consent

Ellen M. Robinson

LEARNING OBJECTIVES

After reading this chapter, the nurse or student nurse should be able to:

1. Describe the importance of informed consent in patient education.

2. Discuss the legal and ethical bases of informed consent.

3. Describe legal cases that relate to the nurse's role in informed consent.

4. Identify the elements of informed consent.

5. Discuss exceptions to informed consent and how they apply to a nurse's role.

6. Develop awareness of the impact of informed consent on special patient groups (eg, culturally diverse patients, children, adolescents, older patients, and patients at the end of life).

7. Discuss a philosophical position on informed consent relative to the independent and collaborative practice roles of nurses.

INTRODUCTION

Informed consent is important in today's health care environment. Patients are faced with complex decisions involving many interventions, including new drug treatments, surgical and related procedures, and the use of advanced technology. Independent nursing practice has advanced and has led to development of nursing interventions in which the patient's informed consent may be needed. This chapter provides an overview of the doctrine of informed consent, so that nurses can understand the importance of this process and integrate it in their collaborative and independent practices.

Informed Consent in Nursing Practice

In nursing practice, educating patients and their families is closely linked to informed consent. As educators, nurses continuously assess a client's understanding of his or her disease state and of the proposed medical or nursing intervention. Patient education often involves disclosure of information to patients and families that will help them make decisions about their health care. A thorough understanding of informed consent is important for nurses as patient educators.

The doctrine of informed consent is applicable to both *collaborative* and *independent* nursing practice and research. The *collaborative* role of nurses involves an active partnership with physicians in the assessment and management of a patient's medical problems. The *independent* practice of nurses is concerned with a patient's responses to actual or potential health problems (American Nurses Association, 1995).

In collaborative practice with physicians, nurses frequently perform medical therapies or assist with procedures that require informed consent; examples include ventilator management or assistance in the insertion of invasive monitoring devices (eg, Swan Ganz catheters). Nurses are often in the best position to assess a patient's understanding of medical treatments, and if the patient has chosen freely to accept treatment. In independent practice, nurses increasingly prescribe and implement interventions that may warrant consent from patients; examples include therapeutic touch, guided imagery, and interventions to restore skin integrity (Bulechek & McCloskey, 1999).

The collaborative and independent research roles of nurses also require expertise in informed consent, which is the process by which the rights of patients who are approached to participate in research are protected. Many authors and professional position statements have considered this important topic in detail (Alderson, 1995a; Bok, 1995; McCabe, 1999; Dalhousie, 1999; Davis, 1996; Flanagin, 1997; Katz, 1993; Kleinman, Brown & Librach, 1994; Macklin, 1999; Marwick, 1997; McCarthy, 1995; Rogero-Anaya, Carpintero-Avellaneda & Vila-Blasco, 1994; Shuster, 1997; Silva, 1995; Truog & Robinson, 1999).

This chapter provides information to help nurses meet the challenge of incorporating informed consent into their roles as patient educators. An overview of the legal and ethical foundations of informed consent are provided, legal cases pertinent to nursing are presented, the five elements of informed consent are defined, research on informed consent is presented, exceptions to informed consent is covered, and informed consent in the context of special patient populations is discussed. Finally, we present an argument for a philosophical position for nursing on informed consent.

 Informed consent is the provision of enough truthful information about a treatment (ie, it's nature, alternatives, risks, and benefits) to a patient so that the recipient of the therapy can decide, through logical reason and free of coercion, whether he or she wants to receive the intervention (Friedlander, 1995). The members of the President's Commission for the Study of Ethical Problems in Biomedical and Behavioral Research thought the issue so important that three volumes were dedicated to the topic (President's Commission, 1982). The Commission decided to address informed consent from a context of relations and communications between patients and health care providers. The goal was to promote a fuller understanding by patients and professionals of their common enterprise, so that patients could participate on an informed basis and, to the extent they could do so, make decisions regarding their health care. Because of the attention that informed consent has received, clinicians have begun to accept the process as an important dimension of their practice. ■

LEGAL THEORY AND ISSUES IN INFORMED CONSENT

Tort Law, Constitutional Law, and Liability

According to Faden and Beauchamp (1986), two areas of law are relevant to the concept of informed consent—*tort law* and *constitutional law*—with the former being most prevalent. A *tort* is a civil injury to one's person or property that is intentionally or negligently inflicted by another and that is measured in terms of and compensated by monetary damages. *Constitutional laws* are that set of laws that have been established in the U.S. Constitution, such as a personal right to freedom and equality.

Battery and *negligence* are the theories of liability that have been applied to court cases on informed consent. *Battery* is defined as the act of offensive touching that is done without the consent of the person being touched, however benign the motive or effects of touching (Prosser, 1971). The source of liability in *negligence* theory is unintended harmful action or omission (Faden & Beauchamp, 1986). *Battery* theory was applied frequently in the past, and *negligence* theory is more commonly applied today.

Landmark Cases

Schloendorff v. Society of New York Hospitals (1914) is a landmark case that demonstrates application of *battery* theory and recognition of the legal principle of self-determination. This case involved a physician who surgically removed a fibroid tumor from a woman who had consented to a laparotomy. The woman had consented to a laparotomy, but not to the removal of the fibroid tumor. Justice Cardoza's opinion is widely quoted and stands as a classic statement regarding a patient's right to self-determination: "Every human being of adult years and sound mind has a right to determine what shall be done with his own body; and a surgeon who performs an operation without his patient's consent commits an assault, for which he is liable in damages" (Schloendorff, 1914, p. 127). This notion of self-determination has proved important in future cases. However, consent is expressed through this right of self-determination; the notion of "informed" was not yet included.

Salgo v. Leland Stanford University Board of Trustees (1957), an important case, added the *informed* to informed consent. In this case, Martin Salgo had undergone a translumbar aortography and sustained permanent paralysis. Salgo sued his physicians for negligence because they failed to disclose this risk, which Salgo argued would have entered his decision-making whether to undergo the procedure. This case emphasized the components of informed consent (ie, the nature of the treatment and its consequences, harms, benefits, risks, and alternatives) as information required by patients to make meaningful decisions regarding treatment (Faden and Beauchamp, 1986).

Application of negligence theory was pioneered in the case of *Natanson v. Kline* (1960). Although she consented to the intervention, Mrs. Natanson sued her physician for administering cobalt radiation treatment to her after a mastectomy, claiming that the physician had not disclosed to her the risks inherent in the therapy. After suffering radiation burns, she sued Dr. Kline for negligence, claiming that he did not obtain her informed consent for a new treatment because he did not warn her of the risks. The decision in the *Natanson* case offered additional support for disclosure as an obligation and continued recognition of self-determination.

Self-determination as the sole justification

and goal of informed consent was further affirmed in *Canterbury v. Spence* (1972). This case shifted focus from the professional practice standard of disclosure to a reasonable person standard. In this case, a patient had undergone a laminectomy for severe back pain, and after falling from bed became paralyzed. The patient sued the physician, claiming that he had not been warned of the possibility of paralysis.

Regarding constitutional law, the right to privacy is relevant to informed consent. This right is based on the first, ninth, and fourteenth amendments of the Constitution. The common theme is prevention of governmental interference with personal health care issues (eg, abortion, treatment refusal) (Purtilo, 1984). Currently, many states have enacted legislation for informed consent, reflecting the importance of the concept. According to informed consent legal experts Meisel and Kabnick (1980), the doctrine has been largely unchanged in statutory reform as compared to common law.

Recent Legal Cases Involving Nurses

The role of the nurse has been scrutinized in several recent legal cases involving informed consent (Tammelleo, 1985, 1990, 1993a, 1993b, 1995, 1997a, 1997b). The first two cases described the nurse's role in collaboration with a physician in the context of patient surgery, the second two cases relate to organ donation, and the final three cases presented relate to poor judgment for that which the nurse was clearly accountable.

Legal Cases Involving Surgery

Obtaining a patient's signature on a consent form for a procedure that a physician will perform is a controversial responsibility sometimes assigned to the nurse in an acute care or same-day-surgery facility. The case of *Foflygen v. R. Zemel, M.D.* (1992; Tammelleo, 1993a) demonstrates the complex nature of informed consent for nurses. Janice Foflygen went to a

physician seeking a gastric diversion, a surgical procedure she read about in a newspaper as being an effective treatment to alleviate obesity. The physician had instructed a nurse to obtain the patient's signature on a standard hospital consent form entitled "Consent for Operation, Anesthetics, and Special Procedures." The nurse obtained the signature as requested by the physician. The patient underwent the surgery, sustained several complications, including pulmonary embolism, acute respiratory distress, phlebitis of the arm, acute bronchitis, stroke, and a right carotid artery occlusion. Ms. Foflygen brought suit against all health care providers, including the nurse, claiming that she had never been apprised of the risks of the surgery or of any alternatives to surgery that would treat the obesity. The court, regarding the case as a battery to the patient, removed the action against the nurse, because the nurse did not perform the operation. Although the nurse was not convicted, Tammelleo (1993a) urges nurses not to lead or to mislead a patient into signing a consent form unless satisfied that the patient has been properly informed. Tammelleo further adds that the physician performing the procedure has the duty to obtain the patient's informed consent (p.4).

Another case related to surgery is described in the Pennsylvania case of *Davis v. Hoffman* (1997; Tammelleo, 1997a). Ms. Roberta Davis sought diagnosis and treatment for her lower abdominal pain from her physician, Dr. Hoffman. Dr. Hoffman diagnosed fibroid uterus, and recommended a laparoscopy and possible hysteroscopy. Ms. Davis agreed, although she stated that she did not want a hysterectomy. Nurse Puchini thoroughly conducted a preoperative teaching session with Ms. Davis. Dr. Hoffman promised Ms. Davis that should a hysterectomy be indicated, he would awaken her and obtain her consent before proceeding. The physician performed the hysterectomy without obtaining Ms. Davis' consent. The patient sued Dr. Hoffman, Nurse Puchini, and the hospital. The plaintiff's complaint against Nurse Puchini was that she, in conjunction with Dr. Hoffman, did not obtain the patient's informed consent for hysterectomy, and that Nurse Puchini did not advise the patient, Ms. Davis, of alternative testing, treatment, or procedures during the preoperative teaching session.

Under Pennsylvania law, the court ruled that a nurse has no legal duty to obtain informed consent for a physician-performed procedure, therefore absolving Nurse Puchini of the complaint related to informed consent. In addition, the plaintiff could not produce substantive proof that Nurse Puchini's preoperative teaching session fell below a professional nurse's standard of care. This case suggests that the public may hold nurses to a standard of preoperative teaching that extends beyond explanation of the pre- and postoperative nursing care related to the surgical procedure. Nurses define professional standards and not take on that which is within a medical purview of practice.

 These two cases alert practicing nurses to understand the boundaries of their responsibilities in obtaining informed consent for surgical procedures, which are performed by physicians. Nurses should focus their efforts for that which they are accountable, the preoperative teaching process, and be clear about the professional practice standard related to such. ■

Legal Cases Involving Organ Donation

Request for organ donation is frequently earmarked as a nursing responsibility in the acute care setting. In the case of *Brown v. Delaware Valley Transplant Program* (1992; Tammelleo, 1993b), a patient named Lawrence Brown was brought to the emergency room of a hospital with a gunshot wound. Within 24 hours of his arrival, Mr. Brown was declared to be brain dead, and noted to be a candidate for organ donation. His next of kin, sister Virginia Brown, was not notified until after Mr. Brown's organs were removed. She sued the hospital, arguing that a good faith effort to notify her was not made. Although the hospital was granted immunity based on the Uniform Anatomical Gift Act (1987), legal expert Tammelleo (1993b)

warns nurses that their participation in procedures, such as harvesting organs from a patient when informed consent has not been obtained or attempted to be obtained, is not advisable (p. 1).

Tammelleo related the organ donation case of *Perry v. St. Francis Hospital and Medical Center* (1994; Tammelleo, 1995). After a heart attack, Kenneth Perry was pronounced brain dead. Family members were approached by Nurse McDonald, who requested organ donation. The Perry family refused initially, because they feared body disfigurement of the deceased. After discussion with Nurse McDonald, the Perry family agreed to cornea and bone marrow donation, with the understanding that retrieval of these organs would not leave the deceased disfigured. The consent form was modified to reflect this discussion between the nurse and the family. A hospital team and Red Cross agents harvested the approved organs, and the deceased was transferred to his undertaker. The mortician informed the family that Kenneth Perry's eyes had been enucleated, and that his long bones had been removed. The family brought suit, citing that they had not agreed to organ donation under conditions of body disfigurement. Although the Kansas court denied both practitioner and hospital liability, the case points to the need for nurses to be fully informed regarding organ retrieval procedures in their agencies before discussing this option with family members.

 Nurses must clearly describe the degree of disfigurement involved, if any, in organ procurement and other involved procedures. Nurses should contact the organ bank in their area for frequent updates and consultation regarding organ donation procedures. ■

Legal Cases Involving Poor Judgment

The following two cases summarized by Tammelleo (1985, 1990) emphasize poor judgment related to activities for which the nurse is clearly responsible. In *Juneau v. Board. of Elementary Secondary Education* (1984–85), a nurse named Jane Juneau was practicing in a special education center and was responsible for the care of a 12-year-old child with an orthopedic disability. The child's behavior became disruptive, and rather than implement the institution's policy (to place the child in a quiet, secluded area for observation), Ms. Juneau instituted a cold shower for the child. A cold shower is considered an aversive therapy in which the goal is to discourage disruptive behavior. Ms. Juneau was dismissed from her nursing position. She appealed her case to the Court Appeals of Louisiana, which upheld the decision, stating that the nurse had used aversive stimuli, which can only be used if approved by the institution's human rights committee and if consented to by the patient's parent or legal guardian (Tammelleo, 1985, p. 4). Neither of these two conditions had been fulfilled. This case emphasizes that nursing interventions, particularly controversial ones, ought not to be instituted without clear institutional guidelines and informed consent.

In *Roberson v. Provident House* (1990; Tammelleo, 1990), a quadriplegic patient named James Roberson was in a nursing home. He told a nurse not to insert a Foley catheter, because in the past these catheters had caused him to have bleeding and infection. Rather than heed the patient's objections, the nurse instructed the patient to "shut up." The patient developed infection and bleeding and was hospitalized for several days. Roberson brought suit against the nursing home. The court voted in favor of the nursing home, even on appeal, explained by the lack of expert testimony to an applicable standard of care.

A dissenting opinion by a Louisiana justice, however, clearly noted that this patient's right to informed consent was violated, drawing on Justice Cardoza's statement (1914) that "every adult human being of sound mind has a right to determine what shall be done to his own body." Clearly, the nurse violated this legal precedent in this patient's care. Both the *Juneau* and the *Roberson* cases (1985, 1990) emphasize that any intervention without baseline assessment and informed consent is not judicious and can be harmful to pa-

tients. Nurses, as independent practitioners, will be responsible for their actions.

The final case demonstrates nursing and medical malpractice, of which patient education and informed consent are one component. In 1988, a group of patients and some of their legal guardians from the state psychiatric hospitals in North Carolina filed a class action suit against the Secretary for Human Resources in the state of North Carolina in the case titled *Thomas S. v. Flaherty* (1988). Amongst the many complaints involving substandard care was one related to lack of education and inappropriate administration of antipsychotic drugs to patients in these state psychiatric facilities.

Professional and institutional nursing and medical standards clearly delineated a gap, thus pointing to the abhorrent practices around this medication issue. Physical examination of several patients in these state institutions by a physician expert in pharmacology revealed side effects caused by the antipsychotic drugs. Chart review further confirmed that these patients and/or patients' guardians were not informed about the risks, side effects, or benefits of the psychotropic medications. In addition, many of the patients who received these medications were not documented to have diagnoses in which antipsychotic drugs would even be indicated.

The court found that professional and institutional standards that provide that the patients and or patients' legal guardians be informed about the risks, side effects, and benefits of specific medications, including psychotropics, and that evidence of this instruction and the patient's response to it be documented in the patient's medical record, was not upheld. In fact, the care of these patients around the administration of and education regarding these medications was a gross violation of institutional and national professional standards. This case represents both medical and nursing malpractice. Clearly the nurse's role to educate patients and families was not upheld as evidenced by both the care delivered and by the lack of documentation regarding patient education and patient response to these medications.

The nurse's legal responsibility to educate and inform patients is contained within the Nurse Practice Acts, which have been developed by all 50 states. Not only do the Nurse Practice Acts protect the lay public from incompetent practitioners by establishing procedures for licensure, but most also define the practice of nursing. Six basic functions are covered by most Nurse Practice Acts; the one pertaining to the provision of health guidance and participation in health education establishes the foundation for the professional nurse's involvement in patient education.

ETHICAL FOUNDATION OF INFORMED CONSENT

The doctrine of informed consent has strong ethical bases. Principalism (specifically the principle of autonomy), care ethics, and character ethics (virtue ethics) provide an ethical foundation to the doctrine (Box 6-1).

Principalism

Faden and Beauchamp (1986), acknowledged experts on the doctrine of informed consent, discuss the ethical foundation in detail. Autonomy and beneficence are the two principles that form the ethical foundation of informed consent. However, autonomy, or the right to self determination, is the major ethical foundation of informed consent. Each human being has a right to make an autonomous choice in the true sense of being informed (Powers, 1993). In health care provider-patient relationships, a duty exists based on the individual's right to make autonomous choices. For nurses, this means that patients have a right to be educated about their choices. Therefore, the principle of respect for autonomy is the primary ethical principle that drives the theory and process of informed consent.

Autonomy

Autonomy is associated with terminology, such as *privacy, voluntariness, self-mastery, choosing freely,* and *accepting responsibility for one's choices* (Faden & Beauchamp, 1986; Beauchamp & Childress, 1989). Informed consent has its roots in the principle of respect for patient autonomy. However, the definition of an *autonomous person* poses a challenge: no specific defining characteristics can be observed in every alleged autonomous person. Some general consensus exists that autonomous persons demonstrate self-directness, a sense of purpose, and act without the control of others. Thus, an autonomous person would make autonomous decisions; however, this is not always the case. A person with the assumed supposed capacity to act autonomously may or may not choose to make him or herself aware of critical information, or may be the victim of some temporary mental or physical disorder that prevents the execution of an autonomous act. Therefore, Faden and Beauchamp (1986) distinguish between *autonomous persons* and *autonomous actions.* Because informed consent and informed refusal represent actions, the focus with informed consent is on autonomous action rather than on autonomous persons. Faden and Beauchamp (1986) and Beauchamp and Childress (1989) further analyze autonomous action according to the concepts of intentionality, understanding, and control.

BOX 6-1. Ethical Foundations of Informed Consent

Principalism
  Autonomy
  Beneficence
Care Ethics
  Consider particulars, context, and relationships
Character (Virtue) Ethics
  Compassion
  Discernment
  Trustworthiness
  Integrity

Intentionality

Intentionality is defined in two parts: The first is the idea of a thought or an intention, which is explained as a desire by a person to perform a particular action. However, desire alone does not constitute entirely the definition of intentionality. Persons may intend to do many things, and never proceed to do so. This leads to the second component of the definition, which is the action. Faden and Beauchamp (1986) say that only if an action occurs with an intention to perform the action, is the action an intentional action (p. 242). An intentional action is deliberate and is performed after being consciously planned by the executioner of the action.

Understanding

Autonomous actions are also analyzed in terms of understanding, suggesting that persons who perform autonomous actions have a reasonable grasp of the specific features of the action and of the possible consequences. This condition can be considered on a continuum from *perfect understanding* to *no understanding*. One may argue that most patients can never achieve total understanding. Even patients who are health care providers cannot be versed in the theoretical and technical knowledge of all medical specialties. Thus, a health care provider who offers treatment may possibly only understand the intervention to the degree that knowledge has been discovered and made available in that field. For patients, there must be a substantial satisfaction of this condition of understanding, meaning that enough information is understood by the patient to make a reasonably informed choice (Beauchamp & Childress, 1989). The amount of information to satisfy the substantial satisfaction standard is probably context dependent.

Control

Autonomous actions also are analyzed by the external control to which the person making the decision is subject. The health care provider must be comfortable that the patient making the decision is doing so of his or her own volition. As participants in society, people are influenced by the institutions (eg, religious group, family, ethnic group, government) to which they belong. We have degrees of control to which we, as members of a society, are subject. Human beings are social and have a desire to be independent and a part of institutions or groups. Therefore, some degree of external influence may always influence informed consent decisions. This, too, is a context-dependent variable, and an autonomous action occurs with reasonable affirmation of the absence of external control on the individual who makes the decision (Beauchamp & Childress, 1989).

Unlike understanding and control, which can be analyzed in terms of reasonable degree on a continuum, intentionality must be a Yes or a No. Intentionality is not a matter of degree; it is either present or it is not (Faden & Beauchamp, 1986). Fulfillment of all three criteria constitute what Faden and Beauchamp (1986) regard as the moral definition of informed consent. That is, informed consent is the autonomous authorization of an intervention by a patient, which occurs when the patient with substantial understanding, and in substantial lack of control by others, intentionally authorizes a professional to do something (p. 278). Effective consent, however, is defined as fulfilling the policy requirements of institutions, which have rules and regulations governing informed consent (Beauchamp & Childress, 1989, p. 280).

Beneficence

Beneficence is the second ethical principle that constitutes moral grounding for informed consent. Essentially, beneficence is the idea that health care providers ought to do good for patients. Beneficence has been a mainstay in the health professions. As nurses, we assume an obligation to do good. Before the patient rights' movement, the actions of all health care providers were primarily governed by the principle of beneficence. Beauchamp and Childress (1989) outline four elements of this principle:

1. One ought not to inflict evil or harm.
2. One ought to prevent evil or harm.
3. One ought to remove evil or harm.
4. One ought to do or promote good.

Reliance on the beneficence principle alone regarding informed consent welcomes paternalism to run amok. Paternalism is defined as the health care provider deciding what is best for the patient, as a parent would decide what is best for a child. In the past, health care delivery based on beneficence was considered acceptable and well-intentioned care. However, in the age of patient rights (1972), the principle of beneficence cannot stand as the sole principle by which members of the health professions guide their practice (Madder, 1997).

Although beneficence is a foundational value, in most cases autonomy is considered the primary principle, particularly when dealing with the conscious competent patient or the incompetent patient who has left evidence of his or her intentions regarding health care decisions via an advance directive or health care proxy (1990). In addition, exceptions to the informed consent doctrine, which are outlined later in the chapter, wherein it can be seen that beneficence plays a *prima facie* (ie, overriding or primary) role.

The American Nurses Association Code for Nurses with Interpretive Statements (1985) reflects evidence of development based on the principles of autonomy and beneficence (Box 6-2). Patient education is a cornerstone nursing intervention and provides an avenue for the nurse to fulfill the tenets of the Code for Nurses. In the role of patient educator, the nurse can assess the patient and family's level of knowledge about a particular health care issue, and proceed to provide information that fills in the gaps for the patient and family.

BOX 6-2. American Nurses Association Code for Nurses

1. The nurse provides services with respect for human dignity and the uniqueness of the client, unrestricted by considerations of social or economic status, personal attributes, or the nature of the health problems.
2. The nurse safeguards the client's right to privacy by judiciously protecting confidential information.
3. The nurse safeguards the client and the public when health care and safety are affected by the incompetent, unethical, or illegal practice of any person.
4. The nurse assumes responsibility and accountability for individual nursing judgments and actions.
5. The nurse maintains competence in nursing.
6. The nurse exercises informed judgment and uses individual competence and qualifications as criteria in seeking consultation, accepting responsibilities, and delegating nursing activities to others.
7. The nurse participates in activities that contribute to the ongoing development of the profession's body of knowledge.
8. The nurse participates in the profession's efforts to implement and improve standards of nursing.
9. The nurse participates in the profession's efforts to establish and maintain conditions of employment conducive to high quality nursing care.
10. The nurse participates in the profession's effort to protect the public from misinformation and misrepresentation and to maintain the integrity of nursing.
11. The nurse collaborates with members of the health professions and other citizens to promote community and national efforts to meet the health needs of the public.

Note. From *Code for Nurses With Interpretive Statements,* American Nurses Association, 1985, Washington, D.C.: Author. Reprinted with permission.

Patients can make autonomous decisions only if given the information that they need to do so. Whether it is in the role of facilitator in respect to medical interventions, or as primary practitioner for independent nursing interventions, the nurse plays a key role in assisting patients and families to arrive at informed decisions.

Care Ethics

Beyond principalism (Beachump & Childress, 1986), a care ethic (Fry, 1994; Gilligan, 1987; Noddings, 1984; VanHooft, 1999) offers additional support to the ethical and philosophical foundation to informed consent. Caring has been described as the essence of nursing practice (Watson, 1985). Nurses are concerned with a patient's response to his or her illnesses (Gordon, 1993). A caring framework emphasizes the aspects of a patient's life situation and how these aspects are affected and influenced by their clinical diagnoses. Relationships are valued in a care ethic. These relationships include those that exist between patients and their family members and those among patients, families, and health care providers.

The particulars of a patient's situation and the relationships in which a patient finds him or herself play a role in the informed consent process. Nurses and other health care providers must be aware of the influence that they and the family may have on a patient's decisions. A case described by Mallary, Gert, and Culver (1986) alerts nurses to the coercive effects that a family member may have on a patient's decision regarding electroconvulsive therapy. What role are such influential persons having on patients? What role ought nurses to play in guarding against the coercive effects of family members to patients? Many of these questions are difficult to answer, and must be considered on a case by case basis.

Character Ethics (Virtue Ethics)

Character ethics, or virtue ethics, described in full by Pellegrino (1993, 1995) refers to an ethic of the good person (i.e., a person who can be relied upon habitually to be good and to do good under all circumstances). The emphasis in virtue ethics is on the agent and his or her possession of virtues. A virtue is a character trait under rational control, a conscious disposition to act in a certain way. Pellegrino (1995) states that health care providers who execute their activities with thought and care make their professions good, or virtuous.

Virtuous Traits

Health care providers should have many desirable character traits. Four character traits that are considered virtuous and that have an impact on the ethical nature of how the informed consent process is performed include the following:

- Compassion
- Discernment
- Trustworthiness
- Integrity

Compassion combines an attitude of active concern for a person with a simultaneous sympathy and discomfort regarding the individual's suffering. Compassion is expressed outwardly by the nurse and is experienced by the recipient. Compassion, although perhaps difficult to measure, makes an important moral difference in the care of patients. The recipient of compassion feels reassured. As applied to the process of informed consent, compassion allows us to appreciate the patient's circumstance, and to consider how the proposed treatment (nursing, medical, or surgical) would fit, given the patient's unique situation.

Discernment combines sensitive insight with judgment and understanding, leading to decisive action on the part of the nurse. The discerning nurse is not distracted by his or her own personal attachments, fears, or other extraneous circumstances. A discerning nurse recognizes what is called for in a situation, and responds accordingly. Relative to informed consent: Does the patient need more information than another might? Does the patient need some private time to reflect upon the information provided? Would it benefit the patient to meet another person who has had a heart transplant or who has survived the side effects of the proposed chemotherapy? Would the patient benefit from gentle persuasion given his or her fears? These questions are raised by a discerning nurse who can truly help the patient and family in making the best decision for the patient's unique circumstances.

Trustworthiness is a virtue that patients might fear is dwindling between health care providers and themselves, given the conflicts that health care providers experience in managed care. To trust another means that one can expect that the other will act with the right motives in accord with moral norms. Is the procedure or therapy being proposed the best one for the patient? Is cost a factor and one of which the patient is unaware? Does the nurse know that another health care provider has a better track record with a particular proposed treatment for a patient? In considering these questions, the nurse must ask: *To whom am I accountable?*

Moral integrity as a virtue provides a summary description of the virtuous health care provider. An individual with moral integrity manifests a balanced integration of self (eg, emotions, knowledge, and aspirations). A person of integrity stands faithful to moral values and is sensitive to threat of such values for the patients for whom he or she cares. Sensitivity alone is not enough. The nurse must manifest one's integrity through actions to defend the vulnerable other; for the nurse, the vulnerable other is the patient in his or her charge. As patient advocates, nurses must support the ethical process of informed consent with patients and their families. Nurses must recognize when they are being asked to violate established trust with patients and/or breach their own integrity to protect wrongdoing on the part of another professional.

A Wisconsin court case provides an example of a breach in moral integrity (Tammelleo, 1997b). Amy Mathias had a Caesarian section under general anesthesia. After the baby was delivered, the obstetrician, Dr. Witt, asked the operating room nurses for instruments to perform a tubal ligation. Operating room nurses Snyder and Perri searched the chart for a signed informed consent for tubal ligation, and found none. They informed Dr. Witt, who acknowledged their statement. Dr. Witt went ahead and performed the tubal ligation. Three days after the procedure, Nurse Paula Yurchak brought an informed consent document to Ms. Mathias, which was backdated to the day of the tubal ligation, and asked Ms. Mathias to sign it, to "just close up our records" (p.1). Nurse Yurchak had forged the signature of Nurse Perri in the witness section of the consent form. The patient brought suit against Dr. Witt and others, claiming that the tubal ligation procedure was performed without her consent.

The Wisconsin court was clear that informed consent for medical and surgical procedures is the physician's responsibility, and that the nurses fulfilled their responsibilities of ordinary care by informing Dr. Witt that the consent for tubal ligation was not in the record. The decision of the Wisconsin court in *Mathias v. St. Catherine's Hosp.* (1997, Tammelleo, 1997b) demonstrated that nurses are not legally bound to obtain informed consent from patients for procedures clearly within the domain of medicine and surgery. However, the conduct of Nurse Yurchak in participating in a cover-up, although ignored by the court, was "unethical, illegal and unconscionable" (Tammelleo, 1997b). Nurse Yurchak unfortunately compromised her own moral integrity by participating in a cover-up, for which she and other nurses had no responsibility. Nurses and other health care providers must remain strong when faced with unethical forces.

THE FIVE ELEMENTS OF INFORMED CONSENT

Beauchamp and Childress (1989) define informed consent as described in the President's Commission Report on Making Health Care Decisions (1982) as consisting of five elements:

1. Competence
2. Disclosure

3. Understanding
4. Voluntariness
5. Consent

Fig. 6-1 depicts the interrelationship between the process of informed consent in terms of its five elements to the process of patient education.

Competence

The concept of competence has generated a great deal of discussion as it relates to informed consent. Jurchak (1990) summarizes four general categories of competency as described by Applebaum and Grisso (1988) (the ability to communicate choices, the ability to understand relevant information, the ability to appreciate the situation and its consequences, and the ability to manipulate information rationally). Nurses as patient educators are familiar with these conceptual areas. Baseline assessment of the patient's mental status and ability to understand and manage new information is an essential first step for the nurse who is planning to educate and inform patients.

The landmark work of Roth, Meisel, and Lidz (1977) on competency identified five categories of competency tests commonly used in practice: making a choice, reasonable outcome of choice, choice based on rational reasons, ability to understand, and actual understanding. In addition, their work has demonstrated that the same subject may be found competent or incompetent depending on the measure used.

Research on the element of competence assessment has been conducted. Cohen, McCue, and Green (1993) demonstrated that intensive care unit nurses' and physician residents' clinical assessments of competency of critically ill patients correlated with one another's assessments, and those of researchers who administered the Mini Mental Status Exam to 200 crit-

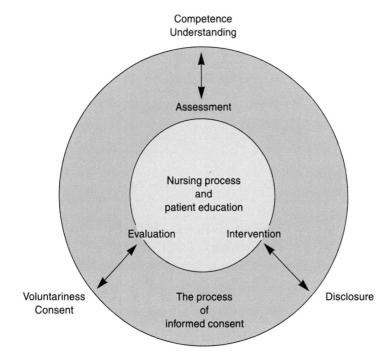

FIGURE 6-1. The relationship of patient education to informed consent.

ically ill patients. Further study of clinical assessment of patient competence that employed specific questions to assess capacity compared to assessment with the Mini Mental Status Exam, was evaluated on 100 inpatients who faced a major medical treatment decision or an invasive medical procedure (Etchells, Darzins, Silberfeld, Singer, McKenny, Naglie, Katz, Guyatt, Molloy, & Strang, 1999). The researchers found that assessment of capacity with both approaches highly correlated. They recommend focused questions to guide in capacity assessment. Such questions should generally include an assessment of the patient's understanding of the problem, the proposed treatment, alternatives to proposed treatment, the option to refuse treatment, fore-seeable consequences of accepting treatment, and finally, the ability to reach a decision that is not substantially based on hallucinations, delusions or cognitive signs of depression.

A study conducted by Fowles and Fox (1995) concerned practices related to reassessment and documentation of competence as the initial element of informed consent doctrine in chronic care facilities. These researchers surveyed 200 facilities that cared for brain-injured patients to learn about the facilities' procedures and practices to obtain competency assessment of patients as related to procedures performed on patients. Only 25% of the facilities surveyed stated that they reassessed and documented patient competence on a regular basis.

Brabbins, Butler, and Bentall (1996) discussed the dilemma of administering neuroleptic medications to acute psychiatric patients when their competence to provide consent to such treatment is in question. This dilemma weighs the benefits of symptom reduction against the burdens of side effects. An ethical justification in this scenario is the exercise of therapeutic privilege described by Faden and Beauchamp (1986) as the right of a health care provider to withhold information because of the harmful effects of the disclosure on the patient. Another justification is the fact that the patient is incompetent to make a rational decision. A risk-benefit analysis exists for the health care providers to consider in the administration of neuroleptic medications. Tardive dyskinesia, a side effect of these drugs, manifests as involuntary motor movements especially of the face, lips, and tongue, and can be permanent. However, Rachlin (1974) addresses the fact the person who is psychotic has no freedom, suggesting that paternalistic intervention preserves a wider range of freedom from psychosis. The problem of autonomy conflicting with beneficence is not readily solved, even after the objective of treatment (ie, no acute psychiatric episode) is achieved. Is the patient now competent to make a decision regarding continued pharmacological treatment? Is the therapeutic privilege still justified? Difficult as these cases may be, psychiatric nurses, in conjunction with patients' family members, are in an important position to assess the competency of psychiatric patients, given their constant attendance with the patient.

Disclosure

Disclosure is defined as the legal obligation of professionals to share information that professionals and patients usually consider material in deciding whether to consent to or to refuse an intervention. Disclosure includes the health care professional's recommendation, the purpose of seeking consent, and the nature of consent as authorization (Beauchamp & Childress, 1994). Three standards of disclosure have been described: the *professional practice standard,* the *reasonable person standard* and the *subjective standard.*

Professional Practice Standard

This standard states that adequate disclosure is determined by traditional practices of the professional community. Faden and Beauchamp (1986) articulate three problems with this standard of disclosure:

1. It may be questionable to what degree a standard exists.
2. A negligent standard could exist and be upheld.
3. A practice standard can undermine a patient's autonomous choice, because an individual's unique situation cannot be reduced to what the professional community holds as sacred.

Application of this standard in court would require expert professional testimony.

Reasonable Person Standard

This standard (Beauchamp & Childress, 1989) states that the type of and amount of information to be disclosed is determined by reference to a hypothetical reasonable person. This standard shifts the focus from the health care provider to the patient. The difficulty lies in ascertaining what a reasonable person would want to know. Interpretation of the reasonable person standard in court leaves the practitioner at the mercy of the jury, who in a particular case would be in the position to judge the adequacy of this standard (Faden & Beauchamp, 1986).

Subjective Standard

This standard (Beauchamp & Childress, 1989) describes information disclosure specific to the needs of the individual patient. This is a preferable moral standard of disclosure, because it espouses the principle of respect for autonomy. The subjective standard considers individual needs, which are crucial in decision-making. Those who oppose this standard claim it places an unfair burden on the practitioner, leaving the practitioner at the mercy of the patient.

In our opinion, the subjective standard is consistent with the philosophical position of nurses. Nurses are concerned with the impact of illness on the lifestyles of their patients. The holistic patient assessment framework espoused by nursing addresses the subjective standard of disclosure. That is, the nurse assesses with the patient the impact of illness on that patient's lifestyle and, therefore, is in a position to tailor disclosure to the individual patient and family in collaboration with medicine.

Research on Disclosure

Research studies that address disclosure have been reported. Farkas (1992) reported on a study of informed consent in utilizing therapeutic paradox as an approach to therapy. Farkas (1992) defined therapeutic paradox as reverse psychology in which a client is told not to change, as a way to get the client to change. This author cited several cases in which this approach has been successful, such as in school phobia, marital therapy, and therapy for the chronically mentally ill. The concern with this type of therapy is the lack of informed consent that is inherent in the paradoxical procedure. If the therapist informs the patient, the therapy is not as likely to be effective. Farkas designed an exploratory study that examined the responses of 34 non-psychiatric outpatients to a request for hypothetical informed consent for therapeutic paradox. Sixty-six percent of this sample never had sought counseling, and 27% were currently in counseling. After reviewing the detailed consent form and a vignette describing a successful case, in which therapeutic paradox was used, 81% agreed to consent to therapy using this technique. Their qualitative comments, however, revealed internal reservations. The results of this study raise questions regarding the reservations that patients may have when they sign informed consent documents.

Studies on physicians' beliefs and practices regarding disclosure suggest discrepancies in point of view regarding what information ought to be disclosed to patients. Newton, Hawes, Jamidar, Harig, and Lehman (1994) surveyed members of a gastrointestinal physicians' organization regarding disclosure practices regarding endoscopic retrograde cholangiopancreatography (ERCP). These researchers found that although physicians agreed that risks (eg, bleeding, perforation, pancreatitis) should be disclosed, physicians did not agree whether risks for surgery, prolonged hospital stay, or risk of death ought to be shared. In their survey of 39 hip specialists regarding a particular hip replacement procedure, Dodd, Donegan, Kernohan, Geary, and Mollan (1993) found that consensus did not exist in terms of the amount of information to share with patients considering this hip replacement procedure. These discrepancies in agreement point to the importance of nurses, in their collaborative role, to be present with the physician whenever possible while he or she discloses information to patients.

Understanding

Beauchamp and Childress (1994) identify understanding as the third element defining informed consent. Powers (1993) argues that decisions made without understanding cannot be autonomous in the true sense. This component of informed consent has been addressed in research.

Hughes (1993), in an exploratory study, examined the relationship between information about breast cancer treatment alternatives and patients' choices of treatment. A convenience sample of 71 females with stage I or II breast cancer was drawn from a breast clinic affiliated with a large tertiary care medical center. The amount of information provided to each subject and the nature of its presentation was tracked using an observer checklist. To determine recall of information and final decision for treatment, the researcher conducted telephone interviews 6 weeks to 8 weeks after surgery. Results indicated that treatment decision was related to the information that the women gained from sources other than health care providers, such as lay media, relatives, and educational brochures before the clinic visit. The results also indicated that patients' recall of information about treatments and related risks was abysmal. Results of this study strongly support the importance of assess-

ing the patient's current level of knowledge and understanding before intervening with information.

Meade and Howser (1992) investigated the reading level estimates of cancer clinical trial consent forms from 44 active studies of the National Cancer Institute. Readability estimates for each consent form were calculated by the Minnesota Interactive Readability Approximation computer program, a standardized program that randomly evaluates the readability of passages from a document. Regarding the consent forms analyzed, readability estimates were from grade 12 to grade 17.5, with a mean grade level of 14.3. These study results have implications for nursing in that nurses frequently assume a role in management and implementation of research protocols. Nurses must play a more active role in developing readable forms, assisting patients to understand what is being explained to them and ultimately asked of them to participate in research.

Sorrell (1991) conducted a study that reviewed the effects of writing and speaking on comprehension of information for informed consent. A posttest-only control group design was used. Eighty participants were randomly assigned to one of three groups: a writing group, a speaking group, and a comparison group. Those in the writing and speaking groups were asked to write or speak, respectively, regarding their impressions, questions, and concerns after reading an informed consent document requesting them to participate in a breast self examination treatment program. After completing their assigned task (or in the case of the control group, 45 minutes after reading the consent form), subjects were asked to complete a 20-item posttest. Results were statistically significant: The writing group scored the highest (range 11–20); the speaking group scores ranged from 8 to 20 and the comparison group scores ranged 7 to 19. Results of this study indicate that the modalities of writing and speaking may be effective and practical interventions to enhance the patient's understanding of the content of informed consent.

Silva (1993) summarized her empirical research on patient comprehension of information for informed consent. Provider-specific factors that promoted comprehension included presentation in a brief and direct manner, information presented by a nurse or health care team, allowing subjects to keep information from 1 day to 3 days, and provider requests for immediate patient recall of information. Subject-specific factors that promoted comprehension included: 1) the perception that the amount of information was "just right," and that the information was presented clearly; 2) higher educational and vocabulary levels; 3) not being confined to bed; and 4) a positive opinion toward the need for informed consent forms. Provider-specific factors that inhibited comprehension included presentation of complex or threatening information and presentation of information by the physician alone. Subject-specific factors that inhibited comprehension included being confined to bed because of illness, erroneous and or selective recall, no strong opinions about the need for informed consent forms, lower educational and vocabulary levels, perception that the amount of information received was too much or too little, and a perception that the explanation was unclear.

Meade (1999) provides a research-based review of those factors that affect a patient's comprehension of informed consent information. These factors include the patient's amount of formal education, vocabulary level, age, literacy skills, and cognitive biases of quantitative and qualitative probability, and the method of presentation and the nature of the information presented. Neptune, Hopper, and Matthews (1994) add that previous experience with a procedure promotes the patient's understanding when faced with it again. Meade (1999) also made several suggestions to improve a patient's understanding. These suggestions include integration of teaching principles when designing informational sessions for patients, building relationships with patients that foster assessment of the patient's knowledge and attitudes toward treatment, and including a family member or a friend in the informational session. Nurses who practice with a holistic philosophy are particularly attuned to Meade's suggestions.

Voluntariness and Consent

The remaining two elements specified by Beauchamp and Childress (1989) include voluntariness and consent, or authorization. Voluntariness is the patient's ability to act independently of manipulation or coercion. Consent, the final element in informed consent, is the patient giving the practitioner permission to perform the specific procedure or therapy. Relative to voluntariness, patients may be unduly influenced by health care providers, family members, or both to consent to procedures or research.

Hewlett (1996) studied patient perception of pressure to participate in clinical trials. Patients diagnosed with rheumatoid arthritis were asked to participate in a clinical trial. Those who agreed to participate were asked to rate, on a visual analog scale, the difficulty they anticipated in receiving their usual care if they did not consent. Conversely, those who did not consent were asked to rate the difficulty they experienced in receiving their usual care given that they had refused participation. Patients who refused to consent to the trial reported less difficulty than those who agreed thought they would have experienced if they refused to participate. The results suggest that at least some patients who consent to research trials may not do so based on a psychological process free from perceptions of coercion.

Mallary, Gert, and Culver conducted a case study (1986) regarding a woman who thought she could not refuse electroshock treatment despite her husband's desire that she have the treatment. The study raises the question of the impact of family coercion. The health care providers in this case believed, based on reports from the patient, that the patient's husband coerced her to have the treatments. Health care providers questioned the validity of the informed consent for this woman. They wondered to what degree were they obligated to impose upon, perhaps longstanding patterns of relationship, with the patient and her husband.

Some published research has addressed the entire process of informed consent. Nusbaum and Chenitz (1990) conducted a qualitative study examining the observed process of informed consent to ascertain if the process fit with the five elements. Subjects in the study were 16 dyads of researcher and research subjects, consisting of four physicians, seven registered nurses, and five research assistants. The findings revealed a poor fit between the elements of informed consent and the interactions during the formal consent interviews. Only the theoretical concept of disclosure was recognizable during an early stage in the researcher-subject interview. The results of this study raise serious questions regarding the implementation of the theoretical elements of informed consent to real life practice.

An anecdotal report in the literature provides a clinical example of the absent theoretical elements in actual practice. Erde (1999) provided the personal account of a medical ethicist, who served as his own case example, by living through the process of informed consent. Although knowledgeable in the theoretical elements of informed consent, the ethicist chose to experience how the physician and other health care providers actualized the doctrine in their practice, specifically related to his case. The ethicist found that the theoretical doctrine of informed consent was hardly noticeable in his case. Minimal information was disclosed to him in terms of what the procedure (nasal septoplasty) would be like and the discomfort he was likely to experience postoperatively. This was coupled with little attempt on the physician's part to establish a trusting, caring relationship, and availability for questions. Overall, this patient's experience was abysmal, largely because of the lack of relationship and inattention to the ethical requirements of the informed consent process.

Agre, McKee, Gargon, & Kurtz (1997) studied patient satisfaction with the process of informed consent in a group of patients scheduled for colonoscopy and endoscopy. Their sample consisted of 204 patients and 102 family members. The study intervention was a videotape and physician discussion before their procedures, followed by a questionnaire that sought to compare this experience of informed consent with past experiences. Most participants reported that they preferred both methods, rather than one.

The process of informed consent is just that—a process. Nurses who see it as a process can best assist patients and families with internalizing the information needed to make decisions that are consonant with their lifestyles and best interests. Berry, Dodd, Hinds, & Ferrell (1996) emphasized that informed consent is not simply a signature on a form, but an ongoing process that nurses can facilitate in a positive way for patients and families through attentiveness to the uniqueness of each patient's needs in the process of patient education.

EXCEPTIONS TO INFORMED CONSENT

Wear (1998) outlined four exceptions to the doctrine of informed consent:

1. Emergency
2. Incompetence
3. Waiver
4. Therapeutic privilege

These exceptions are important for the nurse to consider in his or her role as patient educator, so that he or she can recognize appropriate and inappropriate applications of these exceptions. Wear presented each of these exceptions in terms of how specific evaluative approaches for each exception either preserve or pose threats to self-determination or the ability to gain informed consent. By keeping the purpose of informed consent (ie, enabling patients and families to decide on therapy based on clear, accurate information of risks and benefits) in the forefront, the health care provider can clearly evaluate exceptions to the doctrine in the context of preserving patient autonomy.

Emergency

In an emergency, it is generally thought that a patient would desire the type of medical care that would return that patient to a healthy state. Meisel (1979) differentiated emergency situations from those when the patient is competent (eg, if a limb were severed yet the patient can communicate) to those when the patient is incompetent (eg, when the patient is unconscious because of a motor vehicle accident).

Health care providers also must struggle with how much to disclose to a patient who is competent, yet severely injured and in need of immediate treatment with serious risks. Meisel (1979) used the term *urgency* to assist the health care provider in further delineating an emergency. The concept of urgency helps professionals focus on the consequences that a person would endure if he or she were delayed treatment. Meisel advocated a narrow definition of the emergency exception to those circumstances when the delay of treatment until informed consent could be obtained would result in serious harm to the patient. By advising a narrow definition, Meisel felt that individual patient autonomy is best preserved.

Legal Cases

Tamelleo (1998) reports a case (*Connelly v. Warner*, 670 N.Y.S. 2d 293 1998) involving a man who was intubated emergently, and who subsequently developed adult respiratory distress syndrome from aspiration of stomach contents. The patient sued, claiming that he was not informed of the risks inherent in the procedures. The court contended that the procedure was performed in an emergency, so the physician and hospital were not held liable.

A case currently on appeal challenges the right of a physician to impose treatment in an emergency when a patient refuses treatment. In the case of *Estate of Catherine Shine v. Jose Vega and Massachusetts General Hospital* (*1993*) (Medical Staff Registry, 1999), Ms. Shine, a 29-year-old with asthma, went to the Massachusetts General Hospital emergency room seeking medical care for an asthma at-

tack. A physician treated Ms. Shine initially with conservative measures, which he believed were unsuccessful. The physician then proceeded with intubation, despite the patient's refusals, because he believed that her condition was life-threatening. An initial court ruling favored the physician and the hospital, citing the emergency exception. This ruling was not upheld, however, at the Massachusetts State Supreme Court. The reasoning provided at the Supreme Court level was that the emergency exception applies only in cases when the patient is unable to provide informed consent. In this case, Ms. Shine had refused treatment. The case has been ordered back to the trial court to decide disposition, given the Massachusetts Supreme Court's ruling (Davis, 1999).

When considering the emergency exception coupled with incompetence, the role of the family cannot be underestimated as providers of information regarding what the patient might want. With the implementation of the Patient Self-Determination Act in 1990, some patients have stated their wishes for care in the form of an Advance Directive or through a designated health care proxy who is frequently, although not always, a family member. If the patient's wishes are known, it is the obligation of the health care provider to honor such wishes.

Waiver

Patient waiver is another exception to the informed consent doctrine identified by Meisel (1979). He reported that for at least four decades, the Supreme Court has defined *waiver* as a voluntary and temporary relinquishment of a known right. In patient education and informed consent, a waiver might apply if it were recommended by a physician that a patient have open heart surgery, and the patient agreed to the surgery but declined learning about the risks, benefits, and postoperative care. With waivers, it is crucial that the patient clearly understands that he or she has the right to information regarding proposed treatments, risks and benefits, and alternatives to therapy, with the right to accept or refuse such therapy. Again, the patient's family can be a useful resource in these situations.

Savulescu and Momeyer (1997) argued that health care providers have a responsibility to convince patients that rational deliberation about their options is important, and necessary, thus negating waiver as an option. Beauchamp and Childress (1989) presented the potential solution of setting up rules against waivers for the purposes of protecting patients, with committees to determine the appropriateness of allowing a waiver in a specific patient context. Again, the intent is to preserve patient autonomy by keeping limits around the waiver exception.

Therapeutic Privilege

Therapeutic privilege is invoked when a health care provider, most frequently a physician, decides that disclosure of information to a patient would prove to be more harmful than helpful to the patient in coming to an informed decision, and proceeds to carry out an intervention or withholds an intervention without the patient's consent. This paternalistic practice violates the patient's autonomy. Acceptance of this practice constitutes an abuse of Patient's Rights (1972). This approach also has tremendous potential for abuse because it shifts the decision-making power from the patient to the provider. With increased recognition of patient involvement in decision-making, therapeutic privilege as an exception to informed consent has diminished; when practiced, it is difficult to justify.

SPECIAL CONSIDERATIONS IN INFORMED CONSENT

The Impact of Culture

Respect for autonomy as the main ethical basis for informed consent may conflict with the norms of various cultural groups. The right to self-determination has served as an ethical and legal justification of the clinical practice of informed consent and, through the past several decades, the American health care system has honored the value of self-determination (Friedlander, 1995).

However, cultural groups who have recently immigrated to the United States, or those who have lived here, but perhaps have not assimilated entirely into American culture, may require unique assessment of their needs in relation to informed consent. Research and case study report have demonstrated that autonomy may not be a predominant value in some groups when making health care decisions. Agard, Finkelstein, & Wallach (1998) presented the case of a recently-immigrated, young, highly educated, financially sound Eastern European couple confronted with decisions about intervention to treat the wife's chronic pelvic condition (an intervention that could alter her ability to conceive). Health care providers assessed that the wife was concerned with the potential of the surgical procedure rendering her sterile, but that she was influenced by her husband's strong opinion to proceed with the surgery and to not consider other possible options. In such a case, what should the nurse do? Should the nurse indicate the wife's expressed concern regarding the surgery in the setting of a happy marriage that recognizes and accepts the husband as the major decision-maker? Would the nurse compromise the marriage in doing so? How does an assimilated American nurse reconcile his or her own values in such a situation? Nurses must carefully consider cultural issues that affect the process of informed consent as they educate patients and families regarding proposed procedures.

Blackhall, Murphy, Frank, Michel, & Azen (1995) found that a discrepancy in desire for health care information was present in European Americans and African Americans as opposed to Mexican Americans and Korean Americans. The two former groups were more likely to believe that patients should be truthfully informed and involved in decisions regarding their diagnosis, prognosis, and choices for life-sustaining treatment, whereas the latter two groups showed less value for truth in prognosis or participation in choices related to life-sustaining treatment. In a study of the Navajo Indian culture, Carrese and Rhodes (1995) found that the concepts of beauty, order, goodness, and harmony were important considerations for this group in learning about their illnesses and potential treatments. How, then, might the nurse and physician proceed as a team, in apprising such groups of their options for treatment—honestly, directly, or couched within the contexts of their cultures? Would such couching represent an enactment of the subjective standard of disclosure? Would the nurse's and physician's judgment hold up in the American justice system, which prizes self-determination as the standard?

Through their research with Latino, Chinese, and Anglo American patients, Barnes, Davis, Moran, Portillo, & Koenig (1998) emphasized that language barriers alleviated by interpreters are imperfect, because the interpreter's values and interpretations are interposed between the patient and health care provider. These researchers recommend that interpreters and health care providers, whenever possible, convene several times around a specific patient case to learn one another's approach and to identify strategies to minimize interpreter and health care provider bias. Barnes et al. (1998) also caution health care providers to recognize that their own values (and thus goals for care) may not coincide with specific cultural groups. Health care providers must make every effort to learn the patient's goals of care and those of his or her family system.

The Tuskegee Syphilis Study

Care of African Americans in the American health care system, even today, has been profoundly influenced by the Tuskegee Syphilis Study, described in detail by Brandt (1997). This study, which proposed to learn the natural course of syphilis in black males, was initiated in 1932 by the United States Public Health Service, and spanned 40 years before being halted. Subjects in the study were illiterate males from Macon County, Alabama. A

black nurse, Eunice Rivers Laurie, was employed as research nurse for the study, and was instrumental in recruitment and follow-up of the men. Nurse Rivers' role is critically analyzed by Reverby (1999).

The Tuskegee Syphilis Study is noted for its egregious lack of respect of the self determination of the men who participated. The participants were deceived, even when penicillin, a known treatment for syphilis, became available. When the U.S. government finally halted the study, a class action suit was brought against the government. Although some compensation was made, it was far short of the damages to these poor black men and their families (Jones, 1993). This study, amongst others, will forever be a negative mark on the record of the United States Public Health Service, and has been thought to contribute to a lack of trust of African Americans toward the white-dominated health care system (Dula, 1994; Gamble, 1997).

Americans are enriched by a multicultural society. However, as professionals we must realize the impact that our cultural history has on the evolution of informed consent in the United States, particularly as perceived by those whose heritage was victimized by prejudice. Because of this and the differing values held by various cultures, nurses must rely on an ethic of care and virtue that supports moral justification for the doctrine of informed consent. Nurses and other health care providers must work hard to learn the particulars, important relationships, and context within which the patients of non-American cultures come to the health care system, and through the process of patient education, support the doctrine of informed consent.

Informed Consent for Children and Adolescents

 Parents and legal guardians have legal responsibility for the children and adolescents for whom they are charged to care. As understood, ethical obligations sometimes surpass that for which we are legally responsible. Nurses and physicians who care for pediatric patients may not be satisfied with the legal requirement, and many parents and guardians also experience this lack of satisfaction. Children ought to be recognized, through the process of informed consent, through a developmental model.

A developmental model recognizes the importance of a child's assent to care and is a standard set forth by the American Academy of Pediatrics, Committee on Bioethics (1995). This standard is specific in that it provides practical applications regarding developmental level and accompanying procedures for which physicians ought to obtain informed permission from parents or guardians, assent of the pediatric patient and informed permission of parents, and informed consent of the teenage adolescent patient. Ross' (1997) critique of the document suggests that it might give too much power to pediatric patients. She argues that physicians and nurses involved in pediatric care should collaborate with parents and health care providers to provide the pediatric patient with age-appropriate explanations and the dignity of hearing their concerns. Children are on a continuum of development and thus should be seen as children evolving to adolescence, and then to young adulthood. Children are counted as persons, and therefore, consistent with changes in the evolution of doctrine of informed consent (Friedlander, 1995), which has moved from its paternalistic history; children are not just seen, but ought to be heard in a respectful way. ■

Weir and Peters (1997) provide some powerful case examples of adolescents who lived with chronic, terminal diseases and faced end of life decisions that required the legal informed consent of their parents or guardians. A brief summary of two cases illustrate the value of incorporating the adolescent's wishes into the care plan. A 15-year-old boy who lived courageously with cystic fibrosis required intensive respiratory care several times during his last year of life. He expressed his fear of suffocating and of dying an agonizing death on a respirator. Despite his expressed concerns, his parents insisted that he be intubated for his last decline; thus the boy spent a prolonged time experiencing that which he feared and that for which he did not assent. Conversely, an adolescent girl who heroically battled leukemia for approximately 4 years, when reaching the final stages, had her previous wishes honored by her parents when life-sustaining treatment was withdrawn after a short trial to assess reversal of body system failure.

The first case raises perceptions of moral distress for the boy's health care providers. Nurses, in their collaborative role, are the implementers of most of the life-sustaining technological interventions required by patients. Nurses are the ones who most directly experience the patient's distress, both physical and psychological, as aggressive care is implemented. Whenever possible, nurses ought to work closely with parents and physicians to devise a care plan that is reasonable and that reflects the goals of the child or adolescent patient. Through patient education, nurses can help pediatric patients and their parents to understand the particulars of the therapies under consideration.

Older Patients and Informed Consent

Ensuring that older patients truly understand proposed therapies poses a special consideration to nurses and health care providers. Sugarman, McCrory, & Hubal (1998) conducted a comprehensive review of literature regarding the process of informed consent as employed with older patients. Through their analysis, they concluded that a wide range of decision-making capacity exists amongst elders, but no effective strategy exists to quickly screen for patients who cannot participate in meaningful informed consent.

Disclosure is affected by multiple factors, such as the patient-provider relationship, the time available for disclosure, preliminary decisions made by elders, their perceived vulnerability, and no other available treatment choices. Sugarman, McCrory, & Hubal (1998) plead that, in terms of disclosure, all patients should be asked formally if they have further questions about a proposed intervention before the closure of a patient-provider session. Alt-White (1995) summarized factors that may impede the process of informed consent with elders, such as a perceived lack of freedom to decide for oneself, lack of clarity of information, and impaired decision-making capacity. Older age and less formal education are repeatedly associated with impaired understanding (Agre, Kurtz, & Krauss, 1994; Daugherty, Ratain, & Grochowski, 1995).

Interventions that may facilitate the disclosure process with elders include providing the older patients with more time to absorb disclosed information; making allowances for the fatigue factor by scheduling shorter, more frequent sessions; providing written information in larger typeset to account for visual deficits; and frequent assessment of comprehension (Alt-White, 1995; Sugarman, McCrory, & Hubal, 1998). Most importantly, nurses and physicians must incorporate shared decision-making (Thomasma, 1999) into their interactions with elders. Older patients may require more in-depth nursing assessment to determine decision-making capacity and additional time for patient education to understand and appreciate the meaning of the procedures to which they, or their surrogates, have agreed. Nurses can be elder advocates through careful attention to the process of patient education.

End of Life Treatment

End of life treatment has gained an increasing amount of attention in medical and ethics literature. The Patient Self Determination Act [PSDA] (1990) has formally recognized, by law, the right of individuals to have their wishes for end of life treatment honored, if they cannot speak on their own behalf. End of life treatment requires the process of informed consent, because much life-sustaining technologies are often offered to patients directly or through their surrogates.

It is impossible to anticipate every scenario that may be encountered at end of life situations. Many diagnoses and accompanying aggressive or palliative measures might be proposed. Aggressive life-sustaining treatments include, but are not limited to, cardiopulmonary resuscitation, dialysis, artificial feeding and hydration, and antibiotic treatment. A growing body of research literature documents

the use and misuse of these life-sustaining treatments at end of life (Mahoney, Riley, Fry, & Field, 1999; Phillips, Wenger, Teno, Oye, Younger, Califf, Layde, Desbiens, Connors, & Lynn, 1996; Volicer, Brandeis, & Hurley, 1998).

Palliative Care

Palliative care nursing and medicine have become specialized, and options in this field address the holistic patient (World Health Organization, 1990; Hing-Mak & Clinton, 1999). Patients who reach this point are entitled to be informed about the benefits and burdens of aggressive therapies and the benefits of palliative care. Nurses who provide both aggressive and palliative care therapies to patients at end of life should have a working knowledge of the benefits and burdens, so that they can help patients and/or surrogates make informed decisions regarding treatment options. For example, in the case of artificial nutrition, does the patient realize that tube feedings, during the long term, are generally administered through a gastric tube, which requires surgery for placement? Does the patient and/or surrogate realize that the risk of aspiration pneumonia in some patient populations is not reduced with tube feedings (Meyers & Grodin, 1991)? Does the patient and family understand that long-term mechanical ventilation requires the surgical creation of a tracheostomy?

Cardiopulmonary Resuscitation

Cardiopulmonary resuscitation (CPR) deserves special mention as a life-sustaining treatment. The public often does not realize that admission to an acute care institution ensures the use of CPR as an intervention in the event of cardiac arrest. Even those who recognize the possibility of its use do not fully understand the complexity, and sequelae of this intervention. This was evidenced by findings in which investigators examined patients' preferences for level of life-sustaining treatment and found that most study participants responded that they would opt for resuscitation, but not mechanical ventilation, thus not realizing that the two are essential aspects of CPR (Everhart & Pearlman, 1990). In addition, the public is influenced by the portrayal of CPR on television, which provides an overly optimistic view of success and recovery (Diem, Lantos, & Tulsky, 1996). Most persons do not enter the hospital anticipating a cardiac arrest. However, the possibility exists, particularly with advancing age, increased number of comorbidities, and lengthy hospital stays (Schneidermayer, 1988).

Proxy Consent

Patients who can no longer speak on their own behalf are represented by a designated proxy whom they have selected before their incompetence; if they have not selected a proxy, their next of kin is named. Proxy consent is represented through surrogate decision-making models of substituted judgment and best interest.

The substituted judgment standard requires that the surrogate attempts to make decisions that the incapacitated person would make if he or she could make decisions on his or her own behalf (President's Commission, 1983). The ideal substituted judgment is one in which the patient's self determination is reflected, because the now-incompetent patient has previously stated that which he or she would want done relative to life-sustaining treatment. Making one's wishes known can be accomplished explicitly in writing or through previous verbal communication. A less satisfying form of substituted judgment is that which the proxy invokes when he or she does not know explicitly what the now-incompetent patient might want. The proxy applies the patient's preferences and values to treatment decisions based on knowledge of the person and his or her values in other contexts.

The best interests standard is invoked when a now-incapacitated person has failed to tell a surrogate his or her thoughts on treatment preferences, given any potential or actual condition. Unlike the substituted judgment standard, which rests in the principle of self-determination, the best interests standard expresses the principle of beneficence, or promotion of the patient's welfare through

decision-making by the surrogate. Factors that the surrogate ought to consider when making decisions for patients based on best interest include relief of suffering, preservation or restoration of functioning, and quality and extent of life sustained (President's Commission, 1983).

To operationalize the doctrine of informed consent with surrogates for the patients' benefit, nurses must be aware that the surrogate role is burdensome (Brock, 1996). Surrogates choose more aggressive treatment for their loved ones than they would for themselves (Pearlman, Uhlman, & Jecker, 1992). Nurses are in the best position to assist surrogates in sorting out these issues. In addition, nurses must advocate for the involvement of surrogates, particularly in long-term care. Auerswald, Charpentier, & Inouye (1997) evaluated the competence of 84 older patients in an institutional setting, and then reviewed their records to learn if procedures were performed on these patients, and if so, who provided informed consent. The researchers learned two important pieces of information: First, for the incompetent patients, there was poor documentation regarding assessment of incompetence. Second, surrogate consent was not obtained for procedures performed on the incompetent patient. Barton, Dennis, Harminder, Mallik & Orr (1996) found similar results of lack of surrogate involvement for procedures performed on elders institutionalized in long-term care. These study results suggest that attention to patient's dignity through involvement of surrogate decision-makers when appropriate was lacking.

A PHILOSOPHICAL POSITION FOR NURSING

The Collaborative Role

The nursing profession currently grapples with important issues related to informed consent (issues that are significant to the theoretical and scientific growth of the nursing profession). The dual role of nurses in collaborative and independent practice requires a unique and critical examination of current practices and future directions in the context of informed consent. In our collaborative role with physicians, the overemphasis on the act of witnessing (and in some cases obtaining) the signature of patients for physician performed treatments has blinded nursing to the real concerns (eg, the patient's true understanding of that disclosed to him or her). Nurses must conceptualize a new philosophy of informed consent (Davis & Underwood, 1989). It is not within the purview of the nurse to obtain consent from patients for a medical or surgical procedure that the physician will perform to satisfy the institution's policy for effective consent. The physician who will perform the procedure on the patient is responsible for obtaining the patient's informed consent, as demonstrated in the cases of *Foflygen v. R. Zemel, M. D.* (1992; Tammelleo, 1993a) and *Davis v. Hoffman* (1997; Tammelleo, 1997a) and supported by others in nursing (Richardson, 1993; Alderson, 1995).

More importantly, nurses who practice in the collaborative realm play a vital role in assuring that patients have a clear understanding of therapies (including risks and benefits) such that patients can make autonomous choices specific to their individual situation. The existential advocacy model described by Gadow (1983) is instructive in delineating a philosophical approach that may be applied to informed consent in the collaborative realm of nursing. Gadow conceptualizes the patient as if on a continuum, between consumerism and paternalism. When health care providers opt to take a consumerist view, they present the patient with a range of options with little regard to the patient's values and knowledge. The paternalistic view is at the other extreme, essentially making the choice for the patient who is vulnerable secondary to his or her plight.

The Existential Advocacy Model

The position of advocacy is based on the freedom of individual self determination as the highest value in the nurse-patient relationship. As a partner with the patient, the advocacy nurse comes to know the patient. The advocacy nurse can then help the patient learn what is needed to empower oneself as patient and make the best possible decision. This approach is essentially an operationalization of the subjective standard of disclosure.

The author believes that this philosophical position for the nurse regarding informed consent is consistent with the principle of self determination, the legal and ethical grounding of informed consent and patient education, and is supported by others in nursing (Albarran, 1996; Cameron, 1996). Adoption of this philosophical approach in nursing will clarify collaborative practice of nurses with physicians. Nurses can contribute to the informed consent process in a meaningful way that is consistent with their philosophical underpinnings and their professional roles.

The importance of informed consent in treatment is gaining increasing recognition in professions other than the medical profession (Clawson, 1994; Davis & Underwood, 1989; Rule & Veatch, 1993; Scofield, 1993). Nursing is one of those professions. Three reasons for informed consent becoming more recognized in nursing are the following:

1. Patients are much more aware of their active role in health care decision-making. This active role has been delineated in the President's Commission (1982) and through the Patient Self-Determination Act (1990).
2. Nursing interventions are becoming increasingly sophisticated, with the goal of achieving specific outcomes for patients.
3. Economic forces in health care will make patients more conscious of services they obtain from all health care providers.

Although less clear at this point, nurses are beginning to explore the ramifications of informed consent in their independent domain of practice. Davis and Underwood (1989) argued that attention to this issue will have positive outcomes that will enhance the autonomous nursing role in practice.

From a theoretical standpoint, the existential advocacy model (Gadow, 1983; 1989a; 1989b) fits well with informed consent in nursing practice in both the collaborative and independent domains. Clarification of this philosophical approach to informed consent will enhance the added value of nurses in collaboration with physicians. Attention to the implications of informed consent in our independent practice as nurses will contribute to a clearer definition of nursing practice for patients and nurses. Continued research using quantitative and qualitative methods to examine the elements of informed consent, as they relate to the subjective standard of disclosure and the connection of informed consent to the existential advocacy model, are recommended for the advancement of nursing science, and to nursing practice based on that science. Meade (1999) delineates several research questions that nurses might ask relative to the doctrine of informed consent. As patient and family educators, nurses will continue to be in the best position to evaluate the knowledge and comprehension that patients and families have regarding their health status and proposed interventions, and therefore inform and educate these clients accordingly (Cummings, 1996).

STRATEGIES FOR CRITICAL ANALYSIS

1. Discuss the principles of autonomy and beneficence as the ethical foundations of informed consent. Give an example of when one principle might override the other. Explain how the ethical frameworks of caring and virtue affect the nurse's role in supporting the process of informed consent.

2. A cardiologist asks you to obtain Mr. Brown's signature on an informed consent form. Mr. Brown is an 84-year-old man who is scheduled to have a palliative angioplasty the next day. You know that Mr. Brown and his wife have several questions regarding the procedure (eg, Can he can expect to be free from angina? Is there a risk of heart attack in undergoing the procedure?). You try to tell the cardiologist that Mr. and Mrs. Brown have these questions. The cardiologist tells you to "get the signature, and I'll be back later to talk with the patient." Based on past observations, you are doubtful that the cardiologist will return. Discuss your short-term and long-term actions.

3. As a nurse, what might you take into special consideration when ensuring that an older patient (or a child) understands the risks and benefits of a certain procedure?

4. Name two exceptions to informed consent. From an ethical and legal standpoint, describe the nurse's role for each exception.

5. Discuss the importance of documentation as it relates to patient education and informed consent.

REFERENCES

Agard, E., Finkelstein, D., & Wallach, E. (1998). Cultural diversity and informed consent. *Journal of Clinical Ethics, 9*(2), 173–176.

Agre, P., Kurtz, R. C., & Krauss, B. J. (1994). A randomized control trial using videotape to present consent information for colonoscopy. *Gastrointestinal Endoscopy, 40*, 271–276.

Albarran, J. W. (1996). Exploring the nature of informed consent in coronary care practice. *Nursing In Critical Care. 1*(3), 127–133.

Alderson, P. (1995a). Consent and the social context. *Nursing Ethics, 2*(4), 347–350.

Alderson, P. (1995b). Consent to surgery: The role of the nurse. *Nursing Standard, 9*(35), 38–40.

Alt-White, A. C. (1995). Obtaining Informed Consent from the Elderly. *Western Journal of Nursing Research, 17*(6), 700–705.

American Academy of Pediatrics, Committee on Bioethics. (1995). Informed consent, parental permission, and assent in pediatric practice. *Pediatrics, 95*(2), 314–317.

American Hospital Association. (1972). *A patient's bill of rights.* Chicago: Author.

American Nurses Association. (1985). *Code for Nurses with Interpretive Statements.* Washington, DC: ANA.

American Nurses Association. (1995). Nursing: A Social Policy Statement. Kansas City: MO, ANA.

Applebaum, P. S., & Grisso, T. (1988). Assessing patients' capacities to consent to treatment. *New England Journal of Medicine, 319*(25), 1635–1638.

Auerswald, K. B., Charpentier, P. A., & Inouye, S. K. (1997). The informed consent process in older patients who developed delirium: A clinical epidemiologic study. *American Journal of Medicine, 103*(5), 410–418.

Barnes, D., Davis, A. J., Moran, T., Portillo, C., & Koenig, B. A. (1998). Informed consent in a multicultural cancer patient population: Implications for nursing practice. *Nursing Ethics, 5*(5), 412–423.

Barton, C., Harminder, S., Mallik, H. S., & Orr, W. (1996). Clinicians' judgment of capacity of nursing home patients to give informed consent. *Psychiatric Services, 47*(9), 956–960.

Beauchamp, T. L., & Childress, J. (1989). *Principles of biomedical ethics* (3rd ed.) New York: Oxford.

Beauchamp, T. L., & Childress, J. (1994). Principles of biomedical ethics. (4th ed.). New York, NY: Oxford.

Blackhall, L. J., Murphy, S.T., Frank, G., Michel, V., & Azen, S. (1995). Ethnicity and attitudes toward patient autonomy. *Journal of the American Medical Association, 274*(10), 820–825.

Berry, D., Dodd, M., Hinds, P. & Ferrell, B. (1996). Informed consent: Process and clinical issues. *Oncology Nursing Forum, 23*(3), 507–512.

Bok, S. (1995). Shading the truth in seeking informed consent for research purposes. *Kennedy Institute of Ethics Journal, 5*(1), 1–17.

Brabbins, C., Butler, J., & Bentall, R. (1996). Consent to neuroleptic medication for schizophrenia: Clinical, ethical and legal issues. *British Journal of Psychiatry, 168*(5), 540–544.

Brandt, A. (1997). Racism and research: The case of the Tuskegee syphilis study. In J. W. Leavitt & R. L. Numbers (Eds.), *Sickness and health in America: Readings in the history of medicine and public health* (3rd ed.), Madison, WI: University of Wisconsin Press.

Brock, D. (1996). What is the moral authority of family members to act as surrogates for incompetent patients? *Milbank Quarterly, 74*(4), 599–618.

Bulecheck, G. M., & McCloskey, J. C. (1999). Nursing interventions: Effective nursing treatments (3rd ed.). Philadelphia: W. B. Saunders.

Cameron, C. (1996). Patient advocacy: A role for nurses. *European Journal of Cancer Care, 5*(2), 81–89.

Canterbury v. Spence, 414, F. 2d 772, 775 (D. C. Circ. 1972).

Carrese, J. A., & Rhodes, L. A. (1995). Western bioethics on the Navajo reservation: Benefit or harm? *Journal of the American Medical Association, 274*(10), 826–829.

Clawson, A. L. (1994). The relationship between clinical decision making and ethical decision making. *Physiotherapy, 80*(1), 10–14.

Cohen, L., McCue, J., & Green, G. (1993). Do clinical and formal assessments of the capacity of patients in the intensive care unit to make decisions agree?. *Archives Internal Medicine, 153*(21), 2481–2485.

Cummings, C. (1996). More on informed consent doctrine. *Advance for Nurse Practitioners, 4*(5), 18.

Dalhousie, W. W. (1999). Selecting subjects for participation in clinical research: One sphere of justice. *Journal of Medical Ethics, 25*(1), 31–36.

Daugherty, C., Ratain, M. J., Grochowski, E., Stocking, C., Kodish, E., Mick, R., & Siegler, M. (1995). Perceptions of cancer patients and their physicians involved in phase I trials. *Journal of Clinical Oncology, 13*(5), 1062–1072.

Davis, A. J., & Underwood, P. R. (1989). The competency quagmire: Clarification of the nursing perspective concerning the issues of competence and informed consent. *International Journal of Nursing Studies, 26*(3), 271–279.

Davis, D. (1999). Legal trends in bioethics: Physician-patient relationship. *Journal of Clinical Ethics, 10*(4), 345–346.

Davis, T. (1996). Responsible conduct in research: Recent policy developments in the area of research integrity. *Canadian Journal of Cardiovascular Nursing, 7*(2), 21–24.

Diem, S., Lantos, J., & Tulsky, J. (1996). Cardiopulmonary resuscitation on television: Miracles and misinformation. *New England Journal of Medicine, 334*(24), 1578–1582.

Dodd, F., Donegan, H., Kernohan, W., Geary, R., & Mollan, R. (1993). Consensus in medical communication. *Social Science and Medicine, 37*(4), 565–569.

Dula, A. (1994). African American suspicion of the health care system is justified: What do we do about it? *Cambridge Quarterly of Healthcare Ethics, 3*, 347–357.

Etchells, E., Darzins, P., Silberfeld, M., Singer, P., McKenny, J., Naglie, G., Katz, M., Guyatt, G., Molloy, D., & Strang, D. (1999). Assessment of patient capacity to consent to treatment. *Journal of General Internal Medicine, (14)*1, 27–34.

Erde, E. L. (1999). Informed consent to septoplasty: An anecdote from the field. *Journal of Medicine and Philosophy,* 24(1), 11–17.

Everhart, M. A., & Pearlman, R. A. (1990). Stability of patient preferences regarding life-sustaining treatments. *Chest, 97,* 159–164.

Faden, R. R., & Beauchamp, T. L. (1986). *A history and theory of informed consent.* New York: Oxford.

Farkas, M. M. (1992). Use of informed consent with therapeutic paradox. *Issues in Mental Health Nursing, 13,* 161–176.

Flanagin, A. (1997). World Medical Association Declaration of Helsinki/Who wrote the declaration of Helsinki?. *Journal of the American Medical Association,* 277(11), 925–926.

Fowles, G., & Fox, B. (1995). Competency to consent to treatment and informed consent in neurobehavioral rehabilitation. *Clinical Neuropsychologist, 9*(3), 251–257.

Friedlander, W. J. (1995). The evolution of informed consent in American medicine. *Perspectives in Biology and Medicine,* 38(3), 498– 510.

Fry, S. T. (1994). *Ethics in nursing practice: A guide to ethical decision making.* Geneva: International Council of Nurses.

Gadow, S. (1983). Existential advocacy: Philosophical foundation of nursing. In C. P. Murphy & H. Hunter (Eds.), *Ethical problems in the nurse-patient relationship* (pp. 40–60). Newton, Mass: Allyn & Bacon.

Gadow, S. (1989a). Clinical subjectivity: Advocacy with silent patients. *Nursing Clinics of North America,* 24(2), 535–541.

Gadow, S. (1989b). An ethical case for patient self-determination. *Seminars in Oncology Nursing,* 5(2), 99–101.

Gamble, V. N. (1997). Under the shadow of Tuskegee: African Americans and health care. *American Journal of Public Health,* 87(11), 1773–1778.

Gilligan, C. (1987). Moral orientation and moral development. In Kittay, E. F., & Meyers, D. T. (Eds.). *Women and Moral Theory.* Totowa, NJ: Rowan & Littlefield.

Gordon, M. (1993). *Manual of nursing diagnoses.* St. Louis: Mosby.

Hewlett, S. E. (1996). Is consent to participate in research voluntary? *Arthritis Care Research* 9(5), 400–404.

Hing-Mak, J. M., & Clinton, M. (1999). Promoting a good death: An agenda for outcomes research—a review of the literature. *Nursing Ethics,* 6(2), 97–106.

Hughes, K. K. (1993). Decision making by patients with breast cancer: The role of information in treatment selection, *Oncology Nursing Forum,* 20(4), 623–628.

Ian Shine v. Jose Vega and Massachusetts General Hospital (1993). Massachusetts Superior Court, Suffolk County. Medical Staff Registry, September 16, 1999.

Jurchak, M. (1990). Competence and the nurse-patient relationship. *Critical Care Nursing Clinics of North America,* 2(3), 453–459.

Jones, J. H. (1993). *Bad blood.* New York: Free Press.

Katz, J. (1993). Ethics and clinical research revisited. *Hastings Center Report,* 23(5), 31–39.

Kleinman, I., Brown, P., & Librach, L. (1994). Placebo pain medication. *Archives Family Medicine,* 3(5), 453–457.

Macklin, R. (1999). Understanding informed consent. *Acta Oncologica,* 38(1), 83–87.

Madder, H. (1997). Existential autonomy: Why patients should make their own choices. *Journal of Medical Ethics, 23,* 221–225.

Mahoney, M. A., Riley, J. M., Fry, S. T., & Feild, L. (1999). Factors related to providers' decisions for and against withholding or withdrawing nutrition and/or hydration in adult patient care. *The Online Journal of Knowledge Synthesis for Nursing,* 6(4). Available on-line.

Mallary, S., Gert, B., & Culver, C. (1986). Family coercion and valid consent. *Theoretical Medicine, 7,* 123–126.

Marwick, C. (1997). Assessment of exception to informed consent. *Journal of the American Medical Association,* 278(17), 1392–1393.

McCabe, M. S. (1999). The ethical foundation of informed consent in clinical research. *Seminars in Oncology Nursing,* 15(2), 76–80.

McCarthy, C. (1995). To be or not to be: Waiving informed consent in emergency research. *Kennedy Institute of Ethics Journal,* 5(2), 155–162.

Meade, C. D. (1999). Improving understanding of the informed consent process and document. *Seminars in Oncology Nursing,* 15(2), 124–137.

Meade, C. D., & Howser, D. M. (1992). Consent forms: How to determine and improve their readability, *Oncology Nursing Forum,* 19(10), 1523–1528.

Meisel, A. (1979). The "exceptions" the informed consent doctrine: Striking a balance between competing values in medical decision making. *Wisconson Law Review, 1979(2),* 413–488.

Meisel, A., & Kabnick, L. (1980). Informed consent to medical treatment: An analysis of recent legislation. *University of Pittsburgh Law Review 41*, 407.

Meyers, R. M., & Grodin, M. A. (1991). Decision making regarding the initiation of tube feedings in the demented elderly: A review. *Journal of the American Geriatrics Society, 39*(5), 526–531.

Natanson v. Kline, 350 P 2d 1093 (1960).

Neptune, S., Hopper, K., & Matthews, Y. (1994). Risks associated with the use of IV contrast material: Analysis of patients' awareness. *American Journal of Roentgenology, 162*(2), 451–454.

Newton, J., Hawes, R., Jamidar, P., Harig, J., & Lehman, G. (1994). Survey of informed consent for endoscopic retrograde cholangiopancreatography. *Digestive Diseases and Sciences, 39*(8), 1714–1718.

Noddings, N. (1984). *Caring: A feminine approach to ethics and moral education.* Berkeley, CA: University of California Press.

Nusbaum, J. G., & Chenitz, W. C. (1990). A grounded theory study of the informed consent process for pharmacologic research, *Western Journal of Nursing Research, 12*(2), 215–228.

Omnibus Budget Reconciliation Act of 1990. Public Law No. 101-508.

Pearlman, R. A., Uhlman, R. F., & Jecker, N.S. (1992). Spousal understanding of patient quality of life: Implications for surrogate decisions. *Journal of Clinical Ethics, 3*(2), 114–121.

Pellegrino, E. (1995). Toward a virtue-based normative ethics for the health professions. *Kennedy Institute of Ethics Journal, 5*(3), 253–277.

Pellegrino, E., & Thomasma, D. (1993). *The virtues in medical practice.* New York: Oxford University Press.

Phillips, R., Wenger, N., Teno, J., Oye, R., Younger, S., Califf, R., Laycle, P., Desbiens, N., Connors, A. & Lynn, J. (1996). *Choices of seriously ill patients about cardiopulmonary resuscitation: Correlates and outcomes.* American Journal of Medicine, 100(1), 128–137.

Powers, M. (June 1993). Lecture on Autonomy, *Kennedy Institute of Ethics, Intensive Bioethics XIX.* Georgetown University, Washington, D.C.

President's Commission for the Study of Ethical Problems in Biomedical and Behavioral Research. (1982). *Making health care decisions. 1, 2, & 3.* Washington D.C.: U.S. Government Printing Office.

President's Commission for the Study of Ethical Problems in Biomedical and Behavioral Research (1983). *Deciding to forego life-sustaining treatment.* Washington D.C.: U.S. Government Printing Office.

Prosser, W. L. (1971). *Handbook of law and torts.* (4th ed.) St. Paul, MN: West.

Purtilo, R. B. (1984). Applying the principles of informed consent to patient care: Legal and ethical considerations for physical therapy, *Physical Therapy, 64*(6), 934–937.

Rachlin, S. (1974). With liberty and psychosis for all. *Psychiatric Quarterly, 60,* 410–420.

Reverby, S. M. (1999). Rethinking the Tuskegee Syphilis Study: Nurse Rivers, silence and the meaning of treatment. *Nursing History Review,* 7(1), 3–28.

Richardson, J. I. (1993). Informed consent: Whose responsibility? *Texas Nurse, 67*(2), 3, 15.

Rogero-Anaya, P., Carpintero-Avellaneda, J. L., & Vila-Blasco, B. (1994). Ethics and research in nursing. *Nursing Ethics, 1*(4), 216–223.

Ross, L. F. (1997). Health care decision-making by children: Is it in their best interest? *Hastings Center Report, 27*(6), 41–45.

Roth, L., Meisel, A., & Lidz, C. (1977). Tests of competency to consent to treatment. *American Journal of Psychiatry, 134*(3), 279–284.

Rule, J. T., & Veatch, R. M. (1993). *Ethical Questions in Dentistry.* Chicago: Quintessence Publishing.

Salgo v. Leland Stanford University Board of Trustees, 154, Cal. App. 2d 560, 317 p2d 170 (1957).

Savulescu, J., & Momeyer, R. (1997). Should informed consent be based on rational beliefs? *Journal of Medical Ethics 23,* 282–288.

Schloendorff v. Society of New York Hospitals, 211 N. Y. 125, 128, 105 N. E. 92, 93 (1914).

Schneidermayer, D. L. (1988). The decision to forgo CPR in the elderly patient. *Journal of the American Medical Association, 260*(14), 2096–2097.

Scofield, G. R. (1993). Ethical considerations in rehabilitation medicine, *Archives Physical Medicine Rehabilitation, 74,* 341–346.

Shuster, E. (1997). Fifty years later: The significance of the Nuremberg code. *New England Journal of Medicine, 337*(20), 1436–1440.

Silva, M. C. (1993). Competency, comprehension, and the ethics of informed consent. *Nursing Connections, 6*(3), 47–51.

Silva, M. C. (1995). *Ethical guidelines in the conduct, dissemination, and implementation of nursing research.* Washington D.C.: ANA Publishing.

Sorrell, J. M. (1991). Effects of writing/speaking on comprehension of information for informed consent, *Western Journal of Nursing Research,* *13*(1), 110–122.

Sugarman, J., McCrory, D. C., & Hubal, R. (1998). Getting meaningful informed consent from older adults: A structured literature review of empirical research. *Journal of the American Geriatrics Society, 46,* 517–524.

Tammelleo, A. D. (1985). Nurse uses aversive therapy: Dismissal. Case in point: Juneau v Bd. of Elem. secondary Ed, 506 So.2d 756-LA. *Regan Report on Nursing Law, 28*(2), 4.

Tammelleo, A. D. (1990). Nurse orders objecting patient to "shut up." Case in point: Roberson v Provident House, 559 So.2d 838-LA (1990). *Regan Report on Nursing Law, 31*(3), 4.

Tammelleo, A. D. (1993a). Patient sues nurse for failure to obtain informed consent. Case in point: Foflygen v R. Zemel, MD, 615A, 2d 1345-PA (1992). *Regan Report on Nursing Law, 33*(10), 4.

Tammelleo, A. D. (1993b). Caveat to nurses in "John Doe" organ harvests: Brown v Delaware Valley Transplant Program, 615A, 2d 1379-PA (1992). *Regan Report on Nursing Law, 33*(10), 1.

Tammelleo, A. D. (1995). When nurses obtain consent for organ donations: Perry v. St. Francis Hospital & Medical Center, 865 F. Supp 724-KS (1994). *Regan Report on Nursing Law, 35*(8), 1.

Tammelleo, A. D. (1997a). PA: No liability for informed consent: "Prudent Nurse" explanation standard applies: Davis v. Hoffman-972 F. Supp 308 (1997). *Regan Report on Nursing Law, 38*(6), 3.

Tamelleo, A. D. (1997b). Nurses "Cover Up" lack of informed consent for hysterectomy: Mathias v. St. Catherine's Hosp.-569 N.W. 2d 330-WI (1997). *Regan Report on Nursing Law, 38*(6), 1.

Thomasma, D. C. (1999). Stewardship of the aged: Meeting the ethical challenge of ageism. *Cambridge Quarterly of Healthcare Ethics 8,* 148–159.

Truog, R., & Robinson, W. (1999). Informed consent for research. *Anesthesiology, 90*(6), 1499–1501.

Uniform Anatomical Gift Act of 1987, 1–17, 8A U.L.A. (1989).

VanHooft, S. (1999). Acting from the virtue of caring in nursing. *Nursing Ethics, 6*(3), 189– 201.

Volicer, L., Brandeis, G., & Hurley, A. (1998). Infections in advanced dementia. In L. Volicer & A. Hurley (Eds.). *Hospice care for patients with advanced, progressive dementia.* New York: Springer.

Watson, J. (1985). *Nursing: The philosophy and science of caring.* Boulder, CO: Colorado Associated University Press.

Wear, S. (1998). *Informed consent: Patient autonomy and clinician beneficence within health care* (2nd ed.). Washington D.C.: Georgetown University Press.

Weir, R. F., & Peters, C. (1997). Affirming the decisions adolescents make about life and death. *Hastings Center Report, 27*(6), 29–40.

World Health Organization. (1990). *Cancer pain relief and palliative care.* (Report of a WHO Expert Committee). Geneva, Switzerland.

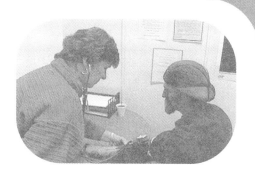

Community Health Promotion:

Assessment and Intervention

Ronna E. Krozy

LEARNING OBJECTIVES

After reading this chapter, the nurse or nursing student should be able to:

1. Describe the interrelationship between community assessment and identification of community health education issues.

2. Utilize several approaches to data collection as the basis for developing a needs assessment.

3. Apply marketing techniques to improve the success of a health education program.

4. Incorporate empowerment strategies in health promotion programs.

5. Implement health promotion strategies that facilitate behavioral change in families, aggregate populations, or community groups.

INTRODUCTION

Patient health promotion represents an integral part of the health professional's role. Health promotion addresses activities that decrease the impact of risk factors and facilitate well-being and self-actualization. *Healthy People 2000,* recently expanded to *Healthy People 2010,* are major national initiatives to improve the health of the nation. Initiated by the United States Department of Health and Human Services (U.S. Department of Health and Human Services, 1990), *Healthy People 2000* was built on objectives set in 1980. Priorities were established around health promotion, health protection, and preventive services. Issues addressed included smoking, violence, physical fitness, mental health, occupational safety, environmental health, human immunodeficiency virus (HIV) and other sexually transmitted diseases (STDs), cancer, and immunizations. The overall goal was to help Americans change behaviors that were unhealthy or a risk to health, to eliminate unequal access to comprehensive health services, and to eradicate many chronic, costly conditions that are essentially preventable. Ultimately, prevention of disability and suffering also improves quality of life.

Notable differences expressed in the goals for this decade in *Healthy People 2010: Understanding and Improving Health* (U.S. Department of Health and Human Services, 2000) include strengthening the scientific basis for health promotion and disease prevention programs, improving methods for collecting comprehensive health statistics, and increasing the government's commitment and provision of services to provide quality care for all citizens. To raise the standard of care for the consumer, increased consumer participation also will be needed (Bastian, 1996).

Health education comprises an important aspect of health promotion. Community health education differs from patient or family education in that its focus may extend to global, national, state, or local needs. The clients of community health strategies include groups and aggregates that cross all age, socioeconomic, and cultural strata. These clients are in homes, schools, occupational settings, shelters, prisons, or on the street. Health promotion initiatives may be aimed at an entire country or a small village; the learners may be comprised of people who are homogeneous or extremely dissimilar. Health educators must develop proficiency in group or aggregate teaching; many participants must be reached efficiently, and groups serve as more potential sources of support and sharing.

This chapter discusses factors that must be considered in promoting health in aggregate populations. Two health education projects in which the author was involved are described. In each of these two projects, the demographic factors and health promotion focus are different; therefore, the approaches to needs assessment and intervention also vary. In the first example, Gordon's 11 functional health patterns (Gordon, 1991, 1997) are used as the framework to assess the health education needs of a culturally diverse population in a poor Ecuadorian community. The second example demonstrates the use of force field analysis and behavioral change strategies with staff attending a university health promotion program.

COMMUNITY HEALTH PROMOTION AND EDUCATION

Definitions

Health education is a helping process using learning theories and teaching techniques that promote the client's knowledge, attitudes and skill to voluntarily engage in a wellness lifestyle. Part of this process requires mobilizing resources and developing supportive relationships with clients. Another aspect is assuming the role of client advocate or political activist for the disenfranchised in whom health education may be a means of empowerment. The health educator must use learning theories and teaching techniques that have been tested, are based on the population's specific needs, and are incorporated into the overall plan.

Health education outcomes include the

client's learning factual information, developing self-confidence, reexamining or changing values, decreasing fear, and developing competence to make informed decisions and perform desired behaviors autonomously. Another important goal is to help clients develop resilience—the ability to withstand internal and external stress without adverse effects (Lindenberg, Solorzano, Krantz, Galvis, Baroni, & Strickland, 1998). The overall goals are aimed at enhancing, maintaining, or restoring health and preventing disease.

Challenges to the Health of a Community

Poor Habits, Chronic Illness, Disability

Poor health habits, chronic illness, and disability are costly to communities in terms of lost work and school days, financing of health care and service agencies, and unnecessary suffering. Therefore, primary prevention is considered the best way to preserve the health of any community. Primary prevention is defined as the activities that prevent an illness or negative condition from beginning. Approaches to community health education often focus on the role of individual responsibility, recognizing that many health problems result from diverse personal habits (eg, smoking, unprotected sexual activity, or overexposure to sun). These habits represent complex behaviors arising from internal and external stimuli; they are not easily amenable to medical intervention or a health professional's advice. Despite potential or real disease, many people have difficulty changing their behavior.

For example, there are many young people who begin or continue smoking despite multifocused antismoking strategies. A 1994 report by the United States Surgeon General notes that most smokers are hooked by age 20. The tobacco industry spends $4 million on advertising to indoctrinate youngsters to smoke by making teenagers think that more people smoke than actually do and that it is a means to an enhanced self-image. Smoking is made to look glamorous, with models and cartoon characters conveying

independence, healthfulness, and adventure. Cigarette displays, billboards, free samples, and trademarks prominent on clothing and at sporting events provide constant reinforcement of prosmoking messages (U.S. Department of Health and Human Services, 1994). The use of sophisticated marketing strategies poses considerable challenge to public health campaigns in which outreach funds are severely limited.

Resistance and Barriers

Resistance occurs when specific populations believe a health behavior change interferes with their perceived quality of life, when it requires resources that are lacking, or when the population sees the change as unimportant.

Barriers also may arise from the health system. Health professionals are expected to establish trusting relationships with clients and act as role models. However, some health care professionals display negative attitudes or behaviors that prevent clients from following advice. Health professionals may hold beliefs that certain people (especially those from different socioeconomic classes) do not value health, do not want to get well, enjoy their sick role, are too unintelligent to learn new behaviors, and are taking up valuable time of the health professionals. Incongruent or ineffective messages also may be transmitted when a health professional engages in the unhealthy behaviors being discouraged (eg, a health care worker who smokes, is overweight, or who drives without a seat belt).

IMPROVING THE SUCCESS OF COMMUNITY HEALTH PROGRAMS

Chapter 4 describes specific teaching and learning principles that can be applied to health promotion programs. Rainey and Lindsay (1994) present a comprehensive list of 101 questions to use in health promotion program planning. However, the following are general questions aimed at increasing the success of any health education campaign.

Identifying the Need

Has a needs assessment been performed to determine the community's perception of the problem? Specific issues can be identified using current vital statistics, public opinion polls, discussions with professionals and lay community leaders. Organizing focus groups, informal discussions with representatives of the target population, and written surveys also are helpful. The use of prevalence data, which increases the community's awareness of the extent of a problem, has been shown to increase the likelihood of a successful intervention (Healey, 1998).

Acceptance by the Majority

Are the health promotion goals and objectives clear? Will most of the target community accept the idea or method? Can they implement the idea and is it congruent with their lifestyle, needs, and resources? Have barriers and facilitators of behavior change been considered? Are the behavior changes considered practical and realistic? Does the health innovation take into consideration local resources, customs, and environment? Are the positive healthy habits of people capitalized upon even if they seem strange?

Involvement in Planning

Has the community (or representatives of subgroups) been involved in identifying the health problem or goal or in developing the approach or the evaluation? It is not uncommon to be confronted by many more opponents than proponents. Therefore, opposing views must be considered. Conflict must be seen as a factor requiring discussion and compromise, so that energy is not expended negatively but rather conjointly.

Cost Benefit and Cost Effectiveness

Is the expenditure of time, energy, money, or other resources required to carry out the action worth the effort, yield, rewards, or inconveniences? Have competing demands that influence learning or behaviors been considered?

Community Enhancement

Will the process enhance the community regarding job opportunities, environmental protection, equalizing wealth? Is there enough consumer orientation reflecting the target audience's specific concerns? Consider the resistance that arises from tobacco farmers whose livelihood is the product that causes cancer and heart disease.

Self-Help

Are self-help and/or self-determination the ultimate goals? Will those in greatest need be included and not just those who can take advantage because of sophistication, education, money, and maturity? Is there a plan for those who cannot act because of physical, emotional, or social impairments?

Use of Theory

Are various theories used that help guide the design, implementation, and evaluation of the health promotion effort (Kreps & Kunimoto, 1994)? Hochbaum and Rosenstock's Health Belief Model, Pender's Health Promotion Model, or Bandura's Self-Efficacy Theory are examples cited in other chapters.

Media Effectiveness

Are the media that have been used attractive and interesting, understandable, geared to different learning styles and rates, inoffensive and tasteful, personally engaging, and persuasive (Windsor, Baranowski, Clark, & Cutter, 1994)?

POLITICAL AND LEGAL INFLUENCES ON HEALTH PROMOTION

Political and legal influences refer to formal and informal sources of decision-making and control. Policymakers or special interest groups can influence withholding health promotion programs from segments of society. For example, as a result of selection bias, researchers have underrepresented older people, the poor, and ethnic minorities from study protocols. These populations must be included because they respond differently to diseases and interventions (Larson, 1994). Drug companies and manufacturers have withheld information on adverse outcomes to gain a profit. Legislators in tobacco-growing states have supported subsidies to tobacco growers and have opposed smoking restriction regulations, despite the evidence of showing the association of tobacco smoking with cancer. In context of the AIDS epidemic, needle exchange programs have been barred and parents and religious leaders have influenced school committees to vote down comprehensive sex education curricula.

These examples suggest that decision-makers may have vested interests or religious proscriptions. They may be unconcerned or opposed to the issues or approaches needed to prevent certain health problems or they may fear offending others and losing status; they may also be uninformed. The influence of decision-makers can be assessed by asking:

- Is health promotion a value?
- Who is permitted to learn?
- Who controls what is taught?
- Who is permitted to teach?
- Are sufficient resources allocated?

A needs assessment must be undertaken to answer these questions and to determine whether the allocated budget, human resources, time, space, and materials are sufficient to address the health problem.

Professionals can influence health policy by developing knowledge of political process, establishing power, and creating support (Clark, 1999). Health professionals must understand the political structure, how change is effected, and who has the authority to implement change. Political decision-makers must be apprised of the health needs of the community using both factual data (such as published vital statistics) and personal testimony. The proposed educational intervention must be presented persuasively with the expected outcomes. Support is garnered through campaigning, lobbying, or establishing a coalition or temporary alliance to work toward a common goal.

COMMUNITY EMPOWERMENT

General Considerations

Community empowerment (also termed community self-determination or community self-help) is a process of decision-making and problem solving. It is one of the most effective ways to effect positive behavioral change in aggregate populations (Wallerstein & Bernstein, 1998) (Box 7-1).

Community empowerment requires active community involvement, ownership of the changes to take place (Armbruster, Gale, Brady, & Thompson, 1999; Covington, 1999), and community organization. The latter is a process of uniting various segments of the community who act in their own behalf and whose aims are to establish legitimacy, to identify and to analyze a problem, to identify goals and the means to achieve them, to select marketing strategies, and to establish eval-uation criteria (Clark, 1999). Health professionals, especially nurses, can facilitate community involvement and decision-making by listening, providing factual information, identifying sources of assistance, advocating, and assisting with evaluation. Shields and Lindsey (1998) suggest a need to prepare nurses as specialists in community health promotion nursing practice, which incorporates an analysis of power relations, critical reflection, acceptance of divergent reasoning, tolerance of ambiguity, and action aimed at creating social change. These skills can be developed while students are learning to provide community-based care as part of their curricula (Green & Adderley-Kelly, 1999; Juhn, Tang, Piessens, Grant, Johnson, & Murray, 1999).

Examples of Community Participation in Health Promotion Programs

Consortium for the Immunization of Norfolk's Children (CINCH)

In recent years, many successful health promotion programs have resulted from broad community participation of diverse citizens and institutions. According to Butterfoss,

BOX 7-1. Community Empowerment Case Study

From Blight to Blossom Park: A Case Study of Community Empowerment

Alice Samuels, a public health nurse, walked along *Blossom Street,* past the boarded up delapidated house sitting back from the street in a yard filled with refuse. Despite the *Do Not Enter* sign posted on the rusting barrier fence, she noted several teenagers sitting on the rotting front stairs smoking and laughing. She had heard that small groups of teenagers entered the house at night through a broken window, using candles for heat and light. Just recently, one had fallen down the stairs in the dark, requiring emergency room treatment for a fractured leg.

Two houses away lived Ms. Jordan, an elderly client. Ms. Jordan had remarked on several occasions how unsightly and dangerous this property was. In addition, the teenagers became rowdy and made people feel uncomfortable. She mused, "What we need there is a little park for children to play in or for us old folk to sit in." The nurse replied, "Let's see if we can do this."

Empowerment Component	Application to the Community
Sufficient knowledge to make rational informed decisions	The nurse identifies key community persons and groups who will "own" the project, which is called Friends of Blossom Park. Multiple community assessment strategies are used to identify awareness of health hazards; impact on neighborhood—eg, sense of identity, safety, property values; and community goals, resources, and needs. All data are shared with the planning group. A Blossom Park Media Campaign is initiated; posted and written notices are placed in churches, schools, supermarkets, health centers, and local news and TV. Participants of a school poster contest, "Paint the Park," will receive free ice cream, and the posters will be displayed at the Park's opening.
Sufficient control and resources to implement decisions	Government support from legal, building, and health departments is required to approve demolition of abandoned property. Voluntary assistance is solicited from Scouts and the local high school; local trash removal company/municipality, landscaping, and construction companies; and personal and business donors, for cleanup, blueprints, plantings, equipment, and funds. A Blossom Park Bash fundraiser is established with a community dance, supper, and raffle. All decisions result from collaboration among community membership.
Sufficient experience to evaluate the effectiveness of the decision	After the park is created, Friends of Blossom Park decide to create other beautification projects and will collaborate with City Park and Recreation Department. Nurse remains as resource.

Morrow, Rosenthal, Dini, Crews, Webster, and Louis (1998), in Norfolk, Virginia, the urban coalition CINCH improved immunization access and increased the rate of immunization for two-year-olds by involving the community in assessment, planning, and intervention. Lynagh, Knight, Schofield, and Paras (1999) describe a health-promoting schools project with a model of intervention based on community organization theory. They identify guiding principles (ie, gaining strong community support, involving key people, providing a specific data-based profile of the target population, and maintaining consistent reporting) that influenced the adoption of health promotion activities by their target schools.

The Falmouth Safe Skin Project

A multidimensional skin cancer prevention program for parents and children through age 13 was launched in an ocean community of Cape Cod, Massachusetts. Goals of the Falmouth Safe Skin Project included educating parents about sun protection for their children and themselves and the dangers of early childhood sunburn. The project used community activism, specific learning activities, and a broad educational initiative that included providing information at maternity hospitals, day care programs, schools, beaches, recreation programs, and through the media. A follow-up survey 3 years after the initiation of the project showed an improvement in community knowledge, attitudes, and behaviors and a reduction in reported childhood sunburns (Miller, Geller, Wood, Lew, & Koh, 1999).

Project Salsa

Project Salsa is a community-based nutritional health promotion project "planned by and for the community to help residents live healthier lives" [and] "promote nutritional health through community development" (Elder, Campbell, Candelaria, Talavera, Mayer, Moreno, Medel, & Lyons, 1998, p. 397). The project was initiated in San Ysidro, which is contiguous to San Diego, California, and adjacent to Tijuana. The intervention community group was composed of 14,500 residents, 83% of whom were primarily low-income Latinos. It was initially funded by the Kaiser Family Foundation with the goal of creating community ownership and a permanent infrastructure. The authors discuss the steps that were taken to implement the project: organizing for change; developing an advisory council; needs assessment via telephone survey,

archival research, and interviews of key informants; setting priorities; establishing interventions; and developing a multifocused evaluation plan.

The project aimed to improve nutrition among several community subpopulations, including:

- Increasing breast-feeding among new mothers
- Making breakfast available for elementary school children
- Instituting "heart healthy" diet education in all school programs
- Providing similar "heart healthy" material for adults in supermarkets, churches, and the media
- Offering cooking classes and establishing programs for coronary heart disease screening, counseling, and referral

An impact evaluation revealed that not all objectives could be achieved. However, the school health program, coronary heart disease risk factor screening, cooking training, and innovative media approaches have been retained by the community five years after the grant period ended. This has been attributed to "true grass-roots organization (p. 400)."

Partnership With the Client

Several authors suggest that bringing a significant impact on health requires a partnership with the client (Courtney, Ballard, Fauver, Gariota, & Holland, 1996). Hedelin and Svensson (1999) discuss a community mental health promotion partnership that involved public and voluntary organizations and a community group of elders. By determining the need for and establishing resources that included social support networks, the community perceived itself better able to meet its own needs. Another approach to community health promotion and empowerment endorses the use of a lay health educator model (Lowe, Barg, & Stephens, 1998). The Healthy Neighborhoods Project, conducted in a low-income urban San Francisco Bay-area neighborhood, suggests that local health departments may play a vital role to increase community participation. The partnership of the health department with housing project residents resulted in construction of street speed bumps, increased lighting, and removal of a tobacco billboard (El-Askari, Freestone, Irizarry, Kraut, Mashiyama, Morgan, & Walton, 1998).

Finally, the Mentoring Mothers Program (Navaie-Waliser, Gordon, & Hibberd, 1996) was developed as an empowering strategy to prevent premature births. The project demonstrated that partnerships between community groups and health professionals improved knowledge and decreased social isolation, a contributing factor in infant mortality. Although using a small sample of pregnant women, 95% of those linked with a community mentor delivered healthy babies with normal birth weight.

THE INFLUENCE OF MARKETING

General Considerations

Marketing is the process of determining a consumer need and meeting the need with a product or service (Tilbury & Fisk, 1989). Through advertising, the product or service is presented in a way that increases usage and loyalty by as many segments of the population as possible. Drexler (Boston Globe, October 23, 1994, p. 18) notes that the alcohol industry is waging an aggressive and successful marketing campaign toward the 21- to 24-year-old, using seductive methods; for example, a well-known liquor company hosts parties at local college pubs. In Massachusetts alone, the tobacco industry spends $70 million yearly in cigarette advertising (Cohen, Lederman, Connolly, & Danley, 1991). Unfortunately, unlike the tobacco or alcohol industries, which have extensive marketing budgets, sponsors of health education programs frequently have limited finances. Nevertheless, health promoters have been advised to use similar strategies to identify target populations and their needs, and to market health behavior accordingly.

Social Marketing

When applied to health, the term *social marketing* is often used and is well described in Andreasen's book, *Marketing Social Change: Changing Behavior to Promote Health, Social Development, and the Environment.* Andreasen emphasizes that behavior change requires more than just promoting the benefits of a new action; the real or perceived cost to the consumer must be considered. Moreover, decisions to change behaviors often evolve slowly, so that a target population may not change its risky behavior immediately, (Andreasen, 1995).

Marketing Example: The Massachusetts Tobacco Control Program

Examples of marketing strategy may be seen in Massachusetts, a state that funds tobacco control programs with taxes from tobacco products. Despite a heavily funded counterattack by the tobacco industry, supporters have achieved a 25-cent state excise tax increase on each package of cigarettes, generating $91 million in 1992. The Massachusetts Tobacco Control Program (MTCP) is a comprehensive statewide initiative that incorporates advertising and community relations, statewide smoking cessation and education programs, and grants to local boards of health, schools, community agencies, and health advocacy organizations. The MTCP's aim is to decrease 50% of the state's tobacco use by 1999 (Massachusetts Tobacco Control Program, 1994a).

With the referendum won by tobacco opponents, the tobacco industry began buying whole-page newspaper advertisements, that cost almost $30,000 each. The tobacco industry's messages suggested a need for compromise or for solving the problem amicably, but also implied that government control overstepped its bounds and will ultimately rob the public of freedom. Another tactic of the tobacco industry was refuting the Environmental Protection Agency's findings on the danger of exposure to secondhand smoke. The MTCP allocated $14 million to launch the State's single largest anti-smoking advertising campaign (Massachusetts Tobacco Control Program, 1994b). One MTCP advertisement cleverly depicts a package of light cigarettes with the message, *"Next, the tobacco industry will want us to believe there's such a thing as light cancer"* (Boston Globe, June 23, 1994, p.19).

The MTCP campaign slogan is, *It's Time We Made Smoking History.* The MTCP's strategies include support of legislation and ordinances to ban smoking in most public places (eg, malls, schools, restaurants, and worksites) and extensive exposure in newspapers, public and cable television, and radio (which reached more than 5 million people). The MTCP targets youth, pregnant women, and persons from culturally diverse communities, who may be left out of the education loop and exposed to many more conflicting messages.

Evaluation of the impact of the MTCP has shown impressive results, despite a 15% decrease in funding since the program began: A 30% decrease in cigarette purchases, exceeded that of the rest of the country; a sharp decrease in smoking during pregnancy; a slight decrease in high school smoking in contrast to a nationwide increase; and a significant increase in indoor smoking bans protecting patrons from second-hand smoke. Results also show that media campaigns have increased smokers' knowledge of tobacco risks (Hamilton & Norton, 1999). According to Biener (1999), smoking reduction in Massachusetts has not only surpassed all other states but may be attributed to the combined effect of policies, media, and cessation programs.

Kreps and Kunimoto's (1994) suggestions for multicultural health communication can be applied to smoking prevention and cessation and other areas. Messages of health should appear in all channels of communication, especially those that are popular with the target group (eg, television shows, soap operas, and age- or gender-oriented magazines). Endorsement from public figures or role models are also helpful. A successful media project in Brazil's anti-smoking campaign was based on the notion that people are more concerned for social acceptability than health. Five posters were developed by a famous cartoonist, depicting the ludicrous and socially inadequate features of smoking. Descriptions of smoking included old-fashioned, tacky, in bad taste, corny, and pathetic. A significant decrease in smoking has been reported since the campaign began in 1986 (da Costa e Silva, 1993). A similar brochure by Journeyworks Publishing is entitled *The Filthy, Disgusting, Ugly, Foul, Hideous, Horrible, Ghastly, Nasty, Nauseating Tobacco Quiz* (Leonard, 1996).

Community health promotion aims to foster behavior that maximizes wellness and minimizes the development of disease. Health promotion at the community level requires an understanding of the needs and desires of the target population. It is important to consider the behavioral lifestyles and values of the various groups that make up the community and to maximize community involvement. Socioeconomic status, educational level, culture and language, formal and informal power structures, occupation, and marketing forces are some of the important factors that must be accounted for if a health promotion initiative is to be successful. The influence of these factors is demonstrated in the health promotion programs presented in the following section.

GLOBAL HEALTH PROMOTION

Despite growing international concern toward health promotion and disease prevention, there are many barriers to promoting global health. These barriers include overpopulation, social injustice, social disorganization, increasing poverty, and population shifts from rural areas to overcrowded shanty towns in which children are born into unsanitary, polluted environments (Kark, Kark, & Abramson, 1993). Thus future health professionals must be prepared "to make decisions at social, economic, and political levels . . . to practice in . . . settings where environmental factors are adversely affecting the population's health . . . [and to direct practice toward] altering global, national and community environments in order to prevent risks to populations" (Kleffel, 1991, p.50).

The Por Cristo-BCSON Health Project

In 1991, a collaborative venture between the Boston College School of Nursing (BCSON) and Por Cristo, a medical missionary group, was initiated by the author of this chapter. From a self-supported voluntary health education mission, the Por Cristo-BCSON Health Project has evolved into a credit-granting undergraduate clinical experience in Community Health Nursing. This project takes place in Isla Verde, an impoverished South American community. Nursing students work with Father Fred, a British missionary priest, who also is a registered nurse, and with the chapter author, a professor of community health nursing at Boston College.

Students assess and care for families in the home, conduct community assessments, and present community health education programs. Students have set up temporary clinics, diagnosed illnesses, prescribed interventions, counseled, and referred. A simple dispensary now exists, and students work with a lay community health worker and part-time physician. This project also has established relationships with two local university schools of nursing. Both Boston College and Ecuadorian nursing students present seminars to one another and a small group of Ecuadorian students accompany the BCSON students to work in the Isla. The goals of this project are the following:

1. To provide basic health education and services to an underserved population
2. To develop creative teaching approaches
3. To be immersed in a linguistically and culturally diverse community
4. To develop sensitivity and awareness of cultural diversity and universality
5. To recognize the dignity of a person, regardless of his or her socioeconomic status
6. To help empower the community through enhancing its self-help capabilities
7. To observe firsthand the effects of poverty
8. To demonstrate the role of the community health nurse and family nurse practitioner

Assessing the Community

An official community assessment and census have not been done in Isla Verde. Although the demographic characteristics appear the same as those in neighboring squatter communities, we realize that an individualized assessment uncovers specific needs, interests, resources, and community capabilities (Lundeen, 1992; Urrutia-Rojas & Aday, 1991). These data form the basis for community diagnoses and educational interventions. A descriptive approach to community assessment was planned with the approval of Fr. Fred and community leaders.

Choosing an Assessment Tool

For many years, the students of this program have used an assessment tool based on Gordon's Eleven Functional Health Patterns (1991, 1997) applied to the community (McCarthy, 1994) [Box 7-2]. Other faculty members support this approach as a comprehensive and standardized method of collecting and organizing data (Kriegler & Harton, 1992).

To account for language and lifestyle differences, the assessment tool required adaptation and a Spanish version was developed (Krozy & McCarthy, 1999). A bilingual health professional and students (several of whom were bilingual), families, groups, faculty and students in the host country, helped to develop and test the tools. Back translations and testing assured that both nurse and client would exchange exact meanings in their communication (Hatton & Webb, 1993). McDermott and Palchanes (1993) assert that validity in translations would account for colloquialisms, idioms, and other sources of misinterpretation.

Conducting the Assessment

Students conduct a walking assessment, speak with community residents and leaders, and tour the institutions in the surrounding city. This approach allows the students to observe and record many aspects of community life. The following are selected examples of data collected:

Isla Verde is a poor coastal community of squatters who live on government-owned property. The community began in 1985 and is

BOX 7-2. Community Assessment Guide*

I. Health Perception-Health Management Pattern

1. History (community representatives)
   a. In general, what is the health/wellness level of the population on a scale of 1–5, with 5 being the highest level of health/wellness? Any major health problems?
   b. Any strong cultural patterns that influence health practices?
   c. Do people think they have access to health services?
   d. Is there a demand for particular health services or prevention programs?
   e. Do people think fire, police, safety programs are sufficient?
2. Objective data (community records)
   a. Morbidity, mortality, disability rates (by age group, if appropriate)
   b. Accident rates (by district, if appropriate)
   c. Current operating health facilities (types)
   d. Ongoing health promotion/ prevention programs; utilization rates
   e. Ratio of health professionals to population
   f. Laws regarding drinking age
   g. Arrest statistics for drugs, drunk driving by age groups

II. Nutritional-Metabolic Pattern

1. History (community representatives)
   a. In general, do most people seem well nourished? Children? Older people?
   b. Are there food supplement programs? Food stamps: rate of use?
   c. Are foods reasonably priced in this area relative to income?
   d. Are stores accessible for most? Meals On Wheels available?
2. Objective data
   a. What is the general appearance of the population (nutritional appearance; teeth; clothing appropriate to climate)? Children? Adults? Older people?
   b. What food do people purchase (observations of food store check-out counters)?
   c. Are "junk" food machines in schools, fast food restaurants, etc.?

III. Elimination Pattern

1. History (community representatives)
   a. What are the major kinds of wastes (industrial, sewage, etc)? Are there disposal systems? Recycling programs? Any problems perceived by community?
   b. Is there pest control? Food service inspection (restaurants, street vendors, etc.)?
   c. How is water supplied and what is the quality? Are there testing services? What does water usage cost? Are there drought restrictions?
   d. Is there concern that community growth will exceed good water supply?
   e. Are heating/cooling costs manageable for most? Do help programs exist?
2. Objective data
   a. Communicable disease statistics
   b. Air pollution statistics

IV. Activity-Exercise Pattern

1. History (community representatives)
   a. How do people find the transportation here? To work? To recreation? To health care?
   b. Do people have/use community centers (seniors, others)? Are there recreation facilities for children? Adults? Seniors?
   c. Is housing adequate (availability, cost, size)? Is there public housing?
2. Objective data
   a. Recreation/cultural programs
   b. Aids for the disabled
   c. Residential centers, nursing homes, rehabilitation facilities relative to population needs
   d. External maintenance of homes, yards, apartment houses
   e. General activity level

(box continues on page 180)

V. Sleep-Rest Pattern
1. History (community representatives)
   a. Is it generally quiet at night in most neighborhoods? If not, why?
   b. What are usual business hours? Are there industries operating around-the-clock?
2. Objective data
   a. What are the activity-noise levels in business districts? In residential districts?

VI. Cognitive-Perceptual Pattern
1. History (community representatives)
   a. Do most groups speak English? Are they bilingual? Other dominant languages?
   b. What is the educational level of population?
   c. Are schools seen as good/needing improving? Is adult education available/desired? Is vocational training available/desired?
   d. What types of problems require community decisions? How are decisions made? What is the best way to get things done/changed here?
2. Objective data
   a. Describe the school facilities. What is the dropout rate?
   b. How is the community government structured? Describe the decision-making lines.

VII. Self-Perception-Self-Concept Pattern
1. History (community representatives)
   a. Do people think this is a good community to live in? Is it going up in status, down, about the same?
   b. Is this an old community? Fairly new?
   c. Does an age group predominate?
   d. What are people's moods in general? Do people appear to be enjoying life, stressed, feeling "down"?
   e. Do people generally have the kind of abilities needed in this community?
   f. Are there community/neighborhood functions?

2. Objective data
   a. Racial, ethnic mix (if appropriate)
   b. Socioeconomic level
   c. General observations of mood

VIII. Role Relationship Pattern
1. History (community representatives)
   a. Do people seem to get along well together here? Are there places where people go to socialize?
   b. Do people think they are heard by government? Is participation in meetings high or low?
   c. Are there enough jobs for everyone? Are wages good/fair? Do people like the kind of work available? Do they seem happy in their jobs or appear to have job stress?
   d. Are there problems in the neighborhood with riots? Violence? Family violence? Child, spouse, or elder abuse?
   e. Does this community get along with adjacent communities? Do they collaborate on any projects?
   f. Do neighbors seem to support each other?
   g. Are there community get-togethers?
2. Objective data
   a. Observation of interactions (generally or at specific meetings)
   b. Statistics on interpersonal violence
   c. Statistics on employment, income/poverty
   d. Divorce rate

IX. Sexuality-Reproductive Pattern
1. History (community representatives)
   a. What is the average family size?
   b. Do people think there are any problems with pornogaphy, prostitution? Other?
   c. Do people want/support sex education in schools or in the community?
2. Objective data
   a. Family size and types of households
   b. Male-female ratio
   c. Statistics on average maternal age,

maternal mortality rate, and infant mortality rate
   d. Teen pregnancy rate
   e. Abortion rate
   f. Sexual violence statistics
   g. Laws/regulations regarding information on birth control

X. Coping-Stress Pattern
1. History (community representatives)
   a. Are there any groups that seem to be under stress?
   b. What is the need/availability of telephone help lines or support groups (health-related, other)?
2. Objective data
   a. Statistics on delinquency, drug abuse, alcoholism, suicide, psychiatric illness
   b. Unemployment rate by race/ethnicity/sex

XI. Value-Belief Pattern
1. History (community representatives)
   a. Community values: What are the top four issues that people living here see as important in their lives (note health-related values, priorities)?
   b. Do people tend to get involved in causes/local fund raising campaigns?
   c. What religious groups live in the community? What religious institutions are available?
   d. To what extent do people tolerate differences or socially deviant behavior?
2. Objective data
   a. Zoning laws
   b. Scan of public health department reports (goals, priorities)
   c. Health budget relative to total budget

*Adapted with permission from McCarthy, N. C. (1994). The 11 functional health patterns assessment guidelines for communities. Health promotion and the community. In Edelman, C. L., & Mandle, C. L., (Eds.), *Health promotion throughout the lifespan*, (3rd ed.), pp. 209–210. St. Louis, Mosby-Year Book.

divided into cooperatives, each run by a council and president. The community has continually expanded and it is estimated that 400,000 people live in the Isla. The community lacks running water, electricity, sanitation services, and fire or police protection. Illness is rampant, and there is little employment and great educational disadvantage. Many children are malnourished, have multiple frequent parasitic diseases, and frequently die.

The birth rate in the Isla and surrounding areas is high. Some deliveries occur at home, and other births take place at a local maternity hospital. This hospital is considered the second or third largest maternity hospital in South America (approximately 120 births daily and more than 500 prenatal visits daily for problem pregnancies only). One student with a special interest in maternal-child nursing was permitted to return to this hospital for a portion of a day. She observed 16 births within 2 hours, with many differences noted in maternity nursing practices. One example was very limited use of pain medication.

Many children do not or cannot afford to go to school. These children play in the streets; swim or play in polluted waters; urinate and defecate on the ground without handwashing; and run barefoot. Children as young as 5 years of age are left in charge of other much younger children while a parent works. A 1-year-old child was observed left in a house alone, unfed and dirty; other small children may be locked in from the outside. Many children and adults have lice, fungus, and other skin infections.

Living quarters are frequently one-room shacks built on sand or on stilts over the river's edge, reached by a network of rickety, narrow, broken catwalks. Accidental injuries and drownings have resulted from falls into the water. The shacks are constructed of new or salvaged materials, such as bamboo, wood, cement block, or cardboard. These shacks frequently do not prevent water or insects from entering. In heavy flooding, the shacks may collapse into the river. As many as 15 children and adults may live in one room, sleeping on rags on the floor or six in one bed. Chickens live in some homes.

Injuries and deaths from burns are considered a major hazard. They occur frequently because people cook on open flames situated next to bamboo walls; small children pull over pans of hot grease; rubbish is burned in the street, often injuring children who play nearby; and adults get electrical burns and shocks while pirating electricity from main lines.

Without a sanitation system, the people who live on the water have used the tidewaters in place of latrines to carry away human and material waste. The government has begun to permit people to live in this area and have filled in parts of the area with tons of sand, permitting housing to be built on a landfill base. The government contends that the sand is the foundation for water pipes to be laid in the future. However, the sand has prevented the natural clearing of waste by tidewater. Groundwater levels have increased particularly after tropical rains and ground waste is accumulating around the homes of families without latrines, increasing the medium for disease transmission.

There is currently no piped-in water system and water is delivered by truck and stored in a covered (or uncovered) barrel outside. Water is used for drinking, cooking, bathing, and cleaning. To be potable, water must be boiled for 20 minutes. If a lack of funds precludes buying fuel, water is often boiled for less than the recommended time or ingested from the barrel. Dysentery, cholera, and typhoid result from ingesting water contaminated with human and animal feces and often cause fatal diarrhea and dehydration. Some families cannot afford to purchase water.

Extreme poverty makes food purchase and safe storage equally difficult. Food is often eaten with soiled hands or left out uncovered, where flies contaminate it. Many houses have no food. One mother admitted to only eating a handful of peanuts the day before. Children are given cola drinks instead of the more costly milk; maternal nutritional deprivation often leads to ineffective breast-feeding; babies may be given coffee or diluted formula to drink. There is a large outdoor market in the city where vendors sell domestic goods, items in bulk, fresh fruits and vegetables, and meat. Students observed chickens being freshly killed and then left out without refrigeration. Unfortunately, the market is inaccessible to Isla residents, who must find and pay for public transportation to get there. This forces residents to buy goods at small stores in the community, where prices and quality of products are problematic.

Health care for the Isla is highly inadequate, although it has improved since the small dispensary was constructed in 1994. Many people cannot afford to pay the equivalent of 50 cents for a visit or for prescriptions. Home remedies, some of which are dangerous, may be used for a sick person. Even hospitalized patients may not receive medication, plasma, or bandages until the family prepays.

There are few avenues for rest and recreation in the community. Adults admit they are too poor or tired to do much that can be considered fun. Children have few toys. A day care center was established to assist working parents and provide socialization for some children. However, 35 children and infants are tended by 3 adults. Stress levels are admittedly high and many people, particularly men, use alcohol as a relaxant. Many families attend Sunday religious services or other activities held at the church. The church plays a prominent part in many of the residents' lives. They hold Fr. Fred in great esteem and frequently turn to him for spiritual, emotional, and economic assistance. Fr. Fred has also developed training programs to try to create job skills for interested residents.

Establishing Community Diagnoses

A community assessment by each student group demonstrates the numerous health hazards in the Isla Verde community, many of which are related to poor hygiene practices and risk-taking behavior. Students choose a functional health pattern, identify associated community diagnoses, and prioritize them according to community strengths and deficits. The students then establish health promotion projects.

Box 7-3 is a selective list of community diagnoses identified by students.

Establishing a Community Health Promotion Intervention

It is challenging to develop successful health promotion programs for culturally and ethnically diverse populations. Language differences, poverty, prejudice, low literacy levels, traditional teaching and learning styles, alternative treatment modes and practices, and beliefs about illness are some of the many factors that must be considered if a program is to be effective (DeSantis & Thomas, 1992; El-Katsha & Watts, 1993; Pinzon & Perez, 1997; Shadick, 1993; Williamson, Stecchi, Allen, & Coppens, 1997). The students in the Por Cristo-BCSON project try to incorporate the community's needs, interests, values, beliefs, and resources into the health promotion programs while recognizing their own time limitations.

Preparing the Health Promotion Projects

Before arriving in the host country, students arrange themselves in teaching groups and begin planning their health promotion projects based on Fr. Fred's feedback and the priority community diagnoses identified by former students. They also incorporate many of the helpful suggestions found in *Where There Is No Doctor* (Werner, 1998) and *Helping Health Workers Learn* (Werner & Bower, 1995) into their teaching activities and materials. (Spanish versions of these books are also used.)

Teaching groups are organized around various health issues, including infant and child care, nutrition, immunization, diarrhea and dehydration, breast-feeding, hygiene, and accident prevention. Adolescence and women's health issues addressed include education about and prevention of STDs and HIV/AIDS and sex education to prevent adolescent pregnancy. General health and safety issues, such as burn prevention and treatment, first aid for choking, when to seek medical attention, and principles of nutrition adapted to the customs, income, and available products of the region, are also addressed.

Developing Relationships and Gaining Acceptance

Fr. Fred has helped the students gain acceptance by securing support of community leaders and residents (Michielutte, & Beal, 1990). Students are warmly welcomed, because of their willingness to roll up their sleeves and dig in. Students have paid for and helped construct latrines, cleaned a poor mother's backyard of broken glass where young children were running around barefoot, and even built a table out of new and used wood for a family who ate on the floor. Students have brought medical supplies, school books, and other items to distribute to the neediest. The Isla Verde community looks forward to the arrival of students and many people attend the community *charlas*, or chats, run by the students.

Implementing the Health Promotion Projects

Once the students are in the Isla Verde community, focus groups are formed to promote community participation, to self-select topics, and to provide insight on the dimensions of problems (Windsor et al, 1994). This approach works well with the Latino population (Anderson, Goddard, Garcia, Guzman, & Vazquez, 1998; Ludwig-Beymer, Blankemeir, Casas-Byots, & Suarez-Balcazar, 1996; Perilla, Wilson, Wold, & Spencer, 1998), and attendees welcome the opportunity to offer suggestions, admitting that few people ever ask for their input. Through the community suggestions, students of the Por Cristo-BCSON project conduct daily *charlas* (afternoon talks), which are publicized by word of mouth and posted notices. Classes take place in either the dispensary or adjoining church and are well attended. Most attendees are women, many with children, and it is not unusual to see a standing-room-only crowd.

BOX 7-3. Community Diagnoses in Isla Verde

Health Perception-Health Management Pattern

Health Seeking Behaviors related to (r/t) faithful attendance at classes, active questioning, attentiveness

Injury: Actual and Potential r/t multiple sources of burns, abuse, drowning, broken glass and syringes on road, bare feet, broken boards in houses on stilts, getting hit by cars, violence (rock throwing, guns, etc.)

Altered Protection r/t wife abuse, child abuse, sexual abuse, lack of police or social protection

Impaired Home Maintenance r/t sense of hopelessness, lack of structural integrity, and inability to purchase repair materials

Infection: Actual and Potential r/t not cleaning wounds, bug bites, using inappropriate remedies for burns (i.e., toothpaste, mud, sputum), multiple sex partners and prostitution, and lack of condom use

Pain r/t lack of medicine, conservative use of analgesics

Nutritional-Metabolic Pattern

Altered Growth and Development r/t altered nutrition and sensory deprivation

Altered Nutrition: Nutritional Deficit r/t inability to purchase food, inability to obtain quality food, knowledge deficit in best use and preparation of local foods, diarrhea

Fatigue r/t nutritional deficit, overworking, etc.

Fluid Volume Deficit r/t diarrhea and knowledge deficit

Elimination Pattern

Alteration in Elimination: Diarrhea r/t environmental pollution, poor hygiene practices, barriers to implementing prevention strategies

Activity-Exercise Pattern

Diversional Activity Deficit r/t small overcrowded living situations and neighborhoods, deficit of play space or equipment

Ineffective Breathing Pattern r/t environmental dust, untreated asthma

Sleep-Rest Pattern

Sleep Disturbance r/t overcrowding, lack of adequate space, noise

Cognitive-Perceptual Pattern

Knowledge Deficit r/t AIDS transmission, basic hygiene

Cognitive Impairment: Potential r/t malnourishment before and after birth, child neglect, lack of stimulation

Self-Concept-Self-Perception Pattern

Fear r/t robbery, rape, abandonment, inability to support family units

Powerlessness: Severe r/t lack of education, social control, abuse of women and children

Role Relationship Pattern

Impaired Social Interaction r/t lack of community cohesiveness, inability to request help despite need

Altered Parenting r/t young pregnancies, no resources, unemployment, abuse cycles, single female-headed families of many closely spaced children

Violence: Potential for r/t dispiritedness, lack of protection against abuse and injustice, reports of weapons in community

Sexuality-Reproductive Pattern

Altered Sexuality Patterns r/t lack of sex education, frequent unplanned pregnancies, rape, prostitution, unprotected sex

Coping-Stress Tolerance Pattern

Family Coping: Potential for Growth r/t observation and report of families supporting and caring for one another and unselfishly sharing all their goods

Anxiety r/t deaths and debilitating diseases

Defensive Coping r/t deplorable living conditions

Value-Brief Pattern

Spiritual Distress r/t lack of basic human needs, human rights abuse, expressions of hopelessness

Teaching Strategies

The students use various approaches (eg, models, posters) in their teaching projects. A large toothbrush and a set of teeth have been used to demonstrate oral hygiene to children. Each child receives a toothbrush for return demonstration and a sample of toothpaste. A doll is used to demonstrate infant care and breast-feeding positions. A realistic breast model worn over the chest permits the attendees to learn about appropriate positions for breast self-exam. Verbal instructions, posters, and handouts are used to teach how to prevent diarrhea in children and how to prepare and administer oral rehydration therapy. Donated microscopes permit the students to teach about sources of bacterial contamination; children and adults are fascinated to see teeming microbes living in samples taken from an ordinary water barrel. By visualizing the organisms that make people sick, the community understands the basis for teaching them to cover food and to boil water.

Discussion groups have been organized by students and include coeducational adolescent support groups to discuss sexual development and prevention of unplanned pregnancy and rape; a parents' support group, with men attending, discusses community issues (eg, stress reduction, domestic abuse, empowerment strategies).

Burn Prevention and Treatment Program

The burn prevention and treatment program is a crucial community-wide project for the Isla Verde. Nursing students present this program to children, adults, health providers and teachers, using the clinic, school, church, and day-care center for settings. The objectives of this program are for participants to identify sources of burn injuries and deaths, practice preventive strategies, and treat burns appropriately. Small groups of children are gathered and the nursing students appear in brightly colored clothing (eg, orange gloves, red shirts, yellow tights) that simulate fire colors. Participation is encouraged by a question and answer period before and after the program. The children are asked if they know anyone who has

been burned. What happened to that person? What caused the burn? What could have been done to prevent it?

The children usually know a burn victim and mention pain and scarring. The causes of burns range from playing with matches to being scalded with hot liquid. Their knowledge of preventive methods is often limited. They are asked what they should do if their clothing catches on fire. Some of the students know the correct answer and are complimented. The student teachers role play with props, actually rolling on the ground or floor, while others recite the Spanish version of "Stop, Drop, and Roll." Volunteers from the audience are then selected.

Posters emphasizing burn prevention strategies depict storing matches away from children, turning pot handles inward, observing children when a trash or other type of fire is burning, and securing a metal shield behind a cooking fire.

Proper burn treatment includes understanding how to treat pain, keeping the wound clean, assessing severity, and knowing when to seek medical treatment. Posters depict first-, second-, and third-degree burns. Students emphasize protecting the burn from dirt, excreta, and insects; they also emphasize using clean cool water on first-degree burns and warm salt water as compresses for second-degree burns (Werner, 1998). They explain why grease, mud, oil, coffee, feces, urine, or toothpaste should never be used and that severe burns, signs of infection, or extended burns on small children should be treated at the clinic.

An oral quiz is given at the end of each session, and questions from the audience are answered. Children are instructed to share what they have learned with their siblings and parents. Teachers are also given materials for reinforcing the lessons.

Water Purification

Lack of potable water is a major public health problem in many poor countries that causes many deaths, especially to young children because of diarrheal disease and dehydration. Therefore, students now teach a water purification process, using an empty plastic soda bottle with half of its surface painted black from top to bottom. A bottle is filled with water that is filtered first if it comes directly from a river. It is then left under direct sun for 5 hours, painted side down. All microbes are killed and the water becomes safe to drink. The procedure has been shared with community residents, staff, and nursing students.

Outcomes

Evaluation of the various health promotion activities must be ongoing, and there are no statistics to demonstrate the outcomes. However, each year the Por Cristo-BCSON project has tried to reach as many children and families as possible. They continue to teach burn prevention and treatment and collaborate with a community pediatrician who has begun to collect data on burns; in a system in which people frequently self-treat except in major crises, data collection is a challenge. Teacher and learner satisfaction have been rated as high, and the community has consistently demonstrated the desire to learn and to promote self-help.

The author believes that the Por Cristo-BCSON Health Project has helped create a vehicle for health promotion by sharing all of our teaching projects with the staff of the dispensary and the students and faculty with whom we affiliate. In this way, we promote continuity in health teaching and nursing intervention from within the population. In 1999, the chapter author facilitated the first nursing diagnosis conference to take place in an Andean country. Dr. Marjory Gordon, the featured speaker, addressed the need for a thorough assessment to guide diagnosis and intervention at all levels. Particular emphasis was placed on the nurse's health teaching role. This conference and other workshops with nurses in practice aimed to increase the commitment of professional nurses to include health promotion and primary prevention in their patient care.

Most of the U.S. population will soon be comprised of people originating from Africa, Latin America, and Asia. An overseas immersion experience provides a milieu for health professionals to develop and incorporate cultural competence and language fluency into clinical practice. Successful health promotion strategies must be congruent with the health beliefs and practices of the target population, based on the population's fundamental concerns and needs, and aimed at results that are desirable and ultimately achievable (Kreps & Kunimoto, 1994, p. 122). Nurses, irrespective of their clinical specialty, must accept health promotion and counseling as an integral part of their nursing practice. These principles will continue to guide our missions to Isla Verde.

Health Promotion Programs in the Workplace: Boston College "The Challenge"

General Considerations

Promoting healthy lifestyles is both a humanistic and an economic concern to employers and those who provide occupational health promotion programs. The American Association of Occupational Health Nurses recognized this need and recommended that by the year 2000, 90% of workplaces would provide their employees with risk reduction and health promotion services (Swanson & Nies, 1997). Although not mandated by federal regulation, many companies take a proactive approach to health promotion and offer employees various services that promote wellness.

Successful workplace programs must promote health practice skills, provide peer support, promote the notion that health is controllable, involve the employee in planning both personal behavior modification and change in the work environment, and define health as wellness rather than risk reduction (Pender, Walker, Sechrist, & Frank-Stromberg, 1990). Moreover, Salazar (1991) contends that successful outcomes increase when programs use a theoretical base for planning and development of interventions.

Description of "The Challenge"

The Challenge is an ongoing health promotion program for university faculty and staff at Boston College. It takes place during the spring semester and includes weekly discussions on health, diet, and exercise; organized exercise activities; and establishment of support groups. The model is based on a team approach, and points are awarded to those teams who lose weight within a predetermined range, engage in specific exercises, and attend weekly 55-minute presentations on a relevant topic. Each team consists of at least five members, headed by a team captain who tallies individual weight and exercise points weekly. Programs include a nominal registration fee and various prizes and "perks," such as a tee-shirt with the program logo.

The School of Nursing faculty and students of the participating university provide consultation on various aspects of the overall program, conduct height and weight measurement and blood pressure screening at the first and last sessions, and conduct some of the seminars. Topics include principles of behavior modification, choosing the right exercises, understanding one's relationship to food, principles of nutrition, stress management, and maintaining one's health promotion program. Additional nutritional and health counseling and referrals are made available.

Force Field Analysis

As a member of Boston College's health promotion team, the author of this chapter incorporated Lewin's force field analysis and various health promotion strategies to teach participants how to plan and maintain wellness behaviors. Lewin's force field analysis has two main components. First, compliance increases when people identify both the stumbling blocks to their own behavioral change and the strategies for change they would find most acceptable. Second, knowledge of the forces that promote positive behavioral change and the strategies that are more likely to effect change help the health professional improve the target population's health outcomes.

Force field analysis, although developed in the 1940s by Lewin and associates, is still considered an important approach to planned change (Lewin, Dembo, Festinger, & Sears,

1944). The behavioral change strategies consist of the following (Lewin et al, 1944):

- **Unfreezing**—making one aware of the need for change or increasing a person's readiness or willingness to change
- **Moving**—using various cognitive, affective, or regulatory strategies to implement the change
- **Refreezing**—that phase of the change when the new behavior is internalized

Force field analysis refers to a major part of the unfreezing stage. It addresses those forces (ie, factors or determinants) that will assist the change (ie, driving forces) and those that will impede change (ie, restraining forces). Change may be effected in three ways: adding forces that promote change, reducing forces that impede change, or redirecting forces that support change (Lewin et al, 1944). Forces that promote or impede change frequently are of unequal strength; for example, resistance to change may be weakened when the behavior is deemed as culturally appropriate, pleasurable, or easy to maintain. When the suggested action is deemed as a loss, painful, culturally incorrect, expensive, beyond the resources of the target population, or without value, resistance will be stronger.

Health Promotion Strategies

Various health promotion techniques for the community have been suggested in the literature. Successful interventions often incorporate various approaches, because no single technique has been found superior. A combination of strategies that provide factual information, stimulate motivation, help change attitudes and behavior, and promote competence may better address the multifaceted nature of health behavior (see the Appendix: Behavioral Change Strategies).

Identifying Personal Barriers, Enhancers, and Strategies for Change

The Challenge program was introduced with the notion of how challenging it is to advise people to change lifelong habits. In considering stress reduction, health professionals often simply suggest changing one's lifestyle without assessing the availability of options or resources for making these lifestyle changes. However, the interest in improving health and fitness shown by Challenge participants was a positive sign of motivation. The attitudinal framework for Challenge sessions would therefore be positive thinking and positive reinforcement rather than negative thinking and reinforcement.

It was explained in multiple Challenge sessions that behavior (ie, what people do) is a result of what people believe or value and the meaning attached to the behavior. The more value (ie, pleasure, reward, satisfaction, or relief of emotional or physical pain) attached to the behavior, the more difficult it is to change the behavior. This connection between behavior and value leads to habits, both good and bad (eg, buckling your seat belt every time you get into a car, reaching for snacks every time you sit in front of a television). Therefore, changing attitudes and customary behaviors requires knowledge, motivation, resources, and skill.

The purpose of these sessions was to help participants identify their particular strengths and weaknesses, uncover their values, examine the bases for their actions, and identify some of the strategies they could use in reaching and maintaining their individual goals. Force field analysis was explained as a method that helps people identify the forces that promote or prevent their own behavior change. Many of these forces are common to all of us. Participants began to identify barriers to change (eg, fear of failure, sense of loss).

For the Challenge, forces that promote or impede change were combined into three categories: biologic-physiologic, emotional-cognitive, and social-cultural-economic. Examples of biologic-physiologic factors included genetic makeup (eg, body type, metabolism), gender, existing disease processes, and age. Emotional-cognitive factors address coping styles, mental status, long- and short-term health goals, and knowledge deficits. Social-cultural-economic factors included cultural food patterns, job-related activity patterns (eg, sedentary work, frequent restaurant dining), and access to health services.

As the beginning step in self-knowledge, participants in the Challenge were instructed to identify a realistic goal and note on an assessment form the positive and negative factors particularly relevant to them (Figure 7-1). Participants were then instructed to assign a level of importance to each factor in accordance with how easy or difficult it would be to accomplish. These steps were based on numerous research reports suggesting that self-efficacy (ie, the belief one is capable of carrying out the action) is one of the strongest determinants of successful behavior change (Bandura, 1982; Lawrance & McElroy, 1986; Merritt, 1989; Witte, Berkowitz, Cameron & McKeon, 1998). Finally, each participant received a worksheet to list the factors perceived as barriers and the behavioral strategies he or she thought would help.

Because of the group's diverse makeup, many different health-related issues, diets, and types of exercise were identified. Participants viewed the university's commitment to health promotion, the availability of excellent resources, and supportive fellow staff as external motivators. Written evaluations indicated that self-assessment of behavioral barriers and motivators provided insight into behavior patterns that had not been considered.

Given the success of this approach with the Challenge, this method has been taught to nursing students for use with individuals or community groups. It remains important that follow-up be done to identify stumbling blocks that may arise and to ascertain that the intervention(s) selected are appropriate, realistic, accessible and used.

SUMMARY

Health professionals are often responsible for helping clients learn new ways to improve their health and to achieve a higher level of wellness. Earlier chapters in this book provide

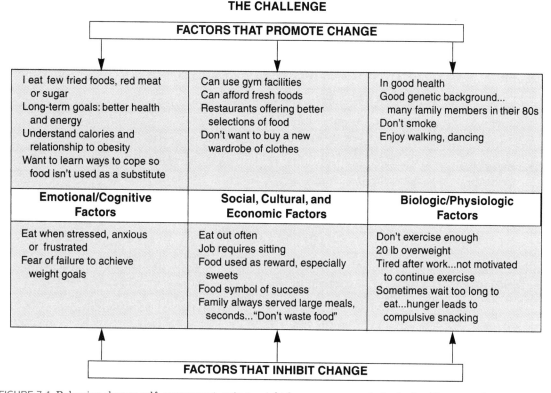

FIGURE 7-1. Behavior change self-assessment, using weight loss as an example in the health promotion program *The Challenge.*

theoretical models for developing patient education programs. This chapter presents two health promotion projects that demonstrate how to assess areas in which health education is needed, how to teach people to identify their own behavioral barriers and enhancers to change, and how to promote clients' health through techniques of behavior change. Health promotion occurs in many different settings with diverse population groups. The health educator must therefore develop cultural competence and the ability to act as advocate to promote the community's acquiring necessary resources and successfully achieving health promotion goals. Although personal responsibility for health is recognized, consideration is given to external factors that arise from the political climate, the social environment, the economy, and the resources that may or may not be available from the health system.

STRATEGIES FOR CRITICAL ANALYSIS AND APPLICATION

1. Compare the differences in planning a health promotion program for a person, a family, or an entire community. What are the advantages and disadvantages of each approach?
2. You work in a community comprised of many low-income families and older people. How would these demographic variables be used to develop a health promotion campaign? What other information would you obtain to prioritize the community's needs?

3. What are the goals of health promotion programs in accordance with the developmental stage?

4. Discuss how culture and language influence health education programs in a community.

5. Identify the persuasive methods that advertisers use to convince consumers to buy such products as tobacco or alcoholic beverages. How could these same methods be used to foster health-promoting behaviors (eg, use of seat belts)?

6. What strategies are necessary to achieve a smoke-free society by the year 2010?

REFERENCES

Anderson, R. M., Goddard, C. E., Garcia, R., Guzman, J. R., & Vazquez, F. (1998). Using focus groups to identify diabetes care and education issues for Latinos with diabetes. *The Diabetes Educator, 24,* 618–625.

Andreasen, A. R. (1995). *Marketing social change: Changing behavior to promote health, social development, and the environment.* San Francisco, CA: Jossey-Bass.

Armbruster, C., Gale, B., Brady, J., & Thompson, N. (1999). Perceived ownership in a community coalition. *Public Health Nursing, 16*(1), 17–22.

Bandura, A. (1982). Self-efficacy mechanism in human agency. *American Psychologist, 37,* 122–147.

Barth, R. P. (1993). *Reducing the risks: Building skills to prevent STD & HIV* (2nd ed.). Santa Cruz, CA: ETR Associates.

Bastian, H. (1996). Raising the standard: Practice guidelines and consumer participation. *International Journal for Quality in Health Care, 8,* 485–490.

Biener, L. (1999). *Progress towards reducing smoking in the Commonwealth of Massachusetts: 1993 to FY 1999.* Boston, MA: Center for Survey Research, University of Massachusetts. *Boston Globe.* June 24, 1994, p. 19, V245 #174.

Butterfoss, F. D., Morrow, A. L., Rosenthal, J., Dini, E., Crews, R. C., Webster, J. D., & Louis, P. (1998). CINCH: An urban coalition for empowerment and action. *Health Education and Behavior, 25,* 212–215.

Chapman, S., Long, W. L, & Smith, W. (1993). Self-exempting beliefs about smoking and health: Differences between smokers and ex-smokers. *American Journal of Public Health, 83,* 215–219.

Clark, M. J. (1999). *Nursing in the community: Dimensions of community health nursing* (3rd ed.). Norwalk, CT: Appleton & Lange.

Cohen, B. B., Lederman, R. I., Connolly, G. N., & Danley, R. A. (1991). *Smoking: Death, disease and dollars.* Boston: Massachusetts Department of Public Health, Chronic Disease Surveillance Program, Bureau of Health Statistics, Research and Evaluation, and Office for Nonsmoking and Health, Bureau of Parent, Child and Adolescent Health.

Courtney, R., Ballard, E., Fauver, S., Gariota, M., & Holland, L. (1996). The partnership model: Working with individuals, families, and communities toward a new vision of health. *Public Health Nursing, 3,* 177–186.

Covington, H. (1999). Community involvement. *Nursing and Health Care Perspectives, 20*(2), 82–86.

da Costa e Silva, V. L. (1993). Anti-tobacco posters in Brazil: Fighting smoking with humour, satire, and ridicule. *Tobacco Control, 2,* 189–190.

DeSantis, L., & Thomas, J. T. (1992). Health education and the immigrant Haitian mother: Cultural insights for community health nurses. *Public Health Nursing, 9,* 87–96.

Drexler, M. (1994). Tapping the youth market. *The Boston Globe Magazine,* October 23, 1994 V246 #15 17–24, 30–31.

Edwards, C. C., Elder, J. P., de Moor, C., Wildey, M. B., Mayer, J. A., & Senn, K. L. (1992). Predictors of participation in a school-based anti-tobacco activism program. *Journal of Community Health, 17,* 283–289.

Elder, J. P., Campbell, N. R., Candelaria, J. I., Talavera, G. A., Mayer, J. A., Moreno, C., Medel, Y. R., & Lyons, G. K. (1998). Project Salsa: Development and institutionalization of a nutritional health promotion project in a Latino community. *American Journal of Health Promotion, 12,* 391–401.

El-Askari, G., Freestone, J., Irizarry, C., Kraut, K. L., Mashiyama, S. T., Morgan, M. A., & Walton, S. (1998). *Health Education and Behavior, 25,* 146–159.

El-Katsha, S., & Watts, S. (1993). A multifaceted approach to health education: A case study from rural Egypt. *International Quarterly of Community Health Education, 13,* 139–149.

Green, P. M., & Adderley-Kelly, B. (1999). Partnership for health promotion in an urban community. *Nursing and Health Care Perspectives, 20*(2), 76–81.

Gordon, M. (1991). *Nursing diagnosis: Process and application* (3rd ed.). St. Louis: Mosby—Year Book.

Gordon, M. (1997). *Manual of nursing diagnosis: 1997–1998.* St. Louis: Mosby—Year Book.

Hamilton, W. L., & Norton, G. D. (1999). *Independent evaluation of the Massachusetts tobacco control program: Fifth annual report summary-January 1994 to June 1998.* Cambridge, MA: Abt Associates, Inc.

Hatton, D. C., & Webb, T. (1993). Information transmission in bilingual, bicultural contexts: A field study of community health nurses and interpreters. *Journal of Community Health Nursing, 10*, 137–147.

Healey, B. J. (1998). The use of prevalence data to unite the community in prevention programs. *Journal of Public Health Management Practice, 4*(6), 88–92.

Hedelin, B., & Svensson, P. (1999). Psychiatric nursing for promotion of mental health and prevention of depression in the elderly: A case study. *Journal of Psychiatric and Mental Health Nursing, 6*, 115–124.

Hovell, M., Blumberg, E., Sipan, C., Hofstetter, C. R., Burkham, S., Atkins, C., & Felice, M. (1998). Skills training for pregnancy and AIDS prevention in Anglo and Latino youth. *Journal of Adolescent Health, 23*, 139–149.

Juhn, G., Tang, J., Piessens, P., Grant, U., Johnson, N., & Murray, H. (1999). Community learning: The Reach for Health nursing program-middle school collaboration. *Journal of Nursing Education, 38*, 215–221.

Kark, S. L., Kark, E., & Abramson, J. H. (1993). Commentary: In search of innovative approaches to international health. *American Journal of Public Health, 83*, 1533–1536.

Kleffel, D. (1991). Rethinking the environment as a domain of nursing knowledge. *Advances in Nursing Science, 14*(1), 40–51.

Kreps, G. L., & Kunimoto, E. N. (1994). *Effective communication in multicultural health care settings.* Thousand Oaks, CA: Sage.

Kriegler, N. F., & Harton, M. K. (1992). Community health assessment tool: A patterns approach to data collection and diagnosis. *Journal of Community Health Nursing, 9*, 229–234.

Krozy, R. E., & McCarthy, N. C. (1999). Developing bilingual tools to assess functional health patterns. *Nursing Diagnosis: The Journal of Nursing Language and Classification, 10*(1), 21–29, 34.

Larson, E. (1994). Exclusion of certain groups from clinical research. *Image—The Journal of Nursing Scholarship, 26*, 185–190.

Lawrance, L., & McElroy, K. (1986). Self-efficacy and health education. *Journal of School Health, 56*, 37–321.

Leonard, T. (1996). *The Filthy, Disgusting, Ugly, Foul, Hideous, Horrible, Ghastly, Nasty, Nauseating Tobacco Quiz (Title # 5060),* Santa Cruz, CA: Journeyworks Publishing

Lewin, K., Dembo, T., Festinger, L., & Sears, P. S. (1944). Level of aspiration. In J. Hunt (Ed.), *Personality and the behavioral disorders: A handbook based on experimental and clinical research.* New York: Ronald Press.

Lindenberg, C. S., Solorzano, R. M., Krantz, M. S., Galvis, C., Baroni, G., & Strickland, O. (1998). Risk and resilience: Building protective factors. *MCN; American Journal of Maternal Child Nursing, 23*, 99–104.

Lowe, J. I., Barg, F. K., & Stephens, K. (1999). Community residents as lay health educators in a neighborhood cancer prevention program. *Journal of Community Practice, 5*(4), 39–52.

Ludwig-Beymer, P., Blankemeir, J. R., Casas-Byots, C., & Suarez-Balcazar, Y. (1996). Community assessment in a suburban Hispanic community: A description of method. *Journal of Transcultural Nursing, 8*(1), 19–27.

Lundeen, S. P. (1992). Health needs of a suburban community: A nursing assessment approach. *Journal of Community Health Nursing, 9*, 235–244.

Lynagh, M., Knight, J., Schofield, M. J., & Paras, L. (1999). Lessons learned from the Hunter Region Health Promoting Schools Project in New South Wales, Australia. *Journal of School Health, 69*, 227–232.

Massachusetts Tobacco Control Program. (1994a). *Fact sheet.* Boston: Massachusetts Tobacco Control Program, Massachusetts Department of Public Health.

Massachusetts Tobacco Control Program. (1994b). *Preliminary report on the impact of the cigarette tax increase on cigarette consumption in Massachusetts and first wave results of tracking study of the Massachusetts Tobacco Control Media Campaign.* Boston: Massachusetts Tobacco Control Program, Massachusetts Department of Public Health.

McCarthy, N. C. (1994). The 11 functional health assessment guidelines for communities. Health promotion and the community. In C. L. Edelman & C. L. Mandle (Eds.), *Health promotion throughout the lifespan* (3rd ed.). St. Louis: Mosby-Year Book.

McDermott, M. A. N., & Palchanes, K. (1993). A literature review of the critical elements in translation theory. *Image — The Journal of Nursing Scholarship, 26*, 113–117.

Merritt, S. (1989). Patient self-efficacy: A framework for designing patient education. *Focus on Critical Care, 16*, 68–73.

Michielutte, R., & Beal, P. (1990). Identification of community leadership in the development of public health education programs. *Journal of Community Health, 15*, 59–68.

Miller, D. R., Geller, A. C., Wood, M. C., Lew, R. A., & Koh, H. K. (1999). Falmouth Safe Skin Project: Evaluation of a community program to promote sun protection in youth. *Health Education and Behavior, 26*, 369–384.

Navaie-Waliser, M., Gordon, S. K., & Hibberd, M. E. (1996). The Mentoring Mothers Program: A community-empowering approach to reducing infant mortality. *Journal of Perinatal Education, 5*(4), 47–61.

Pender, N. J., Walker, S. N., Sechrist, K. R., & Frank-Stromberg, M. (1990). Predicting health-promoting lifestyles in the workplace. *Nursing Research, 39*, 326–332.

Perilla, J. L., Wilson, A. H., Wold, J. L., & Spencer, L. (1998). Listening to migrant voices: Focus groups on health issues in South Georgia. *Journal of Community Health Nursing, 15*, 251–263.

Pinzon, H. L., & Perez, M. A. (1997). Multicultural issues in health education programs for Hispanic-Latino populations in the United States. *Journal of Health Education, 28*, 314–316.

Popham, W. J., Potter, L. D., Bal, D. G., Johnson, M. D., Duerr, J. M., & Quinn, V. (1993). Do anti-smoking media campaigns help smokers quit? *Public Health Reports, 108*, 510–513.

Rainey, J., & Lindsay, G. (1994). 101 questions for community health promotion planning. *Journal of Health Education, 25*, 309–312.

Salazar, M. K. (1991). Comparison of four behavioral theories: A literature review. *AAOHN Journal, 39*, 128–135.

Shadick, K. M. (1993). Development of a transcultural health education program for the Hmong. *Clinical Nurse Specialist, 7*, 48–53.

Shields, L. E., & Lindsey, E. (1998). Community health promotion nursing practice. *Advances in Nursing Science, 20*(4), 23–29.

Stehr-Green, P. A., Dini, E. F., Lindegren, M. L., & Patriarca, P. A. (1993). Evaluation of telephoned computer-generated reminders to improve immunization coverage at inner city clinics. *Public Health Reports, 108*, 426–430.

Swanson, J. M., & Nies, M. A. (1997). *Community health nursing: Promoting the health of aggregates* (2nd ed.). Philadelphia: Saunders.

Tilbury, M., & Fisk, T. (1989). *Marketing and nursing: A contemporary view.* Owings Mills, MD: National Health Publishing.

Urrutia-Rojas, X., & Aday, L. A. (1991). A framework for community assessment: Designing and conducting a survey in a Hispanic immigrant and refugee community. *Public Health Nursing, 8*(1), 20–26.

U.S. Department of Health and Human Services. (1990). *Healthy People 2000.* Washington, D. C.: U. S. Government Printing Office.

U.S. Department of Health and Human Services. (2000). *Healthy People 2010: Understanding and improvoing health.* Washington, D. C.: U.S. Government Printing Office.

U.S. Department of Health and Human Services. (1994). *Preventing tobacco use among young people: A report of the Surgeon General.* U.S. Department of Health and Human Services, Public Health Service, Centers for Disease Control and Prevention, National Center for Chronic Disease Prevention and Health Promotion, Office on Smoking and Health.

Wallerstein, N., & Bernstein, E. (1998). Empowerment education: Friere's ideas adapted to health. *Health Education Quarterly, 15*, 379–394.

Werner, D. (1998). *Where there is no doctor: A village health care handbook* (Rev. ed.). Palo Alto, CA: Hesperian Foundation.

Werner, D., & Bower, B. (1995). *Helping health workers learn.* Palo Alto, CA: Hesperian Foundation.

Weston, C., & Cranton, P. A. (1986). Selecting instructional strategies. *Journal of Higher Education, 57*, 263–268.

Williamson, E., Stecchi, J. M., Allen, B. B., & Coppens, N. M. (1997). The development of culturally appropriate health education materials. *Journal of Nursing Staff Development, 13*(1), 19–23.

Windsor, R. A., Lowe, J. B., Perkins, L. L., Smith-Yoder, D., Artz, L., Crawford, M., Amburgy, K., & Boyd, N. R., Jr. (1993). Health education for pregnant smokers: Its behavioral impact and cost benefit. *American Journal of Public Health, 83,* 201–206.

Windsor, R., Baranowski, T., Clark, N., & Cutter, G. (1994). *Evaluation of health promotion, health education, and disease prevention programs* (2nd ed.). Mountain View, CA: Mayfield.

Witte, K., Berkowitz, J. M., Cameron, K. A., & McKeon, J. K. (1998). Preventing the spread of genital warts: Using fear appeals to promote self-protective behaviors. *Health Education and Behavior, 25,* 571–585.

Application of the Principles in Nursing Practice

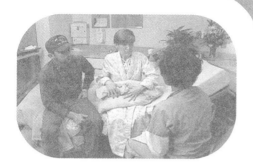

Assessment for Patient Education

LEARNING OBJECTIVES

After reading this chapter, the nurse or student nurse should be able to:

1. List red flags used to identify patients with complex discharge planning needs as part of the assessment process.

2. Identify the four steps of the assessment process and describe how they relate to patient education.

3. List four questions a nurse should answer to gain vital assessment data.

4. State two benefits of using a Patient and Family Assessment Guide.

5. Discuss how patient education relates to all nursing diagnoses and the limited circumstances in which you might select the following nursing diagnoses: knowledge deficit, noncompliance.

6. Describe benefits of home visits for patient assessment.

INTRODUCTION

Nursing Process and Patient Education

Patient education plans are part of the total plan for patient care. Patient education is an integral part of each of the four phases of the nursing process: assessment, planning, intervention, and evaluation (Figure 8-1). The medical diagnosis begins with early screening on admission to determine what is likely to cause trouble for the patient and to anticipate functional problems. That is, shift the focus from medical diagnosis to functional problems. Ask, How does the medical diagnosis affect *this* patient?

The nurse also looks realistically at anticipated length of stay and determines how much and when to teach each patient. The nursing process helps the nurse examine his or her relationship to the patient. Use of the nursing process encourages the application of protocols and standards that will direct, rather than dictate, patient care. The components of the nursing process offer a framework for modifying care so that nurses and patients grow in a cooperative relationship. When this cooper-

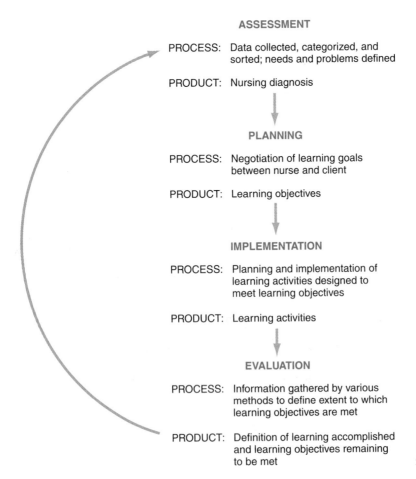

ASSESSMENT

PROCESS: Data collected, categorized, and sorted; needs and problems defined

PRODUCT: Nursing diagnosis

PLANNING

PROCESS: Negotiation of learning goals between nurse and client

PRODUCT: Learning objectives

IMPLEMENTATION

PROCESS: Planning and implementation of learning activities designed to meet learning objectives

PRODUCT: Learning activities

EVALUATION

PROCESS: Information gathered by various methods to define extent to which learning objectives are met

PRODUCT: Definition of learning accomplished and learning objectives remaining to be met

FIGURE 8-1. The nursing process in patient education.

ative relationship exists, patients are cared for as individuals and can learn to participate in their own care in a meaningful and satisfying manner.

This chapter illustrates the use of the nursing process as a model for patient education, highlighting the important skills of assessment, planning, implementation, and evaluation. Although the principles may appear simple, application of the nursing process involves a broad understanding of the patient, family, and considerable clinical expertise to provide individualized care. Individualized care fulfills the following criteria:

- Includes a care plan that is specific to the individual patient
- Requires critical thinking to meet the patient's unique needs
- Cannot be accomplished in a cookbook approach

The case studies offered in this chapter illustrate principles of patient education, but are not intended to be used as a cookbook. As nurses continue training in their specialty areas and continue learning more about patient problems they encounter, they can use this text to complement their education of patient and family and to develop individualized teaching plans.

Discharge Planning

As soon as patients are admitted to the hospital, assessment of the potential for discharge begins. Discharge planning occurs not just in inpatient acute care settings, but also in emergency rooms, home health care, surgical centers, and long-term care. Discharge planning is an important evaluation of actual or potential problems that must be dealt with before a safe discharge is made. Ideally, all members of the health care team contribute to the discharge assessment process. For many patients, discharge planning and patient education are intertwined. The patient and family will be taught survival skills and will assume functions of health care management. For some patients, postdischarge needs are complex.

Early detection of special assistance and resources and making timely arrangements for continuing care are essential, especially in light of decreased lengths of stay (Menke, 1993; Miller & Capps, 1997).

One method of ensuring coordinated care is use of an admission database that contains questions to screen for discharge concerns. These concerns are referred to as *red flags*. Interdisciplinary case conferences are common on hospital units to pick up red flags. Nursing rounds have become increasingly popular to continue the screening, and to coordinate discharge planning and patient teaching efforts. Discharge planning, a part of routine patient care, also is an interdisciplinary process to help patients and their families develop and implement a feasible post-hospital plan of care.

Nurses often organize the health care team in regularly scheduled meetings to review patient cases. Depending on the identified patient needs, the following disciplines are also represented: medicine, nutrition, social work, pharmacy, physical therapy, occupational therapy, recreational therapy, and home health. Sometimes patients and family members are included.

Box 8-1 provides examples of red flag patients who are high risk and in need of intensive discharge planning. Red flag patients may be identified before or during admission, during routine patient care, or through the expressed concerns of significant others. The plan of care for these patients usually requires social services and a highly individualized approach. In addition to picking up red flag patients, the nurse addresses four key questions related to discharge planning to obtain vital information (Box 8-2).

Patient and family education, which must include teaching about physical care and how it can be performed at home, is critical to successful discharge planning. Nursing assessment and counseling must prepare patients throughout hospitalization to evaluate their family resources, understand their illness and treatment, help them make behavioral changes, and manage their continuing care.

BOX 8-1. "Red Flag" Patients

Older patients (older than 70; may include
  younger patients with disabilities)
Older patients suspected of being abused
  or neglected
Patients living alone
Children abused, neglected, or with birth
  anomalies
Patients transferred from other institutions
Recent admissions
Multiple readmissions
Patients who depend heavily on community
  resources
Patients with financial problems
Patients with terminal illnesses
Patients who live out of state or out of the
  country
Patients with care-intensive disease,
  catastrophic illness, or chronic illness
Patients with multiple chronic illnesses
Patients with newly diagnosed disease
Patients who receive few or no visitors
Substance abusers
Patients suspected of being abused,
  including domestic violence
Patients with family problems
Patients with psychiatric disorders
Patients with poor living conditions
Patients who speak little or no English
Patients with recent disabilities

BOX 8-2. Assessment: Vital Information

- What information does the patient need?
- What attitudes should be explored?
- What skills does the patient need to
  perform health care behaviors?
- What factors in the patient's environment
  may pose barriers to the performance of
  desired behaviors?
  1. Is the patient likely to return home?
  2. Can the family or significant others
     handle the care that will be needed?
  3. Is the home situation (or environ-
     ment) adequate or appropriate for the
     type of care needed?
  4. What kinds of assistance (eg, financial
     resources, medical equipment,
     manpower, community support) will
     be needed?

At-Risk Patients

In complex situations, strategies should be developed to follow-up with the patient, family,
and community services to determine the outcomes of discharge planning. High-risk situations, such as domestic violence or other forms
of abuse, require skilled observation and appropriate questioning on the part of the nurse
(Warner, Rowe, & Whipple, 1999; Campbell,
1999).

During the assessment process, the patient
often hides the signs of abuse or makes excuses
for injuries, which may be life-threatening.

Domestic violence, a pattern of assault and
coercion, includes physical, sexual, and psychological attacks. The patient may attribute
recurrent episodes of injury to being "accident-
prone." There may be substantial delay between onset of injury and presentation for
treatment. Suicidal thoughts and depression
are also common. Patient groups at special risk
for abuse are children, pregnant women, and
older people (Chez, 1994; Campbell, 1998).

Assess the patient alone in a safe and private environment. The following questions,
asked in a nonjudgmental way, can help patients break the silence about abuse. Acknowledge that violence is not the victim's fault
(McAfee, 1993, 1994; Bash & Jones, 1994; Miles,
1999; Campbell, 1998).

"At any time, has a partner or parent kicked,
  hit, or otherwise hurt or frightened you?"
"Have you ever been emotionally or
  physically abused by your partner or by
  someone important to you?"
"I noticed your bruise. How did your injury
  occur? Did someone hurt you?"

"Often patients with these types of symptoms have a history of having been hurt by another person. Has that ever happened to you?"

It is important to document the findings of suspected domestic violence with objective data. Use the patient's own words regarding the injury and abuse and include the name of the assailant and his or her relationship to the patient. Legibly document all injuries using a body map and take photographs of the injuries. Notify the patient's physician immediately. In states with a reporting law, any person who suspects abuse or neglect of a child is required by law to report this suspicion to the county Department of Social Services. This includes instances of physical abuse causing physical harm; neglect causing failure to provide for the child's basic physical, medical, educational, and emotional needs; sexual abuse, such as fondling, intercourse, incest, rape, sodomy, and exhibition; and emotional maltreatment, such as bizarre punishment, belittling, or psychological rejection. Be certain to assess a patient's safety in returning home. Ask if weapons are kept in the house and determine if children are in danger (Brown & Runyan, 1994; Campbell, 1998). The same types of abuse can apply to all patients, including older patients (Chez, 1994; Fulmer, 1999).

THE ASSESSMENT PROCESS

The first step of the nursing process is *assessment:* the collection of data to identify actual or potential health problems. Other members of the health care team also gather data. The primary source of information is the patient, and a strong assessment process sets the stage for ensuring that patient's role as a member of the health care team. Families play an important role in helping the nurse assess a patient, especially when the patient is sedated, in pain, or unable to provide crucial information. Families can cue a nurse about the patient's typical behavior and responses, daily patterns, and sources of comfort. A spouse may inform the nurse of a particular fear the patient is un-willing to disclose, thus helping the nurse to address it and promote the patient's readiness to learn (Tanner, Benner, Chesla, & Gordon, 1993).

Children and adolescents, ages 10 years to 19 years, who are taking on responsibilities of caring for adults with cancer, are also caregivers; it is important to include their perspectives and needs (Gates & Lackey, 1998). In the assessment process, nurses continuously collect information from different sources, validate these data, and sort, categorize, and summarize or interpret the information. The end-products of the assessment are nursing diagnoses—judgments based on sound data that have been systematically collected and analyzed.

The practice of nursing is founded on the ability of nurses to carry out nursing interventions based on the assessment of individual situations. Nurses respond to patients and their families who cannot meet their own needs. The goals of nursing care are to reinforce the patient's strengths, assist the patient in meeting basic human needs, and help the patient regain the ability to meet these needs to the greatest degree possible. To provide appropriate nursing care, we must define strengths and needs accurately and state patient problems clearly.

Nursing assessment is not guesswork. It is a conscious, deliberate process, consisting of three steps. We make assessments every day in our personal and professional lives, often without realizing it. While driving to work, we quickly note that the fuel gauge is almost empty, and drive to a gas station. We take inventory in the pantry and make a list before grocery shopping. We walk into a patient's room, notice shortness of breath, and elevate the head of the bed. All of these actions are based on assessment. It is vitally important in patient education for the nurse to make an accurate assessment of strengths and problems, so that learning may be tailored to the specific situation. This assessment is based on collecting specific data from various sources, sorting the data, and writing a summary statement of problems or needs, which we call *nursing diagnosis*. Assessment should be documented to ensure accountability.

In patient education, the nurse's goal is to ensure that the patient is guaranteed the right to information and that he or she is taught the skills that will help him or her meet basic human needs. Therefore, making a thorough assessment is essential for accomplishing nursing goals. The three steps of the assessment process are the following:

1. Gathering data
2. Sorting and categorizing data
3. Writing a summary statement (nursing diagnosis or diagnoses)

We now look at each step in the assessment process as it is applied to patient education.

Gathering Data

Nurses are especially aware of the need to collect data in an organized and efficient manner. Because data collection is time consuming, it is imperative to collect only useful information in the assessment process. Nurses must avoid the common mistake of gathering too much data, because they then overlook how the information is to be used.

Learning needs are defined when a nurse assesses the patient. The assessment for patient education does not have to be separate from other patient assessment activities. Information about the learning needs of the patient and family is gathered with other data about the patient's condition. To collect information vital to an assessment of learning needs, the nurse must consider the questions listed in Box 8-2.

Assessment Guides

Data should be gathered using criteria that directs the nurse to the areas to be assessed. Many guides are helpful in assessing the learning needs of patients and families. Some are directed toward a particular patient population (eg, patients with diabetes, stroke, or ostomy). Some nurses construct their own assessment tools, which may better meet individual situations. The important point about assessment tools is that the tool should guide the nurse in a holistic view of the patient within the contexts of the family and environment. The instrument should help the nurse focus on the total person and direct him or her in collecting data in specific areas related to what the patient must learn.

The health assessment instrument often begins with physiologic data: chief complaint, history of the present illness or problem, and a review of systems. It is also important to note the informant, if other than the patient. Assessment often uses many informants, including other nurses and health professionals, and, of course, the patient and family. During or after physical appraisal, the nurse also gathers psychosocial data that affect the educational process. Taking a patient's history is a skill that improves with practice and experience. Nurses learn to fine-tune the reporting of problems and to look for "significant negatives," ruling out possible problems. (Rawly, 1998). For example, a nurse told us about her experience assessing an older patient in a long-term care setting. The patient's daughter reported: "My mother can't walk." When the nurse had the patient attempt to walk, she found the patient could balance herself but was short of breath and dizzy. The problems were dehydration and shortness of breath rather than a musculoskeletal weakness. Other problems to be ruled out include depression, social isolation, pain, and functional dependence.

The assessment instrument may be a checklist with space included for responses, or it may be in guide form with an accompanying flow sheet for summary in the patient's chart. Hand-held or bedside computers are frequently used to document assessment data. The tool that seems most helpful to the nurse and most appropriate to the care setting is the one that should be used (JCAHO, 1998).

Depending on the setting and the amount of time the nurse spends with the client, the assessment is completed in several phases. Data are gathered at different times and are used to update the plan of care. At the first encounter, the nurse screens for the most obvious and acute needs. This is a starting point for beginning care. As time permits, a more comprehensive assessment can be made, and some data-gathering may be delegated to other nurses working with the patient. During assessment, nurses should also look for potential problems that can be anticipated in the plan of care. Particularly in the hospital setting, registered nurses often ask how nursing assistants and licensed practical nurses can participate in this process. Both can contribute observations; however, the registered nurse should help them know what to look for and should validate their data, rather than use them as the only source of information.

We constructed our own guide for assessment in patient and family teaching and demonstrate its application in this chapter. This guide applies to various situations and prompts a thorough consideration of factors that will either promote learning or pose barriers to behavioral change.

Patient and Family Education Assessment Guide

Various guides have been drawn up for assessment of individual learner's needs, and family assessment guides are abundant in the literature as well. Box 8-3 is an assessment guide we developed—*Patient and Family Education Assessment Guide*. This guide is based on material contained in educational, nursing, psychological, and sociologic writings. The guide considers the patient and family as a system in a potential learning environment. It also illustrates the importance of evaluating the family as a system, while considering the impacts of the community, the health care industry, and sociocultural influences as suprasystems. A model of patient and family education was constructed to help the reader visualize the related components that influence learning. Figure 8-2 illustrates the components of assessment found in the assessment guide. This model represents a healthy educational situation, in which the family has reasonable resources and an assessment of family functioning demonstrates strengths.

We believe that patients who have the support of family members in the learning process cooperate better with the medical regimen. We have witnessed this correlation in our clinical experience. As patient education clearly

becomes recognized as being within the domain of the nurse, questions arise as to who will be taught.

In the past, the nursing profession centered its interest on the hospitalized patient. Any teaching that was done with a patient's family members tended to be peripheral or owing to a particular necessity (eg, if the patient was blind and could not draw up insulin or if the patient had sensory aphasia). Most health professionals now include families in the process of patient education. A systems approach to patient education mandates the inclusion of family members, and teaching one isolated subsystem without dealing with the important family system can, in some instances, negate all teaching efforts.

We believe that educating the patient without including the family frequently results in poor rehabilitation and poor cooperation with self-care measures, whether the patient is acutely ill or faces life with a long-term chronic illness. We firmly believe that patient education should be conducted with the family present, whether in the hospital, ambulatory care setting, or at home. We developed the assessment guide to set the stage for such a teaching environment. It was first used for an adult patient and his family who were dealing with a chronic illness. With some minor changes, the guide in Box 8-3 can be adapted to a family dealing with a patient who has just suffered an acute illness or to a family trying to establish everyday health maintenance, such as one with a newborn.

Systems Theory Applied to Patient Education

Using a systems perspective, this guide moves from the family system, its structure, function, and processes, and how the family relates to education, to the patient as a subsystem of the family, and to some of his or her educational needs. Integrated in the guide are factors that commonly affect the teaching of older patients (Deakins, 1994).

Systems theory has gained prominence among family therapists as a method of understanding the effects of family members on

BOX 8-3. Patient and Family Education Assessment Guide

I. Physiologic data
  A. Chief complaint
  B. History of present illness or problem
  C. Review of systems
  D. Functional, cognitive, and sensory abilities (anxiety, ability to concentrate)

II. Family profile: a word picture of the family
  A. Household composition
  B. Gender and age of members
  C. Occupations of family members
  D. Health status of family members; physical limitations
  E. Genogram: a diagram showing family relationships

III. Resources available to the family
  A. Ability to provide for physical needs
    1. Home: space, comfort, safety?
    2. Income: sufficient for basic needs and important extras?
    3. Overall ability to perform self-care
    4. Health insurance: available to the family?
  B. Neighborhood/community resources: friends, neighbors, church, and community organizations helpful and involved?
    1. What kinds of support are provided?

IV. Family education, lifestyle, and beliefs
  A. Educational backgrounds and attitudes toward education
    1. Do all adult family members have basic reading and writing abilities? Check ability to read aloud from patient education material.
    2. To what extent is education, formal or informal, valued? How much education does each family member have?
    3. Are there language barriers to verbal communication among the patient, family members, community, and medical personnel?
  B. Lifestyle and cultural background
    1. Does the family subscribe to folk medicine beliefs?
    2. Is there a conflict between cultural and lifestyle approach and the health professional's teaching?

    3. What are the normal diet patterns of the family?
    4. What are the family's sleep habits?
    5. What are the activities, exercises, occupations, and hobbies of family members?
  C. Learning abilities of family members
    1. Do they assimilate information easily?
    2. Are they able to apply what is taught?
  D. The family's self-concept
    1. Are family members lacking in self esteem?
    2. Do they have feelings of powerlessness as a result of either life situation or patient's sick role?

V. Adequacy of family functioning
  A. Ability to be sensitive to the needs of the family members
    1. How is the identified patient perceived?
    2. What are the relationships of other family members to the identified patient and to each other?
  B. Ability to communicate effectively with each other
  C. Ability to provide support, security, and encouragement, especially pertaining to the learning environment
  D. Ability for self-help and acceptance of help from others when needed
    1. How open is the family to the health professional's teaching?
    2. How likely are family members to request help in the future, if needed?
  E. Ability of perform roles flexibly
  F. Ability to make effective decisions
  G. Ability of the family to readjust ideas about family status, goals, and relationships
  H. Ability to the family to handle crisis situations
    1. Has the family been confronted with chronic illness in the past?
    2. How have family members reacted to situations, such as accidental injury or death? Who helped them through it?

VI. Family understanding of the present event
  A. Current knowledge about the problem; ask these eight questions:

1. What do you think has caused your problem?
2. Why do you think it happened when it did?
3. What do you think your illness does to you? How does it work?
4. How severe is your illness? Will it have a short course?
5. What kind of treatment do you think you should receive?
6. What are the most important results you hope to receive from this treatment?
7. What are the chief problems your illness has caused for you?
8. What do you fear most about your illness?

B. Point in the life cycle of the family at which the problem occurred
C. Type of onset of the illness or problem: gradual or sudden?
D. Prognosis for survival or prognosis for restorative training
E. Nature and degree of limitations imposed on the patient's functioning
F. Level of the family's confidence in the health system with which it affiliates

VII. The identified patient, health problem, and educational needs
   A. The patient's educational and cultural background, especially if different from the family's
   B. The patient's self-concept and reaction to stress
   C. Physical limitations that are barriers to learning or self-care
   D. Information base of the patient
      1. Does he or she understand the health team management and the health team's advice?
      2. Does he or shed know others with the same problem and have knowledge of their treatment?
      3. What are his or her position and role in the family?
      4. Has he or she had past illnesses?
      5. What kind of physiologic feedback does he or she use?
   E. Are the patient and family members willing to negotiate goals with the health care team?
   F. Are the patient's perceptions and expectations congruent with those of family members?

one another during their ongoing interactions. The product of the interactions of the individual members, or *subsystems*, are the beliefs, goals, roles, and norms that form the *family system*. One of the tenets of systems theory is that the system is more than the sum of its parts. What this means to the patient educator is that the family system must be assessed and intervention provided if the patient (subsystem) is to learn to adapt. For example, if the spouse and children of a patient with hypertension are unwilling to prepare and eat low-sodium, low-fat meals, the patient will have difficulty complying with the medical regimen.

Another aspect of systems theory that is important to the patient educator is the concept of the *suprasystem*. When we consider the family as a system, the suprasystem is the community to which the family relates (eg, school, church, economic, legal, and health in-

stitutions). Assessment of the suprasystem is important in patient education, because it provides the patient educator with information about support systems that may be implemented to aid in rehabilitation and financial assistance.

Family Structure and Function

Families, like other social systems, have structures and functions. The effectiveness of a family's organization can affect the extent to which new health behavior is assumed. Problems with family organization and role definition often pose obstacles to learning. Differentiation and specialization of roles are important in assessment. For example, the patient's roles may have to change with the onset of a chronic illness, and the provider must recognize this to assist the family to adapt (MacVicar & Archbold, 1976).

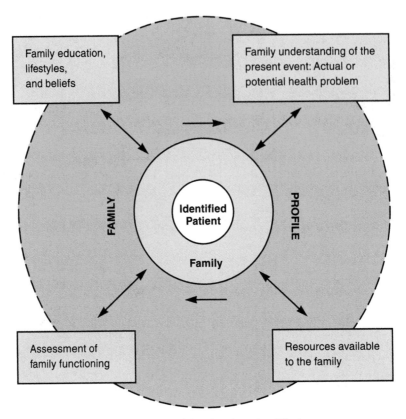

FIGURE 8-2. A model of patient and family education. The two-way arrows between each component and the family system demonstrate their dual effects on each other. The broken line indicates the interactions among all of the components; the family encircles the entire model.

Family functions are closely related to family structure, as pointed out by Horton (1977). The functions that remain in the family " . . . are the maintenance of the household and the intimate personal relations of the family members." Family strengths relate closely to family functions and are covered in Part V of Box 8-3. If the desired family strengths are absent, the wisdom of including the family in patient education must be reconsidered or planned in a careful way, because the family may be more destructive than beneficial, posing barriers to the patient's learning process.

The family processes of adaptation, integration, and decision-making are important to patient and family education. A family faced with the illness of one of its members must adapt and change in a healthy fashion. The ability of the family to handle a crisis situation is a strong indication of family adaptation (Eliopoulos, 1997; MacVicar & Archbold, 1976; Otto, 1963). Boundary maintenance, or the ability to meet needs by obtaining, containing, retaining, and disposing of resources, reflects important data about the ability to adapt. Assessment questions pertaining especially to obtaining and containing resources are found throughout the assessment guide. Dealing with neighborhood and community resources is of special importance. Human resources outside the family are necessary during illness or stress, and they also are indicative of the family's ability to form trusting, caring relationships with others outside of the family.

The family process of integration is covered mainly in parts IV and VI of Box 8-3 and chiefly refer to the family norms and beliefs that help to form the bonds in well-integrated families. A high degree of family integration, built through cultural beliefs and lifestyles, may complicate the learning process if the beliefs and values differ widely from those of the health care provider (Gragg & Rees, 1980; Leininger, 1994; Redman, 1997).

Culture and Beliefs

The cultural assessment in section IV B of Box 8-3 brings to light the diversity of backgrounds among patients. Values and beliefs influence health and the patient's care. When nurses encounter patients with beliefs and values different from their own, the cultural assessment section must be expanded to include the following significant variables:

1. **Time.** In some cultures, there is a "right time" to do things, and the Western concept of time and clocks is disregarded. Patients may not arrive for appointments at the scheduled time, but when the time seems right to do so.
2. **Religious beliefs.** Some religious beliefs may prevent the patient from seeking health care or accepting treatments and must be considered.
3. **Cultural remedies and healers.** It is important to know about any remedies or healers the patient currently uses or consults and their meaning to the patient. Fully explore diet and dietary remedies.
4. **Language and communication.** Note what language is spoken and what nonverbal signals are used.

Cultural differences make each patient unique and, when ignored, lead nurses to treat all patients in a similar way, often resulting in a failure of patient education. Nurses who develop a broad knowledge base and become sensitive to the patient populations they serve can plan care creatively and are more likely to achieve successes in patient and family education (Orgue, Bloch, & Monroy, 1983; Rehm, 1999; O'Neill & Kenny, 1998; Andrews & Boyle, 1995). If customs and beliefs are ignored, the patient may have difficulties making recommended changes in the diet. To communicate effectively in patient education, nurses should never make assumptions without validation from their patients. They should also be active listeners and teach other staff what they learn about the culture from patients (Patient Education Management, 1998). Chapter 3 addresses challenges and approaches to working with patients whose cultural and belief systems differ from those of the nurse. Additionally, we recommend that nurses seek continuing education to prepare for assessment of the diversity of cultures encountered.

Decision-making in the family during events of stress or illness can affect the family's future. If decision-making is not organized adequately, the family may be unable to make important choices related to health care plans or unable to assume responsibility in health care practices. When patient education is involved, it is frequently necessary for the family to decide, whether by consensus, accommodation, or de facto decision-making, who will learn the required skills (eg, how to irrigate a colostomy or give an insulin injection). The importance of assessing the patient as a subsystem of the family is covered in part VI of Box 8-3, drawn partially from Robinson (1974).

The patient's perception of his relationship to the family, whether realistic or unrealistic, can alter the educational process and should be determined before the teaching plan is begun. The work of Kleinman (Kleinman, Eisenberg, & Good, 1978), which was introduced in Chapter 4, is integrated in the guide with eight questions listed in part VI of Box 8-3.

Data should be gathered as objectively as possible. Collecting these data (using fact or measurement, rather than feelings or judgments) will guide the nurse to define needs or problems accurately. Words such as *seems, appears, acts,* and *looks* should be avoided. More useful data would note direct observations or actual behaviors. Whenever possible, note what the patient said in his or her own words.

Describe what you hear, smell, see, and feel. Share your observations with the patient to validate what you observe. Note the source of the information.

Several effective methods of gathering data exist:

1. Observation
2. Interviews with patient, family, and significant others
3. Review of patient records and literature; continuing education
4. Collaboration with the health care team

Observation

Much information can be collected through the senses. Assessments can be made of the patient's abilities to perform self-care activities, and maintain physical appearance, and of his affect. The nurse can gather valuable information in the home by observing the interactions of family members, the comfort and safety afforded by the patient's dwelling, and the facilities available to meet basic needs. Observation will also provide information about the patient's literacy level, leisure activities, and the role assumed within the family.

Although the most common method of observation is through sight, nurses also rely on information from things they hear, feel, and smell. Verbal and nonverbal cues gathered by observation provide us with valuable information about what the patient thinks, feels, and believes. Questionnaires and tests are often used to assess a patient's knowledge of facts and to explore attitudes.

Interview

Taking a patient history or performing a patient and family interview is the most reliable method of obtaining data. When patients cannot supply information about their physical or emotional condition, family members are asked to supply as much information as possible. Whether the nurse interviews the patient or one of the family members, he or she has guidelines and suggestions for interviewing effectively.

Establishing a Trusting Environment

Patients must feel secure to confide information. They must feel that their concerns are taken seriously and that their needs are important and respected. Communicate trust and respect to patients by concentrating attention on them, maintaining eye contact, and being an active listener. The necessity of establishing a trusting environment is illustrated by the situation that develops when a nurse deals with a patient with a sexually transmitted disease (STD). The nurse must assure the patient that all information will be held in strict confidence. After the nurse has assured the patient of confidentiality, he or she must then explain the importance of notifying the patient's sexual contacts so that they can be treated. Such situations are delicate, and if the client does not trust the nurse, it will be impossible for the nurse to provide assistance.

Use Open-Ended Questions

Help the patient to provide more complete information by using the principles of active listening. Use phrases such as *"Go on"*, or ask: *"Can you tell me more about that?"* Repeat the last words of what the patient said. This approach communicates interest in what the person has to say and a desire to understand how he or she feels. Open-ended questions that ask for descriptions allow the patient to give information about how he or she perceives needs. If we continue with our example of the client with an STD, the nurse can use open-ended questions, such as, "can you tell me what you know about STDs?" If the nurse states to the client, "You know how you got this, don't you?" the client will probably simply respond, "Yes," because he or she is embarrassed, does not want to admit ignorance, and feels generally uncomfortable with a nurse present. In such situations, and in many other patient education settings, avoid judgmental behaviors. The use of open-ended questions allows the client to present what he or she knows so that the nurse can assess what else must be taught.

The nurse also can use open-ended questions to determine what is most important to the patient or what troubles him or her most by asking, "Please tell me what is troubling you the most," or "If you could change one thing, what would it be?"

Effective interviewing occurs in a setting where the patient and interviewer can be free of distractions and where information can be shared privately. Obstacles to effective interviewing arise when the patient is too tired or ill to share his thoughts comfortably, or when the interviewer is distracted. Extremely lengthy interviews are difficult for both the patient and interviewer. Plan the interview so that critical information is obtained first; perhaps it will be necessary to have several short sessions. For example, counseling related to STDs must be accomplished discreetly and without family members or anyone else present. The client should be alone with the nurse in a private room where there will be no interruptions.

Family members can be included in assessment when they visit the patient, or if this is not practical, by telephone. The nurse might say: "Staff members are devising a plan of care for your mother, and we would like your input. Can you answer a few questions to help us?"

Allow the patient to tell you how he or she perceives his or her needs and problems. Maintain objectivity about what the patient says and try not to make judgments about his or her perceptions of pain or of his or her needs. Speak to the patient using language he or she can understand, rather than using medical terminology and abbreviations. Remember that children misinterpret adult language easily and nurses must tailor explanations to a child's level of understanding (Rogers & White, 1998). When interviewing, speak slowly and clearly, allowing time to think about your questions. If the patient wanders off-track, gently repeat your question. Explain the purpose of the interview to the patient. Explain that you want to get to know him or her better to provide care in the best manner possible. For example, let the adult patient with chronic obstructive pulmonary disease (COPD) and asthma explain his or her perception of the problem. The patient may believe that the recent onset of severe symptoms is related to a specific activity (eg, walking or sexual intercourse) when, in fact, the blood level for the medication is not in the therapeutic range. Once we learn what the patient believes, we may correct some important misconceptions.

Notes from the interview make documentation more accurate and efficient. However, avoid writing too many notes during the interview, because this may disturb the patient. Facts, symptoms, times, names, and short quotes from the patient may be recorded quickly and can be used when you are ready to document the results of the interview. Before beginning to record data during an interview, it is imperative to say to the patient: "I am going to write down a few things you say so that I don't forget anything important." Taking notes during an interview frequently makes clients uncomfortable; an explanation can alleviate such discomfort and prevent misunderstandings. With the growing use of computers at the patient's bedside, it is important to keep in mind that eye contact with the patient is essential. The focus is the patient, not the computer.

Review of Patient Records

The patient's medical records are often the nurse's first source of information. Although information can be gathered quickly from the patient's chart, it should be supplemented by information from other sources. Medical records supply data about the patient's health history, previous hospitalizations, past experience with the health care system, and observations others have made. They can give us clues to finding additional sources of information, such as a public health nurse or community agencies that have worked with the patient. Observation and the patient interview should validate information gathered from the patient record.

Review of the Literature: Continuing Education

Reading texts and journals to update knowledge and skills is a professional responsibility.

Basic nursing education is a foundation for practice, but the ability to anticipate and intervene in areas of need depends on willingness to increase that original knowledge base through continuing education.

To intervene responsibly with patients and their families, be prepared with an understanding of the disease or health problem, its medical management, and its impact on lifestyles. Nursing fundamentals textbooks are valuable resources. Many journal articles describe new approaches to teaching patients and their families or increase our awareness of self-help groups and other resources that assist in preventing, resolving, or coping with health problems. Workshops and other continuing education programs offer good opportunities for learning from experienced colleagues about patients' problems and the causes and management of these problems. The Internet has the potential to provide much valuable information and resources (see Chapter 11).

Collaboration With the Health Care Team

Data gathered by other nurses, physicians, dietitians, pharmacists, physical therapists, and various other health care professionals, can validate and supplement information gathered from the sources previously mentioned. Whenever possible, team members should contribute to planning the care of the patient and family. Patient education is a concern of the team. Coordination of learning goals and activities is important for ensuring that the time of the professional, the patient, and the family is used productively.

Collaboration is facilitated by good verbal and written communication, team conferences, updated nursing care plans, and effective use of such opportunities as physician and nurse rounds to discuss the patient teaching plan. For example, the hospital social worker who interviews the family is frequently given lists of medications that the patient has received from various physicians. The social worker will then give this list of medications and prescribing physicians to the nurse, who is responsible

for sharing the list with the patient's admitting physician. "Think big. Who else can you involve in the patient and family education process? Go beyond traditional organizations and boundaries. Who can you invite to join the health care team?" (London, 1999, p. 68.)

Sorting and Categorizing Data

Data gathered from various sources must be carefully considered, validated, and grouped into problem areas. In optimal circumstances, the health care team agrees on assessment of patient problems, learning needs, and factors affecting behavioral change for health promotion.

*P*atients are often overwhelmed by the barrage of information they receive upon discharge from the hospital, particularly if they suffer from an illness that requires permanent lifestyle modification (eg, cardiovascular disease). They are expected to make many changes at once, which is difficult for most people. A dietician, physical therapist, lipid specialist, and nurse might all advise a patient. A good assessment can help identify the one or two most important modifications a patient can make to reduce risk factors. By helping patients prioritize and focus on short-term goals, the recovery plan seems more manageable.

(STALLINGS, 1996)

Writing the Nursing Diagnoses

The summary statements that describe problem areas in which the nurse can intervene are called *nursing diagnoses*. A nursing diagnosis is different from a medical diagnosis because it focuses on a patient's response to a health problem that can be prevented or altered by nursing intervention. A medical diagnosis, by contrast, describes the illness, focuses on its pathology, and guides medical orders or protocols (Eggland & Heinemann, 1994). Nursing diagnoses, statements of actual or potential health problems, are derived from the data collected in assessment. The patient and family who, while doing so, become prepared to negotiate goals with the nurse, should validate these diagnoses.

The North American Nursing Diagnosis Association (NANDA) provides a standardized list of nursing diagnoses. Nurses in all specialties, working together since 1973 to develop the scientific basis of nursing practice, have developed this taxonomy. Each diagnostic category contains descriptions of etiology, contributing factors, and definitive characteristics that help the nurse select the correct nursing diagnosis. Many health care organizations have established policies and procedures supporting the use of nursing diagnoses and incorporating them in documentation systems. In 1992, NANDA updated the taxonomy of nursing diagnosis by including high-risk diagnoses (supported by risk factors that make a person vulnerable for the condition) and wellness nursing diagnoses, such as *family coping, potential for growth* (Eggland & Heinemann, 1994; NANDA, 1990; Carpenito, 2000).

Nursing Diagnoses

All nursing diagnoses have implications for patient and family education. The diagnosis *knowledge deficit* is frequently selected to incorporate all patient learning needs related to knowledge or skills needed for self-care. We believe, however, that patient education is better integrated in the total plan of care by referring to educational needs as they relate to each nursing diagnosis. Knowledge deficit may be best used for preoperative teaching, prenatal education, parenting skills, and so forth.

The diagnosis *noncompliance* should be used carefully and specifically after a thorough assessment to describe the patient who wishes to follow a recommended plan, but cannot do so because of physiologic or situational reasons. This diagnosis should not be used if the patient has made an informed decision not to

comply (Carpenito, 2000). Nurses must be detectives about readmissions related to medication noncompliance. If a patient has not taken medications correctly or does not have a therapeutic level of drug in his or her system, nurses can help the patient and family determine what went wrong. Did the patient take the medicine as prescribed? Ask the patient to recall, in the last day or week, when and how much of the medication was taken. Was financial assistance found to obtain the medication? Were there unanticipated side effects, causing the patient to stop taking the medicine without calling for assistance? Instead of only teaching the patient about the medicine, the appropriate educational intervention might be to work with the prescribing physician. Without a good assessment, the teaching may be misdirected.

Management of the Assessment Process

Prioritizing Needs and Problems

It is often difficult to set priorities when faced with problems in several areas. A consideration of a hierarchy of human needs helps the nurse rank the priority of problem areas and offers guidance in how and where to begin patient teaching.

All people have common needs that must be satisfied. The ability of patients and their families to survive depends on their effectiveness in meeting these basic human needs. When they cannot meet basic needs, problems arise that they often cannot resolve alone. At that point, health professionals are called on to intervene. The nurse's goal is to help clients regain the ability to meet their own needs and to foster their maximum development, both as individuals and in their relationships with others.

Maslow suggests that needs exist in various levels, and that these groups of needs can be visualized as a hierarchy in which lower-level needs must be at least partially met before a person can meet higher-level needs (Maslow, 1992). A consideration of these needs helps us to prioritize needs in nursing care and in patient teaching. Many of us have discovered that learning is hampered when the family faces problems with housing, finances, or threatened self esteem. Patients who are in pain or are fearful of pain place high priority on managing it; they will learn little else until this need is met. Because the assessment process involves not only a listing of needs but also a consideration of priorities, it is helpful to use Maslow's hierarchy of needs as a guide in doing so. Figure 8-3 illustrates examples of nursing assessment for individuals, families, and communities based on Maslow's work.

Learning During the Assessment Process

When the patient and family have an active role in defining their problems, family learn-

ing occurs. Self-care activities depend on the ability of the patient and family to solve problems by gathering information and categorizing signs and symptoms into problem areas. Nurses can help them build skills by verbally sharing thoughts during the assessment process. Let the patient and the family witness and contribute to a systematic collection of data and definition of problems. Inform them about the rationales for collecting certain kinds of data and the best ways for discovering and documenting them. The promotion of learning during assessment builds problem-solving skills, encourages validation of data with the patient and family, and serves as a motivator for future learning.

Adults are more motivated to learn when they can identify their own needs and con-

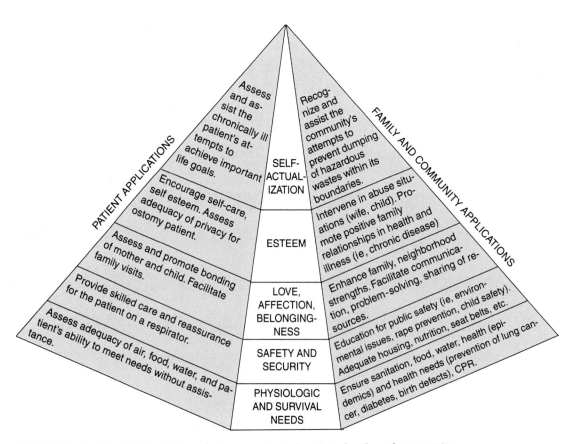

FIGURE 8-3. Applying Maslow's hierarchy in assessment of patient, family and community.

tribute toward planning a program tailored to their particular circumstances. The questions asked by the nurse provide families with a sense of what is important and what they will need to do to prepare for discharge.

Time Management

Time management issues are often mentioned as impediments to the assessment process. It seldom seems feasible to dedicate an hour to collecting information in an interview or to making a detailed assessment. We emphasize a few points related to time issues:

1. **A good assessment is a time-saver.** Although assessment requires spending time in astute observation and active listening, time will be lost if the care plan is constructed without input from the patient and family. In these cases, interventions are often ineffective, and additional time is spent going back to the assessment process to discover barriers to change that were preventing progress all along.
2. **The patient and family must have time to tell their story.** They must be given time to offer their perceptions of their own problems. The nurse must take time to help them understand what is expected of them if they are to eventually take charge of self-care activities. This is critical in the management of chronic illnesses that affect children, such as asthma.
3. **Assessment can be made any time a nurse interacts with a patient and family.** Gathering information need not be restricted to a 60-minute interview. Bath time, meal time, rounds, visiting hours, and medication times are all potential opportunities for assessment.
4. **Patients are sensitive to the time pressures of health professionals.** They often do not know what is expected of them, whether (or for how long) they will have your attention, or how to contribute important information. Nurses can teach them to help with time restraints by offering statements such as the following: "Mrs.

Wise, I have set aside 15 minutes this morning at about 10:00. I will ask you and your husband to answer some specific questions for me about your health problems so I can better plan your care with Dr. Mason and the nursing staff." This gives the patient an idea of what is expected and informs her that she will be asked specific questions instead of being put in the position of not knowing what information is important. In some instances, a questionnaire can be given ahead of time to collect initial data, which will be discussed during the interview. Whatever can be done to minimize interruptions and distractions during the interview will help to maximize productivity. Fifteen minutes of well-planned, well-used time accomplishes more toward assessment than does an hour with interruptions and lack of direction.

5. **Assessment varies based on the setting and the patient.** Even in the most brief encounter, the nurse can ask "What brought you here at this time?" and gain a wealth of information that is outlined in the assessment guide. In outpatient clinics, patients and families may be asked to complete brief written or computerized assessment instruments.

 Children are a higher risk population than adults. They have less control, and they account for a higher percentage of hospitalizations and ER visits.

(ELLIS & WESTON, 1997).

Nurses in a pediatric clinic recognize that the best time for patient education is during well-child visits. So during the first visit, they assess the home environment as part of the initial history. Teaching at each immunization visit is based on the age of the child and key information from the assessment, such as whether guns, lead paint, or poisonous houseplants are found in the home. Education is focused on safety and prevention. The nurse practitioner continues further assessment and teaching during the examination of the child. For instance, she might ask about pets in the home, stressing that pet dander is a cause of child allergies (Speros, 1999).

Two California nurses set in place a program for pediatric asthma patients including one-on-one and group classes, individualized peak flow meter monitoring (based on green, yellow, and red zones), and follow-up phone calls to discuss how things are working out at home and school. The information gained is key to an accurate assessment and ongoing care, and extends the impact of the emergency room (ER) visit or hospitalization (Ellis & Weston, 1997).

CASE STUDIES

How can the wealth of information offered by patients and families be used during short inpatient experiences in the hospital?

The assessment guide in Box 8-3 is a comprehensive tool for identifying barriers to learning and clues for individualizing the teaching plan. Even with this tool, it is difficult to gather all pertinent information at one time, and nurses often cannot cover every aspect. The more information to which a nurse has access, the better able the nurse will be to understand and influence patient behaviors. The guide offers direction for discovering such information during the initial assessment and throughout ongoing assessment as part of the relationships among the provider, the patient, and family.

Nurses who work on hospital inpatient units typically do not have the time and opportunity for extensive patient and family education assessments. Patients are often so ill and families so stressed in an acute episode that assessment must be conducted at various times throughout the hospitalization. This information is helpful, not just in planning, but during the inpatient phase. With good documentation and continuity of care, the information benefits other providers, such as home health nurses, who can build on the assessment data

during home visits. The following case study is an example.

C A S E   S T U D Y

THE SMITH FAMILY

PHYSIOLOGIC DATA

The Smith family was in the Newborn Intensive Care Unit. The wife recently gave birth to 34-week premature twins, Joshua and Sarah. Both babies do well and are soon discharged after 2 weeks of birth.

At the initial encounter with the nurse, Mrs. Smith says she wakes up every 3 hours to breast-feed Joshua and console him. Sarah is still learning to suck and swallow, and is working on feeding with the nurse so that the mother can concentrate on Joshua. They both receive initial respiratory assistance.

Joshua goes home first and Sarah soon follows, but she still cannot breast-feed. Mrs. Smith appears determined to learn the skills required in caring for these two infants. After the twins discharge, the nurse follows up with them for 6 months to assess their needs and coping abilities.

Pertinent History

Joshua and Sarah: Normal pregnancy until 8 months, when Mrs. Smith's membranes ruptured prematurely and the babies were delivered the same day, 2 hours apart. Joshua is intubated initially and Sarah is put on continuous positive airway pressure (CPAP). Overall, Joshua's recovery is quicker and smoother. Sarah is sicker and required oxygenation for a longer time, delaying her ability to latch and suck at the breast. The mother has two lactation consultations since Sarah's discharge. She believes they "didn't tell me anything new, they just said I was doing everything right."

At the nurse's first home visit, however, the mother plans to bathe with Sarah that

(case study continues on page 215)

evening to "recreate the womb," because of a suggestion given to her from the lactation consultant.

The Smiths have been married for 12 years, with 6 moves during that time. Both families of origin live on the East Coast. The Smiths moved to the West Coast 2 years ago and are happy in their location.

Family Profile

Family Structure (Figure 8-4)

The family is composed of the husband, Lad, 52, a successful businessman; wife, Karen, 38, a full-time mother; and children, Max, 3, and Joshua and Sarah, 3 weeks. Health status for all is well with the exception of a lack of sleep for both parents, lack of patience for Max, and occasional colds acquired by Max at school. Both newborns are healthy and growing, but Sarah continues to have difficulty breast-feeding and both twins are on different sleep/feed schedules.

Resources Available to the Family

The family can meet its physical needs. They live in a modest home in the suburbs that provides enough space for three children and two adults. It is child-safe and appears comfortable, although the mother complains about the disorganization and clutter around the house. Lad's income is sufficient for basic needs, but the family can also access some community resources for additional needs. These resources include twin and breast-feeding support groups, friends and neighbors who bring over meals in the evenings, Max's school friends, and Jewish community center contacts. These support networks help the Smiths with babysitting and house cleaning.

Karen expresses concern about the extent of their family's needs and her support network's ability to maintain this intensive amount of help. Health insurance is available to all family members and has paid for the few lactation consultant visits at the home and several at the hospital. The Smiths' overall ability to perform self-care is limited because Lad is gone all day and Karen cannot meet all the children's needs alone. Max attends preschool 8 hours a day, 5 days a week, which reduces Karen's workload. Still, she needs help with the twins during the day and at night, because neither she nor Lad sleeps longer than 2 to 3 hours at a time during the night. Karen has presently organized a schedule for help she receives 3 days a week from a college-aged neighbor in the afternoons when Max gets home from preschool, but still feels overburdened and overwhelmed.

(case study continues on page 216)

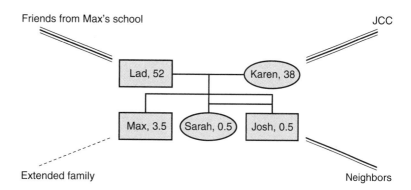

FIGURE 8-4. Ecomap of the Smith family.

Family Education, Lifestyle, and Beliefs

Both parents have college degrees, and Lad has a graduate degree. Education appears to be important in this family. The parents have no language barriers between them, but they are still teaching Max how to communicate his needs and are learning how to understand the twins' communication of their needs. Karen emphasizes her needs with anyone: friends, medical personnel, or family. Lad is more reserved than Karen, but does communicate when asked. This family subscribes to Western medical ideals, and their cultural and lifestyle approach agrees with their health professional's recommendations, although Karen did express frustration with Sarah's inability to breast-feed and the health profession's lack of help in this area. Normal diets include food from the four basic food groups, eaten generally three times a day with snacks throughout the day. Karen often drinks large amounts of fluids to help her with breast-feeding.

The family's sleep patterns are a concern. Lad has been sleeping on the first-floor couch to get some sleep, although Karen is up every 2 hours breast-feeding Joshua and Sarah. Lad is in charge of Max in the evenings and nighttime; recently, Max has been waking up during the night. Consequently, no one in the house is getting enough sleep. Lad has continued to maintain his exercise routine, but now must wake at 5:00 A.M. to get his workout in. He then helps get Max ready for school, and then takes the ferry to work. He works in the city, approximately 45 minutes from home.

Karen is too exhausted to exercise, and is concerned whether she is eating enough because of her current stress level. She worked in retail for years before having children and always believed she would return, but never did, once she had Max. She enjoys being a mother, has Max involved in many community programs (eg, art classes), and encourages him to be creative. The family is active in the Jewish temple and enjoys many friendships from this association.

Both Karen and Lad are bright, assimilate information easily, and apply what they learn. For instance, Karen took the information a lactation consultant gave her and attempted to breast-feed in the bath with Sarah, which was successful. Both parents and Max present with strong self-esteem. Karen feels overwhelmed with her situation at times, but she always tries to learn new ways to make things work and is receptive to new ideas. She stated: "I know that this is temporary, so I am trying to enjoy this time because I know it will fly by quickly."

Adequacy of Family Functioning

Because of the lack of sleep, no one is particularly sensitive to the needs of the other family members at present. Karen and Lad often take things out on each other and sometimes even on Max. Max has been biting children at school. In addition, he was home for a week with a bad cold, and felt sick and neglected. Both Karen and Lad are aware of their lack of patience with each other and they are also aware of Max's need for attention. Max has never acted angrily toward either twin, but will do anything to get Karen's attention when she is breast-feeding. One solution she discovered was to breast-feed wherever Max was playing, so that they could talk to each other without her having to choose between Max or one of the twins. She also left the twins once a week with a babysitter for an hour and spent that time with Max. Since Karen and Max began having one-on-one time together, Max has stopped acting out and is more independent of his mother. Karen believes this is because he feels more secure in his relationship with her. During the weekends, Lad spends most of his time with Max.

Lad and Karen's relationship has suffered the most since the twins came

(case study continues on page 217)

home. They have not slept in the same bed since that time. Karen considers Lad's job a vacation compared with being at home; Lad disagrees. They are both sleep-deprived, impatient with each other, and severely in need of time alone. Karen copes well, but with all her overwhelming responsibilities, she is presently in survival mode. She told me that the only people who could visit were those that would help. This was one of the reasons her family had not been to visit, because she believed they would not be helpful to her and she could not handle it. Karen is adept at asking for help and would be likely to ask for future help if someone could provide assistance. Lad is less likely to ask for help and at times doesn't understand why Karen is so needy.

Karen and Lad have had numerous discussions about seeking help from a community-based program called Mother's Help, which sends someone to the house night or day to assist with infant care. Lad has offered to stay at home 2 days a week, but Karen says she would rather have him at work, because he would be bored and unhappy. She also says she would rather have someone else, such as a nursing assistant or a trained babysitter, helping her rather than he. Lad has tried to be flexible in his role as a father, but is less so in his role as manager of the family budget. Karen would rather spend money on extra help and have him go to work to make up the difference. She thought that they both would be happier if they had outside help. Both parents can make effective decisions, but it became apparent that they had different values that caused difficulty in making this decision.

The Smiths had a great ability to readjust ideas about family status, goals, and relationships. Both parents realize that Lad won't sleep on the couch forever, that Sarah and Joshua will one day sleep through the night, and that Max will soon enjoy a relationship with his siblings

without feeling threatened about his current relationship with his parents. Overall, the Smiths exhibited a good response while handling this crisis situation. Karen's positive outlook extends to all of the family members.

When the nurse commented that it was surprising in only a year and a half of living in the neighborhood that this family has built such a strong support system and awareness of community resources, Lad smiled and said: "You wouldn't be surprised if you knew Karen. This is how she handles everything."

Family Understanding of the Present Event

All family members are aware of how dramatically their lives changed when Joshua and Sarah were brought home from the Newborn Intensive Care Unit 2 weeks after their delivery. Their present challenge is to figure out what will work out for them emotionally, physically, and financially as far as getting more help during the day or night, getting more sleep, and meeting each other's needs during this temporary crisis. Considering how well the Smiths have handled the situation thus far, their survival prognosis is excellent. One aspect of this event that is different than in other health care settings is that the changes are happy changes and the family is happy and enthusiastic about working out the problems, despite the stress. In addition, these choices were made consciously, so they could prepare for the changes. The level of the Smiths' confidence in their affiliate health system is high, and they receive frequent pediatric and obstetric visits.

Health Problems and Educational Needs

Nursing Diagnoses:

1. Knowledge deficit related to care of premature newborn twins

(case study continues on page 218)

2. Ineffective breast-feeding related to unsatisfactory breast-feeding process, secondary to inability to attach
3. Altered family process related to gain of new family members, secondary to need to meet physical needs of all family members and seek help appropriately
4. Fatigue related to interrupted sleep patterns secondary to feeding and care needs of newborns
5. Altered nutrition (less than body requirements) related to increased maternal needs during breast-feeding

Both babies must be placed on a consistent schedule. Sarah must continue practicing breast-feeding until she no longer needs supplementing, if Karen continues to have the patience and desire to do so. The twins' are progressing appropriately and growing with each pediatric visit. The nurse addressed concern to the family about Karen not taking care of herself (ie, lack of sleep, nutrition, and stimulation). By educating both parents about Karen's physical needs for breast-feeding alone, the nurse could discuss Karen's desire for outside help and weigh this possibility against the challenge of meeting financial obligations. The nurse discusses with Lad and Karen the possibility of getting away together for just 1 night or 1 day and letting someone else care for the children. The nurse encouraged them to let family members help with the children, if possible, and stay for extended periods.

Conclusion

By the end of 6 months, Karen had help during the nights and several days during the week. Both she and Lad were sleeping better and feeling better emotionally and physically, although they were still sleeping in separate rooms. They did allow their family to visit and were surprised at how helpful they were. With this extra support, Lad and Karen left for 2 nights together while the grandmother watched the children. Sarah learned how to breast-feed, and both babies were well established with breast-feeding and gained an enormous amount of weight, which helped them sleep through most nights. Max established relationships with both siblings, and couldn't wait for them to play with him and be more mobile. Karen was feeling better, and was meeting her physical and emotional needs as well.

How can nursing students gain practice in assessing patients and families for the purposes of patient education? We recommend home visits as a helpful way to learn assessment skills. The authors worked with students who identified a patient in the family medicine clinic and then conducted a follow-up visit at home. A pair of students made each visit, and then wrote a summary based on the assessment guide.

CASE STUDY

The Dawe Family
HISTORY

Mrs. Dawe comes to an outpatient clinic for her regular appointment. She tells the nurse she has "to keep check on my sugar and have my blood pressure checked." She states that she has diabetes and needs help with her "weight problem." The physician shares with the nurse some of his frustration in caring for Mrs. Dawe. He refers to her as a "delightful lady" who is just "not compliant," despite numerous patient education efforts.

The nurse suggests a home visit as a means of identifying factors that might influence Mrs. Dawe's cooperation with her self-care management in the areas of diet, exercise, medication, and blood glucose monitoring. The physician agrees that this is

(case study continues on page 219)

a good idea and together the physician and nurse suggest it to the patient. The following information is collected using *the assessment guide.*

Family Profile

Family Structure

Mrs. Dawe is a 73-year-old, Caucasian, obese woman. At 157.5 cm (5 ft 3 in), she weighs 77 kg (169 lb), 30% more than her ideal weight of 52.3 kg (115 lb). Her manner in the outpatient clinic is matter of fact. Mrs. Dawe is a retired RN. She makes certain that the nurse immediately recognizes her status and competence.

An appointment for the first home visit is made during the visit to the outpatient clinic. The following information is obtained during the home visit.

Mrs. Dawe meets the nurse at the door in a house dress with sandals and no stockings, her white hair neatly combed. Mr. Dawe is dressed in denim overalls. He is smaller than his wife and considerably outweighed by her. He is slightly deaf, but makes every effort to keep up with the conversation, although he is neither as verbal nor as articulate as his wife. Mr. and Mrs. Dawe were both born in the South and lived there all their lives.

Mr. and Mrs. Dawe are both retired. Their last jobs were at a medical center, where Mrs. Dawe worked as an RN floater and where Mr. Dawe was a maintenance worker. Mr. Dawe's occupational history included various skilled and semiskilled jobs; he had worked for railroads, textile mills, and during World War II, for the Army at a military camp.

The household once included the Dawes' four children. The oldest child (and only daughter) is presently employed at a local government agency. She was educated at a local private university, and was married and widowed within 4 years. A daughter from this marriage, now 20 years old, was presently a freshman at a local state university. The Dawes' daughter remarried, and the second marriage was unhappy, involving physical abuse and separations. The Dawes' second child is married with three children, and lives and works in the same county as his parents. He is employed in the electronics industry. The third child seems to be the "fair-haired boy." He graduated from a local state university, and then went to work for a large insurance company, which had steadily promoted him and transferred him around the country. This son, his wife, and three of their four children are living in Arizona, and are greatly missed by Mrs. Dawe. The Dawes' youngest child is living nearby with his wife and son. He works as a painter, and recently painted the exterior of his parents' house.

The health status of the Dawes is important to consider in assessment because it influences other areas in the analysis. Both Mr. and Mrs. Dawe are in robust good health well into their 50s. After that, however, Mrs. Dawe's genetic heritage and the effects of Mr. Dawe's physically demanding work caught up with them.

At age 56, Mr. Dawe had a power-tool accident that resulted in permanent loss of function of his left hand. Ten years after surgery, Mr. Dawe suffered a myocardial infarction, from which he fully recovered. Two years later, emphysema developed and persisted, limiting Mr. Dawe's ability to engage in yard work or gardening. Mr. Dawe had smoked approximately a pack-and-a-half of cigarettes per day, but quit. Glaucoma had been a problem, but was arrested by medications. Mr. Dawe is amazingly spry considering his ailments.

Mrs. Dawe's health history is not as long and complicated, but its implications for the future are probably more negative. Mrs. Dawe's diabetes was first diagnosed at age 56, and she was placed on insulin (premixed 70% intermediate and 30% long acting) at the time of diagnosis. Her insulin

(case study continues on page 220)

requirements have steadily increased, and she has been on a long-term regimen of 44 U/day. She takes 29 U in the morning and 15 U each evening. Her weight has steadily increased from 65.9 kg (145 lb) to 74 kg (163 lb), and her attempts at weight reduction using an American Diabetes Association (ADA) diet have been fruitless. Retinopathies and a cataract requiring removal had developed since the onset of diabetes. Mrs. Dawe's written records of home blood-glucose monitoring show few periods of diabetic control. Hypertension was diagnosed about 8 years earlier. She currently takes Prinivil (30 mg/day) and enteric-coated aspirin daily. She has exercised progressively less during the years, and the combination of obesity, diabetes, and coronary artery disease has left her in poor physical health. The slightest amount of exertion makes her short of breath, and she states that she cannot participate in any guided exercise program.

Resources Available to the Family

The Dawes' seven-room home, which they own outright, is situated in a small, rural community and has aged comfortably during its 30 years. The interior is well kept, with additions such as carpeting and a new furnace added since they first built the house themselves "piece by piece." The furniture is comfortable and in good repair, and provides a homey feeling, accentuated by a pleasant clutter of family photographs, trophies, and knick-knacks. Prominently displayed on a table is a photo of their second oldest son and his family, who are now located in Arizona. Photos of other children and grandchildren are in less prominent places. Mrs. Dawe gives the nurse a tour of the home, pointing out the large size of the rooms and explaining that the candy in the dining room is not for her but for the visiting children. The nurse notes three boxes of cake mix in Mrs. Dawe's kitchen cupboards and a cake plate sitting out in the dining room. The home is

larger than necessary for their present needs. The Dawes' previous lack of financial resources seems to have been surmounted.

Income for the family is derived mainly from Social Security benefits and two pensions from the medical center. Although the Dawes' income is limited, it does allow for travel; the previous summer they drove to Arizona to visit their son and his family. Limited financial help is received from their children in the form of home improvements and money for traveling. Recognizing the limitations of Medicare, Mr. and Mrs. Dawe paid for additional medical insurance; the premiums are a rather large expenditure for them.

Neighborhood and community resources are informal but supportive. Neighbors watch the homes of one another, and they all keep keys to one another's homes. In the summer and fall, the Dawes enjoyed their neighbors' garden produce. The family faithfully attends a local Methodist church, because it is convenient and they like the parishioners, but both hastened to add that they are not members of the church. When questioned about involvement in community organizations, Mrs. Dawe speaks with pride of her work in the local school system when they were both employed. She tells the nurse about her initiation of an immunization program at a local elementary school. She remarks that she still had a feeling of accomplishment every time she saw the school. The family has informal and unstructured interface with community agencies and resources. In times of personal need, however, they obtain services from the church, which has also helped their daughter through some difficult times.

Family Education, Lifestyles, and Beliefs

Education is highly valued by the family, especially Mrs. Dawe. She graduated from nurses' training program. She prides herself on keeping current with medical matters, gaining most of her knowledge from *Family*

(case study continues on page 221)

Health magazine, to which she subscribes. Mr. Dawe graduated from high school. All four of the Dawe children graduated from high school, and two completed college. Books, magazines, and newspapers are evident in the household.

The learning abilities of Mr. and Mrs. Dawe are adequate, although Mrs. Dawe cannot follow her ADA diet. The self-concept of this couple appear healthy. Together they express the view that they had worked hard in life "but had come through in good shape." As a couple, they both seemed to have achieved psychologist Erikson's various stages and were in the eighth developmental stage, completing the tasks of ego integrity (Erikson, 1993).

Adequacy of Family Functioning

The adequacy of family functioning is assessed on the basis of the self-report. Mrs. Dawe appears to be viewed by her husband with fondness and warmth that developed during 47 years of a marriage marked by economic and personal tribulations. Mrs. Dawe is quick to say that the marriage has been good and that they are happy together now. Mr. Dawe laughs in a somewhat embarrassed fashion, but nonverbal clues such as nods of agreement and appropriate smiles indicate that he agrees with her assessment. Relationships with their children seem healthy and supportive on the basis of Mr. and Mrs. Dawe's reports. Communication between husband and wife is adequate. Mr. Dawe is not as verbal as his wife, and he tends to let her finish his sentences for him. Support and encouragement for each other are communicated in important nonverbal ways, such as Mr. Dawe's willingness to take his wife to the outpatient clinic to talk with the nurses and his willingness to be available when the nurse arrives for the home visit. Another sign of mutual support and security is the fact that they still sleep in the same double bed together. Mr. and Mrs. Dawe maintain their emotional and financial resources carefully, sharing them mainly with their children.

The family's ability to accept help, especially in areas of health care, is limited. This is mainly because of Mrs. Dawe's background as a nurse; she must feel competent and self-sufficient in all medical areas. Other family members place demands on her that make it difficult for her to follow her health care plan. This is the area that caused the greatest difficulty in patient and family education. Because Mrs. Dawe is not following her ADA diet, she is placed in a constant state of jeopardy—she knew what she should do but could not, or would not, comply. As a result, her weight continues to increase, and she is left in the rather untenable position of having to justify her situation by claiming she has "a strange case of diabetes." Unfortunately, her choices have negative outcomes for the family system.

Role flexibility is not of imminent importance to this family in its life cycle. The family has a traditional delineation of work: Mrs. Dawe did the household chores, and Mr. Dawe supervised a neighborhood teenager who did the yard work.

Decision-making in this family tends to fall primarily to Mrs. Dawe, as had discipline of the children in the past. Although some of the decisions are made in a de facto manner by Mrs. Dawe, there were also instances when decisions are made by the process of accommodation (ie, a process of begrudging compromise and a questionable commitment to the decisions).

In the Dawes' viewpoint, family status, goals, and relationships are not seriously impaired by chronic illness. Adjustments to Mrs. Dawe's diabetes and to Mr. Dawe's emphysema have been smooth. The concurrent onset of chronic illness and onset of aging has, perhaps, made acceptance of the illnesses easier.

(case study continues on page 222)

Relationships have changed as the children grew up and moved out, but overall the family seems to have adjusted well.

With an immediate mobilization of energies, the Dawes respond to crisis situations, especially serious injury or death. Because of Mrs. Dawe's background as a nurse, she immediately was called on in times of illness or injury. Besides caring for the ill or injured family member, she also carried messages from the rest of the family. Mr. and Mrs. Dawe both indicate that although they became distressed in such situations, they felt they could respond appropriately.

Family Understanding and the Present Event: Chronic Illness

This family has a long association with diabetes through relatives on both sides of the family. The Dawe family genogram (Figure 8–5) shows the remarkably high incidence of diabetes and diabetes-related deaths on both sides of the family. Both partners seemed to accept diabetes philosophically, even fatalistically. When asked how he felt 17 years before about the diagnosis of his wife's diabetes, Mr. Dawe states, "It's just something that happens." He feels that the only way her diabetes has affected him had been in her cooking: "it's not as good as it used to be."

This chronic illness was not diagnosed until late middle age, and relatively few restrictions were imposed on the family's ability to function at a pre-illness level, which probably accounts for the relative ease with which they had handled it. Although Mrs. Dawe had to contend with a limited menu and portions, insulin injection, blood glucose monitoring, and other medically prescribed guidelines, her role within the family was initially undisturbed. The complications of diabetes (retinopathies and hypertension) that were found in Mrs. Dawe are of concern to the family and interfere with daily activities. Mrs. Dawe cannot drive, which makes her more dependent on her husband. Based on this information, the nurse asks her to show how she performs her blood-glucose testing and insulin injection preparation. She is happy to do so, because she sees herself as "teaching" the visiting nurse. She draws up her insulin accurately with the assistance of a specially marked syringe. Her blood-glucose testing is done with a digital read-out designed for patients with impaired vision. Her reading is 250 mg/dL, 2 hours after eating. This reading validated Mrs. Dawe's poor diabetic control. The nurse takes her blood pressure, which is 170/94 mm Hg, indicating hypertension. As her activity level declines and her weight increases, she cannot move around easily, which limits the mobility the couple enjoyed during the past few years. Mrs. Dawe's role as provider of nursing-care and child care provider for grandchildren and other family members is restricted.

The couple's children recognize the hereditary nature of diabetes and have their blood checked occasionally for glucose, Mrs. Dawe reported. As far as the parents knew, however, their children have no pervasive fear of diabetes.

Health Problem and Educational Needs

Mrs. Dawe's educational background as an RN occasionally becomes a problem. Her self-concept involves an image of herself as one who should cope with diabetes management problems and, at times, she hesitates to ask for support or advice. "I just don't feel I can ask these young guys about things the way I used to when I knew them from working with them," she states. Further complicating the problem of daily diabetes management is her hypertension. The physiologic feedback she receives (headache, occasional nausea) is symptomatic for both conditions and therefore confusing.

The principles of diabetic self-care (diet, exercise, medication, response to hypoglycemic and hyperglycemic reactions, prevention of complications) are outlined for Mrs. Dawe by the nurse. She is proud of her medical knowledge and skills. It becomes clear, however, that in this case (as

(case study continues on page 224)

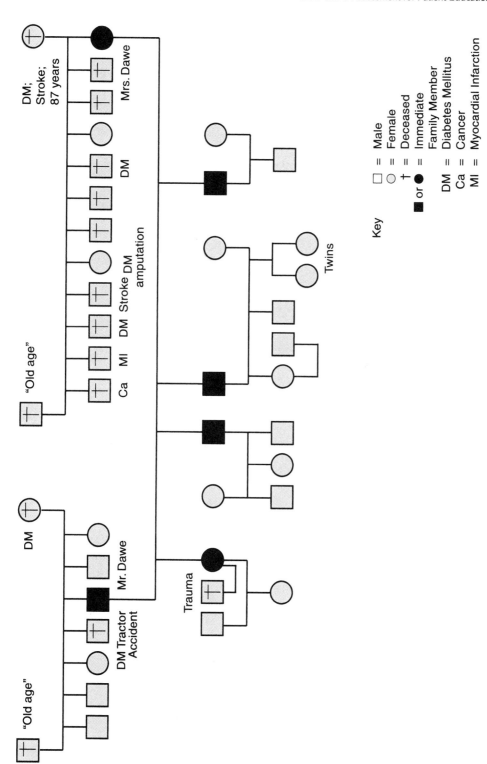

FIGURE 8-5. Genogram of the Dawe family

with many other health professionals under medical care themselves), knowledge and skills are often not enough to promote healing behaviors. To assess Mrs. Dawe's learning needs accurately, the nurse encourages Mrs. Dawe to talk about problems with her treatment plan and her lifestyle. Mrs. Dawe's responses to questions defined the following areas that she saw as problems:

1. Weight gain—diet is too restrictive; cannot eat "normally"; always hungry
2. Cannot follow exercise program because of fatigue, shortness of breath
3. Poor control of blood pressure because of an inability to follow low-sodium, low-fat diet; salt substitute "tastes awful"; husband likes salt used in cooking
4. Poor control of diabetes, resulting in hyperglycemia, retinopathies

Mr. Dawe displays a lack of knowledge about diabetes and its management when questioned. He "left it up to her" to know what to do because she is a nurse. Mrs. Dawe did not talk about her diet with him, but he noticed that her "cooking had changed some."

The visiting nurse concludes the assessment for patient education by discussing and validating the problem areas with Mrs. Dawe.

Conclusion

1. Altered Nutrition: More than body requirements related to nonadherence to diabetic low-salt, low-fat diet
2. Educational Needs: Negotiate and coach behavior modification related to ADA diet
3. Positive factors affecting behavioral change
   Patient is knowledgeable about health problems
   Patient cooks
   Patient makes decisions
4. Negative factors affecting behavioral change
   Self-concept is decreased
   Environment includes availability of restricted foods
   Patient feels hungry

Patient feels diet is too restrictive
Husband is not impressed with seriousness of health problem
Activity Intolerance related to decreased mobility and obesity
6. Educational Needs: Negotiate and instruct to increase activity with consistent exercise program
7. Positive factors affecting behavioral change
   Interferes with role of caring for others, including grandchildren
   Patient wants to be independent and more mobile
   Symptoms bother patient
8. Negative factors affecting behavioral change
   Patient is obese
   Patient's dependence on husband has increased
   Patient cannot follow diet

SUMMARY

Patient education is an integral part of nursing care. Although the steps of the nursing process are always the same (assessment, planning, implementation, evaluation), the nurse must tailor practice to meet the needs of patients and the constraints of the patient care setting. Assessment, using an assessment guide, is as detailed and thorough as possible to determine accurate nursing diagnoses and factors that will affect patient and family learning. Thus, assessment reflects both process and product.

Two case studies illustrated how patient education begins in the hospital or clinic, but then must extend into the home, where true learning takes place. Home visits can provide an opportunity to assess problems related to behavior management of chronic problems and to better appreciate family strengths. Even with limited time for assessment of a newly admitted patient, the nursing diagnoses and educational needs that are formulated in the hospital or clinic can later be refined as more detailed information is gathered.

In both cases, assessment highlighted problems commonly encountered by patients and families. An ongoing need exists for education of patients and families that extends beyond the walls of the hospital or the outpatient clinic. The nurse assesses the patient's and the family's basic knowledge about the problem and its management. The nurse also looks for educational needs to help the client cope with the recommended treatment plan and solve problems that arise at home. She encourages the family to seek appropriate assistance from community classes, clinical experts (dietitians, lactation consultants, etc.), and to maximize its own support systems.

Patient education involves much more than simply sharing the medical information we have with the patient by communicating it in a vocabulary he or she can understand. We recognize the importance of assessing individual situations to see the patient as he or she sees himself or herself. Only then can we assist the patient in recognizing and overcoming obstacles that prevent the desired behaviors. This requires a skilled approach to patients for which health professionals must be prepared.

STRATEGIES FOR CRITICAL ANALYSIS AND APPLICATION

1. Using the Patient and Family Education Assessment Guide, conduct a home visit. Write a summary of your assessment similar to the summary of the Smith Family or the Dawe Family, illustrated in this chapter.
2. Have students role-play being a person with diabetes. Some students should be assigned the role of being a non-insulin-taking patient with diabetes who has to go onto a strict dietary regimen. The calories should be appropriate for the student; the idea is to follow a meal plan precisely for one week, adding no extra treats. Other students can be assigned roles with different levels of insulin therapy. For instance, a two-injection-per-day regimen, a three-injection-per-day regimen, and a four-injection-per-day regimen. They all need to perform self-monitoring of blood

glucose, follow the diabetic meal plan, record all blood sugars and dietary intake, and inject saline in the appropriate doses per instructions. The sales product representatives from the various diabetes product companies will often provide the materials necessary for this exercise. Debriefing these experiences at the end of a week can add a great deal of insight into the problems of living with a chronic illness that requires self management practices.
3. Have students play the roles of educator and patient. During the conversations, have some dyads use judgmental language asking why patients comply rarely or at all with suggestions. Have students practice asking questions to assess the personal meaning of the illness or condition to the individual. Compare the kinds of information received from the two types of communication used to assess patients and families.
4. Listen for references to "noncompliance" in your clinical practice setting. Use these reports in seminar discussions or post-clinical conferences to ask students to suggest other ways to describe the problem. Practice speaking up to other professionals in these circumstances, pointing out the need to consider the context in which the patient is functioning.

REFERENCES

(1998). To work with culturally diverse patients, tailor lessons to individual. *Patient Education Management, 5*(3), 29–33.

Andrews, M., & Boyle, J. (1995). *Transcultural concepts in nursing care* (2nd ed.). Philadelphia: J. B. Lippincott.

Bash, K., & Jones, F. (1994). Domestic violence in America. *North Carolina Medical Journal, 55*(3), 400–403.

Brown, G., & Runyan, D. (1994). Diagnosing child maltreatment. *North Carolina Medical Journal, 55*(9), 404–408.

Campbell, J. (1998). *Empowering Survivors of Abuse: Health care, battered women and their children.* Newbury Park, London, England: Sage.

Campbell, J. (1999). If I can't have you no one

can: murder linked to battery during pregnancy. *Reflections, 25*(3), 8–12.

Carpenito, L. (2000). *Nursing diagnosis: Application to clinical practice* (8th ed). Philadelphia: Lippincott Williams & Wilkins.

Chez, N. (1994). Helping the victim of domestic violence. *American Journal of Nursing, 94*(7), 33–37.

Deakins, D. (1994). Teaching elderly patients about diabetes. *American Journal of Nursing, 94*(4), 39–42.

Eggland, E., & Heinemann, D. (1994). *Nursing documentation: Charting, recording, and reporting.* Philadelphia: J.B. Lippincott.

Eliopoulos, C. (1997). *Gerontological nursing* (4th ed.). Philadelphia: Lippincott-Raven.

Ellis, R., & Weston, C. (1997). Management controls pediatric asthma. *Patient Education Management.* Suppl, Nov. 1997.

Erikson, E. (1993). *Childhood and society.* New York: W. W. Norton.

Fulmer, T. (1999). Our elderly: harmed, exploited, abandoned. *Reflections, 25*(3), 16–18.

Gates, M., & Lackey, N. (1998). Youngsters caring for adults with cancer. *Image—The Journal of Nursing Scholarship, 30*(19), 11–16.

Gragg, S., & Rees, O. (1980). *Scientific principles in nursing.* St. Louis: C. V. Mosby.

Horton, T. (1977). Conceptual basis for nursing intervention with human systems: Families. In J. Hall, & B. Weaver (Eds.), *Distributive nursing practice: A systems approach to community health* (pp. 101[a], 104[b], 105[c], 112 [d]). Philadelphia: J. B. Lippincott.

Joint Commission on the Accreditation of Healthcare Organizations. (1998). *Comprehensive Accreditation Manual for Hospitals.* Oakbrook Terrace, IL: JCAHO.

Kleinman, A., Eisenberg, L., & Good, B. (1978). Culture, illness, and care: Clinical lessons from anthropologic and cross-cultural research. *Annals of Internal Medicine, 88*(2), 251–258.

Leininger, M. (1994). *Transcultural nursing: Concepts, theories, and practices.* New York: Greyden Press.

London, F. (1999). *No Time to Teach.* Philadelphia: Lippincott Williams & Wilkins.

MacVicar, M., & Archbold, P. (1976). A framework for family assessment in chronic illness. *Nursing Forum, 15*(3), 180–194.

Maslow, A. (1992). *Motivation and personality.* New York: Cambridge University Press.

McAfee, R. (1993). Doing something about violence. *Ross Roundtable Report—Family Violence* (pp. 1–12).

McAfee, R. (1994). Physicians' role in the fight against family violence. *North Carolina Journal of Medicine, 55*(9), 398–399.

Menke, K. (1993). Linking patient education with discharge planning. In Giloth, B. (Ed.), *Managing Hospital Based Patient Education.* Chicago, IL: American Hospital Association, 153–164.

Miles, A. (1999). When faith is used to justify. *American Journal of Nursing, 99*(5), 32–35.

Miller, B., & Capps, E. (1997). Meeting JCAHO patient-education standards. *Nursing Management, 28*(5), 55–58.

NANDA (North American Nursing Diagnosis Association (1990). *Taxonomy of nursing diagnoses.* St. Louis: NANDA.

O'Neill, D., & Kenny, E. (1998). Spirituality and Chronic Illness. *Image—The Journal of Nursing Scholarship, 30*(3), 275–280.

Orgue, M., Bloch, B., & Monroy, L. (1983). *Ethnic nursing care: A multicultural approach.* St Louis: C. V. Mosby.

Otto, H. (1963). Criteria for assessing family strengths. *Family Process, 2,* 329–337.

Patient Education Management (1998). To work with culturally diverse patients, tailor lesson to the individual. (5)3, 29–32.

Rawly, E. (1998). Review of the literature on falls among the elderly. *Image—The Journal of Nursing Scholarship, 30*(1), 47–52.

Redman, B. (1997). *The process of patient education* (8th ed.). St. Louis: Mosby–Year Book.

Rehm, R. (1999). Religious faith in Mexican-American families dealing with chronic childhood illness. *Image—The Journal of Nursing Scholarship, 31*(1), 33–38.

Robinson, L. (1974). Patients' information base: A key to care. *Canadian Nurse, 10*(12), 34–36.

Rogers, J., & White, B. (1998). Medical terms not always clear to kids. *Patient Education Management, Suppl,* May 1998.

Speros, C. (1999). Well-child visits provide teachable moment. *Patient Education Management, Suppl.,* Mar. 1999.

Stallings, K. (1996). *Integrating patient education in your nursing practice.* [Video]. Reproduced with permission of Glaxo Wellcome Inc. (Produced by Horizon Video Productions, 4222 Emperor Blvd., Durham, NC 27703.

Tanner, C., Benner, P., Chesla, C., & Gordon, D. The phenomenology of knowing the patient. (1993). *Image—The Journal of Nursing Scholarship, 25*(4), 273–280.

Warner, P., Rowe, T., & Whipple, B. (1999). Shedding light on the sexual history. *American Journal of Nursing 99*(6), 34–40.

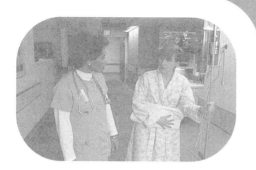

Planning: Shared Goals
for Patient Education

LEARNING OBJECTIVES

After reading this chapter, the nurse or student nurse should be able to:

1. List four characteristics of effective patient educators.

2. Describe three characteristics of the adult learner that are important to consider in planning patient education.

3. Discuss the importance of constructing learning objectives before developing learning interventions.

4. Briefly define cognitive learning, affective learning, and psychomotor learning.

5. List the key components of a learning contract and describe its benefits in goal setting with patients, family, and staff.

6. List two methods for increasing multidisciplinary collaboration in patient education.

INTRODUCTION

Goal Setting: Targeting Outcomes for Learning

Once nursing diagnoses are formulated and validated with the patient and family, the nurse incorporates the diagnoses in the patient care plan. If a computerized care planning system is used, the nurse tailors a critical pathway based on the problem or on the diagnosis-related group to reflect the needs of the patient. The planning process can now begin. Nursing diagnoses or functional problems must be reviewed, and critical learning needs associated with resolving each problem are considered. Nurses must look beyond the medical diagnosis and pinpoint functional problems (eg, *What problems does the patient experience as a result of his or her disease or condition?*). Patient education should be tailored to address functional problems rather than a disease state. For example, not all patients with diabetes have the same functional problems; therefore, the patient education will not be the same for every patient with diabetes.

In planning patient teaching, nurses should ask, *How does this diagnosis affect this patient?* Answering that question helps determine the teaching priorities. Learning needs are prioritized by asking, *What is most critical to the safety of this patient?* Short- and long-term goals are then negotiated. Finally, specific behavioral objectives for patient education help the nurse and other health care providers work with the patient and family to make the learning experience outcome oriented. Care maps, which are discussed in Chapter 13, also help providers and patients to sequence learning goals within an estimated length of stay as part of the diagnosis-specific critical pathway.

Patient learning occurs during goal setting, as the proposed treatment plan is reviewed and the patient's readiness to learn is assessed. Therefore, teaching is not a separate intervention but an integral part of every aspect of nursing care. If patients are in denial about their problems, they cannot participate in goal setting. In managed care, patient education trends attempt to dictate the teaching schedule. Readiness is a variable that must be considered in individualizing patient education; however, it is sometimes necessary to proceed with teaching even if the patient does not seem ready, because teaching and coaching are embedded in expert nursing care and are not limited to formal, planned teaching sessions (Benner, 1984).

Using Data From the Assessment

We teach patients and families, and they teach us. They know their bodies so well that no matter what the textbook on anatomy and physiology says or what the pharmacology textbook says about a certain medication, the patient knows how their chest pain feels or how that medication makes them feel. When they share their perceptions, they teach us an awful lot.

E. W. (STALLINGS, 1996)

In Chapter 8 we discussed the process of assessment. The more comprehensive the assessment, the more aware a nurse becomes about the patient's problems and needs. This awareness facilitates counseling and helps the nurse provide clients with learning experiences in which they may gain knowledge, attitudes, and skills to promote health.

Assessment provides nurses with information about what the patient and the family know and what they want or need to know (e.g., informed consent) to prepare them to make informed choices. Assessing a client's learning needs includes assessing barriers to behavior change and expanding knowledge, attitudes, and skills related to diagnosis, complications, management, prognosis, prevention, and resources for assistance. The authors encourage actively involving patients and their families in assessment. A nurse's task is to help them articulate their perceptions of their needs and problems.

Skills Needed by the Nurse

Although the planning process for patient education is a responsibility shared by the nurse with the patient and family, it is directed by the nurse. The nurse is ultimately responsible for determining priorities, sorting out *need-to-know* versus *nice-to-know* facts, and helping clients master skills critical to their future safety. Patients expect nurses to exhibit certain strengths in this process. The authors interviewed many patients to determine how they would describe a nurse who is an excellent teacher. Patients were articulate in accounting the teacher-learner relationship. The authors identified four characteristics of excellent nurse-teachers from these conversations (Box 9-1): confidence, competence, communication, caring.

Goals of Patient and Family Education

Goals for patient and family education must embrace the concerns of both the client and the nurse. The nurse must be sensitive to the patient, yet he or she must provide direction and firm priorities for discharge teaching. Patients have told the authors that they depend on nurses to do this. Therefore, goal setting is shared with the patient and family. Goals target patient education to address survival skills, to teach the patient to recognize problems, and to help the patient and family develop decision-making skills.

Goals are accomplished by mastering learning objectives that refer to the patient's ability to demonstrate or perform health behaviors. Setting goals is an important step in the nursing process, but it is too often ignored. Goals and objectives help the nurse focus on what is critical and keep patient teaching on track. Throughout this chapter, the nurse will learn how to work with the patient and family to negotiate goals. The authors demonstrate how learning objectives are constructed and how they direct the entire learning process. Components of a learning contract are outlined and its use as a motivator for learning, a mechanism for communication, and a source of standards for evaluating the teaching and learning process are discussed. Strategies to promote planning with the interdisciplinary team are considered.

BOX 9-1. The Four Characteristics of the Excellent Nurse-Teacher

Confidence
- Selects what to teach
- Alleviates the patient's anxiety
- Provides appropriate learning environment
- Prepares appropriate teaching plan and material

Competence
- Decides what is important to teach
- Ensures the patient's safety
- Provides individualized written instructions

- Teaches home management of special problems

Communication
- Gives clear directions
- Uses simple pictures or models
- Speaks the patient's language

Caring
- Has empathy
- Recognizes patient concerns
- Provides encouragement
- Ensures adequate time
- Shows sensitivity to patient's mood

Learning About the Diagnosis

Every patient who enters into the health care system should know why he is there at that time. This fact may seem obvious, but patients often know their symptoms but not how the symptoms relate to a diagnosis. Patients often do not know how a group of symptoms relates to the current problem. By learning why they are "here, in this place, at this time," patients gain perspective on health management. Learning can be taken a step further by considering whether the presenting problem could have been prevented. If so, what might the patient and family have done differently to avoid an acute episode of illness?

Patients and their families typically want simple explanations about the diagnosis, in terms they can remember and repeat to other family and friends. Even before they are ready to engage in formal learning activities, they want to know what will be expected of them when they are discharged. Patients and families want to know about common trouble signs (e.g., difficulty breathing, increased bleeding postsurgery, dizziness, fever, pain, swelling) and how to get emergency care.

PATIENT-CENTERED GOALS FOR TEACHING AND LEARNING

Understanding Patient Concerns During Hospitalization

Although nurses place greater emphasis on discharge teaching, they also must be aware that patient concerns during hospitalization often interfere with discharge teaching. The nurse must anticipate and address a patient's concerns during hospitalization. For example, a patient may be concerned with the following questions:

- Am I going to be all right?
- What is going on? What are they planning to do to me?
- Is this going to cost me my job? Will I be fired?
- Is my wife worried? Who is going to tell her what is going on?
- Do these doctors know what they are doing? My own doctor knows my condition, but what about all the other doctors?
- Am I going to be in a lot of pain after this surgery?
- There are so many staff members here. Who is really in charge of me?

Fear can be a barrier to learning, and lessening anxiety is always a goal of patient education. It is important to remember that the patient and family may interpret the seriousness of the illness differently from the nurse and may experience one or more of the concerns listed in Box 9-2.

Feelings of shame, anger, and grief commonly arise when a patient is faced with altered body image. Nurses should let patients know that these feelings are to be expected, even though they are difficult to confront. One nurse illustrates this need when working with adolescents who have inflammatory bowel disease and who face surgery. Their concerns may include the appearance of the stoma, whether the pouch will be seen under clothes, how to empty the pouch, and how to deal with leaking or odor (O'Brien, 1999).

Patients and families may also feel guilty for how they have related to one another in the past; they may feel angry about becoming ill or the problems the illness brings to the family; or they may feel helpless to cope with the illness. When family members have been

---

BOX 9-2. Potential Barriers to Learning

Patient Concerns During Hospitalization
- Fear of pain
- Fear that the illness cannot be cured
- Fear of scarring or deformity
- Fear of being a burden on others
- Fear of dying
- Fear of cost of hospitalization

caregivers, the experience of control (or lack thereof) in their stressful and complex lives brings an added dimension and additional needs to patient and family education. Nurses should be attuned to language and behaviors of these caregivers so they can determine when interventions are needed, including possible support from community agencies (Szabo & Strang, 1999).

> *The role of the family is incredibly important in all aspects of cardiovascular disease. Anyone who works with patients can see the impact that a supportive family can have on the situation. However, I also spend a lot of time stressing to patients who have the disease that it is their disease. The heart disease does not belong to the spouse. If the wife learns everything that the husband is supposed to do and the husband never takes responsibility for it, you have conflict built right into the recovery process.*
>
> **L. P. (STALLINGS, 1996)**

During the planning process, the nurse must attend to the issues causing greatest concern for the patient and family. What to expect, how to get help, and how to manage pain are questions addressed through patient education.

Critical Learning Needs: Preparing for Discharge

Nurses bring pressing concerns to patient education encounters. Nurses are aware that patients must know many things and do them correctly to survive independently of the health care team (eg, how to take medications, ambulate on crutches, change a sterile dressing), and these things must be learned before discharge. The nurse must determine what learning is critical by asking four key questions:

1. What potential problems are likely to prevent a safe discharge?

2. What potential problems are likely to cause complications or readmission?
3. What prior knowledge or experience does the patient and family have with this illness or surgical recovery?
4. What skills and equipment are needed to manage the illness or surgical recovery at home?

Ensuring patient safety through teaching is not just an ethical necessity but also legal necessity (see Chapter 6).

Learning Overload

Health professionals often try to teach too much during a short time. This occurs most often in the inpatient setting, in which patients are overwhelmed with instructions before discharge. Reinforcement and evaluation of learning are often neglected. Patient and family learning needs should be carefully prioritized and creatively met in various settings. Although teaching about chronic illness often occurs in the hospital setting, it must be followed-up and reinforced in the home or in the outpatient clinic. It is important for nurses to use telephone or written communication to inform nurses and physicians in health departments, offices, clinics, and nursing homes about the teaching plan and the patient's progress. Learning overload also occurs in outpatient settings, in which patients are given many instructions related to self-care and prevention. Review and reinforcement are often lacking when the patient attempts to integrate the learning into daily behavioral changes.

Considering the Patient's Needs

Nurses who teach patients with diabetes struggle with priorities because so much content must be taught and skills must be learned in a short time. A staff nurse in a diabetes clinic recommends that the nurse considers the patient's needs before beginning teaching. The nurse may be ready to begin teaching the client about the pathophysiology of diabetes when all the client wants to know is whether he or she can return to work. If pressed for time, concentrate on survival skills—injection techniques, the signs and symptoms of hypoglycemia and hyperglycemia, basic dietary instruction, and the importance of regular exercise. This nurse emphasizes that further teaching can be done when the patient is followed as an outpatient (Lumley, 1988).

Always consider the patient's chief complaint or reason for admission. If the patient has a diabetic ulcer, wound management and healing are the teaching priorities. When we take into account the survival data for patients with diabetes who have lower extremity amputations, foot ulcer prevention and treatment of ulcers are considered survival skills (Halpin-Landry & Goldsmith, 1999).

A certified diabetes educator offers additional tips for teaching patients about insulin when "the clock is ticking" (Hurxthal, 1988):

- Assess the patient's strengths, resources, and daily schedule.
- Call in the family to learn even the most basic skills.
- Teach survival skills, including:
  - How to draw up insulin and inject it
  - How to self-monitor blood glucose
  - How to manage hypoglycemia and hyperglycemia
  - What and when to eat in relation to insulin timing
  - When and how to call for help
  - Formulate the follow-up plan

When caring for older patients who have diabetes, Deakins (1994) reminds us of the importance of repetition in patient teaching. Patients must learn about the disease and master specific skills, as well as integrate the cornerstones of management—medication, activity, and diet—into their daily lives.

Prioritizing Needs and Setting Realistic Goals

The following four points support the importance of prioritizing learning needs and setting attainable goals in each patient situation. They also highlight the need for cooperation among professionals in many health care settings.

Length of hospitalization has shortened dramatically in recent years because of rising health care costs, bed shortages, improved technology, and the advent of prospective payment systems. Patients are discharged when they are physiologically stable rather than when teaching is completed. Patients are often acutely ill during most of the hospital stay and have physical and emotional restrictions that prevent learning. They may leave the hospital having had little opportunity to practice skills, review information, or ask questions. Nurses are often informed of the patient's discharge with only a few hours' notice, and they worry that the client has not been taught enough to manage self-care.

Patients who are overloaded with learning materials and activities feel a sense of frustration and failure when they cannot perform all behaviors successfully. This makes them feel powerless, defeated, and dependent. Many adults would rather deny failure than admit to it, and they will revert to old behaviors instead of asking for assistance.

Patients need to know what self-care activities are most important in their individual situations. When time and energy are at a premium, they need to know what learning must be achieved for survival.

Health professionals have limited time and energy. Setting priorities for teaching helps to structure their time for its best use and ensures that acute learning needs are met. Professionals can discharge patients more confidently when they know that learning will be continued and reinforced.

The difficult task of assigning priority to learning needs is helped by considering the individual within the context of Maslow's hierarchy of needs (see Chapter 8). Because five different levels of needs exist, needs that are lower on the hierarchy must be at least partially met before needs on the next level can be satisfied. This approach helps nurses to prioritize learning needs and to recognize the patient's reliance on others to help satisfy higher needs.

In acute and chronic illness, patient education is often limited to physiologic and survival needs (Box 9-3). To assist in prioritizing

---

BOX 9-3. Basic Needs of Patients

Physiologic and Survival Needs
Care and use of oxygen
Recognition of health problems, danger
  signs, and how to respond to them
Knowledge of nutrition and hydration
Comfort with sexuality
Management of pain
Recognition of depression and how to deal
  with it
Administration of insulin and other
  medications or treatments
Care of ostomy or Foley catheter

Safety and Security Needs
Poison prevention for parents
Ability to hold job
Competence in handling hazards on job or in
  environment (eg, toxins, dangerous
  machinery, stress)
Ability to deal with family violence
Financial capabilities in meeting basic needs
  of food, shelter, medication

Affection and Belongingness Needs
Adaptation to peer pressure
Maintenance of family role
Ability to contribute to family, work group,
  community
Need to feel lovable and desirable despite
  illness or problem
Ability to deal with body image,
  disfigurement

Esteem or Recognition Needs
Need to succeed
Need to make choices, control own destiny
Need to be recognized as a valuable individual
Need for privacy, dignity
Ability to deal with lack of respect, abuse, ill
  treatment on job or in family

Self-Actualization: Self-Determining Needs
Success through own definition of what is
  desirable
Ability to meet developmental milestones
Independence in meeting lower needs

---

learning needs, the nurse must ask the following questions: What are the most acute needs of the client? What does the client already know? What behaviors can the client perform? What learning needs are unmet? Which problems are life-threatening? Box 9-4 provides a useful framework for assessing individual patient learning needs and educational goals.

Empowering the Adult Learner

How can I motivate patients to learn?

This question is commonly asked by nurses who attend workshops we have conducted. Nurses know from experience that the learners must play an active role in the teaching process (ie, nurses cannot *make* patients learn, but they can *help* patients learn.)

Many nurses teach patients and families in the way they were taught as children: The learner assumes a passive role, and the nurse

lectures and demonstrates. If the nurse tries to imagine himself or herself as an adult student seated in a fifth grade classroom, he or she will understand why adult patients need a different environment. The nurse might imagine feeling anxious about what the teacher expects, concerned that the material may be repetitious and boring and that the class schedule is rigid and the chair uncomfortable. He or she knows not to speak without permission, thinks that past experience is not important and that he or she may have to learn things that are not relevant to his or her interests.

When the nurse considers his or her own positive learning experiences as an adult (eg, a well-liked teacher in nursing school, an effective preceptor), he or she is likely to recall an environment of physical and psychological comfort in which he or she felt accepted, valued, and encouraged to contribute thoughts, ideas, and past experiences. The subject matter

---

BOX 9-4. Scope of Patient Education Needs in Acute and Chronic Illness

1. Diagnosis: explained in ways understandable to patient
   a. Etiology
   b. Contagiousness, malignance, premalignance, heredity
   c. Anatomy, physiology involved (limit to basic facts)

2. Complications: provide meaning to patient symptoms or possible symptoms
   a. Causes
   b. Prevention
   c. Early signals

3. Management: "big picture" of treatment plan, including discussion of patient self-care behaviors needed after discharge
   a. Surgery
   b. Radiation
   c. Diet
   d. Exercise, relaxation programs
   e. Medication
   f. Behavior modification and controls
   g. Environmental control
   h. Counseling
   i. Appliances (e.g., pacemaker, braces, crutches, traction)
   j. Consultation and referral
   k. Soaks, hot packs, dressings, treatments

4. Aggravating factors
   a. Foods
   b. Tobacco
   c. Drugs, alcohol
   d. Schedule of work and rest
   e. Interpersonal relationships
   f. Environmental aspects

5. Prognosis
   a. Short-term
   b. Signs of trouble, complications
   c. Long-term

6. Prevention of recurrence of acute problems

7. Resources for assistance
   a. Continuing care plan
   b. Economic, transportation
   c. Self-help groups
   d. Printed patient education materials
   e. Patient videotapes, CAI, Internet sites
   f. Group or community classes

Note. From Society of Teachers of Family Medicine. (1979). *Patient education: A handbook for teachers.* Kansas City, MO. Adapted with permission.

---

was of interest and would help in his or her job or role (eg, as a spouse or parent). With help, the nurse defined his or her own learning goals and then evaluated the result of the learning activities. There were opportunities for role playing or trying new behaviors. He or she felt free to ask questions without embarrassment.

Adult patients have similar needs as learners. Physical and emotional comfort and active participation in defining their own needs and goals motivate patients to learn. Nurses who are aware that adult patients and their family members learn best in the same kind of environment that would be personally comfortable for the nurses themselves tend to provide such an environment for patient education.

Malcolm Knowles: Andragogy (Adult Learning)

Malcolm Knowles contributes four reasonable assumptions about adult learners that distinguish them from children. Readers are strongly encouraged to read his book, *The Modern Practice of Adult Education,* for more information on the role of the adult educator and on strategies for helping adults learn (Knowles, 1970, 1998). Table 9-1 provides applications of each of the four assumptions to patient and family teaching.

Knowles' assumptions about the adult learner are as follows. As a person matures:

1. His or her self-concept moves from dependency to self-direction. He or she

TABLE 9-1. Application of Adult Learning Theory to Patient and Family Education

ASSUMPTIONS ABOUT LEARNER	APPLICATIONS
Self-concept moves from dependency toward self direction; sees self as capable of making own decisions, taking responsibility for consequences, managing own life.	Acknowledge learner's desire to articulate own needs, make choices, and gain respect for own ability to manage life; create psychological climate that communicates acceptance and support; help learner to feel comfortable taking chances, expressing thoughts and ideas without fear of shame or embarrassment; remember that adults are motivated to learn when they realize that they have a need to learn.
Growing reservoir of life experience is a resource for learning.	Use past experiences as a resource for learning; remember that adults experience positive feelings of support and recognition when their experience is acknowledged; relate new learning to old; have adults teach other adults in a group setting; be aware that negative past experiences may pose barriers for learner and teacher.
Readiness to learn is strongly influenced by social roles and developmental tasks.	Recognize social role of patient (eg, father, mother, husband, wife, worker) and developmental tasks; relate learning to ability to become, to succeed in these roles.
Time perspective changes; orientation to learning shifts; needs immediate application of new knowledge and problem-centered learning.	Give adults practical answers to their problems; help them to apply new knowledge immediately through role play or hands-on practice (eg, return demonstration); remember that adults are particularly motivated to learn at times of crisis or when problems arise; prioritize learning activities by immediacy of need and patient-family perception of need; reinforce learning and promote problem-solving skills.

Note. From *The modern practice of adult education,* by Knowles, M. S., 1970. New York: Association Press. Adapted with permission.

feels capable of making decisions, taking responsibility for their consequences, and managing his or her own life.

2. He or she accumulates life experiences that are an increasing resource for learning.
3. His or her readiness to learn is increasingly oriented to their developmental tasks and social roles.
4. His or her time perspective changes and orientation to learning shifts. He or she needs immediate application (rather than postponed application) of knowledge, and learning is problem centered rather than subject centered.

The following points made by Knowles offer additional guidance in goal setting with the patient and family:

1. Adults see themselves as producers, or doers, and derive self esteem from their contributions.
2. Adults need to be perceived by others as self-directing.

3. Adults respond in an informal and friendly environment, one in which they are known by name and valued as individuals (Knowles, 1988b).

To summarize, adults are performance centered and seek information that helps them in their daily lives. Patients listen for the bottom line and want health professionals to tell them what they need to know versus what is nice to know. Patients rarely want a detailed description of anatomy and pathophysiology related to their body systems. They want to know how to perform a prescribed regimen of survival skills once they go home and how to adapt current lifestyles to include healthy behaviors. Perceived benefits that encourage these behaviors are often related to performing roles as spouse, parent, and worker (Knowles, 1988a).

Because, as Knowles suggests, the adult's readiness to learn (thus, motivation to try out new behaviors) is influenced by developmental tasks, the patient educator will want to be familiar with Erik Erikson's writings on the

TABLE 9-2. Erikson's Eight Stages of Man	
STAGE	**ISSUE**
Oral-sensory: birth to 1 yr of age	Trust vs. mistrust
Muscular-anal: ages 1–2 y	Autonomy vs. shame
Locomotion-genital: ages 3–5 y	Initiative vs. guilt
Latency: age 6 to puberty	Industry vs. inferiority
Puberty, adolescence: puberty to late teens	Identity vs. role confusion
Young adulthood: late teens to mid twenties	Intimacy vs. isolation
Adulthood: variable	Generativity vs. stagnation
Maturity: variable	Ego integrity vs. despair

eight stages of man (Erikson, 1993). Table 9-2 briefly outlines the eight stages as Erikson identifies them.

The Health Belief Model Applied to Goal Setting

The Health Belief Model is helpful in understanding patient motivation to adopt health behaviors and follow a treatment plan. As explained in Chapter 4, the Health Belief Model suggests that understanding the process of patient reasoning and sequencing provider-patient interactions to support this reasoning promote patient engagement in the patient education process. Table 9-3 outlines how the steps of the model can be applied to goal setting.

Gaining the patient's commitment to learn healthy behaviors and incorporate them into daily life should precede patient education interventions. Nurses should not approach patients as passive learners who are obligated to change their behaviors based solely on direction. The Health Belief Model illustrates that patients will calculate their perceptions of a return on investment. Performing health behaviors commonly involves cost, discomfort, shifting of time and priorities, social isolation (eg, a person on a special diet may feel isolated from events focused on eating or food), and breaking long-standing habits. By following the goal-setting process of the Health Belief Model, nurses can help the patient see how the benefits outweigh these costs. Ongoing support and assistance from family and health

care providers can be an important benefit that helps patients perform health behaviors. The process may reveal that the patient is unwilling to change or perform some behaviors. Smoking is frequently a behavior that a patient is unwilling to change, despite evidence presented by the health care system.

A review of research testing the Health Belief Model suggests that the barriers and costs are the most salient reasons that prevent individuals from engaging in preventive health behaviors or behaviors related to the recommended illness care (Janz & Becker, 1984). Susceptibility to and severity of an illness were not as powerful predictors of behavior as barriers and costs, except for persons who already have an illness (eg, coronary artery disease). To achieve better outcomes, nurses must encourage patients to discuss perceived barriers and identify possible resources to confront these barriers.

If a patient cannot afford to purchase the prescribed medication, financial assistance or a less costly medication is needed. If the patient has been unsuccessful with a therapeutic diet because it is too confining, negotiating the list of forbidden foods and helping the patient's entire family adapt meal preparation will set the stage for more effective patient teaching. Resources for cooking and preparing good-tasting food may also break down barriers to long-term health behaviors (Polin & Giedt, 1993). The American Diabetes Association (ADA) meal planning for patients with diabetes has updated its guidelines to provide more flexibility for patients and less strict calorie restrictions. Because many patients with diabetes also have heart disease, the diet must target blood sugar levels and fat intake (Gershoff, 1994). Rather than a standardized diet approach, the ADA guidelines now call for individual assessment, goal setting, problem solving, and ongoing evaluation (American Diabetes Association, 1996).

Challenges of Chronic Illness and Goal Setting

Another challenge in patient education is helping a patient who needs to change two or more behaviors simultaneously (eg, diet, exercise,

STEPS	APPLICATION
I. The patient perceives that he or she has a condition or is likely to contract it.	I. a. Discuss the problem and symptoms. b. Explore patient's prior knowledge and experience. c. Assess obstacles to understanding (anxiety, fear, misconceptions).
II. The patient perceives that the disease or condition is harmful and has serious consequences for him or her.	II. a. Patient's perception of consequences (includes lifestyle) b. Discuss prognosis. c. Discuss beliefs and attitudes; trust of providers and health care system. d. Discuss experiences of family/friends with similar problem.
III. The patient believes that the suggested health intervention is of value to him or her.	III. a. Understands proposed treatment plan (including medications). b. Discuss what may happen with or without proposed treatment. c. Is this a cure? d. Discuss financial costs, life-style changes, side effects.
IV. The patient believes that the effectiveness of the treatment is worth the cost and barriers he or she must confront.	IV. a. Contract (agreement) with the patient on the treatment plan. b. Outline provider responsibilities. c. Outline patient responsibilities. d. Outline patient education plan for developing needed knowledge, attitudes, and skills.

TABLE 9-3. The Health Belief Model Used in the Interview to Identify Patient Goals and Decisions

The Health Belief Model was constructed to predict health behaviors. It provides a tool for understanding the patient's perception of disease and his or her decision-making process in the consumption of health services. In each of the four steps, family members and significant others should be considered.

References
1. Hochbaum, G. M. (1958). *Public participation in medical screening programs.* (U.S. Public Health Service Publication No. 572). Washington, DC: U.S. Government Printing Office.
2. Rosenstock, I. M. (1975). Patient's compliance with health regimens. *Journal of the American Medical Association, 234,* 402–403.
3. Rankin, S. H., Stallings, K. D. (1990). *Patient education: Issues, principles, and practices.* Philadelphia: J. B. Lippincott.

smoking cessation, taking medications, maintaining treatments). Patients are often unsuccessful because they cannot make such profound changes and may be labeled as noncompliant. Setting priorities and establishing long-term plans of support, follow-up, and reinforcement are critical for patients with many recommended changes. Realistic approaches and sequencing of learning, combined with support that extends beyond the hospital or clinic walls, can enhance the patient's commitment to engage in patient education interventions and promote self-efficacy in the management of health and illness (Strecher, DeVellis, & Becker, 1986; Bandura, 1982).

One way nurses engage in goal setting with cardiac patients is by sharing a list of eight topics of common concern, including how the heart works, activity restrictions, sex, medications, and diet. The nurse uses the list to begin discussion; the patient may add to the list, based on what he or she expects to achieve. The nurse then serves as a clinical expert, pulling out the patient's knowledge, concerns, lifestyle, and past experience to make an individualized and realistic set of goals.

Focus groups of patients who have experienced a particular health problem can teach health care providers how to develop patient-centered teaching plans. In Chapter 13, an example of cardiac education is described based on a product line model that follows the patient across various settings. By examining what the patient needs and wants to know at each stage of the illness, learning goals and objectives can be accomplished when it is most important or applicable for the patient.

Using this approach, information overload is avoided, retention is accomplished, and patient learning is tied to his or her readiness (Hanisch, 1993).

Stating Goals

Adults are motivated to learn when they recognize a gap between what they know and what they want to know (Knowles, 1970, 1998). Assessment provides the nurse with information about the patient's knowledge, attitudes, and skills for self-care. Goal setting is an activity in which the patient educator makes a contract with the patient for what he or she wants to accomplish. Patient educators should never force their own goals on the patient and family. They should try to meet the patient and family "on their own ground," encourage whatever participation the patient and family can make, and consider ways to support and reinforce the patient and family strengths.

CASE STUDY

MR. STANLEY

PHYSIOLOGIC DATA

A medical-surgical nurse begins an admission data base for Mr. Stanley, a 60-year-old patient, gathering assessment information critical to his care. Mr. Stanley is admitted to the hospital with a medical diagnosis of asthma. His wife and daughter supply most of the assessment information, because Mr. Stanley is puffing and coughing. The initial assessment is conducted in approximately 30 minutes.

The patient was diagnosed with asthma 15 years ago. The primary nurse knows that she should gear her questioning toward self-care management: preventing acute episodes, using controlled breathing techniques, avoiding bronchial irritants, and using medications correctly. Asthma and chronic obstructive pulmonary disease are among the top diagnosis-related groups at the hospital, and a special patient education effort is aimed at improving the correct use of inhalers. It is estimated that more than 50% of patients who use inhalers experience therapeutic failure because of incorrect technique.

Family Profile

The nurse learns that Mr. and Mrs. Stanley lived in a ranch-style house. Their 38-year-old daughter lives 2 miles away. Mr. Stanley is a retired groundskeeper for the city and spends much of his time planning his home garden. He also likes to fish and is active in his church. Mrs. Stanley reports that, aside from discomfort from her arthritis, she is in good health.

Understanding the Current Event

Mr. Stanley has had progressively worsening attacks of dyspnea for the last month, with occasional tachycardia. Today's episode occurred after working in his garden—"overdoing it," as Mrs. Stanley describes. Mr. Stanley reports a decrease in appetite and difficulty sleeping. The nurse notices that the Stanley's daughter completed Mr. Stanley's admission papers. All three family members appear anxious.

Mrs. Stanley reports that her husband worries her with his frequent use of his inhaler and increasing episodes of breathlessness. When asked to demonstrate controlled breathing techniques, Mrs. Stanley says that he has forgotten how to do them and that he just relies on his "trusty friend" (ie, his inhaler). Mrs. Stanley tells the nurse, "I've been trying to get him to go to the doctor for more than a week. It finally came to this!" Mr. Stanley's three prescribed asthma medications are inhalants: fluticasone propionate (flovent), 220 mcg, 4 inhalations twice daily; salmeterol-xinafoate (serevent), a long-acting bronchodilator, 2 inhalations twice a day; and albuterol (ventolin), taken as needed, but no more than 2 puffs every 4 to 6 hours. Because

(case study continues on page 239)

steroid inhalations can cause osteoporosis, Mr. Stanley also takes alendronate (Fosamax), 10 mg, every morning. Fosamax must be taken on an empty stomach 30 minutes before eating and the patient must stay upright after taking it. Mr. Stanley also takes 500 mg of calcium, three times daily, with meals.

Mr. Stanley admits to using albuterol on a daily basis against the orders of his physician. He admits to smoking "a few cigarettes" lately, despite having quit for 10 months after his last hospitalization.

Mr. Stanley is quickly fatigued. Therefore, the nurse completes an initial screening of systems and flags the assessment data base form so that additional information can be gathered in the following areas:

1. Observation of the patient's inhaler technique
2. Potential environmental irritants
3. Income and health insurance (which often prevents patients from obtaining needed medications)
4. Reading and writing abilities of the Stanleys (to determine appropriate written materials)
5. Typical diet and sleep patterns of the family
6. Daily schedule
7. Ability of family to handle crisis situations
8. Degree of limitation on the patient's and family's functioning
9. Family's desires and needs to know about the illness or problems associated with the illness

The Identified Patient, the Health Problem, and Educational Needs

Mr. Stanley summarizes his problems succinctly: frequent episodes of puffing and fatigue (sometimes with his heart beating too fast). Mrs. Stanley adds that her husband has had a poor appetite lately and that he has not been sleeping well. The nurse explains that poor appetite, rapid

heart rate, and difficulty sleeping may be related to overuse or improper use of the inhaler. The nurse tells Mr. Stanley that she will help him understand how to better manage his asthma at home.

Nursing Diagnoses and Educational Goals
Impaired gas exchange related to chronic airway obstruction

Educational goals. The patient will learn proper use of an inhaler; state the importance of eliminating smoking and other bronchial irritants, including stress; recognize warning signs and prevent exacerbations; and describe the danger of overuse of asthma medications.

Ineffective airway clearance related to reduced cough strength and slowed mucous transport

Educational goals. The patient will perform coughing and breathing techniques; demonstrate ways to increase fluid intake; demonstrate proper use of inhaler; identify ways to avoid infection; and identify signs and symptoms of infection.

Activity intolerance related to dyspnea
Educational goal. The patient can describe how to manage activity and prevent excessive breathlessness. Patient and family express feeling of helplessness; discuss how to handle acute episodes to increase confidence and gain support; suggest methods of relaxation.

Altered nutrition: less than body requirements related to fatigue, weakness, and breathlessness
Educational goal. The patient and his wife will outline a plan of adequate fluid intake, small meals, and frequent snacks.

Risk for noncompliance with therapeutic program related to chronic nature of disease
Educational goal. The patient will participate in the development of an

(case study continues on page 240)

individualized program to integrate all facets of management and consider referrals to a smoking cessation program and other resources that will help family cope with chronic illness.

Factors Influencing Mr. Stanley's Learning
The nurse realizes that she needs to pinpoint teaching priorities and organize them so Mr. Stanley can learn according to his physical ability. She identifies both the positive and negative factors that will influence his learning. Positive factors affecting Mr. Stanley's behavioral change include that he has experience with this disease and its symptoms, that he was smoke-free for 10 months before resuming smoking, and that he wants to continue gardening. Negative factors affecting Mr. Stanley's behavioral change include that he tends to delay seeking treatment for dyspnea, that he resumed smoking, and that both patient and family exhibit anxiety.

Developing Behavioral Objectives

We emphasize that patient education is a process of influencing behavior, not just giving information. Successful patient education must be directed toward accomplishing behavioral change. The patient educator must justify that the material being taught will help the patient perform the desired behavior (Kaluger & Kaluger, 1979). Setting specific behavioral objectives for patient education ensures that learning interventions will be tailored to the client's unique situation and needs. Objectives describe the behaviors (actions) that the patient will perform to meet a goal (Fig. 9-1).

When objectives are clearly stated, the learner knows what his or her role is and what is expected of him or her. The learner can organize his or her energy toward learning. Likewise, when goals and objectives are stated, the teacher knows his or her role. Both teacher and learner know how the results will be measured. Written documentation of learning objectives ensures the patient's straightforward communication with the health care team.

Learning connotes a change in knowledge, attitudes, or skills as a result of an educational experience. Behavioral objectives, also referred to in the patient education context as learning objectives, guide the planning of learning activities and the measurement of learning outcomes. These objectives should state what the learner will *do* as a result of patient teaching (see Figure 9-1). A common mistake of nurses is to define learning objectives in terms of the nurse's rather than of the patient's behavior. For example, a nurse may state, "Review the four signs of a hypoglycemic reaction with the patient." Instead, the objective should state, "The patient will describe or list four signs of a hypoglycemic reaction."

Types of Objectives

Three types of learning objectives are the following:

1. Cognitive objectives, which refer to knowledge
2. Affective objectives, which refer to attitudes
3. Psychomotor objectives, which refer to skills

Cognitive learning refers to rational thought, including basic facts and concepts. For example, cognitive learning is accomplished if the patient can describe his or her health problem in his or her own words, list signs and symptoms associated with the problem, and outline steps in a procedure. Cognitive learning moves from simple to complex concepts, so that the patient can apply facts to different situations. Understanding basic anatomy and physiology addresses the cognitive domain of learning.

Affective learning refers to the patient's feelings and reactions to his or her illness, appreciation of the costs and benefits of treatment, and a willingness to change. Helping patients explore options, gain support of significant others, and explore the relationships

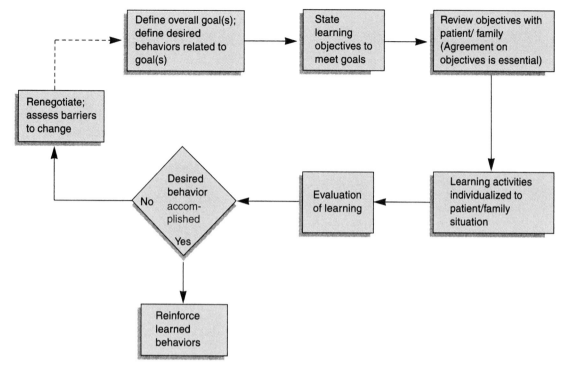

FIGURE 9-1. Using behavioral objectives in the learning process.

of values, culture, and beliefs promote affective learning.

Psychomotor learning refers to musculoskeletal movement, the ability to perform a procedure, skills, and the dexterity to manipulate objects or parts. Mastering psychomotor learning usually involves the need for demonstration, practice, and more practice until the skill is ingrained. Periodic rehearsal or review is needed when skills are not required on a frequent basis.

Components of a Behavioral Objective

According to Mager (1997), a behavioral objective has three components: performance, conditions, and criteria. To write clear learning objectives for patient education in the domains of cognitive, affective, and psychomotor learning, nurses must follow the three steps.

Performance. The learning objective states any activity in which the patient will engage; it describes what the learner will do. The learning objective uses an action verb and denotes an activity that can be measured. The activity may be visible (eg, writing a list) or invisible (eg, solving a problem). Verbs such as *believe, understand, value,* and *know* are not measurable and should be avoided when performance is being described in a learning objective.

When choosing an action verb, the teacher should ask, Can I measure whether the learner can do this? (Box 9-5) The verb should be simple enough that the learner can understand how he or she is expected to show competence. Each learning objective should reflect only one behavior (Bloom, Englehar, Furst, Hill & Krathwohl, 1984).

Conditions. The learning objective states what special circumstances will be included

BOX 9-5. Suggested Verbs for the Three Domains of Learning

Cognitive domain: Developing Knowledge, Facts, and Concepts in Patient Education

*   Identify, define, list, match, name, record, repeat, show, state, select, tell, underline, choose, collect, locate, report

* *   Describe, discuss, explain, outline, restate, review, summarize, give example, prepare, recognize

* * *   Apply, demonstrate, design, implement, measure, modify, prepare, schedule, solve, use, negotiate, compute, practice, write

* * * *   Compare, contrast, diagram, differentiate, sort, test, debate

Affective domain: Developing Appreciation of Benefits and Value in Patient Education

*   Commit, describe, explain, defend, assist

* *   Arrange, choose, combine, compare, explain, express, modify, relate

* * *   Disagree, help, join, initiate, propose, justify

* * * *   Participate, perform, practice, state willingness, reply, try, label, attempt, answer

* * * * *   Accept, accommodate, admit, heed, follow

Psychomotor domain: Developing Skills and Procedures in Patient Education

*   Choose, compare, describe, differentiate, identify, select, separate

* *   Attempt, ask, copy, display, prepare, respond, show, start, volunteer

* * *   Apply, arrange, cleanse, count, connect, cut, demonstrate, examine, find, fold, grasp, guide, hold, insert, lift, locate, open, operate, place, pour, practice, pull, push, raise, remove, separate, shake, squeeze, stand, transfer, walk, wash, weigh, wipe

* * * *   Adapt, modify, correct, rearrange, replace, substitute, vary

* to * * * * * notes increasing levels of complexity and competency.

in the learner's performance. For example, time of day, sterile technique, equipment and tools, place, calorie restrictions, and particular symptoms are all conditions that may be part of a learning objective. For example: Given a list of common foods, Mr. Jones will identify those high in sodium, which should be avoided.

Criteria offer a component of evaluation. They state how the teacher and learner will know when the learning has been accomplished. A criterion states how long or how well the behavior must be performed to be acceptable. Examples of criteria include score or speed, weight, quality, number of times, accuracy, and frequency. For example: Mrs. Harde will draw up and administer 22 units of insulin using sterile technique at 7:00 AM on 3 consec-

utive days. The criteria used in measurement include the number of units of insulin, the time, and the frequency of administration.

Criteria are especially important when teaching psychomotor objectives, such as walking with crutches. How many times does the nurse want to observe a return demonstration to be confident that the patient has mastered the skill? What degree of error or variation in performance is acceptable? For example, when teaching a patient to take his or her pulse, within how many beats of the nurse's measurement must the patient measure to be considered successful?

Mager states it is important for both the teacher and the learner to answer the following three questions about the behavioral objective:

1. **What can the learner do?** What does the learner have to do to show he or she has achieved the learning?
2. **Under what conditions will the learner do it?** Will he or she use special equipment?
3. **What is the performance standard?** How well must it be done? How will the learner know when it is done well enough?

These three questions are the components of a learning objective and are intended to help design a learning objective (Mager, 1997). The nurse should make learning objectives specific, measurable, and attainable. To accomplish this, the nurse must understand the patient's view of what he or she wants to achieve. Although the learner's ability should not be doubted, it is important that goals are not set too high. Learning should be a positive, supportive experience in which the learner gains confidence and self-esteem. Learning should begin with activities that the patient can successfully accomplish, moving from simple behaviors to those that are more complex. Also, learning objectives that are critical for safety (three or four critical behaviors) should be identified and should be reviewed and reinforced throughout the patient's stay.

Learning objectives keep patient education focused on outcomes. For that reason, nurses should relate the objectives to nursing diagnoses and limit the number of learning objectives. We have witnessed exhaustive lists of objectives (30 or more) that look scholarly, but are useless to nurses and patients. To cover the objectives, patient education has become an exercise of rapid fire teaching and little practice on the part of the patient. The number of objectives should be based on what is feasible for a patient to learn in a given phase or setting. Nurses should avoid the temptation of simply teaching the same amount of material in a fraction of the time.

Getting the Patient and the Family Involved

The involvement of the patient and family in setting learning goals affirms their willingness to participate. Criteria for evaluation should be acceptable to and valued by them. For example, "working for one hour in the garden without breathlessness" or "caring for a grandchild" may be more meaningful outcomes to a patient than "22 respirations per minute" or a "10-lb weight loss." The behavioral change involved in these examples, however, may be the same and could satisfy both the provider and the patient. It is important that patients express their own goals verbally or in writing. The patient educator should encourage them to talk about the changes they would like to make and help them to state these in objective form.

Health professionals must share with the patient their goals for the patient. The nurse must be willing to revise these goals and objectives if they are not agreeable to the patient. The patient may understand the hazards of smoking but may not be willing to give up smoking cigarettes during the evening. The patient may understand the need for weight reduction and may want to lose weight, but may be unwilling to sacrifice ice cream. A measurable reduction in smoking or a measurable weight loss using a modified diet plan may be a workable compromise.

Strategies for getting the patient and the family involved include asking them for their perceptions of the patient's problems and what they would like to change. The nurse should share his or her view of the problem and ask the patient if he or she would like help in working on the identified problems. Discuss the priority of needs with the patient and write behavioral objectives using the patient's input. Working together, contract for what you will teach, what the patient will learn, and what your respective responsibilities will be.

C A S E   S T U D Y

MRS. DAWE

In Chapter 8, we introduced Mrs. Dawe who was struggling with her daily management of hypertension and diabetes.

(case study continues on page 244)

Mrs. Dawe identified her greatest problems as her weight and her high blood pressure. She agreed that she would like to work on these problems. She stated that her shortness of breath would decrease if she lost weight and she felt that she could follow her exercise plan. She described the low-fat, diabetic ADA diet she had been prescribed 5 years ago as "too restrictive," but agreed to renegotiate an ADA diet that included one-half of a cup of ice cream each week and limited amounts of other favorite foods. She thought that her weight increase and blood pressure problem were closely related. She also saw her shortness of breath as a problem and stated, "I would be happy if I could keep my granddaughter for the day without getting sick."

The nurses involved in her care shared their perceptions with Mrs. Dawe. The nurses' perceptions were similar to Mrs. Dawe's (eg, about her obesity, hypertension, and shortness of breath). The nurses reinforced her knowledge of her health problems and her positive behaviors of checking her blood glucose and examining her feet regularly. The nurses complimented her dependability in keeping her appointments and in taking her medications. A meal plan was offered to help her lose weight and lower her blood pressure. She agreed with the nurses' suggestions. It was decided to continue a discussion of her diabetes management at her clinic visit scheduled for the next week. Mr. Dawe was present during the discussion but was silent.

The nurses stressed the importance of family support in improving the overall nutrition and health for both partners, because the recommendations for healthy eating and well-planned exercise are important for everyone. The family's focus on healthful eating after a spouse or parent has a heart attack is critical. When all family members make changes to lower fat in their diets, they show the patient that he or she is not alone and that they want him or her to stay alive. That kind of support can be instrumental in helping the patient make necessary long-term changes. Membership in the local chapter of the American Diabetes Association and a subscription to the monthly newsletter *Diabetes News* were also recommended to the Dawes to help establish a new start to the treatment plan.

Learning goals and objectives related to Mrs. Dawe's obesity and hypertension were mutually negotiated. By 24-hour recall, Mrs. Dawe's current intake was estimated at approximately 2,200 calories/day. She agreed to an appointment with the dietitian to learn about the new dietary guidelines and how to plan sample menus. She agreed to limit her use of salt and fat in cooking.

NURSING DIAGNOSIS: ALTERED NUTRITION: MORE THAN BODY REQUIREMENTS RELATED TO NONADHERENCE TO DIABETIC LOW-FAT DIET

Goal. Mrs. Dawe will follow a low-fat, diabetic meal plan by June 1.

Educational needs. With the dietitian, outline food suggestions for breakfast, lunch, and dinner using her meal planning guide. Describe how one-half of a cup of ice cream is worked into the weekly meal plan.

Behavioral objectives. Mrs. Dawe will record in notebook all foods eaten during the week. She will state why weight control is especially important in the management of diabetes. Mrs. Dawe will attend the patient with diabetes luncheon at the hospital.

Goal. Achieve systolic blood pressure below 160 mmHg and diastolic blood pressure below 90 mmHg by June 1.

(case study continues on page 245)

Educational needs. Review high-sodium foods and ways to avoid them.

Behavioral objectives. Mrs. Dawe will omit salt in cooking and name 10 high-sodium foods that should be avoided. Mrs. Dawe will eliminate canned foods from the diet during the week and substitute fresh fruits and vegetables, recording them in notebook.

Mrs. Dawe was willing to keep specific records in a notebook that she would bring to her next office visit. A contract was written up and signed, and Mrs. Dawe kept the contract at home. When the nurses returned to the office, they documented the agreement in the progress notes section of her chart and made an appointment for her with the dietitian; this had been suggested so she would have an opportunity to explore variations in her food choices and receive cooking suggestions. Mrs. Dawe would return to the family practice clinic for a visit 1 week later. Prioritizing problems was not difficult because the problems were closely interrelated physiologic needs. An effort to set achievable goals increased the probability of attaining success and developing a positive self-image. Mr. Dawe was willing to help by supporting Mrs. Dawe's renewed effort to follow her meal plan and to limit her salt intake. He remarked, "It would help me to cut down on my salt, too, and I can use some at the table."

THE LEARNING CONTRACT

The learning contract is a tool used to formalize the agreement between the teacher and learner. It clearly states learning behaviors, the responsibility of the teacher and the learner, and the methods of follow-up and evaluation. The contract is renegotiated as learning is accomplished and new goals are defined. If the patient changes his or her mind or finds the goals too difficult to achieve, the objectives can be revised. Learning contracts can be used in the hospital, home, and clinic settings (Fig. 9-2).

Fig. 9-3 illustrates the essential components of a learning contract for the case study of Mrs. Dawe. It is helpful to type a standard contract form on hospital or clinic stationery and complete it with the patient. A copy can be kept in the nurses' station or in the patient record and a copy should be given to the patient. A bonus clause has been used to denote additional resources available to the patient (eg, self-help groups, classes, and other health professionals). As behaviors are accomplished, it is essential to include a reinforcement as an intervention to support the patient when the contract is revised. The reinforcement may be weekly weight checks in the clinic, an occasional home visit, a telephone call, or a referral to the public health nurse or office nurse.

Learning contracts help patients retain information gained though individual and group teaching. In the case of cardiovascular patients, patients are encouraged to identify their own barriers to behavior change and provide strategies for risk factor management. These strategies include relaxation techniques, smoking cessation, changes in eating patterns, and exercise. They are asked to identify small, attainable goals, and commit these to a verbal or written contract that specifies how these changes will be incorporated in their daily routines (Lai & Cohen, 1999).

The learning contract is a powerful motivator for both patient and staff. Through the contract, goals and objectives become specific, achievable, and clearly defined. The contract provides a mechanism for communication by formalizing conversation. A time limitation exists for renegotiating the contract, the responsibilities of health care team members are outlined, and community resources that may be of assistance to the patient are detailed. The contract provides standards for evaluation of learning by specifying desired behaviors, conditions, and criteria and also provides opportunity for measurement of behavioral change.

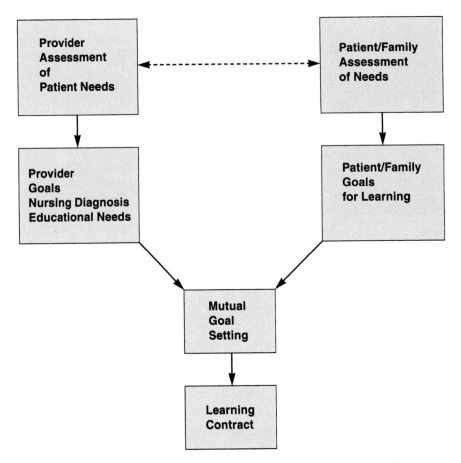

FIGURE 9-2. Designing a learning contract based on client goals for patient education.

CLINICAL RELEVANCE OF PLANNING

Motivating Patients

> *E*xpert nurses have found that the best way to motivate patients to participate in their care and to follow the instructions that are recommended by health care providers is to find out what those patients value. It's different for every patient.
>
> **K. S. (STALLINGS, 1996)**

How can we motivate patients to learn?

Recognizing what motivates a patient is probably the most important factor in having a patient successfully respond to patient education with the desired behavioral changes. Motivating factors can vary significantly. A patient may be motivated by assurance that he or she will be in control of his or her own life; another patient may be motivated by a desire to please the health care professionals.

> *I* had the experience of being a patient on my own unit. I was on the other side, and got a "taste of my own medicine," so to speak.

FAMILY MEDICINE CENTER

Learning Contract

Goals:
To lose 6 lb during the next 2 months.
To achieve systolic blood pressure below 160 mmHg, and diastolic blood pressure below 90 mmHg.

Learner Actions:
Record in notebook all foods eaten each day. Follow recommendations of American Diabetes Association (ADA) meal plan. Take medications daily and record in notebook. Eliminate canned foods this week. Return for clinic visit next week.

Teacher Actions:
Supply diet outline for ADA meal plan.
Check weight and BP weekly.
Label reading models—will review with Mrs. Dawe at clinic visit 4/7. Instruction in reading labels on canned foods done today in the home.

Method of Measurement:
Weight
BP
Patient record in notebook

Length of Contract:
2 months

Bonus Clause:
Diabetic luncheon at hospital
ADA diet plan and instructions for meal preparation and meal spacing
Booklet: "Your Diabetic Meal Plan"
Appointment with dietitian scheduled for 4/7

Signatures:

_____   _____

_____   _____

Date:3/31

FIGURE 9-3. Learning contract for Mrs. Dawe.

What I found out is that what I taught has worked for me. Fortunately, I could do all of the things I taught my patients to do. Miraculously, it worked. It worked for me because my attitude was "I want to get

better!" I wanted to get back into the workforce. I wanted to get back home. Having been in the role of patient, I see things differently now. I understand why patients cry, and why they have some of the concerns that they do. They want to have a good outcome and to feel good about themselves. Now I take that little extra time to listen to what the patient is saying to me.

N. B. (STALLINGS, 1996)

Getting the Health Care Team Together

When the patient comes in, we try to incorporate as many people from the healthcare team as possible in planning the care. That would include the physician, the nurse, the dietitian, the chaplain, the physical therapist, the social worker, the discharge planner, and anyone else, even if that's someone on the outside from a community resource that we can bring in.

N. B. (STALLINGS, 1996)

How can I get the health care team together to coordinate patient education?

Coordinating patient education can be a difficult job when many disciplines are involved. For example, the patient with newly diagnosed diabetes is usually taught by nurses, dietitians, and, in some settings, pharmacists; a physician is also involved and, if a community referral is needed, social workers may join the team. A general planning meeting can be useful in saving time for everyone and avoiding replication of efforts. If this meeting is set up around the physician's scheduled time on the unit or in the agency, the process will be facilitated. Mutually derived goals should be written at the planning meeting. Notifying the patient's family of a time to be present for planning is also helpful. And, because the focus of the team is the patient, the patient should also be present. It is also important that the nurse make the patient's family aware of the times when health team members will teach the patient, so that they can be present, if appropriate.

 Advanced practice nurses gain skill in the art of negotiation with colleagues, both in nursing and other disciplines, and therefore make an important contribution to problem solving in teamwork. Negotiation between physicians and nurses is developed through experience, and depends on having a strong clinical grasp, the judgement that a particular situation needs to be tended to, having developed a trusting relationship with the physician, and an ability to make the case with skill (Benner, Tanner, & Chesla, 1996). ∎

Continuity of care and logical progression of the teaching plan can be accomplished by having all health care team members use the same problem list and document their teaching in the progress notes section of the chart. The team approach, when applied to patient education, is one of the most effective uses of a group management technique. Communication is rendered coherent and concise, teaching efforts are not replicated, and the entire health care team, especially the patient, benefits.

Physical Limitations and Environment: Effects on Patient Education

We encounter various situations in the home that are different from hospital nursing care where everything is kept sterile and clean. The patients may have no running water, or they might not be as clean as we would like them to be. You have to adjust to what's available in the home, and many times you have to change your way of thinking and be more flexible in what you teach. You have to improvise. I think we have to listen to the patients and families. They really do have a lot of good ideas and sometimes we are too quick to say "This is the way you need to do it, and you're going to do it this way." That really doesn't work. We have to listen to them and incorporate what they say into our teaching. You still must get across that the open wound has to be kept clean, and the dressing has to be changed if the wound is going to heal. You review the medications and diet for diabetes. But you have to realize that you cannot change everything about the way a person has lived for a long period of time. You really have to respect the patient's way of life and his or her beliefs.

J. M. (STALLINGS, 1996)

We had a young man on our unit who presented us with a big challenge. He was deaf and legally blind. So when he first came, we had the interpreter come to the unit each time that we needed to explain a procedure to him. We learned to communicate with him. The staff on our unit learned to sign. Where most people you sign to can see your hand movements, he could not. So we had to sign inside his hand. That was a neat experience. He taught us many things once he realized that we truly wanted to communicate with him.

F. B. (STALLINGS, 1996)

How does a patient's pain and fatigue affect patient education?

The effects of pain, illness, and fatigue should be manifest to nurses. However, because we become somewhat inured to these behaviors, we forget to assess them and their effects on planned health teaching. Pain can be an all-encompassing experience. If the client experiences severe pain, our only intervention should be alleviation of pain, either through medications or nonpharmacological techniques. Once pain has been lessened, relaxation

and breathing techniques can be taught for use in the future. Alleviation of pain also ensures that necessary skills can be taught. For example, a nurse may realize the patient needs to learn how to use crutches or cough, turn, and deep breathe, but until the patient enjoys a modicum of comfort, these skills cannot be taught.

Illness and fatigue can deplete a client's physical resources to the extent that he or she has no energy left for learning. If the client is not listening or focusing on the patient education session or cannot retain simple information, it is preferable to plan teaching when he is more rested or when family members are present.

If the patients are feeling nauseous or if they are in pain, or they are worried because they haven't seen their loved one yet today, they don't absorb even our most basic teaching. So first we must get their discomforts and worries under control, and then we can give them the information, little pieces at a time.

E. W. (STALLINGS, 1996)

 Pain experienced by older patients who have been discharged from acute care settings to long-term care facilities is underestimated, underreported, and undertreated. If pain management in the long-term care facility is inadequate, the success of patient education in that setting is certainly affected. The most important indicator to assess is the resident's perception of his or her pain. An effective pain management program can provide pain relief during time, enable the resident to improve sleep, independence in activities of daily living, greater participation in recreation, and heightened feelings of well-being and control over one's health (Loeb, 1999). ■

Acute and chronic pain management is inadequate in all settings and within all age groups. Those especially vulnerable to undertreatment of their pain are small children, older patients, patients who are intubated, people with mental disabilities, non-English speaking patients, and patients with a history of substance abuse (Winslow, 1998; Hughes, 1999). Therefore, patient education with these populations may be compromised if the nurse does not consider that pain management may be a key component of the teaching plan.

Patient Education for Homeless Clients

In our walk-in clinic, we try to get as much information as we can about each patient's situation. We learn from our patients all the time about many things—things we had not thought about, perhaps difficulties or situations they face that we have never experienced. They are just living in a different world, so assessment is a mutually beneficial process. We learn from them about how to help. We bring in services for our clients, such as teaching on foot-care or diabetes, or asthma. I think it is extremely important in our setting to do as much as we can to teach prevention. I think it's difficult for people who are living in difficult circumstances to conduct themselves that way—to do a lot of planning, to think ahead. So we do what we can to help them look at what they are eating, at health habits, to see ways they could make improvements—ways that are actually possible for them, however small. We've learned to measure progress in tiny increments.

M. M. (STALLINGS, 1996)

How can I conduct effective patient education in extreme conditions, such as homelessness?

Situations involving homeless clients with health problems are some of the most difficult in which to intervene. Consider the case of a man with type I diabetes who lives on the street during the day and in a homeless shelter at night. Neuropathies make this client more likely to develop skin breakdown and foot sores, and because of constant walking during the day in poorly fitting shoes, major foot ulcers are more likely to develop than in a non-homeless person with diabetes. Additionally, self-monitoring of blood glucose is almost impossible to accomplish. Added to this are problems related to syringes, which on the streets are frequently shared or stolen for use in injecting intravenous drugs, thus increasing the risk of hepatitis B and human immunodeficiency virus (HIV) infection for a client who has diabetes. Standard teaching regarding diabetes management is not realistic for these clients. At best, the client should be encouraged to come to a health clinic in a shelter daily for insulin injection and occasional blood glucose monitoring.

Psychosocial problems are another factor when considering patient education in situations involving extreme conditions. For example, one nurse practitioner who works in a homeless shelter explained that circadian rhythms and sense of time quickly become confused by homeless people. Those who are newly homeless need constant reorientation to time and place and frequently state that they feel like they are losing it and going crazy. In this type of situation, nurses often cannot provide the same type of patient education to which they aspire. Instead, health care providers try to provide some stability for the homeless client and attempt to address some of the underlying problems related to homelessness, such as unemployment, alcohol and drug abuse, and mental illness.

Homeless women and children have many physical and psychological concerns and may underestimate the health care that is available to them. When asked to describe their health concerns, these women usually identify drug abuse, bipolar disorders, anxiety, depression, suicidal behaviors, self mutilation, and domestic abuse. Shame, fear, need for information, and poverty influence attempts at patient education. Women and children may stay in homeless shelters for a long time, providing nurses an opportunity to intervene with health promotion and patient empowerment strategies (Walker, 1998).

 Migrant workers and their families comprise a vast labor workforce for the American agriculture industry, which is constituted mostly of people of Hispanic, African, and Asian decent. The National Advisory Council on Migrant Health reports that nurse and nurse practitioners are the primary health care providers for these workers. In serving this population, nurses see disease transmission and domestic violence (resulting from cramped and unsanitary housing). The children of these workers receive interrupted schooling, which poses psychosocial and developmental risks.

Data indicate poor immunization rates, lack of dental care, and increased incidence of accidents and injury. Nurses appreciate the cohesive communities of migrant workers based on language, music, food, and religion. Social interaction, folk health practices, and family structure must be considered when planning patient education. Teaching interventions must acknowledge cultural diversity and incorporate social supports. One successful program, the North Carolina Maternal and Child Health Migrant Project, overcame barriers to health care (eg, limited transportation, communication difficulties, and lack of child care) by training women in the migrant camps to serve as lay health advisors, providing health education, medication instruction, and first aid. They also targeted breast-feeding promotion among mothers, offering incentives for women to bring their friends and relatives to nutrition education appointments. Nurse practitioners work closely with this population to gather information about changes in family relationships and acculturation to be used in designing health programs to ensure that the health services match the needs of specific migrant cultures (Sandhaus, 1998.) ∎

Patient Education in the Psychiatric Setting

The challenge for nurses in working with individuals with psychotic disorders is to provide them with information about their illness in a way that will be useful. You need to provide them enough information so the patient can become an active consumer. Just as we would want a patient with diabetes to ask the physician why the dose of insulin is being changed, we want individuals with schizophrenia to be just as confident to ask, "Why are you changing my medication?" And families are asking us, "Give me information that will allow me to talk with the physician in an understandable manner. Teach me the words the physician will use. They realize that when the patient leaves the hospital, or when the patient comes home from the community mental health center, they are the ones who are going to have to take care of them. Families want to be active consumers.

A. C. (STALLINGS, 1996)

How can patient education principles be applied in the psychiatric setting?

Psychiatric patients have the same basic patient education needs as do medical-surgical patients (ie, to function to the best of their ability on the wellness-illness continuum and in a manner consistent with their expressed needs and desires).

Patient education addresses the three goals of survival skills, helping the patient to identify problems and preparing the patient to make appropriate decisions to benefit his or her health. It is the nurse's responsibility to orient patients to the psychiatric environment, whether inpatient or outpatient. This orientation can be crucial to the patient's adjustment to the therapeutic milieu. Hamer's study of psychiatric inpatients demonstrated that patients thought their learning needs soon after hospitalization involved reestablishment of homeostasis (ie, learning how to achieve a balance between sleep, activity, and food consumption needs) (Hamer, 1991). They also recognized their need to learn how to manage anger.

Patients who had been hospitalized for long periods reported needing education in the area of involvement in the community, especially through support groups. Thus, learning needs of psychiatric inpatients change during time just as the learning needs of patients with other chronic illnesses shift.

Many psychiatric patients have had problems structuring their time to meet the demands of daily existence. Therefore, the nurse's role in facilitating the patient's ability to organize his or her time in a meaningful manner is pivotal to the ability to function in the community.

Inpatient psychiatric clients with long histories of institutionalization have problems adapting to the communities into which they are discharged. On admission, these patients already have been recognized as having difficulties with social interaction and problem-solving skills. If reintegration into the community is to be successful, it is imperative that coping skills are taught both before and after discharge. Social interaction and problem-solving skills are frequently learned in group therapy contexts. Other skills, such as the ability to perform the basic activities of daily living, can be taught by nurses in a combination of didactic and practical approaches. In many instances, patients must be taught activities as basic as personal hygiene or how to use a stove; they must be oriented to technology, such as the use of microwave ovens, automated bank machines, and computers.

Stanley (1984) suggests the use of goal attainment scaling to evaluate the psychiatric patient's achievement of treatment goals. The patient decides on the goals that he or she wishes to achieve and weighs the goals in terms of importance. When the patient and nurse review achievement of the goals, a goal attainment score gives the patient and nurse an indication of the progress made. Such ongoing evaluation reinforces patient education with the psychiatric patient.

 Last, teaching a patient's family is always an important aspect of patient education, and it may be even more important with the caregiving family members of psychiatric patients. Family members need assistance in decreasing stigma or guilt and in learning how to explain behaviors of their family member to friends, other relatives, and the public. Other aspects of family education include involvement of the family in the treatment plan if indicated, preparation for hospital discharge to the home, and realistic long-term planning. Patient teaching with psychiatric patients and their families requires creativity and patience, but the rewards can be great. ■

CASE STUDY

CINDY BENJAMIN, BIPOLAR ILLNESS

Cindy is a 32-year-old woman admitted to the acute care psychiatric unit because of a manic episode. She is loud, cannot sleep, and is impulsive. She resists limits set by the staff, and she responds with inappropriate and promiscuous behavior. The milieu is not therapeutic: other patients become angry and she responds with more aggression.

The patient care plan reflects the following approach to Cindy's care. The first step is to reduce the stimulation by confining Cindy to her room with hourly, supervised breaks. She is supervised to take care of basic grooming. A written contract is used to help her take responsibility for her own limits. She has to be reminded to follow the plan, but she does follow it. The plan is explained to the other patients at community meetings so they would reinforce the plan and understand that less stimulation helps Cindy focus on her behavior.

As the manic symptoms decrease, Cindy

(case study continues on page 253)

spends more time out of her room. Eventually the staff sees a mood shift to depression: less activity, loss of appetite, and neglected grooming. A new plan of care is initiated to support and encourage Cindy to spend more time out of her room.

Like most patients with bipolar illness, Cindy begins drug therapy to be used long-term. Nursing diagnoses in her care plan included: inappropriate aggression; manipulation; manic behavior; depressive behavior; alteration in thought process; and self-care deficit: feeding, hygiene (McFarland, Wasli, & Gerety, 1997).

As Cindy's nursing diagnoses were resolved, the care plan is altered to place priority on the nursing diagnosis of *knowledge deficit related to nature and management of bipolar disorder.*

Goal. The patient will accept her illness and take responsibility for her own treatment (including ongoing drug therapy and outpatient psychotherapy).

Educational needs. Instruct Cindy about the nature of the illness, its course and symptoms, the treatment, and how to manage it. Include Cindy's fiancée and roommate in teaching.

LEARNING OBJECTIVE: SURVIVAL SKILLS
Cindy will:

State the diagnosis and describe it in her own words.
Describe symptoms of manic and depressed states.
Outline the three components of the treatment plan she will follow after discharge.
Describe the drug therapy to be used, including dose, schedule, and periodic blood level monitoring.

LEARNING OBJECTIVE: RECOGNIZING PROBLEMS
Cindy will:

State two situations for which she should contact her psychiatrist.
Discuss the reason to avoid alcohol.

LEARNING OBJECTIVE: DECISION-MAKING
Cindy will:

Describe what is meant by relapse and what action plan she should follow if relapse occurs.
State the importance of notifying other health care providers about the medication she takes. (Brenners, Harris, & Weston, 1987).

SUMMARY

Client goals for patient education are derived from nursing diagnoses and associated educational needs. The patient's concerns or fears and the pressing needs of the nurse to ensure a safe discharge must be considered when making goals. Adult learning theory emphasizes the goal directedness of adults and the importance of setting goals for patient education. Learning objectives related to goals were described for the three domains—cognitive (knowledge), affective (attitudes and understanding), and psychomotor (skills). It is important to identify the three or four objectives that are critical to the safety of each patient and reinforce these in each encounter with a patient.

STRATEGIES FOR CRITICAL ANALYSIS

1. Imagine that you are diagnosed with a rare illness that will require treatment for the rest of your life. You are hospitalized after arriving in the emergency room after a fainting episode. What fears or concerns do you experience that may influence your readiness to learn? List your three most pressing questions.
2. You work as a nurse on the maternity unit of the hospital. Six years ago, when you began work on the unit, you participated in a patient education committee that developed the postpartum teaching plan. This plan was based on a 3-day length of

stay. Your average patient stay after a routine vaginal delivery is now 24 hours or less. How can the patient learning objectives be reduced? Which three or four critical objectives could serve as a basis for teaching survival skills?

3. Using the case study of Mr. Stanley, write one learning objective for each of the three learning domains (ie, cognitive, affective, psychomotor).

4. Using the case study of Cindy, develop a learning contract using the format in Figure 9-3.

REFERENCES

American Diabetes Association. (1996). Nutrition recommendations and principles for people with diabetes mellitus. *Diabetes Care, Suppl 19,* S16–19.

Bandura, A. (1982). Self-efficacy mechanism in human agency. *American Psychologist, 37,* 122–147.

Benner, P. (1984). *From novice to expert: Power and excellence in clinical nursing practice.* Menlo Park, CA: Addison-Wesley.

Benner, P., Tanner, C., & Chesla, C. (1996). *Expertise in Nursing Practice: Caring, Judgement, and Ethics.* New York: Springer Publishing Company.

Brenners, D., Harris B., & Weston, P. (1987). Managing manic behavior. *American Journal of Nursing 87*(5), 620–623.

Bloom, B., Englehar, M., Furst, E., Hill, W., & Krathwohl, D. (1984). *Taxonomy of Educational Objectives: The classification of educational goals.* New York: Longman.

Deakins, D. (1994). Teaching elderly patients about diabetes. *American Journal of Nursing, 94*(4), 39–42.

Erikson, E. H. (1993). *Childhood and society.* New York: W. W. Norton.

Gershoff, S. (Ed.). (1994). Rethinking the diabetic diet: The 'rules' ease up. *Tufts University Diet and Nutrition Newsletter, 12*(6), 3–6.

Halpin-Landry, J., & Goldsmith, S. (1999). Feet first: diabetes care. *American Journal of Nursing, 99*(2), 26–33.

Hamer, B. A. (1991). Health teaching needs of psychiatric inpatients. *Canadian Journal of Nursing Administration 91*(4), 6–10.

Hanisch, P. (1993). Informational needs and preferred time to receive information for phase II cardiac rehabilitation patients: What CE instructors need to know. *Journal of Continuing Education in Nursing, 24*(2), 82–89.

Hochbaum, G. M. (1958). Public participation in medical screening programs. *(U.S. Public Health Service Publication No. 572.)* Washington, D.C.: U.S. Government Printing Office.

Hughes, A. (1999). HIV-related pain. *American Journal of Nursing, 99*(6), 20.

Hurxthal, K. (1988). Quick! Teach this patient about insulin. *American Journal of Nursing, 88*(8), 1097–1100.

Janz, N., & Becker, M. (1984). The health belief model: A decade later. *Health Education Quarterly, 11*(1), 1–47.

Kaluger, G., & Kaluger, M. (1979). *Human development: The span of life.* St. Louis: C. V. Mosby.

Kasl, S. (1974). The health belief model and behavior related to chronic illness. *Health Education Monographs, 2,* 433–454.

Knowles, M. S. (1970). *The modern practice of adult education: Andragogy versus pedagogy.* New York: Association Press.

Knowles, M. (1998a). *The Adult Learner: A Neglected Species* (4th ed.). Houston, TX: Gulf Publishing Company.

Knowles, M., Swanson, R., & Holton, E. (1998b). *Adult Learner: the Definitive Classic in Adult Education and Human Resource Development.* Houston, TX: Gulf Publishing Company.

Lai, S., & Cohen, M. (1999). Promoting lifestyle changes. *American Journal of Nursing, 99*(4), 63–67.

Loeb, J. (1999). Pain management in long-term care. *American Journal of Nursing, 99*(2), 48–52.

Lumley, W. (1988). Controlling hypoglycemia and hyperglycemia. *Nursing, 18*(10), 39.

Mager, R. (1997). *Preparing instructional objectives* (3rd ed.). Atlanta, GA: Center for Effective Performance, Inc.

Mc Farland, G., Wasli, E., & Gerety, E. (1997). *Nursing Diagnosis and Process in Psychiatric Mental Health Nursing.* Philadelphia: Lippincott-Raven.

O'Brien, B. (1999). Coming of age with an ostomy. *American Journal of Nursing, 99*(8), 71–73.

Polin, S., & Giedt, F. (1993). *MDUL-The Joslin diabetes gourmet cookbook.* New York: Bantam Books.

Rankin, S. H., & Stallings, K. D. (1990). *Patient education: Issues, principles, and practices.* Philadelphia: J. B. Lippincott.

Rosenstock, I. M. (1975). Patient's compliance with health regimens. *Journal of the American Medical Association, 234,* 402–403.

Sandhaus, S. (1998). Migrant health: a harvest of poverty. *American Journal of Nursing, 98*(9), 52–54.

Stanley, B. (1984). Evaluation of treatment goals: The use of goal attainment scaling. *Journal of Advanced Nursing, 9,* 351–356.

Stallings, K. (1996). *Integrating patient education in your nursing practice.* [Video]. Reproduced with permission of Glaxo Wellcome Inc.

(Produced by Horizon Video Productions, 4222 Emperor Blvd., Durham, NC 27703.

Strecher, V., DeVellis, B., & Becker, M. (1986). The role of self-efficacy in achieving health behavior change. *Health Education Quarterly, 13*(1), 73–92.

Szabo, V., & Strang, V. (1999). Experiencing control in caregiving. *Image—The Journal of Nursing Scholarship 31*(1), 71–75.

Walker, C. (1998). Homeless people and mental health: a nursing concern. *American Journal of Nursing, 98*(11), 26–31.

Winslow, E. (1998). Effective pain management. *American Journal of Nursing, 98*(7), 16. Philadelphia: J. B. Lippincott.

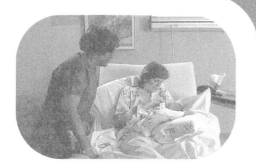

Educational Interventions

for Patients and Families

LEARNING OBJECTIVES

After completing this chapter, the nurse or student nurse should be able to:

1. List the benefits and drawbacks for individual and group teaching formats.

2. Discuss how a teacher can use instructional methods (ie, lecture, discussion, demonstration, role-play, tests, programmed instruction) to achieve learning objectives.

3. Describe ways to increase the effective use of patient education videos.

4. List guidelines for developing effective written patient teaching tools (eg, handouts, one-page discharge instructions).

5. Describe strategies that encourage active patient involvement in patient education interventions for both individual and group teaching programs.

6. Discuss how family roles and expectations can affect learning.

INTRODUCTION

Interventions for Patient Education

Individualized goals set the course for patient education interventions. Between the time goals are agreed on and the time learning activities begin, decisions must be made about content, staff, teaching methods, and tools. The nurse often coordinates this planning through team conferences, contact with the patient's family, hospital, and community resources. A nurse may act as a case manager, promoting patient education as an integral part of the total care plan provided by the health care team.

This chapter offers practical advice and frameworks for designing and implementing educational interventions. Characteristics of a positive learning environment are outlined, teaching and learning styles as they relate to program design are discussed, and the selection of instructional methods and media is explored. There is an emphasis on making patient education realistic, basing it on the patient's length of stay and the survival skills they will need. Suggestions for developing and evaluating both printed patient education materials and educational videotapes are included. This chapter discusses interventions for individual patients and groups and includes case studies to illustrate practical applications.

Scope of Teaching Programs

Planning interventions involves making decisions about the patient education setting, content, resources, and instructors. Although learning interventions must be tailored to each patient, teaching programs planned for target populations (eg, patients with newly diagnosed diabetes) provide guidance and standards for care. We strongly support the development of these programs within hospitals and other health care agencies, tightly linking them to case management and quality improvement systems. A patient education coordinator, hospital-based educator, clinical nurse specialist, or patient care coordinator may organize task forces composed of physicians, nurses, dietitians, pharmacists, and physical therapists to derive teaching plans for special groups. Teaching plans should be an integral part of patient care services and should account for case management tools, quality processes, and the patient experience that crosses service or department lines (Cesta & Falter, 1999). This approach tends to be supported by physicians and other health providers, because they feel confident about the quality of the intervention and the preparation and knowledge of the staff.

Established teaching programs encourage a consistent approach among staff, facilitate a planned interdisciplinary format, and provide populations to be studied (so that the effectiveness of patient education can be measured). We encourage nurses to investigate and promote the programs developed in their institutions. Institution-based programs often provide written and audiovisual teaching tools for the learner and teaching guides for health professionals, such as care maps. (Chapter 13 offers additional information about care maps.)

In institutions in which teaching programs are not developed, the nurse can consult with other health care agencies to learn about teaching programs applied to specific populations. Information about teaching programs may also be obtained from organizations and associations (eg, the American Hospital Association, the National Institutes of Health, the American Cancer Society, and the American Diabetes Association). Another valuable resource for planning patient education programs is a series of *Clinical Practice Guidelines* developed by the Agency for Healthcare Research and Quality (AHRQ). These interdisciplinary guidelines address many health care problems to assist practitioners in the prevention, diagnosis, treatment, and management of clinical conditions, with a focus on patient outcomes. For each clinical practice guideline developed under the sponsorship of AHRQ, several documents are produced to meet different needs. These guidelines contain background information, research findings, a literature review, and bibliography. A patient's guide (or parent guide for pediatric problems) is also available in English and Spanish, providing information to increase patient involvement in health care decision-making. A strong feature of the AHRQ guidelines is their recommendation for patient education. (Guidelines are available by visiting AHRQ's Web site at *www.ahcpr.gov*.)

Patient teaching programs must be continually evaluated to assure that patient outcomes are achieved. Patient education programs can become outdated within a few months of being developed, because of dramatically changing delivery patterns for health care. For example, a new program to teach parents of pediatric bone marrow transplant patients at a large academic medical center became outdated within a few months when the care shifted from the hospital to the outpatient setting. The authors encourage the development of programs that cross settings and providers, focus on patient outcomes, and address patient needs in all settings. These programs are often called product-line models.

SETTING THE STAGE FOR TEACHING AND LEARNING

Effective patient and family education includes finding the right educational materials and making sure they are accurate, age-specific, easily accessible, and appropriate to patient needs. A hospital might create a list of patient education materials that are available and post it throughout the hospital or in a computerized, online version.

(JCAHO, 1998)

Many nurses are confident about the material they teach patients and families. However, some nurses may be unsure of the content and survival skills that must be taught.

Consequently, essential content may be missed, incorrect information may be given, or learning activities may be inappropriate. Some nurses may react to a lack of preparation by avoiding teaching situations and by hoping that someone else will meet the patient's learning needs. Nursing management and staff development must ensure the quality of patient education by preparing all nurses to teach and developing patient care standards that include patient education. Resources (eg, handouts that support learning) should be available for patients, and coaching and modeling should be available to help all nurses become capable teachers.

The education department of a health care facility can create a data base of all patient education media (eg, handouts, booklets, and videos). The data base should itemize the date the material was developed, and the learning outcomes addressed; other factors about the educational media (eg, the literacy level of the material, type size, and target population) should be in the data base. The cost of producing or purchasing the source should be determined. A centralized system is recommended for maintaining adequate supplies and monitoring costs. Clinical nurse specialists and clinical service managers who address common patient diagnoses should collaborate around the possibility of standardizing, eliminating, or procuring of needed materials based on the critical learning needs of patients and their demographics. Patient education materials for non-English speaking patients should be obtained when needed.

 Clinical nurse specialists and other expert nurses can help their colleagues identify what to teach by leading patient care conferences and being available to help others work through difficult teaching situations. Textbooks, reference books, drug handbooks, nursing journals, and books addressing special patient groups also help determine patient education content. Finally, the Internet offers many resources for patient education. Chapter 11 offers guidance in finding and evaluating Internet resources for staff, patient, and family education. ▪

Setting Priorities

To set priorities for the teaching plan, the nurse must consider the patient's ability and readiness to learn. Assess what the patient and the family value as important, the level of their anxiety about a particular topic or skill, the level of need (eg, survival skills), and the time available for implementing teaching activities. If pain management issues preoccupy a patient's attention (eg, with cancer patients), addressing this topic is an educational priority (McCaffery, 1994).

In general, learning should progress from familiar to unfamiliar and from simple to complex. Printed materials intended for patient use often help introduce concepts and relating these concepts to self-care. The nurse should select the three or four most important learning objectives and use these as a basis for evaluation, remembering that the three goals of patient education are to help patients 1) gain survival skills, 2) learn to recognize problems, and 3) have the confidence to make appropriate decisions that benefit health status.

Selecting Instructional Methods and Media

Instructional methods are aligned with the teaching format (eg, self-directed, individual, small group, large group) and the learning activity (eg, lecture, demonstration, discussion, role-play). Instructional media are tools used by the teacher to help the learner to retain, compare, visualize, and reinforce learning. Sometimes too much emphasis is placed on media, and instruction is insufficiently personalized. Health professionals sometimes justify a lack of patient education interventions because of the shortage of funds to purchase videotapes, television equipment, computers, and so forth. Although the effectiveness of instructional media in patient education is emphasized in the literature, it must be tailored to individual situations in planned intervention. If funds are not available for investments in software (eg, videotapes or computer-assisted learning programs) and hardware (eg, video monitors or computers), effective learning can still occur in inpatient and outpatient settings. One-on-one teaching using a clear list of discharge instructions can often provide patient outcomes that are missed when patients are overwhelmed with information from various formats during a short length of stay.

Nurses recognize that low or absent literacy skills pose challenges to the safety and effectiveness of patient instructions (Dixon & Park, 1990; Doak, Doak, & Root, 1995). This chapter also offers tips to improve the effectiveness of written discharge instructions and patient education videos by evaluating them from the patient's perspective.

Creating a Climate for Adult Learning

All nursing staff must individualize the teaching programs that we have put together. As you interact with the patient, and discuss the information with the patient, you listen to what the patient is saying and find a way to make the information usable. Patient education, if it's not usable, is worthless. We have to let the patient teach us as we are teaching them.

A.C. (STALLINGS, 1996)

Adult learners have special needs as they engage in teaching and learning activities, just as they had in the goal-setting process. When these needs are met, learning becomes satisfying and effective. If the teacher fails to acknowledge the patient's needs, barriers arise that slow down or prevent the learning of new behaviors (Iacono & Campbell, 1997).

A climate that promotes adult learning considers the physical and emotional needs of the learner. It uses problem-centered learning, in which the nurse relates material to the patient's life situation and concerns. The learning activities include opportunities for an exchange of ideas between the teacher and learner and for applications of learning in simulated or real exercises (Knowles, 1970; Brookfield, 1986).

Physical Comfort

Pain or anxiety interferes with the exchange of ideas or the ability to listen. Patients who are in the hospital or bedridden may depend on others to assist them with bathing, elimination, dressing changes, medication, and ambulating. A thoughtful teacher is sensitive to these needs and helps the patient achieve as much comfort as possible. Consider whether the patient can physically tolerate a lengthy teaching session or can participate in group learning. Encourage the patient's participation by making certain he or she has eyeglasses or dentures and is positioned comfortably. Watch for signs of hunger, thirst, restlessness, or discomfort.

Capitalize on the time spent helping patients to meet their basic needs by teaching content and skills related to their care. Teach the patient and family members about medication while administering it and then ask them to repeat the information. Talk through the procedure while changing a patient's dressing and ask him or her to direct it the next time it is changed. Discuss the function of insulin with the patient at the time he or she administers it or discuss insulin reactions with the patient after he or she experiences a reaction.

Emotional Needs

Many patients perceive a mystique surrounding the roles of physicians and nurses. Especially in times of illness or change, patients often want to be cared for or to find someone who will perform "magical" acts to restore a previous state of health, erase pain, or remove conflict. Health care personnel have frequently perpetuated this desire by encouraging dependence or by not taking the time to encourage patient learning and partici-

pation in medical management. Patients may hesitate to participate later, feeling incapable of learning the proper skills or of managing aspects of their own care. They may worry that if they become more independent, they may be deprived of necessary help and unable to meet their own needs.

Acknowledge each patient's support needs and anxiety about learning new health behaviors. Patients should know that they would receive necessary help and teaching until new skills are mastered and that medical personnel will support them. Patients may be afraid to disclose their lack of knowledge or to make mistakes. The nurse should structure learning to proceed from simple to complex, so that the patient will feel successful, and provide support and advice as the patient tries out newly learned behaviors. In times of crisis or stress, the patient may need greater support and may test the nurse's willingness to help.

In the current climate of short hospital stays, patients and families frequently feel illprepared for discharge. Some report that they were given "too little information, too late"; whereas some report that they were given "too much information, too soon," causing them to be overwhelmed, insecure, and unable to manage. The key to successful patient education is to focus on three or four critical learning objectives and to teach survival skills. In addition, all patients should know how to recognize problems and how to reach help after their hospital discharge.

The following are two examples that illustrate emotional needs in patient education:

CASE STUDY

PATIENT 1: MR. BENTON

Mr. Benton is a 53-year-old man who has had insulin-dependent diabetes for 6 years. He makes frequent visits to the clinic with

(case study continues on page 262)

various minor complaints and leaves the clinic much improved after each visit. He lives alone and depends on the clinic staff for support. He calls the nurse station almost daily, occasionally stating, "I just can't seem to get going, give myself my insulin, and get to work." Through the teaching and review, the staff members knew he had mastered the necessary skills to do so. The clinic's social worker is called to help Mr. Benton get involved in the local chapter of the American Diabetes Association, thus increasing his support system. In addition, the clinic's nurses schedule regular, monthly, 30-minute visits, during which they support Mr. Benton and occasionally ask him to share his expertise in insulin injection with patients who had newly diagnosed diabetes.

PATIENT 2: MRS. HESTER

Mrs. Hester receives prenatal care at the clinic and looks forward to breast-feeding her baby. She reads books on infant care and attends prenatal classes. Although the classes stressed the importance of being flexible in planning labor and delivery, Mrs. Hester plans to have a vaginal delivery. A breech presentation, however, necessitates cesarean section. Mrs. Hester successfully nurses her baby in the hospital and has good support and teaching from the hospital staff.

Two days after discharge, Mrs. Hester calls the clinic's nurse. She cries, stating that she feels like a failure because the baby "will not take her milk." After supporting her on the telephone, the nurse suggests that Mrs. Hester come to the clinic and feed her baby in the examination room where the nurse can offer assistance. Mrs. Hester happily agrees. When she arrives, the nurse realizes that Mrs. Hester's anxiety and fatigue were causing her difficulty with nursing. Together they review the progressive muscle relaxation exercises done in prenatal classes. Mrs. Hester then relaxes before nursing the baby, and the baby nurses successfully. The nurse compliments Mrs. Hester on how well she cares for the baby. She points out

signs of effective nursing, such as the jaw movement back to the baby's ears with sucking, audible sucking, and the number of wet diapers the mother reported changing in the last day (Burton, 1999).

The nurse weighs the baby so the patient can verify that the baby is gaining weight. The nurse also offers additional visits of this nature if needed. She also reminds Mrs. Hester to nap when the baby naps and to drink plenty of fluids. The patient agrees to call the nurse the next day and let her know how the breast-feeding is progressing. When she did, the report was a positive one. Mrs. Hester remarks, "It is just so good to know I can call you if I need help."

Problem-Centered Learning

Learning activities should be centered on potential problems that the patient may face (eg, asthma episode, hypoglycemic reaction). The teacher will want to assist the learner in recognizing the problem, knowing what to do, and feeling competent in performing the necessary behavior. Patients should describe their diagnosis or health problem and how their symptoms relate to it.

Patient education should help the patient who experiences an acute episode to answer the following questions: *Why am I here at this time? What could I have done to prevent it?* Patients often bring problems or concerns with them to the learning session. Breast-feeding problems are a good example. Similarly, expectant parents may express the following concerns:

- How can I deal with the pain of labor?
- How will I know if the baby is sick?
- What do I do if the baby does not stop crying?

Preoperative patients also want information:

- What will it be like in surgery?
- What will they do to me?
- Will I be in pain?
- What will it be like when I wake up?

Patients with diabetes and their family members also often have questions:

- Why are insulin shots needed?
- How difficult will it be to give myself shots?
- What is an insulin reaction?

Some patients mention their problems and concerns freely, whereas others hesitate to do so. Occasionally, patients with newly diagnosed problems do not know what to ask. The nurse should encourage the patient to verbalize concerns and then address these concerns in learning activities. If the patient and the family need help describing concerns, teachers may begin, for example, by saying: "Patients who are pregnant often have questions about labor and delivery and want to know what to expect. I wonder if you might have concerns about that?"

Application of Learning

Learning activities provide opportunities for the application of learning. Although teaching may include lecture and discussion, it should also pose problems and give the learner a chance to react to them. Application takes place as soon as possible. Simulated situations (eg, a mock labor and delivery used in prenatal classes) may be used.

Participative Learning

Participation must be encouraged at the onset of learning activities, so that patients build confidence. Some patients are more comfortable than others in voicing concerns and attempting new skills; others are reluctant and anxious and may need special attention. With adequate support and realistic learning goals, participation can be gained from even the most reluctant learner.

 Nurses [cannot] evaluate patient learning if the patient has not participated and application of learning has not been observed. This problem may arise if there is not enough time for teaching and learning; if learning activities are restricted to lecture and demonstration; if learning is assumed to be accomplished by media alone; if the nurse is not comfortable with the teaching role; or if the nurse does not like to teach. These problems are alleviated by careful selection of learning activities and preparation of staff members who will serve as teachers. Alternating instruction with return demonstration is also an effective strategy; this approach allows the patient to see incremental learning, receive immediate feedback, and learn through repetition. ■

The Teacher-Learner Relationship

Learning is a shared experience, requiring openness from both the teacher and the learner. The nurse must be willing to establish a relationship with the individual learner. The nurse must be dependable, must encourage the learner until goals are met, must be flexible enough to negotiate, and must provide support and reinforcement. The nurse commits herself in an agreement—a learning contract (see Chapter 9)—whether verbal or written. The nurse must be willing to admit when she does not have an answer and be eager to seek additional information.

As in all therapeutic relationships, the teacher-learner relationship takes time to develop. By giving the patient an opportunity to tell his or her story, the nurse and patient become acquainted. Assessment and problem identification begins. The learner begins a testing phase, in which he or she considers the willingness and ability of the nurse to understand his or her needs, to help and support him or her, and to commit to mutual goals. Eventually, the teacher and learner establish a working relationship and engage in activities together. The teacher provides experiences through which the learner tries new behaviors (Kreigh & Perko, 1979). The teacher must instill in the patient the confidence that he or she can learn to participate in his or her health care and perform survival skills. To do this, the teacher uses repetition, focuses on few priorities, and helps the patient relate teaching to everyday life. The teacher respects the patient's cultural and religious beliefs and acknowledges the patient's right to choose.

Styles of Learners

Patients approach learning in various ways determined by individual lifestyle, personality, and past experience. The patient educator should identify characteristics of the learner's style to help plan teaching interventions. Some patients may read extensively about the health problem and may vocalize many questions; others may want to know only the basic facts. Some patients are comfortable in classroom lectures and others are not. Some patients may be enthusiastic to return demonstrate a procedure taught by the nurse, whereas others may hesitate and ask the nurse to review the procedure several times. Some patients may freely discuss difficulty and confusion, but others may deny problems unless they know they are observed. Some patients may play the informed expert and offer the nurse a challenge during a learning needs assessment; other patients may hold back what they know, wishing to be taken care of rather than to assume responsibility in health management. Patients also learn at different rates, depending on age, intelligence, motor skills, degree of impairment, anxiety, and past experience. Each teaching and learning activity must be adapted to the style and need of the learner.

Styles of Teachers

Nurses who teach have particular teaching styles. Some teachers are comfortable with an expert role in telling or showing; others encourage constant involvement from the patient in a give-and-take fashion. Some teachers may have difficulty dealing with the patient who sees himself or herself as an expert; others may feel comfortable allowing the patient to direct the teaching while they clarify, correct, and supplement knowledge. These same nurses may have problems working with a passive, dependent, or depressed patient.

In patient education, the nurse must be flexible because he or she must respond to the style of the learner despite having a preferred style of teaching. For example, a nurse with high control needs as a teacher may compete with the expert patient, in which case the

learning experience will become frustrating and unproductive. A passive, dependent patient, however, will also learn little if only taught according to the needs he or she verbalizes. For these reasons, a nurse who teaches patients should consider his or her own teaching style and may require training to overcome difficulties adapting to particular learning styles. In addition, the compatibility of the teacher with the learner is an important consideration when selecting patient teaching staff.

For example, we are familiar with a case in which a controlling nurse was assigned to teach tracheostomy suctioning to a patient who had a radical neck dissection and glossectomy. The patient attempted to control his environment in response to his multiple losses and refused to accept any teaching from the nurse who communicated little empathy. His discharge from the hospital was delayed until a new nurse, who understood his attempts to exert control, was assigned as his primary nurse.

Preparing Staff for Teaching

Provide a planned, consistent approach in patient education, while simultaneously avoiding unnecessary repetition and confusing presentation of material. The nurse should not overload the patient and family but must include ample opportunity for review and practice. In addition, the contributions of other members of the health care team (eg, physical therapists, dietitians, and pharmacists) must be considered as part of the teaching plan. Collectively, teaching to the patient by all of these professionals can be overwhelming. Thus, in a short hospital stay, patient education may be more effective if carried out by one or two professionals who are responsible for the entire teaching plan.

In the midst of other patient care planning, few of us are afforded the luxury of time needed to construct such approaches. However, the authors have discovered that teaching protocols may be established in cooperation with other members of the team and then adapted to patient situations. The protocols are targeted toward specific patient groups as part of case management (Lindberg, Hunter, & Kruszewski, 1994). Provider responsibilities are outlined, and staff members are trained in the use of the care map and teaching activities. This type of planned team approach saves time, alleviates confusion, and directs the selection of staff.

Responses to the following questions will also aid in selecting staff members best suited to carry out patient education interventions:

- Does the staff member have ample opportunity to interact with the patient and family?
- Does the staff member understand the goals, objectives, and learning style of the patient?
- Does each staff member understand his or her role and the other providers' roles?
- Does the staff member have adequate preparation and knowledge to perform patient teaching?
- Who will coordinate the teaching plan?

Remember, interdisciplinary care planning does not require that every member of every discipline teach every patient. The team should plan and focus on the overall key learning needs of the patient, based on the prognosis, and distill this into one set of discharge instructions.

Staff development efforts should support staff involvement in patient teaching, eliminating barriers perceived by nurses, such as inadequate knowledge of the content to be taught or lack of preparation to carry out teaching activities (Marchiondo & Kipp, 1987). Suggestions are offered in Chapter 5.

STRATEGIC USE OF INSTRUCTIONAL METHODS

Chapter 9 reviewed three types of learning behavior: cognitive learning (knowledge and information), affective learning (attitudes and values), and psychomotor learning (skills and performance). Learning in each of these three areas contributes to behavior change (Mager, 1997).

For example, for educating a patient with newly diagnosed diabetes, the following behaviors are desirable:

1. **Cognitive learning.** The patient can describe what diabetes is and name three things a patient with diabetes should do to manage his or her care. The patient can state that insulin reactions may be caused by the wrong amount or kind of medication, late or omitted meals or snacks, failure to follow diet plan, and increased activity.
2. **Affective learning.** The patient can discuss why it is important for him or her, the family, the physician, and other health care professionals to work together in medical management. The patient can state why he or she should tell friends and coworkers that he or she has diabetes, explain to them the signs and symptoms of insulin reactions, and tell them how to help if reactions occur.
3. **Psychomotor learning.** The patient can make food choices to plan one breakfast, one lunch, and one dinner within guidelines of an ADA meal plan. The patient can demonstrate proper technique for daily washing and checking of feet.

Learning objectives must be categorized into these three areas to prepare for the selection of teaching and learning formats, methods, and media best suited to patient education needs. The teacher considers whether learning can be accomplished in a large group or whether it is better suited to an individual teaching situation. In many cases, a combination of formats can be used to provide learning experiences, add variety, and meet different types of objectives.

Individual Teaching

Often called one-on-one teaching, individual instruction is ideal for continued assessment of the learner (and family) and technical skill training (eg, urine testing, insulin injection, self-catheterization). Individual teaching promotes sharing of confidential information and problems, tailoring of teaching plans, and learning by persons with a low literacy level, physical impairment, cultural barriers, anxiety, or depression. Individual teaching is often used as an initial intervention, through which basic knowledge and skills are achieved and the patient's confidence in self-care is increased. Advantages of this format include an active learner role that builds motivation, an opportunity for consistent and frequent feedback, and flexibility to create an unstructured, informal atmosphere.

Teachable moments can be capitalized on with one-on-one learning. The teacher can respond to the learner's problems and needs in a timely fashion, helping the learner to build problem-solving skills. Preoperative teaching, initial diabetic teaching, and diet teaching are often performed using the individual format. The obvious disadvantages of individual teaching are a lack of sharing with and support from other patients and their families and the high cost of staff time for instruction. However, especially in ambulatory settings, one-on-one teaching is often most productive because it is intensive, highly individualized, can occur spontaneously during every patient encounter, is culturally sensitive, and provides repetition and review.

Telephone calls initiated by the patient, a family member, or a nurse are used for patient education. Nurse advice lines provide answers to questions, reassurance, clarification, and assistance. They provide a safety net for follow-up after discharge from the hospital. Telephones can be used to accomplish individual preoperative assessment and teaching and are invaluable for reaching learners who live in rural communities or who are homebound. Telephone teaching is also effective for many learners with low literacy skills (London, 1999).

Group Teaching

There are three distinct advantages to group learning: it is economical, it helps patients learn from one another and teach one another through their own experiences, and it fosters positive attitude development. Although group members may have slightly different learning goals, a needs assessment can be done in patient advisory or focus groups or at the time of group teaching by asking patients what they want to learn. Teaching content can be tailored to meet learner objectives.

Small groups (ie, 2 patients to 5 patients) may offer some of the advantages of individual teaching. Nurses in psychiatric acute care settings find small groups an effective format for medication teaching, activities of daily living teaching, and discussion about post-discharge concerns. Small group teaching of older outpatients provides helpful approaches to managing functional problems and strategies for health promotion.

Medium-sized groups (ie, 6 patients to 30 patients) may be used effectively for prenatal care, pediatric care, stress reduction, safety, diabetes review, or self help and support groups. Large groups (ie, 30 patients or more) are appropriate for lectures and videos but should be interspersed with small group experiences or discussion. A medium or large group format is generally unacceptable for skill training and reduces patient-teacher feedback. It is difficult in these groups to evaluate whether individual learning goals have been met. Patients who are physiologically or emotionally unstable are poor candidates for group teaching. The group teacher must be aware of the patient characteristics and must have a flexible approach. The group format is ideal for teaching patients and their families together.

Self help groups are gaining the recognition of professionals and patients. They offer mutual assistance to patients with common health-related learning needs. The groups are often led by patients and may be sponsored by community agencies or health care organizations. Lay persons who recognize the need for mutual support in dealing with prevention, management, and adaptation to chronic illnesses begin some self help groups on the grass-roots level. Some physicians are uncooperative or indifferent toward the self help movement, demonstrating reluctance or refusal to refer patients to such groups. However, as health care costs rise and hospitals face greater barriers to providing free services, health care professionals, especially physicians and nurses, are reconsidering their attitudes toward self help groups. They recognize that many active self help support groups play an important role in educating patients and their families and that they encourage appropriate use of health care services. Because of public interest and demand, most hospitals now sponsor various self help groups open to the community. The authors have found that nurses are generally more aware than physicians of community groups and that nurses tend to make more referrals to them. Chapter 11 offers information about online self help groups.

Combining Individual and Group Formats

In health care delivery systems, the management of patient education encompasses both individual and group teaching. There has been a recent focus on institutional leadership and management of patient education programs. Although teaching plans have continued to develop and patient education is incorporated into critical paths and care maps that guide the sequence and timing of patient progress in many agencies, these structures are not in place to support the delivery of patient education in all settings (Redman, 1993).

Care Maps

More hospitals and health care agencies have developed systematic patient care maps for educating patients with specific diseases or problems. These care maps use individual and group teaching interventions, including self-directed learning. Patients and their families are taught through use of a standard outline, including basic information components that are tailored to the individual situation. (Some items may be deleted, and others may be expanded to address the patient's personal barriers to behavioral change.) Care maps generally include teaching about pathophysiology, treat-

ments, medications, diet, diagnostic tests, procedures, recommended activity, and self care skills. With care maps, hospitals can tailor patient instruction to the specific procedures relevant to the patient's experience in that institution or facility. Patient learning outcomes are tied to each phase of the patient's course, based on an estimated length of stay, thus improving efficiency, quality, and potentially decreasing inpatient days. Staff members are trained through classes and tutors to use the teaching formats and strategies. The roles of various providers are outlined according to subject matter and areas of expertise. Specific provider responsibilities are described with respect to the teaching and learning process. Although nurses often perform the initial assessment, many providers intervene, evaluate, and document teaching and learning.

Teaching materials should be selected based on the patient's interests, abilities, and cultural background. The time required for teaching segments of the content is estimated, and resources are suggested to help patients meet the learning goals. Content, teaching strategies, and activities suitable to meet the goals are preselected and defined by a planning committee when the care map is established. A combined format of individual and group teaching and referral to community resources for support after discharge may be involved. Teaching aids, such as audiovisuals and printed matter, may be purchased or developed by the health care institution to enhance patient teaching. In addition, the care map specifies what types of information should be documented in the medical record and where it will be located. Measures for evaluation of patient learning are specified. (See Chapter 13 for more information about patient care maps.)

We believe that care maps should blend the use of different formats in systematic patient learning experiences. However, we caution that all teaching plans must be individualized to meet patient needs and that an assessment of readiness and barriers to learning is an essential preliminary step in any patient education approach.

STRATEGIC USE OF LEARNING ACTIVITIES

Whether the format for teaching is individual or group, the principle of patient inclusion applies. At the outset, the teacher should introduce each patient to the three or four critical skills he or she needs to learn. By providing this big picture or bottom line, as some patients describe it, the patient acknowledges the need to participate actively in the process of patient education.

Knowing how to use various learning activities to meet educational objectives can make patient education more interesting, challenging, and effective for both the teacher and the learner. The patient educator will want to choose learning activities thoughtfully, so that they will be suitable for particular patient objectives. Box 10-1 offers a guide for selecting activities conducive to cognitive, affective, and psychomotor changes. Some learning activities are appropriate for more than one type of learning objective. Brief descriptions of the major types of learning activities are offered with suggestions for effective and appropriate application.

Self-Directed Learning

Computer-assisted instruction (CAI) and self-directed learning workbooks have become popular resources for patient education. The use of the Internet for patient education is also increasing in popularity (see Chapter 11). A growing trend in health care settings is the creation of patient and family education resource centers—small libraries containing books, videotapes, and pamphlets that discuss health and illness topics (Patient Education Management, July 1999). For example, a hospital-based Cancer Resource Center serves patients and families by providing answers to questions about cancer, information about support groups, and tips on coping with cancer treatment. When patients are first diagnosed with cancer, they usually have numerous questions about the illness, treatment, and prognosis. They are concerned about their insur-

---

BOX 10-1. Selecting Learning Activities for Patient Education

I. Cognitive (Knowledge)
Learning Facts
Lecture
Demonstration
Independent study format
Tests
Discussion—Questions and Answers
Practice
Simulation
Visual Identification
Demonstration
Simulation
Tests
Practice
Independent study
Understanding and Applying Knowledge
Demonstration
Practice
Role-play
Discussion—Questions and Answers
Independent study
Simulation
Tests

II. Affective (Attitudes and Appreciations)
Discussion—questions and answers
Role Play
Simulation

III. Psychomotor (Skills and Performance)
Practice
Role Play
Simulation
Demonstration
Tests
Independent study

---

ance, how surgery or treatment will affect them, and how to talk to their children about the disease. But most important, they want to know that as their questions continue they will have somewhere to turn for answers.

A resource center offers assistance based on

the patient's expressed needs and information about support groups in which experienced facilitators can help patients learn about treatment options, nutrition, coping with cancer, survivorship, and insurance. It even offers a program that pairs newly diagnosed patients with other patients who have the same diagnosis. These resource centers are responsive when patients are ready to learn, and they bridge the gaps often experienced by patients as they receive care in multiple settings from multiple providers. Resource centers are viewed as especially valuable by patients and families who cope with chronic health problems.

Lecture

Lecture is the method most often used by nurses who instruct or transmit information to patients. It is an effective method of teaching cognitive behaviors and is more efficacious when used with discussion. Lecture is enhanced by use of handouts, pictures, and visual aids (eg, overheads and slides) that promote identification. Material presented in a lecture should be prepared according to the patient's level of understanding, and patients should have an opportunity to ask questions. Lengthy lectures may cause loss of attention; patients become bored, distracted, or anxious about the material presented. Patients may be eager to contribute or to try out or apply knowledge; this eagerness may be stifled by a formal lecture approach in which the teacher is the expert. Long lectures may also create the impression that the patient's problem is so complicated that he or she cannot manage it.

It is important to remember that lectures can be highly effective for influencing cognitive behaviors but will not be effective in achieving affective or psychomotor learning objectives. For example, a lecture is often used to give initial knowledge about pathophysiology to patients with diabetes but is ineffective when used alone to teach insulin injection. Lectures may be given in person, televised, or audiotaped. In individual teaching, the amount of total teaching time should include a minimum of lecture and should focus on building survival skills needed to ensure patient safety after discharge.

Group Discussion

Discussion requires two or more people to exchange ideas. It differs from lecture in that it is an excellent method of involving patients in the learning process. This learning activity promotes understanding and application of knowledge (cognitive behaviors) and development of certain attitudes (affective behaviors). The teacher, who asks specific questions or proposes problem situations, frequently directs it. Discussion facilitates learning from the experience of others, fosters a feeling of belongingness, and reinforces previous learning.

Demonstration

Demonstration is useful for cognitive and psychomotor learning. It is most often used to teach skills and to present performance standards. Demonstration may be done in person or in videotaped programs. The sense of sight is used in learning from demonstration, but hearing, smell, and taste may also be stimulated. Demonstration should be performed slowly, and the teacher should be certain that the learner can see and hear well. This strategy shows the learner that the behavior is possible and increases confidence that he or she can perform it. For example, when teaching insulin injection, the nurse may demonstrate injection using sterile water before the patient actually performs an insulin injection. When demonstration is used to teach discharge skills, the actual type of equipment or supplies to be used at home should be used for teaching. Repetition and return demonstration are needed for teaching procedures with multiple steps.

Role-Play and Return Demonstration

Both role-play and return demonstration involve doing or practicing. These activities help the patient apply knowledge or skills, usually after demonstration. When used appropriately, role-play and return demonstration tailor the learning to the patient's past or present life experiences, and the teacher offers guidance and feedback.

In role-play, the learner acts out his own situation or that of another person. This is highly effective in meeting affective objectives. Return demonstration follows exhibition of a skill by the teacher; the patient performs the skill one or more times. In both cases, clear instruction must be given to the learner about what to do and how to do it. Enough practice time should be allowed for the learner to repeat the exercise until he or she has mastered it. Role-play and return demonstration are effective strategies for teaching cognitive, affective, and psychomotor behaviors. Role-playing helps patients learn to recognize and handle problem situations, such as a hypoglycemic reaction or a cardiac arrest, with which they have no first-hand experience.

For patients with complications or readmission, return demonstration can be used to assess skill deficits that may contribute to exacerbations of a chronic condition. For example, nurses in one rural community hospital assessed through return demonstration that there was a high readmission rate for patients with chronic obstructive pulmonary disease who were previously discharged with metered-dose inhalers. Although the patients were taught during hospitalization, the return demonstration identified improper technique using inhalers that prevented patients from getting the prescribed doses of medication at home. Priority in patient teaching was placed on practice and coaching to develop proper technique for using inhalers.

Tests

Tests may be valuable learning experiences, because they indicate current knowledge level and what the patient needs to learn or master. Tests are helpful when used to guide patients and give feedback. They are effective in meeting cognitive and psychomotor objectives, but are obviously inappropriate for affective learning because attitudes and values are not measured with a right-versus-wrong approach.

Patients may become anxious about test-

ing. The nurse should introduce tests positively in patient education and should use the results to reinforce progress toward the learning goal. Tests may use a written, oral, or skill format. They may be used in assessment to determine the patient's initial level of understanding or skill and in evaluation after the lecture or demonstration.

Programmed Instruction

Patients can learn by independent study or by using specially prepared workbooks, textbooks, audiotape, and computer programs. Many commercially prepared programs are available; however, teachers may choose to prepare their own. Programmed self-study units allow learners to work at their own pace for mastering cognitive and psychomotor behaviors. Frequent testing and review are offered during instruction. Knowledge about chronic illness and management, preventive health topics, and diet teaching are commonly offered in programmed instruction packets. The teacher should be aware of the level of motivation or readiness of the learners, their literacy levels, and visual and hearing abilities; these factors are crucial in evaluating the appropriateness of such programs for individual clients. When programmed instruction is used, it must be suited to patient needs and situations. The nurse should set the stage by introducing the three or four critical things the patient needs to learn, and then follow-up teaching with review to ensure that the patient has achieved those outcomes. Patient readiness, physical ability, intellectual and language ability, and patient interest should be considered before programmed instruction is selected for discharge teaching.

STRATEGIC USE OF EDUCATIONAL MEDIA

Media (eg, videotapes, audiotapes, computer programs) are usually used to enhance the previously mentioned learning activities. Media should not be used in place of the teacher but can effectively promote all three types of learning when used in combination with other strategies. A health care professional should be available to discuss, demonstrate, and clarify concepts introduced by media. This role should not be neglected or left to untrained lay volunteers. Media should be carefully selected and should be consistent with instructional objectives.

General Guidelines for Media Use: Prepare, Present, Review

Having cautioned our readers that media should not be used carelessly in patient education, one may ask: What then is the advantage in using media?

Media help to deliver a message. Various media can be used creatively to help patients learn more, to help them retain better what they have learned, and to encourage the development of skills. Nurses seldom have formal training in media selection and application, and they consequently look for guidance in these areas. To avoid some of the common pitfalls of inappropriate or unsuccessful use of media, the teacher should faithfully follow three steps: preparation, presentation, and review.

To prepare, it is necessary to preview the media to be used. A plan for using a medium is constructed, including how it will be introduced, followed-up, and related to other learning experiences. The environment also must be prepared. This includes obtaining physical facilities and equipment needed to display the medium. The learner must be informed of what to expect from the medium, (ie, significant points or upcoming discussion). Presentation of media requires care, so that projection and materials are clear, sound is adjusted, and, in general, the message can be received. Review involves follow-up of the learning experience and evaluation of whether learning objectives were met. Box 10-2 details several generalized principles that can be applied to all types of media.

Posters, Displays, Flipcharts, and Bulletin Boards

Visual displays using drawings and illustrations do not have to be works of art to deliver a

---

BOX 10-2. General Principles for Using Instructional Media

1. **No one medium is best suited to all purposes.** For example, in some cases, visual identification is best accomplished with a picture, cartoon, or slide; in others, three-dimensional images, such as films or videotapes, are most effective.
2. **The application of media should be consistent with learning objectives.** Just as learning activities promote certain types of behaviors, media are also chosen to coincide with objectives.
3. **The teacher must be familiar with the content of the media.** A common mistake made by nurses is to use materials that are inappropriate in message, presentation, or educational level. Media must be previewed and evaluated.
4. **Media must be compatible with learning formats.** Videotapes may be used in a large group (provided that they can be projected adequately), but audiocassettes should not.
5. **Media must be selected with the capabilities and learning styles of the audience in mind.** Printed booklets with few illustrations are poorly suited to the patient who cannot read or who dislikes reading, and the message will fail to reach him or her.
6. **Physical conditions influence the effectiveness of media.** Improper acoustics, lighting, seating, distractions, and room temperature may interfere with the delivery of the message.

---

message. They should be aesthetically appealing, using contrasting colors and large lettering. Posters, displays, flipcharts, and bulletin boards are inexpensive, require little time to prepare, and attract interest. They clarify information, simplify concepts, and summarize teaching. Contributions from participants can be written on flipcharts or chalkboards during a teaching session. Bulletin boards in waiting rooms or hospital corridors can spark curiosity about health care issues and problems.

Use of these types of media is inappropriate in large groups unless the displays are enlarged. They are not well suited to teaching in which movement needs to be demonstrated.

Graphics

Graphics include graphs, charts, diagrams, cartoons, and maps. They can show proportions and relationships that are difficult to understand when presented only by spoken or written material. They emphasize the most important points of a presentation. Drawings and cartoons can deliver a message to patients with limited reading and vocabulary levels and to children. For example, picture pages are often used to teach insulin injection techniques to newly diagnosed patients with diabetes. Cartoons can make learning fun and present thoughts in a humorous but effective fashion (London, 1999). Graphics highlight sequence and also convey general information and key concepts. Some of the main advantages of using graphics for patient education are their abilities to attract attention and to deliver information economically.

Overhead Projection and Slides

Overhead transparencies and slides are popular for teaching both large and small groups. They require a projector and a screen or white wall. They encourage verbal and visual creativity and allow the teacher to control the materials shown and their timing. They can present ideas in a colorful sequence and help the learner focus on thoughts and ideas. Overhead transparencies are easy to make and can be prepared ahead of time in a copy machine or a computer printer. Computer generated slides (such as PowerPoint™) can also be generated and edited quickly. Each overhead or slide should present one idea or topic and should have a limited word count. Overheads can be used in a well lit room as long as there

is dimmed light near the screen; this makes overheads more desirable than slides for keeping learners awake and attentive. Two cautions are offered: First, print should be large and details kept to a minimum. Second, the teacher must be careful not to use overhead transparencies or slides as a temptation to present too much material. A few overheads or slides used to bring out the main points and provide review of what patients need to remember will be most helpful.

Photographs and Drawings

Patients enjoy pictures and learn from them. Visual images promote understanding of facts and ideas by helping the learner to imagine real situations and reflect on past experiences. Still pictures may be presented in printed matter, on slides, or on videos. They may encourage discussion when the learner is asked to describe what he or she sees.

Pictures can attract and maintain the patient's interest. They also help the patient to remember what has been said. Generally, color pictures appeal to learners more than do black and white pictures. The color should be accurate and portray a realistic image. Images should be relevant to the learners, reflecting a familiar environment, similar age of patients, various gender and cultural backgrounds, and familiar geographic locations.

Slide-tape or slide-voice programs include a recorded message that explains the picture and adds content. A synchronized program of still pictures and speech can be made available as a Web-based computer program or more inexpensively with a cassette tape player and a slide projector. These programs may be ideal for self instruction and for group teaching. They are produced commercially or by the teacher and are suited to teaching patients with low literacy skills if the text is concise, simple, and clear with vocabulary restricted to one- and two-syllable words.

Audio Materials

Audiotapes, usually cassette tapes, offer a distinct advantage for some patient teaching occasions. They are small and easy to transport, and they require only an inexpensive recorder for use. They are available on various topics, are economical, and can be used almost anywhere. Audiotapes can be made by the teacher and tailored to the individual situation to reinforce facts, directions, and support. Patients may use them in the home, car, office, hospital, or clinic. Study kits with printed text or pictures are available to accompany the audio component.

Audio materials help deliver a message to patients who enjoy radio and who benefit from repetition and reinforcement. Relaxation and stress reduction exercises also are well suited to delivery by audiotape. For patients who have retinopathies secondary to diabetes, patients with low literacy skills, and patients who do not speak the English language, audiocassettes may be the only practical media. Doak, Doak, and Root (1995) offer detailed instructions on preparing an audiotape.

Videotapes and Closed Circuit Television (CCTV)

Television's popularity and pervasive use among American households promotes learning in many spheres and influences knowledge, attitudes, and skills. It is entertaining and educational. Videotapes present experiences, places, and situations that can recreate life situations, thus encouraging patients to explore attitudes and understandings. Videotaped programs also teach basic facts and how to handle problems. They may be effective for patients with limited reading abilities.

The use of television and videotaped recordings has become an attractive teaching and learning activity in the school, office, and health care setting. Many groups have made significant investments for the purchase of programs (software) and equipment (hardware). Videocassette recorders (VCRs) are now used in all types of health care settings and in patients' homes. Consider how suitable this medium is for specific learning objectives and understand how television is best incorporated into patient education.

Television is best used when the program is carefully selected, introduced, and followed-up as part of patient teaching. It should not be expected to replace the teacher. Hospitals with cable distribution systems may wish to concentrate on video programs because they can be broadcast throughout the hospital and reach more people (Patient Education Management, July 1999). Videotapes may be purchased commercially or prepared by audiovisual departments and teachers.

Videotapes are often a good basis for discussion. They must, however, be carefully previewed and selected. The teacher will want to evaluate the film with consideration of the patient group's actual life situations, levels of understanding and literacy, and learning needs. Films 15 minutes to 20 minutes in length are ideal for most situations; those longer than 30 minutes are difficult for many patients to view. Discussion time should be planned and the presentation should be reinforced. The videotape should be suited to learning objectives, and key points should be covered. The teacher may wish to use a handout that highlights these points so the patient can follow them as the videotape progresses.

Remember that skills must be taught with active learner involvement in return demonstrations. A videotape cannot provide this. Because patient teaching efforts focus on survival skills, videotapes must be carefully balanced with other formats to avoid overloading the patient with information. Making and duplicating your own videos has become a common strategy to combat the pressures of early discharge by supplementing teaching in the patient's home. Sending a video home with the patient may be one of the best applications for this medium because it can continue coaching, provide for continued affective learning, and prevent feelings of isolation (Engelke, 1999). Also, many situations that patients are instructed to handle may not be experienced until the patient goes home. For example, baby care and feeding are often learned best after discharge with the help of a video, provided the patient has a VCR and an interest in using it. Many hospitals also use videotapes for preadmission teaching and preoperative teaching. A video may offer self-care instructions by health professionals and realistic accounts by patients with the same diagnosis. These videotapes may demonstrate self-care, outline warning signs that necessitate physician contact, and answer commonly asked questions. Patients and family members can review a demonstration of self-care procedures as often as needed.

The use of patient education videos has been associated with increased patient satisfaction; increased physician satisfaction; assistance with meeting the requirements of the Joint Commission on the Accreditation of Healthcare Organizations; reduced risk of malpractice, negligent discharge, and inappropriate readmissions; and enhanced community image and cost savings.

Electronic Media

Computer-assisted instruction is now common in hospitals, physician offices, and homes. Many software programs are available to help patients learn how to adopt healthier lifestyles and manage health problems. There are six types of CAI: drill and practice, tutorials, problem-solving, simulation, gaming, and testing. Printed material (eg, workbooks, slides) frequently accompany CAI.

Drill and practice lessons help patients learn or review facts and offer question-and-answer formats to assess understanding. Tutorials use branching options to individualize lessons to the knowledge and needs of the patient. Problem solving, simulations, and gaming help patients gather information and make decisions in hypothetical situations. Testing can be done with CAI as part of tutorials, simulations, and practice to assess knowledge and attitudes, and feedback can also be provided.

A skilled designer can develop software for CAI programs, but it is also readily available commercially. It should be compatible with hardware and evaluated based on each program's instructional objectives and how well the objectives can be met by the CAI lesson. Just as with other media, electronic media lessons should be previewed and evaluated, giving consideration to patient needs, the pa-

tient's actual life situations, level of understanding, and literacy. The nurse should review key points. Patients vary in comfort and experience with computers, and some may be anxious about or disinterested in CAI. Other patients, especially teenagers and young adults, may be reached effectively with CAI lessons on topics such as pregnancy prevention, birth control, drug abuse prevention, and wellness.

In the next decade, experts expect computers will be used much more creatively for patient education. Computer programs can already help patients with diabetes to adjust insulin dosages and plan meals, track data about glucose levels, offer self-paced instruction about knowledge of diabetes, and offer nutritional analysis of foods. Home computers and videos provide increasing opportunities for providers to observe and instruct patients at home and to link home and provider information systems (Redman, 1993).

Objects, Models, and Demonstrations

Having actual objects available during patient teaching helps the learner to become actively involved and to apply knowledge and skills immediately. The patient may observe, handle, manipulate, display, discuss, assemble, and disassemble objects while the teacher provides feedback. For example, breast models are often used to teach patients to examine their breasts. The teacher usually demonstrates the use of the objects or models, and the patient repeats the performance. Some models, such as the resuscitation manikin used to teach cardiopulmonary resuscitation (CPR), are expensive. Pharmaceutical companies may supply others, such as the plastic female pelvic area, free of charge. Through creative experimentation, many nurses find that they can make their own models for teaching various skills. One nurse, who was unable to purchase an expensive breast model, made her own from a nylon stocking stuffed with cotton socks. She simulated a breast mass in another stocking by adding Styrofoam particles and used the two models to teach breast self-examination.

Displays can be used to encourage patient participation. For example, teaching about infant safety becomes more effective when it is accompanied by a display of actual infant car seats. In one-on-one encounters, demonstration and return demonstration can often be performed by the patient without the use of models. Examples of this are blood glucose monitoring, breast examinations performed in the privacy of the patient's room, dressing changes, and baby bathing. Furthermore, these teaching and learning opportunities can occur even if funding for teaching aids is lacking.

Community Resources

Health departments and agencies, businesses, and professional groups (eg, fire and police departments) offer learning experiences for patients. Valuable support and information can be gained through such resources as groups with diabetes, ostomy clubs, hospital health nights, bicycle safety programs, and community infant car seat programs. For example, adolescents who cope with chronic illnesses gain opportunities to share their feelings with other adolescents who have similar conditions and who can promote independence and decision-making through their involvement with support groups (Muscari, 1998).

The patient educator can benefit from knowledge of and referrals to teaching programs that offer skills training. In one outpatient clinic, the staff saw many patients and their families in the rehabilitation phase after myocardial infarction. The authors wanted to give family members CPR training but were unable to do so because there was not enough staff to offer the teaching or the finances to purchase equipment. Many of the family members were unable to pay registration fees for CPR classes at local schools. The authors discovered that a local fire department offered CPR classes free of charge, and the patients were referred to them.

Games and Simulations

Games can be used to involve the patient in teaching and learning. Instructional games can introduce information and offer practice in simulated situations. They are often used with pediatric patients for preoperative parties that introduce them to hospital procedures, environment, and staff before elective surgery. One of the advantages of using games as learning experiences is that actual situations can be viewed in less time. During a game, the patient can take a course of action and view the consequences in a nonthreatening way. Problem solving can be incorporated into the game.

Commercially prepared games should be evaluated for use with individual patients. The patient should succeed, yet be challenged, in the exercise. Games may use flash cards, pictures, or computer programs. They may be modifications of popular games, such as Bingo or crossword puzzles. With the exception of computer games, most games are relatively inexpensive to purchase or to make. Simulations include planning low-fat meals, using food models, and shopping for low-sodium foods in a mock supermarket.

Printed Materials

Pamphlets and information sheets are among the most common teaching tools. Printed materials can help to explain common health problems and their management and make the public more aware of health risks and prevention. Some printed materials are ideal teaching tools because they have large print, use language appropriate for the patient audience, emphasize important points, and reinforce learning. Distributing written information seems, at first glance, to be a quick and easy way to teach without requiring staff time to talk with patients. This is a misconception held by many physicians and nurses. Distributing written materials does not ensure a transfer of knowledge. Many patients are anxious about the information contained in the literature or cannot understand it. Even when printed matter is evaluated and used appropriately, taking into account interest and reading level, the message may not be received. Many well-educated patients do not enjoy reading or do not retain what they read.

Printed patient education materials may be used effectively to enhance patient participation in learning. An individualized teaching plan, designed to use patient assessment data, will guide educators in the appropriate use of books, pamphlets, and information sheets. We have found printed materials especially helpful in contraceptive counseling. After receiving basic teaching in the office, patients may take a booklet home to consider the various methods of contraception. Patients then frequently return for the next visit prepared to ask questions and willing to take responsibility for choosing a method. Although many patients initially come to an office visit with a particular birth control method in mind, we have discovered, through assessment, that the decision is usually based on experience or the advice of friends. A combined approach of one-on-one counseling and written patient education materials promotes enlightened choices.

The use of written materials requires assessment of the readability of each booklet, pamphlet, or handout. The teacher must be certain that the wording and sentence complexity are compatible with the patient's level of understanding. Many formulas can be used to predict readability or the grade level at which patient education materials are written. One of the most popular formulas is the SMOG formula (National Cancer Institute, 1981), as shown in Box 10-3. This formula requires time to count words, sentences, and syllables and to do simple computations. Word processing software for the computer also tests reading levels of text. Another method for limited time involves having the patient read aloud the first paragraph in the booklet and then restate its meaning, in his or her own words, to the nurse. The nurse learns whether the patient's eyesight and ability to read are adequate and whether the content is understood. We have discovered that patients frequently display less comprehension than would be expected from their highest grade of school completed.

BOX 10-3. SMOG Readability Formula

1. Count off 10 consecutive sentences near the beginning, in the middle, and near the end of the text. If the text has fewer than 30 sentences, use as many as are provided.
2. Count the number of words containing 3 or more syllables (polysyllabic) including repetitions of the same words.
   a. Hyphenated words are considered as one word.
   b. Numbers that are written out should be counted. If written in numerical form, they should be pronounced to determine if they are polysyllabic.
   c. Proper nouns, if polysyllabic, should be counted.
   d. Abbreviations should be read as though unabbreviated to determine if they are polysyllabic. However, abbreviations should be avoided unless commonly known.
3. Look up the approximate grade level on the SMOG Conversion Table below:

Total Polysyllabic Word Count	Approx. Grade Level (+1.5 Grades)
0–2	4
3–6	5
7–12	6
13–20	7
21–30	8
31–42	9
43–55	10
56–72	11
73–90	12
91–110	13
111–132	14
133–156	15
157–182	16
183–210	17
211–240	18

Note: From "SMOG grading: A new readability formula," by G. McLaughlin, 1969, *Journal of Reading, 12*(8), pp. 639–646. Adapted with permission.

The One-Page Instruction Sheet

Patients should always be given written discharge instructions to outline medications, treatments, follow-up appointments, and emergency guidelines.

Many nurses find it helpful to organize instructions chronologically. For example, a handout outlines what to do before breakfast, before leaving for work, at lunch, before bed, and so forth. Often instructions are given to both the patient and another family member. They are always reviewed with the patient before discharge. It is common hospital policy to have the patient or family member sign at the bottom of the instruction sheet, indicating that he or she received the information. A duplicate copy is placed in the patient record.

With the widespread use of computerization, nurses find it helpful to prepare basic instructions for patients with a particular diagnosis-related group. These standard instructions can be tailored for each patient and printed out on the nursing unit. Only the most pertinent information should be given, and instruction lists should be only as long as necessary. Box 10-4 offers suggestions for evaluating individualized handouts.

BOX 10-4. Patient Instruction Evaluation Checklist

- Are sentences and item length as short as possible?
- Is unfamiliar jargon avoided?
- Are instructions limited to "must-know" facts?
- Is information organized in a logical way?
- Is a shopping list provided for equipment and medications?
- Do patient and family know how to identify problems, what to look for?
- Do patient and family know what to do if problems arise?
- Who is to be called if problems occur?
- Is emergency plan included?

Brief patient emergency instructions can be printed on refrigerator magnets with a telephone number. Also, patients should be encouraged to post their one-page instructions at one or all of the following locations: on the refrigerator, by the telephone, and at the workplace. Instructions are ineffective if the patient cannot find them or has difficulty remembering the self-care regimen when he or she is away from home.

Patients benefit from instructions that use short, nontechnical words of two syllables or less, that give simple definitions, and that are written in active voice. Tell readers only what they need to know and do.

Special Challenges: Patients with Low Literacy Skills

Nurses must consider that nearly 20% of Americans are functionally illiterate (ie, they lack the necessary literacy skills to benefit from even the simplest handouts or videotaped programs). Patients who are functionally illiterate may be difficult to reach in patient education encounters. Despite attempts to simplify written materials from the typical ninth- or tenth-grade reading level to an improved sixth-grade level, the patient with low literacy skills is still lost.

Doak and colleagues (1995) present the special challenge of patient education with these adults comprehensively in their book *Teaching Patients with Low Literacy Skills*. (This text is a must for all nurses.) It helps nurses understand these patients, how to test their comprehension, and how to test their ability to read current materials; it teaches nurses how to write and rewrite materials and how to develop and incorporate audio and visual aids in patient education. Another valuable resource is a free publication from the U.S. Department of Agriculture, *Guidelines: Writing for Adults With Limited Reading Skills* (U.S. Department of Agriculture, 1988). The authors tell us that videotapes are not a quick answer for these patients. Illiteracy is not just the inability to read. Illiterate adults and those with low literacy skills process information differently than do readers. They may have limited vocabulary, may not understand abbreviations, and usually do not ask questions. Yet they may have average IQs and speak articulately. Identifying many of these individuals can be difficult because they have learned to cope in varying degrees and can hide their limitations from others.

A patient with limited reading skills often has a short attention span; thus, the message should be short, direct, and specific. The patient may depend on visual cues to clarify or interpret words; therefore pictures, illustrations, and graphics must be combined with words. A patient with low literacy skills also has difficulty understanding complex ideas. Information should be condensed into basic points with examples that apply the material to real-life situations he or she is likely to encounter.

For teaching patients with low literacy skills, guidelines are offered to help adapt existing methods and materials for these adults (Box 10-5). Many of the tips for working with these patients should be used with *all* patients. For example, what is critical when the patient is given a medication prescription? Should he or she know how to spell the name of the med-

ication? Is it more important that he or she knows the medication's purpose, what it looks like, when to take it, and possible side effects? To keep instructions as simple as possible, the nurse must ask the following questions:

- What should the patient do?
- What should the patient change or do differently?
- Which one or two points are most critical for the patient to understand?

 We may consider it critical that an older patient takes his or her diuretic medication at the beginning of the day to avoid sleep disturbance from increased urination. The patient should weigh himself or herself daily, record weight, and report dizziness, falls, rapid weight loss or gain, swelling in ankles or fingers, bleeding, bruising, or muscle cramping.

The nurse should use simple messages, familiar words, and pictures. The nurse should organize text in small sections with headings such as *Your Fluid Pill, Every Morning,* and *Call the Doctor If . . .*

Other suggestions for developing useful instructions:

- Always list first what the patient should do; limit the number of *don'ts.*
- Avoid mixing the sequence of *do's* and *dont's*; this may confuse patients.
- When giving instructions for medications, list the exact times the medication should be taken; avoid language such as "take three times a day."
- For PRN medication, list each medication separately with the instruction "take for _____," being specific about which symptom. Also, mention how often it can be taken, how long between doses, and how may times in 24 hours it can be taken. Indicate what the patient should do if the symptom is not relieved.
- List any symptoms for which the doctor should be notified immediately. ■

BOX 10-5. Guidelines for Teaching Patients With Low Literacy Skills

- Focus information on the core of knowledge and skills patients need to survive and to cope with problems.
- Teach the smallest amount possible.
- Make points vivid. Put important information either first or last.
- Sequence information logically, for example, step-by-step (1, 2, 3 . . .), chronological (a time line), or topical (using 3 or 4 main topics).
- Have the patient restate and demonstrate.
- Review.

Writing and Reviewing Instructions

Table 10-1 provides tips for writing medication instruction sheets. A safety hint for all patients: Give a complete list of all medica-

TABLE 10-1. Medication Instructions

USE	RATHER THAN
Take once daily	Take daily
Take at approximately 8 AM and 8 PM	Take twice daily
	Take every 12 h
Take at approximately 8 AM, 2 PM, and 10 PM	Take 3 times daily
	Take every 8 h
Take at approximately 8 AM, 1 PM, 6 PM, and 10 PM	Take 4 times daily
	Take every 6 h
Take 30 min before meals on an empty stomach	Take before meals
Take during meals 3 times a day	Take with meals
Take every _____ h as needed for (symptom)	Take as needed for (symptom)
Do not exceed _____ in a 24-h period	

Do Not Use

Take for (symptom)
Take as directed

tions to be taken after discharge. Patients may have old prescriptions at home or PRN medications that should not be part of the current treatment plan. This discharge list helps to reinforce the medication plan.

Testing the readability of patient education materials before patient use continues to be an important and simple step. Also, have patient education materials reviewed by actual patients, followed by an assessment of their comprehension of the material and suggestions for making the content more "patient friendly." Most nurses believe that every patient who is given printed matter should be asked to read a portion aloud and explain to the nurse what it means in his or her own words; this is the final and most critical test for readability.

Making written patient education materials more readable and effective is only a partial solution. Many patients cannot or will not read written material. This includes not only patients who are functionally illiterate, but those with physical handicaps or language barriers. For these patients, individual teaching, demonstration, coaching, involvement of family and significant others in the community, and novel approaches with "wordless"

patient education materials can improve comprehension of instructions and patient safety (Feldman, Quinlivan, Williford, Bahnson, & Fleischer, 1994). Pictorial care maps designed for patients are also described in Chapter 13.

DESIGNING PATIENT EDUCATION PROGRAMS

Nurses involved in patient education are asked to make choices every day, whether they address individual patient and family situations or design larger, agency-wide programs.

Many variables influence the design of a patient education program, including the numbers of and types of staff, monetary resources, the needs of patients, the health care setting, proximity to instructional design and audiovisual experts, and the availability of hardware and software suitable for use in patient teaching. Thus, there is no one prescription we can offer for designing interventions (patient education programs) that is practical for every situation. As we consider the following frequently asked questions, we draw from our own practice experience and that of our colleagues.

Designing a Patient Education Program: Questions to Consider

In which situations should group teaching be used? In which situations are one-on-one teaching preferable?

There are distinct advantages inherent in both one-on-one and group teaching situations. It is difficult to generalize when one is more effective than the other because of the individual characteristics of patients. All patients should be provided with some individual teaching to help them understand and accept their diagnosis and understand their own role in the management of their health. Every patient in every setting should know why he or she is there, what he or she can contribute to managing his or her health, and what he or she can expect to learn from health care providers that will enable him or her to do this effectively.

Provided that an assessment of the patient and family learning needs is made, group teaching can then be as effective as continued individual teaching for cognitive and affective learning. Important considerations in offering group classes include whether transportation and time are convenient and whether patients and their families can attend. Physicians may be more supportive of group teaching if they are introduced to the class objectives, content, and staff. Some physicians are interested in participating as teachers.

We have determined that individual patient teaching is more effective than group teaching (whether with a family group or a large, unrelated group) in the following situations:

- **When the health professional has little knowledge of the patient and an assessment of the patient for education purposes has not been completed.** Trying to assess individual knowledge in a group situation is difficult and usually impossible because most clients do not want to reveal their knowledge deficits to a group.
- **When family members or friends try to co-opt teaching sessions.** Some family members have been noted to use teaching sessions to make the patient feel guilty for

not following a medical regimen or to attract attention to themselves and their roles as caregivers.

- **When the information to be taught provokes a great deal of anxiety** (eg, teaching related to cardiac surgery) or when the information is sensitive (eg, sexual function, reproduction, or bowel function). Even when a patient seems to be a good prospect for a group learning experience, he or she should first be assessed individually to determine readiness.

 The authors have found group teaching useful both as a helpful adjunct to one-on-one teaching and also as the primary format for patient education. Group teaching sessions help patients with acute and chronic conditions feel less alienated. Patients frequently remark after a group teaching session that it was helpful to hear other people express the same problems and feelings. Groups in which patients are encouraged to formulate their own agenda and conduct the group session seem to be even more motivated to learn. Groups also encourage patient sharing of coping techniques and useful hints. For example, it may be difficult for health professionals who have never had to struggle with an ileostomy or with asthma to understand or be aware of the many problems of daily existence involved with these conditions. The sharing and social support in group sessions can be augmented by technical assistance from health professionals, as long as they do not attempt to co-opt the group.

Another benefit of a group teaching format is the decreased costs (eg, time, money, health professionals). Group teaching also helps families gain added support from health professionals and other patients and their families. Families gaining support from one another is especially evident in pediatric settings and is one of the reasons for the success of the Ronald McDonald Houses for parents of critically ill children. This sharing and support transfers to more structured settings, such as group teaching classes (eg, a spouse of a patient with heart disease may share recipes with another). The feeling that "we're all in this together" is especially gratifying to family members, who are frequently more overwhelmed than the patient with the magnitude of the problem.

All of the data are not yet in on the advantages and disadvantages of group versus individual teaching, and we would like to see more evaluation research conducted in this area. Whether to use one or the other or a combination of the two is at the discretion of the health professional, who must constantly remember the individual needs of the patients. ■

Can hospital-based protocols (eg, critical pathways and care maps) be used in an outpatient clinic? If so, which target populations are most conducive to this?

The use of critical pathways and care maps (typically used in hospitals) can also be effective in an outpatient clinic or home health setting. These systems direct the coordination of the health care team through teaching protocols. Evaluating common learning needs of specific patient populations that require ongoing teaching (eg, patients with asthma) can be accomplished by using computer statistics that list the most common diagnoses. Nurses may also keep a log of patient education encounters for a 6-month period and make their own comparisons. Using this log-keeping method in an outpatient clinic, we discovered that the following situations are ideal for group teaching: weight reduction, hypertension, diabetes, prenatal care, and neonatal care. It may be helpful to start with high-volume or high-risk problems seen in one's own practice setting.

How does the nurse decide what learning activities are best for a given situation?

A combination of learning activities works best in each situation. It will help the patient and family to assume active roles in learning and to enjoy patient education if the following points are kept in mind:

- **Match learning activities with learning objectives.**
- **Keep the patient and the family involved** through discussion, role-play, games, and media.
- Test the patient's new abilities to help him or her feel a sense of accomplishment. Try to build success and reinforcement into patient education.

- **Make learning fun.** Humor and support decrease the patient's anxiety and will help one learn at his or her own pace.
- **Allow ample time to practice skills.** Skill-building exercises should not be last on the agenda. These exercises often determine how safely the patient can perform new skills at home.
- **Incorporate methods other than lecture alone** to teach skills and develop the patient's attitude.

Are there general guidelines that can be used to evaluate different types of media, whether they are written materials, videotapes, slides, or CAI?

Box 10-6 provides a checklist for evaluating written patient education materials. It is adapted from the Society of Teachers of Family Medicine, a group actively involved in promoting patient education (STFM, 1979). Box 10-7 is an evaluation guide used when previewing patient education videos.

How should one prepare to teach a patient education class or session?

Advanced preparation and coaching are important before teaching a group. First, define the target audience, estimate the group size, determine the goals for the session, and estimate the amount of time available for teaching. Then, various teaching methods may be combined, such as lecture and discussion, or perhaps a case study. Hospital staff development coordinators can help with program planning; these individuals are typically experienced in planning classes using adult education models.

Generally, group teaching is used to persuade patients to perform health behaviors. Information and facts are presented to help them understand the need to perform certain health behaviors; then, examples are given to help patients understand how they can accomplish this. These principles apply equally to health promotion or disease-specific management classes.

A strong understanding of the health problem being addressed in the patient education session is important. The nurse teacher may want to review the nursing literature and the AHRQ guidelines. Presenting information per-

BOX 10-6. Checklist for Evaluating Patient Education Materials

The following checklist is designed to be used by health professionals when they review instructional materials for use in patient education. It is adapted from The Society of Teachers of Family Medicine: *Patient Education: A Handbook for Teachers* (1979), Kansas City.

Title
Author
Publication date
Specified intended audience:
Age span: _____ to _____ (years)
Language or ethnic background
Socioeconomic group

I. Accuracy
   A. Are facts, diagrams, pictures, and other visual representations accurate?
   B. Is subject matter up to date?

II. Content
   A. Breadth or scope of coverage
      1. Does the subject matter or content presented address major areas of difficulty/functional problems experienced by many patients with the specific medical problems?
      2. Is content (subject matter or product endorsements/advertising) included that is inappropriate for the intended audience?
   B. Balance of coverage
      1. Is the subject matter balanced in terms of emphasis on various major areas?

III. Educational Methods
   A. Organization of content
      1. Is there an organizational structure or logic that is apparent to the patient?
      2. Are major content areas set off so that material can be put into perspective?
   B. Contribution of organization of content to efficient learning
      1. Are concepts or terms introduced in an appropriate sequence?

   2. Does material start with simple concepts, then move to the more complex?
   3. Is material sequenced in a patient-friendly manner (ie, step-by-step, chronological, or topical)?
   4. Is there a summary?
   C. Educational objectives or goals and methods for assessing learner achievement
      1. Are objectives explicitly stated and included in the educational material in a way that is understandable to the patient?
      2. Is it likely that patients will reach the objectives by study of the material? Is the number of objectives reasonable?
      3. Are learner-assessment methods included that help patients determine whether they have met the objectives (i.e., test questions)?
      4. Do the objectives address areas that are generally of concern *to most physicians* who treat patients with this problem?
      5. Do the objectives address areas that are generally of concern *to most patients* with the particular problem?

IV. Communication
   A. Appropriateness of the reading level for the state audience
      1. Are other key audience characteristics specified?
      2. Whenever possible, are sentences short and simple, containing only commonly used terms, and is medical jargon avoided?
   B. Availability of feedback
      1. Are there appropriate places for the patient to practice?
      2. How will the patient obtain feedback about the mastery of facts, concepts, and principles?

suasively requires a confident teacher, with a lively affect, who can keep the attention of the learners. Observe others who are experienced in group teaching and witness first-hand group teaching techniques. Nurses are usually good group teachers because they are at ease with patients and families and are viewed as credible and sensitive.

<hr>

BOX 10-7. Tool for Evaluation of Patient Education Videotapes

1. Title:
2. Beginning time:
   Ending time:
   Total running time:
3. Vocabulary: List all words with which patients may not be familiar. Are terms defined? Estimate the number of words that exceed two syllables.
4. Purpose of the film: If goals and objectives are stated, list.
5. Intended audience:
6. What types of people are portrayed in the video?
7. Questions answered by the video. Are these questions or problems commonly encountered by patients?
8. Priority areas addressed?
   What must a patient do to manage this problem?
   What decisions should patients be prepared to make?
9. Are sources suggested for further help or information?
10. Technical quality:
11. Cost:
12. Source:

<hr>

It is important for nurses to realize that to truly affect a patient's opinion (ie, in a powerful way that influences behavior), the nurse must think as a patient would think. The Health Belief Model (see Chapter 6) outlines the four steps that lead to a patient's decision about health behaviors. When organizing a group class, the Health Belief model also can be used as a guide. First, patients must believe they have or are likely to be affected by a particular health problem. The nurse can provide evidence that the patient has hypertension or diabetes (or is at risk for these conditions). The nurse can also provide facts about the prevalence of the condition. Patients should understand in their own words a simple defi-

nition of the health problem. Second, the patients must believe the condition discussed is harmful and has adverse consequences. Patients frequently wish to talk about how this problem has affected or may affect their lives, families, work, and social roles. Third, the patients need to understand the proposed treatment plan or health promotion plan and what behaviors the patient is asked to consider integrating in his or her life. These behaviors should be stated clearly, with practical suggestions to help patients overcome barriers they might encounter, including learning skills, finding ongoing support, and perhaps acquiring financial assistance. Fourth, patients weigh the perceived costs and benefits of the proposed health interventions and make decisions about their commitment to act.

Group teaching can motivate patients to adopt new health behaviors or comply with treatment regimens, thus contributing to self-care. Learning should be patient centered, and the learners should have the opportunity to ask questions and share experiences. Therefore, time must be allocated in group teaching for these activities, which may require a limited amount of time in lecture format.

Table 10-2 illustrates how group teaching can be organized following the steps of the Health Belief Model.

CASE STUDY

MRS. FOX'S FRACTURE

Case Presentation

Mrs. Fox is 70 years old. She is well known on the medical surgical unit of the small community hospital. She was admitted 3 months ago because her diabetes was out of control because of poor dietary habits, and her blood sugar was dangerously high. She is physically inactive, watches television and plays bridge for entertainment, and smokes two packs of cigarettes daily.

Her current admission is the result of a fall down the front stairs of her home. Mrs.

(case study continues on page 284)

Fox has a fractured tibia. A cast is applied in the emergency room. Because of poor circulation and immobility, Mrs. Fox is admitted overnight for evaluation. Her physician plans to discharge her within 2 days.

Assessment and Nursing Diagnoses
During the admission assessment, her nurse notes the following important information:

The Foxes live in a one-story ranch home with wood floors and area rugs. Mr. Fox works the evening shift as a security guard for the local shopping mall. Mrs. Fox has not followed her diabetic meal plan. Mr. Fox found Mrs. Fox asleep on the couch with a burning cigarette in her hand last week and is worried about a fire in the home while he is at work.

The nursing staff has a conference to discuss a patient care plan for Mrs. Fox. Considering the short time she will be hospitalized, the nurses are overwhelmed by what must be taught so Mrs. Fox can safely manage her care. Should they immediately get a dietitian involved to repeat diet teaching? What about the smoking and its hazards? The nurses decide to make a list of all nursing diagnoses and then work together to set priorities. Mrs. Fox's nursing diagnoses are the following:

1. Altered tissue perfusion in peripheral system
2. Impaired tissue integrity
3. Risk for injury
4. Impaired physical mobility
5. Altered nutrition: more than body requirements
6. Impaired home maintenance management
7. Activity intolerance
8. Pain

Goals and Implementation
After careful consideration of survival skills and safety issues, the nursing staff confidently places highest priority on *impaired physical mobility, risk for injury, and altered tissue perfusion.* The survival

skills Mrs. Fox needs are the ability to walk on crutches and the ability to check circulation on her affected leg. The goals for Mrs. Fox and her family are the following:

- Properly maintain the cast with adequate circulation.
- Assess the cast and the skin under the cast edges to determine skin condition (four times daily).
- Assess foot and leg for circulatory and neurologic impairment (four times daily).
- Walk safely with the use of crutches and appropriate gait.
- Prevent axillary skin breakdown.
- Administer medication as ordered.
- Adapt home environment to prevent injury caused by falls.
- Provide at-home assistance with activities of daily living.

Skills, such as cast care and crutch walking must be taught with active learner involvement and repeated practice. The nurse should accurately assess and document the patient's abilities in these areas.

The nursing staff caring for Mrs. Fox make the difficult decision to accomplish diabetic teaching and smoking cessation promotion with post-hospital referrals. They decided to focus their immediate efforts on the problems posed by her broken bone injury. They also called a team conference. They speak with the physical therapist to coordinate teaching for crutch-walking skills, they speak with the dietary department about diet reinforcement, and the hospital social worker is brought in to work with the Foxes on the possibility of a home health referral and at-home assistance to assure safety.

Every nurse who enters Mrs. Fox's room for the next 24 hours demonstrates and reinforces circulation checks and crutch-walking skills and receives return demonstration. Mr. Fox also is involved in teaching. A one-page instruction sheet is created, giving priority instructions regarding ambulation and circulation.

TABLE 10-2. The Health Belief Model Used in Planning Patient Education Interventions	
STEPS	**APPLICATION**
I. The patient perceives that he or she has a condition or is likely to contract it. II. The patient perceives that the disease or condition is harmful and has serious consequences for him or her. III. The patient believes that the suggested health intervention is of value to him or her. IV. The patient believes that the effectiveness of the treatment is worth the cost and barriers he or she must confront.	I. a. Discuss problem and symptoms (to be prevented or treated). b. Explore prior knowledge and experience of audience. c. Address obstacles to understanding (anxiety, fear, misconceptions, denial). II. a. Describe potential consequences of the problem. b. Discuss prognosis. c. Explore common beliefs and attitudes. d. Describe experiences of individuals with similar problem (including lifestyle). III. a. Describe proposed treatment plan, health promotion activities, proposed behavior changes (includes medications). b. Discuss what may happen with or without proposed treatment. c. Is this a cure? d. Financial costs, lifestyle changes, side effects discussed. IV. a. Outline provider responsibilities. b. Outline patient responsibilities. c. Outline needed knowledge, attitudes, and skills. d. Suggest and provide resources for knowledge and skills development.

References:

1. Hochbaum, G. M. (1958). *Public participation in medical screening programs* (U.S. Public Health Service Publication No. 572). Washington, DC: U.S. Government Printing Office.

2. Rosenstock, I. M. (1975). *Patient's compliance with health regimens Journal of the American Medical Association, 234*(4), 402–403.

3. Rankin, S. H., & Stallings, K. D. (1996). *Patient education: Issues, principles, and practices* (3rd Ed.). Philadelphia: Lippincott-Raven.

The Health Belief Model was constructed to predict health behaviors. It provides a tool for understanding the patient's perception of disease and his decision-making process in the consumption of health services. In each of the four steps, family members and significant others should be considered.

Discharge and Home Health Care Services

As a result of economic pressures, patients are often discharged while still needing some level of professional health care. Nurses must become familiar with home health care services, so they can assist patients with discharge planning. Nurses must anticipate the needs patients will have at home, what kinds of resources are already available, and what types of services they will need. The case study of Mrs. Fox illustrates critical needs, including patient teaching and safety measures, which remain after discharge. A nurse works with the family to assess the physical layout of the home, how to adapt it if necessary, and how to add needed equipment. The nurse helps the family assess whether the principal caregiver will need to in-

volve other helpers to assist, pick up medications, run errands, and so forth. The nurse must also help the patient determine what insurance will cover; the nurse may consult others to determine this. For patients who qualify, third-party payment will reimburse for at least part of home health care services. The following documentation suggestions facilitate home health care authorization and referral:

1. Clarify the homebound status of the patient. The patient's condition prevents him or her from leaving home without help from others; therefore, leaving home is rarely feasible. Stress functional limitations.
2. Emphasize acute episodes or acute exacerbation of the condition.
3. Reflect the level of current need. For

example, size and appearance of wound should be documented rather than stating, "wound healing well." Provide specific measurements whenever possible.

4. Emphasize the need for reinstruction rather than for reinforced teaching. If the family's ability to master learning is limited, this should be noted.

5. Document whether the patient's condition is unstable. Skilled nursing care to monitor medications or vital signs may not be reimbursed unless the patient's condition is unstable.

Many acute care nurses are unaware that home care nurses must also focus on discharge planning at the time of admission and must skillfully achieve patient learning outcomes rather than simply prolonging care. The prevalence of managed care has resulted in shorter lengths of stays with home health nurses and with nurses in the acute care hospital setting.

Clinical Relevance: Prenatal Education Program

The prenatal education program is an example of group teaching. Both authors were involved in its development, first as a pilot program, and then as an established component of prenatal care for all patients enrolled in the obstetrical practice at the family medicine center. One author (KS) was head nurse in the family medicine center and the other (SR) was a faculty member from the school of nursing.

A program of prenatal education was originally developed as part of a clinical practicum for an advanced practice nursing student doing a clinical practicum at a university family medicine practice. The classes evolved in response to an informal needs assessment conducted at the outpatient clinic of a university's family medicine residency training program. Faculty, residents, and nurses designated prenatal classes as the outstanding patient education need for clinic patients. The clinic served a group of prenatal families who were socioeconomically and culturally diverse.

Teenage parents, single mothers, and international patients did not seem to be served by traditional couple-oriented approaches to childbirth education. The involvement of childbirth coaches was strongly supported, and these individuals included mothers, sisters, friends, and spouses. After a successful pilot program developed by the APN student, the Family Practice Clinic assumed the leadership of the prenatal classes and established the following philosophy about the delivery of prenatal education.

Education is an essential ingredient in the health care delivered to prenatal patients. The family medicine center made a commitment to offer prenatal classes to all of our patients on a regular basis.

Prenatal classes should be attended as early as possible in pregnancy. There are numerous advantages to the patient, her family, the physician, and the nurse.

1. The mother's participation in her own care is essential, especially in the areas of nutrition and care of her body. The classes give parents and significant others the information they need to work in partnership with the physician and nurse.

2. Classes that address the labor and delivery processes give expectant parents an opportunity to verbalize anxieties or fears about childbirth.

3. Expectant parents enter a supportive relationship with other expectant parents.

4. Relaxation and breathing techniques are learned, making both routine obstetric examinations and the labor and delivery better experiences.

5. Expectant mothers and fathers and significant others are encouraged to communicate their feelings effectively with one another and to consider ways to keep the communication lines open during stressful events surrounding the birth of their child.

6. Parents gain knowledge about newborn care and helpful suggestions for dealing with the new baby's siblings and other family members.

7. The prenatal care curriculum offers a blend of general childbirth education and Lamaze techniques. No single approach to

the birth experience or child care is promoted. Instead, the aim is to provide expectant parents with information that enables them to consider their own needs and wishes. Openness and flexibility in planning for labor and delivery and in considering each family's special circumstances are of paramount importance.

8. Expectant parents learn from the health care providers and from each other. Health care providers also learn a great deal from the patients in an informal group, in which all members are supported and encouraged to share their thoughts and feelings with one another.

9. A commitment to patient education is demonstrated by the willingness to become team members in health care with patients. It is a statement of the nurse's respect for patients as consumers. Finally, offering an attractive prenatal care package is an important step toward enrolling new families in the practice. (Duke-Watts Family Medicine Program, Durham, NC.)

This philosophy articulated the benefits to the prenatal client and her support system, as well as the agency. Care was taken to ensure continuity of the prenatal classes regardless of changes in clinic staff and residents. Guidelines and standards were developed to help each staff nurse who would serve as a prenatal class coordinator handle the logistics of the classes, and allay anxiety they might have about the program.

After guidelines were developed, objectives were written for each class (Box 10-8). During the first of four class meetings, a learning needs assessment was filled out by each client and her significant other. These assessment data were then put into the general schema of classes. Thus, the prenatal clients can set their own agenda (ie, the class is taught to meet its needs, not those of the health care professionals). Data from the learning needs assessment were transferred to the client's chart (with her knowledge), so that during routine office visits the physician could discuss her stated con-

cerns. The learning needs assessment included questions about previous pregnancies, who would attend classes and delivery with the patient, previous prenatal education, and what the patient was hoping to learn in the classes.

Group discussions and demonstrations enlivened classes. During the first class, a couple who attended the previous set of classes was enlisted to bring their infant. The expectant parents had many questions for the parent visitors and seeing the outcome of the prenatal period (ie, a healthy baby) focused the class for everyone. Participants were divided into smaller groups of five or six to discuss topics (eg, sexual activity during pregnancy) and to play educational games related to nutrition.

During the fourth class, which discussed the care of the newborn, a family nurse practitioner or a family medicine resident demonstrated physical assessment of a neonate. The couples were invariably amazed to see the newborn's range of behaviors and could anticipate their forthcoming infant, laying the foundation for infant stimulation practices. Demonstration segments break the tedium that can occur with the lecture format and also allow the participants an opportunity to become acquainted with one another.

At the end of the last class, each participant completed an evaluation form rating the classes and teachers and offering suggestions for improvement. Evaluations were useful in planning future classes and in giving specific teachers feedback on their performance in the classes. Another evaluation format, a confidence survey, was used during the first class series to obtain information related to the participants' growth in confidence levels during the five class meetings. One of the purposes of any type of prenatal education is to instill confidence in the couple so that they can to manage self-care practices related to pregnancy and to care for the neonate. Confidence levels on 19 different items were determined on pre- and post-tests (ie, at the beginning of the class series and after the last class).

The confidence level survey used in the classes is shown in Fig. 10-1. Another method of evaluation and feedback used was

BOX 10-8. Objectives for Prenatal Classes

Class I: Nutrition During Pregnancy
At the close of Class I, each participant will be able to do the following:

A. Answer the following questions correctly:
 1. How much weight do you plan to gain during your pregnancy?
 2. Now that you are pregnant, how many more calories do you think you need: 2 times normal, 3 times normal, only 300 calories more, only 100 calories more?
 3. Which of the following foods do pregnant women especially need: dairy products, sweets, fatty foods, fresh vegetables, protein foods?
 4. Which of the following items might be dangerous to eat or use while you are pregnant: alcoholic beverages, salt, sugar, nicotine, caffeine?
 5. In which of the following situations would a pregnant woman be wise to lose weight: if the woman were overweight before pregnancy, if the woman has diabetes and is overweight, if the woman suddenly gains 10 lb that is primarily fluid?
B. List three advantages of breast-feeding.
C. State three advantages of exercise during pregnancy.
D. Choose one type of exercise and describe where and how often it will be done.

Prenatal Class II: Physiologic and Psychological Changes of Pregnancy
By the close of Class II, each participant will be able to do the following:

A. Describe breast changes and care of the breasts during pregnancy.
B. Describe recommendations for the following during pregnancy:
 1. Rest and sleep
 2. Smoking and alcohol
 3. Dental care
 4. Travel and work
C. Name two common discomforts of pregnancy and recommended treatments.

D. State why the doctor should be consulted before *any* medication is taken during pregnancy.
E. Identify three warning signs for which the doctor should be notified immediately.
F. Demonstrate the Kegel exercise for toning pelvic musculature, demonstrate slow, deep chest breathing used during the initial stage of labor.

Prenatal Class III: Labor and Delivery
At the close of Class III, each participant will be able to do the following:

A. Describe the work of the uterus in labor.
B. Describe the changes of the cervix in labor.
C. Describe three signs of labor.
D. Demonstrate the timing of contractions.
E. Describe how and when to contact the doctor when there has been a sign of labor.
F. Describe three stages of labor.
G. Consider own plans for labor and delivery (e.g., birthing room, rooming-in arrangements, early discharge).
H. Describe some variables that make cesarean section necessary.

Prenatal Class IV: The Newborn
At the close of Class IV, each participant/couple will be able to do the following:

A. Describe why fatigue is a problem that most new parents face.
B. Discuss two ways new parents can minimize unnecessary fatigue.
C. Consider which helpers might be staying with patients when they come home from the hospital and describe what helpers can do.
D. Describe three infant care problems for which the doctor should be notified.
E. Describe three needs for which babies depend on their parents.
F. Describe two issues that new parents often confront as a couple.

(box continues on page 289)

Prenatal Class V: The Postpartum Period
At the end of Class V, each participant will be able to do the following:

A. Identify two common postpartum discomforts and describe how to initiate relief measures.
B. Identify two symptoms or problems for which the doctor should be notified.
C. Consider a method of contraception that is acceptable to them.
D. Demonstrate the following in a mock labor and delivery:
   1. Deep chest breathing
   2. Shallow breathing
   3. Panting
   4. Pushing

INSTRUCTIONS

We are interested in knowing how confident you feel about your knowledge associated with pregnancy, labor, and delivery. Please answer these questions carefully by circling the response that refers to your confidence level.
A sample question will help you understand how to fill out the questionnaire.
I know how to fill out this questionnaire.

VC   C   ?   I   VI

VC — I feel very confident and secure in my knowledge of this material.
  C — I feel confident that I can deal adequately with this material.
  ? — I have no particular feelings about this material; I do not know what this material means.
  I — I feel insecure, knowing that I would have a difficult time dealing with this material.
VI — I feel very insecure, knowing that I definitely could not deal with this material at this time.

1. I know which foods a pregnant woman should eat and why.
      VC   C   ?   I   VI

2. I understand the changes in my breasts.
      VC   C   ?   I   VI

3. I know about the possible effects of alcohol on my baby.
      VC   C   ?   I   VI

4. I know how many pounds I can gain during my pregnancy.
      VC   C   ?   I   VI

5. I understand restrictions placed on me because of my job.
      VC   C   ?   I   VI

FIGURE 10-1. Prenatal confidence level survey. *(figure continued)*

6. I know how to do a pelvic tilt.

| VC | C | ? | I | VI |

7. I understand the reasons for frequent urination during pregnancy.

| VC | C | ? | I | VI |

8. I know the danger signs to watch for during pregnancy.

| VC | C | ? | I | VI |

9. I understand the fear—tension—pain cycle.

| VC | C | ? | I | VI |

10. I know how to do breathing exercises to be used during labor.

| VC | C | ? | I | VI |

11. I know what to expect from a newborn baby.

| VC | C | ? | I | VI |

12. I understand the differences between bottle-feeding and breast-feeding for the mother and baby.

| VC | C | ? | I | VI |

13. I know how to give a baby bath.

| VC | C | ? | I | VI |

14. I know what kind of birth control to use while nursing.

| VC | C | ? | I | VI |

15. I know what kinds of pain medications are available during labor.

| VC | C | ? | I | VI |

16. I know at least three signs of beginning labor.

| VC | C | ? | I | VI |

17. I know how to get my body into shape after delivery.

| VC | C | ? | I | VI |

18. I understand the various forms of birth control and the ones best suited for me.

| VC | C | ? | I | VI |

19. I know the types of equipment and clothing necessary for me and my baby.

| VC | C | ? | I | VI |

(figure continued)

> ## BOX 10-9. Suggestions for Writing About the Birth Experience
>
> **Beginning of Labor**
> How and when did it begin? What did you do? How did you feel?
>
> **Admission to the Hospital**
> When were you admitted? What was it like?
>
> **Stages of Labor**
> How long did each stage last? Did you feel that the nurses kept you informed on your progress? Which tools helped the most? Which helped the least? Did you receive medication? If so, what kind, when, how
>
> effective was it? What kind of emotional support did you have?
>
> **Birth**
> What did the baby look like? How did you feel during and immediately after birth?
>
> **Postpartum**
> How long did you stay in the hospital? Describe how you felt during the first week you were at home after delivery. What problems did you have? What people or things were most helpful to you?

asking patients to write a summary of their birth experiences. Patients were given a guide for writing the report (Box 10-9). This is a keepsake for the family and a process to help the mother work through feelings about such a powerful experience. Although not all patients are willing to write a report, most are eager to discuss the birth experience. This provided us with valuable pointers about how to improve childbirth classes to better prepare patients for labor and delivery.

Additions were made to the patient education offerings at the clinic because of evaluations of the prenatal classes. More in-depth classes were provided on breast preparation and breast-feeding for patients in the seventh to eighth month of pregnancy. A room at the clinic was also equipped for patients to view videotapes on cesarean delivery, basics of baby care, and postpartum fatigue and depression. A daily baby care "call-in" telephone hour was proposed to provide information and answer patient questions before the first return visit to the clinic. To achieve successful outcomes of group teaching, nurses must incorporate assessment, preparation, and individualized approaches for non-English speaking patients from different cultural backgrounds.

CASE STUDY

THE VUONG FAMILY

General Considerations:
Cultural Practices and Prenatal Care
Childbirth is an important event in the lives of families, and cultural practices affect how prenatal care is provided. Most nurses do not expect to be experts on all cultural groups and their beliefs about birth. Variations exist even among people in the same cultural group. All nurses should be open and interested in learning about the needs and concerns of patients as influenced by culture (Lester, 1998; Spector, 1996; Andrews & Boyle, 1995). Suggestions are offered in Chapter 3. Nurses should respect each patient's background and through patient education help families form partnerships in prenatal care. In health care settings serving multilingual populations, prenatal teaching should include maternal nutrition materials in other languages (especially Lao, Vietnamese, Cambodian, and Spanish) and "nonlanguage" handouts.

(case study continues on page 292)

Case Presentation

Mai Vuong, a Vietnamese woman, comes for her first clinic visit when she is 12 weeks pregnant. She comes alone, is quiet, and seems withdrawn. The assessment of her learning needs about the pregnancy is difficult. Also, time is limited during an outpatient encounter. A nursing student working at the clinic that day offered to conduct two home visits to help compose a family assessment and identify Mai's needs.

Family Assessment

The family unit is composed of the husband, Tran, age 38, who works in a print shop; Mai, age 28, the wife, who works full-time as a seamstress and is pregnant with their first child; and Li, age 28, who is Tran's sister and works in the same print shop as her brother. Mai states she knows nothing about pregnancy, labor, delivery, or caring for a newborn child and denies having had any role model in these areas.

Mai and Tran are both Vietnamese and immigrated legally from Vietnam. Li has always lived with them. Before leaving Vietnam, Tran was a farmer. This was a difficult life, physically and economically. He came to the United States in hopes of a better and prosperous life. Mai did not complete high school; she left school to work and support her family. All three of them continue to financially support their parents, and Mai sends her brother, who lives in Texas, one-third of her monthly salary. Both sets of parents are supportive of the pregnancy. However, neither mother can come and help with the care of the newborn, a traditional role of Vietnamese grandmothers (Grosso, Barden, Henry, & Vieau, 1981).

The Vuong family is a warm, hospitable Catholic family, with a secure sense of family loyalty, closeness, and strength. Traditional Vietnamese families have a patriarchal structure in which the eldest man is the head of the household and the woman is dutiful and respectful toward her husband (Calhoun, 1985). In the Vuong family, Tran is the head of the family, as is evident in the way he speaks for his wife and appears to be her caretaker. Mai is dutiful to her husband in the way she respects his opinion and serves him and their guest first. However, these roles are also flexible: all three members of this family share the domestic duties of their small two-room flat. They are also emotionally supportive and mutually respectful of each other as is evident in the gentleness Tran and Li showed toward Mai when she has difficulty understanding the questions of the English-speaking interviewer.

The Vuongs live among and work predominantly with Vietnamese immigrants and refugees. This may signal social exclusivity within their ethnic community, because they have few non-Vietnamese friends. Consequently, this results in their being limited in their awareness of community services (ie, childbirth preparation classes). This also decreases their opportunities to assimilate into their new culture and improve their English language skills.

All three state that they do not know what to expect with pregnancy and childbirth, and they show concern regarding their lack of knowledge. They are presently receiving their knowledge from friends and neighbors, because they have no family in the immediate area. This could potentially lead to confusion, fear, and unrealistic expectations of the course of the pregnancy and labor and delivery. Tran and Li seem to have formed an alliance in which they bond to support Mai and relate to her gently. Although culturally understandable, this could foster her dependence on her family to meet her needs of effective communication.

The family anticipates the new baby with pleasure. Having been raised in traditional

(case study continues on page 293)

Vietnamese families, they respect their cultural heritage and believe the family to be important. When asked about raising their child in the American culture, Tran responded, "I think my baby was, born, okay I have to teach her. Sometimes we have to keep the Vietnamese idea in my family. I want to say no anything Vietnamese ideas excellent, but I think American idea something excellent. So we have to keep two of them in my family." Mai echoed, "Together."

In anticipating becoming parents, Tran and Mai seem aware that their child will be raised in a different culture and have some understanding of the challenge before them. Another strength of the potential parent-child system is Tran's involvement in the pregnancy. He speaks about needing to move to a larger home and shopping for the baby's bed. Having no role models regarding pregnancy, childbirth, or the care of the newborn, the Vuong family has a knowledge deficit regarding the role changes and task realignment a new family member will bring into their home.

In traditional Vietnamese culture, the fathers are not expected to participate in childbirth (Hollingsworth, Brown, & Booten, 1980); childbirth is regarded as a thing among women. Tran expresses feeling uncomfortable with entering the labor and delivery room. This may cause a conflict with the American expectation that fathers be involved in coaching the woman through labor and delivery. Because of a knowledge deficit regarding pregnancy, childbirth, and child care, Mai is at risk for difficulty in making the role transition to mother. Mai is reluctant to use her English language skills and has limited comprehension of the English language. This fosters dependency on her family and other members of her ethnic group to communicate for her.

The family members are interested in seeking knowledge in the areas that they feel are lacking and are interested in the child preparation classes offered by the clinic. Because extended family is so important in the Vietnamese culture, having no grandmother in the same geographic location may make the transition of having a newborn more difficult for this family.

Recommendations

Tailoring prenatal group education and individual teaching to the needs of the Vuong family includes the following.

1. The family needs to be encouraged to participate in childbirth preparation classes. This will provide anticipatory guidance in relationship to the labor and delivery process. Li or another woman needs to accompany Mai to the classes even if Tran feels that he wants to be involved in the coaching of Mai's labor and delivery.
2. The family needs to find a trusted friend who might give them reliable information regarding what is normal in pregnancy, labor, delivery, and newborn care. They also need to ask questions of their physician and the clinic nurses.
3. The health providers of this family need to be made aware of the family's cultural differences and work with them within their cultural context. An example of this would be not to pressure Tran to be Mai's labor coach but rather allow a woman to be with her.
4. Mai needs to be encouraged to continue English classes and to use her language skills to decrease her dependency on others to communicate. The clinic should not rely on written learning materials to provide instructions to Mai.

Outcomes

As an outcome of this family assessment, Mai and Li participate in the clinic's childbirth classes. They are also given needed attention when Mai came for her

(case study continues on page 294)

prenatal visits because the clinic staff members were aware of her needs and appreciated cultural norms of the Vietnamese family. Written teaching materials are used selectively because of Mai's limited ability to read and understand English.

SUMMARY

Matching learning objectives to appropriate learning methods and media is important to achieve positive results in patient education. Various examples were offered in this chapter to illustrate the design of interventions based on nursing diagnoses, learning needs, goals, and patient learning objectives. Case studies illustrated interventions for individual patients, including tips for using home health care services to bridge the gap between hospital and home, and using an individualized care plan to accompany group teaching for a Vietnamese patient. Valuable tools for evaluating patient education materials and videos are provided in the chapter.

STRATEGIES FOR CRITICAL ANALYSIS

1. Using the case study of Mrs. Fox (see Chapter 9), describe which instructional format and methods you would choose for discharge teaching. Base the teaching on the patient's length of stay and priorities for patient learning. How would you coordinate your teaching with the physical therapist? Who else besides the patient should be included in teaching?

2. Select a sample patient education handout and a sample video addressing a topic of your choice. Evaluate them using Boxes 10-5 and 10-6. What suggestions would you make for making them more patient centered? How could they be adapted to meet the needs of patients with low literacy skills?

3. If you were asked to teach a 1-hour class to fellow nursing students about the need for their own adequate nutrition and exercise, how could you prepare the class using the Health Belief Model as a guide?

4. Identify resources in your community that could be used to support the learning of non-English speaking patients. Where can interpreter services be found? Where can nurses obtain teaching materials written in other languages? What resources are available for patients to learn how to read and understand the English language?

REFERENCES

(1999). Library empowers families to participate. *Patient Education Management 6*(7), 81.

AHRQ (Agency for Healthcare Research and Quality) www.ahcpr.gov. Accessed 9/29/00. Department of Health and Human Services, 2101 E. Jefferson Street, Suite 501, Rockville, MD, 20852.

Andrews, M., & Boyle, S. (1995). *Transcultural Concepts in Nursing Care.* Philadelphia: Lippincott-Raven.

Brookfield, S. (1986). *Understanding and Facilitating Adult Learning.* San Francisco: Jossey-Bass.

Burton, J. (1999). When your patient is postpartum. *American Journal of Nursing, 99*(2), 64–69.

Calhoun, M. (1985). The Vietnamese women: Health/illness attitudes and behaviors. *Health Care Women International, 6*(1), 61–72.

Cesta, T., & Falter, E. (1999). Case management: its value for staff nurses. *American Journal of Nursing, 99*(5), 48–51.

Coughlin, R. (1965). Pregnancy and childbirth in Vietnam. In D. Hart, P. Rapidhon, & R. Coughlin (Eds.), *Southeast Asian birth customs: Three studies in human reproduction* (pp. 207–270). New Haven, CT: Human Relations Area Files.

Dixon, E., & Park, R. (1990). Do patients understand written health information? *Nursing Outlook, 38*(6), 278–281.

Doak, C., Doak, L., & Root, J. (1995). Teaching patients with low literacy skills. *Nursing, 17*(10), 75–81.

Engelke, Z. (1999). Take-out education extends teaching. *Patient Education Management 6*(7), 78.

Feldman, S., Quinlivan, A., Williford, P., Bahnson, J., & Fleischer, A. (1994). Illiteracy and the readability of patient education materials. *North Carolina Medical Journal, 55*(7), 290–292.

Grosso, C., Barden, M., Henry C., & Vieau, M. (1981). The Vietnamese American family . . . and grandma makes three. *American Journal of Maternal Child Nursing, 6*(2), 177–180.

Hollingsworth, A., Brown, L., & Booten, D. (1980). The refugees and childbearing: What to expect. *RN 4*(1), 45–48.

Iacono, J., & Campbell, A. (1997). *Patient and Family Education: The compliance guide to the JCAHO Standards.* Marblehead, MA: Opus Communications, 25.

Joint Commission on the Accreditation of Healthcare Organizations (1998). *Comprehensive accreditation manual for hospitals,* Chicago: Author.

Knowles, M. (1970). *The modern practice of adult education: Andragogy vs. pedagogy.* New York: Association Press.

Kreigh, H., & Perko, J. (1979). *Psychiatric and mental health nursing: Commitment to care and concern* (pp. 74–77). Reston, VA: Reston Publishing.

Lester, N. (1998). Cultural Competence: A nursing dialogue. *American Journal of Nursing, 98*(9), 36–42.

Lindberg, J., Hunter, M., & Kruszewski, A. (1994). *Introduction to nursing: Concepts, issues, and opportunities* (2nd ed., pp. 229–231). Philadelphia: J. B. Lippincott.

London, F. (1999). *No Time to Teach.* Philadelphia: Lippincott Williams & Wilkins, 138–141.

Mager, R. (1997). *Preparing instructional objectives,* 3rd ed. Atlanta, GA: Center for Effective Performance, Inc.

Marchiondo, K., & Kipp, C., (1987). Establishing a standardized patient educating program. *Critical Care Nurse, 7*(3), 58–66.

McCaffery, M. (1994). How to use the new AHCPR cancer pain guidelines. *American Journal of Nursing, 94*(7), 42–46.

McLaughlin, G. (1969). SMOG grading: A new readability formula. *Journal of Reading, 12*(8), 639–646.

Muscari, M. (1998). Coping with chronic illness. *American Journal of Nursing, 98*(9), 20–22.

National Cancer Institute. (1981). *Readability testing in cancer communications.* (NIH Publication No. 81–1689). Bethesda, MD: Cancer Information Clearinghouse.

Redman, B. (1993). Patient education at 25 years; where we have been and where we are going. *Journal of Advanced Nursing, 18*(8), 725–730.

Society of Teachers of Family Medicine (STFM, 1979). *Patient education: A handbook for teachers.* Kansas City, MO: Author.

Spector, R. (1996). *Cultural Diversity in Health and Illness.* Stanford, CT: Appleton & Lange.

Stallings, K. (1996). *Integrating patient education in your nursing practice.* [Video]. Reproduced with permission of GlaxoWellcome, Inc. (Produced by Horizon Video Productions, 4222 Emperor Boulevard, Durham, NC 27703.

U.S. Department of Agriculture, Office of Information. (1988). *Guidelines: Writing for adults with limited reading skills.* Washington, D.C.: Author.

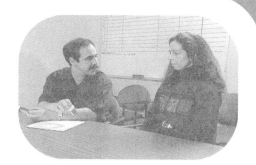

11

Patient Education Resources

on the Internet

Karen S. Zeliff

LEARNING OBJECTIVES

After reading this chapter, the nurse or student nurse should be able to:

1. Describe the three components of a successful Internet search.

2. Describe the communication resources available on the Internet (eg, e-mail, mail lists, newsgroups, chat rooms, video conferencing) and their potential use in patient education.

3. Describe the information resources available on the Internet (eg, search and metasearch engines, subject and review subject directories, databases) and the types of questions these resources can answer.

4. Apply a 10-step search planning and implementation process to locate educational and self-help resources for alternative therapies.

5. Identify six criteria for evaluating the quality of Internet information.

INTRODUCTION

Created in the late 1960s by the Department of Defense (Howe, 1999), the Internet has evolved from a tool designed to safeguard American intelligence secrets into a tool that has ushered in an information age that was, until recently, only imagined in science fiction.

The Internet has grown into a vast and unique publishing tool, offering access to information in multiple formats, from multiple resources from multiple locations in a customizable and in a nonlinear manner that provides the user with both novel opportunities and challenges for information retrieval. Although the aura of chaos that currently pervades Internet publishing sometimes makes retrieving selective and relevant information difficult, continued efforts by librarians, archivists, commercial vendors, and government agencies to organize and classify Internet resources help this medium realize its potential as a unique educational tool. The interaction among people and the resources available on the Internet provides an opportunity for self-directed learning that is not replicated by any other medium. The Internet is both an information resource and a potential educational medium that can be used independently or in tandem with other teaching methodologies. The strategies for locating quality health and medical information on the Internet outlined in this chapter, although primarily directed at the patient educator, can be applied to self-directed learning by the patient, or by any person involved at any level in the delivery of healthcare.

The Internet: A Tool for Patient Education

Managed care is shifting the focus of health care away from disease management and toward disease prevention. Thus, greater personal responsibility by each person for his or her own positive health outcomes is also a focus. The Internet facilitates this by providing access to many resources that help empower the person to take an active role in maintaining physical well-being. The Internet has both mirrored (and been partially responsible for) the shift from *passive patients* to *informed consumers*.

Tom Ferguson, MD, of the Center for Clinical Computing, Harvard Medical School, and author of *Health Online: How to Find Health Information, Support Groups and Self-Help Communities in Cyberspace,* notes that online consumers "want their doctor to be a colleague, not an authority, a consultant, not a parental figure" (Ferguson, 1996). This shift in perspective has affected the relationships that physicians, nurses, and other clinicians develop with their patients. Informed health consumers no longer look solely to their physicians for health advice, passively following instructions with little information and even less questioning. Informed health consumers expect to be active partners in resolving their health care problems. Organizations, such as the Health Commons Institute, seek to increase the use of computer technology to promote informed, shared decision-making in patient-centered healthcare (Health Commons Institute, 1999).

Informed consumers believe that their personal health outcomes are improved by shared decision-making. They seek to engage in informed interactions not only with their physician, but with nurses, social workers, and other people who can add to their knowledge about a health care issue. They consult people from different clinical disciplines and backgrounds and lay persons, many who are themselves experienced health consumers. Frequently, these active health consumers bring information derived from one of these alternative resources to their health caregivers, pointing out alternative therapies and asking that the information be integrated into their treatment (Table 11-1).

With millions of adults turning to the Internet for health and medical information each year (Miller, & Reents, 1998), physicians, nurses, and health educators must accurately access the quality of information delivered through the medium. Professionals in the health care industry think that the rapid growth of the Internet and the lack of quality control of Internet information will lead to the spread

TABLE 11-1. Internet Health and Medical Information Searches*

ONLINE HEALTH TOPIC	(%) SEARCHING ON TOPIC
• Diseases	• 52
— Cancer	— 18
— Heart Disease	— 14
• Diet & Nutrition	• 36
• Pharmaceuticals	• 33
• Health Newsletters	• 32
• Women's Health	• 31
• Fitness	• 29
• Children's Health	• 15
• Illness Support Groups	• 13

*Percentage of 22 million adult Internet health/medical searchers who searched on specific topics

Source: July 1998 Cyber Dialogue Study

http://www.cyberdialogue.com/pdts/whitepapes/intel.pdf

of misinformation, with potential negative effects. This concern is valid given the rapid growth of the Internet. Recent surveys of Internet use suggest that there are more than 179 million users worldwide and that the rate of increase is almost 4% per month (NUA Internet Surveys, 1999). With more than 6 million sites (Netcraft Web Server Surveys, 1999) providing millions of different documents online, there are legitimate concerns about the quality of the information.

The *Journal of the American Medical Association* (JAMA) published an article that described the Internet as a "cocktail conversation rather than a tool for effective health care communication and decision-making" with "vast chunks of incomplete, misleading or inaccurate" information (Silberg, Lundberg, & Musacchio, 1997). Although the Internet has provided misinformation with serious consequences (Weisbord, Soule, & Kimmel, 1997), it also was critical to life-saving treatments (Dearlove, Sharples, & Stone, 1997). Although some studies indicate the lack of quality of much of the medical information available on the Internet (Impicciatore, Pandolfini, Casella, & Bonati, 1997; McClung, Murray, & Heitlinger, 1998), scant clinical evidence exists to indicate

that this has had a serious negative impact on public health outcomes.

Internet searching by patients, health care consumers, and health providers is increasing steadily into a tide that cannot be stymied, even to the point, as some suggest, of radically transforming the delivery of health care (Kassirer, 1995). The challenge for patient educators is to take advantage of the opportunities for consumer and patient education afforded by the Internet, but simultaneously reduce the potential damage of erroneous information. Dr. Frank Sonnenberg, University of Medicine and Dentistry of New Jersey, Robert Wood Foundation (Princeton, NJ), suggests three approaches to incorporating the Internet into health care:

1. Health providers and educators can develop their own Internet resources to point patients to reliable information.
2. Health providers can advocate for endorsement of sites by professional organizations.
3. Health providers can adapt to their new role as intermediary between patients and Internet information (Sonnenberg, 1997).

Many health professionals have followed Sonnenberg's first two recommendations, and the Internet is replete with authoritative resources generated and compiled by qualified professionals. Many government agencies and professional associations are stepping forward to develop guidelines and quality standards for Internet communication and information resources (Jadad & Gagliand, 1998; Kane & Sands, 1998). To be an effective *Internet intermediary* and prevent the proliferation of misinformation, health practitioners and educators must become *discriminating information searchers*. They must know where to locate authoritative information on the Internet, understand which of these resources are appropriate for use under which circumstances, and accurately evaluate the quality of information published. This will enable them not only to guide their patients to information that will enhance their health and well-being, but also to allow them to maximize the vast potential of the Internet for their own professional development and lifelong learning.

The Internet is a unique hybrid of many other information technologies, and it is developing at an accelerated rate. Using it effectively requires that skills used to retrieve information from more traditional resources be adapted to meet the particular requirements of this new medium, and that these skills continued to be modified in response to the rapidly changing context of the Internet.

The Information Retrieval Process

Although searching for information on the Internet or World Wide Web may be new to many people, searching for information is not. Although information needs vary widely from person to person, most people of all ages and educational backgrounds are adept at finding information to meet their primary information needs. They all initiate and complete a process that consists of three general steps that may be comprised of many supporting actions. The three steps in the *information retrieval process* are 1) definition, 2) searching, and 3) evaluation.

Definition

What do I need to know, and where is the best place to find the answer?

The person defines an information need, generally in the form of a question that needs to be answered, before proceeding with an activity or meeting an objective. The person then determines, based on personal experience, the most likely resource that will answer the information needed. Having defined the need and selected the most likely resource for answering that need, the person proceeds to the second step of information retrieval, the searching phase.

Searching

How do I use the resource I have selected to find the information I need?

Each person determines the best way to utilize the selected resource to answer the information need. He or she may adjust searching strategies repeatedly if retrieved answers do not satisfy their information need. He or she may even return to step one and investigate another source of information based on their inability to develop an effective strategy for retrieving information from the originally selected source.

Once a successful strategy for retrieving the information from a selected source has been developed, the information seeker proceeds to step three, evaluation.

Evaluation

Does this information adequately answer my information need?

The information is reviewed by the information seeker and judged for its quality, by applying criteria based upon satisfaction rates that are predetermined (often implicitly) by the searcher. If, however, the results of the information retrieval process are unsatisfactory, the person may go back to any previous step in the process, redefining the information need, looking for a new resource, attempting a new search strategy, or, even determining that the need for information is not worth additional effort and simply discontinuing the quest.

APPLYING THE INFORMATION RETRIEVAL PROCESS TO THE INTERNET

It is possible to apply the information retrieval process to locating information on the Internet. The definition stage requires an ability to determine where to look on the Internet for solutions to different types of information problems. The second stage in the process is to develop a strategy that can be applied to retrieve applicable information quickly and efficiently from these different tools. Stage three of the information retrieval process, evaluation, is completed by establishing criteria that can be used to judge the quality of information retrieved from sites and documents on the Internet.

Defining Internet Resources: Knowing Where to Look for Patient Education Information

Internet health and medical resources can be categorized as one of two types: tools that are primarily used for communication, and tools that are primarily used for data storage and retrieval. *Communication tools* consist of e-mail, mailing lists, newsgroups, and chat rooms. The two major *information tools* for retrieving resources on the World Wide Web are *subject directories* and *search engines,* both of which retrieve data generally indexed by keyword. These two primary Web information tools are comprised of subsets, *review* (or focused subject) directories and *metasearch* engines. The newest resource on the Web is a hybrid called a portal site, which is comprised of a customizable combination of both search engines and directories. Although not truly a Web resource, no discussion of quality health and medical information would be complete without mentioning the information available through proprietary databases that do not index Web sites, but index other selective resources (like peer-reviewed journals) and provide access to these databases through a Web interface. Each of these tools is distinguishable not only by its operational structure, but by its types of information and how it can be used as a patient education tool.

Communication Tools

Internet communication tools come in two formats: asynchronous and synchronous. People who communicate asynchronously with one another via e-mail, mail lists, and newsgroups do so during separate times. Synchronous or real-time communication occurs over the Internet by using chat or web conferencing.

Electronic Mail (E-mail)

E-mail is one of the oldest Internet communication tools and generally represents the first exposure most people have to the Internet. Many users begin communicating with family, friends, and coworkers via the Internet and then begin to branch out to communication with strangers with common interests.

Healtheon Corporation's most recent Internet Survey of Medicine, an ongoing research project to track the computer needs of more than 10,000 physicians reports that 33% of physicians have used e-mail to communicate with patients, a 200% increase in just the past year (CyberAtlas, 1999). This survey contrasts a study conducted in the previous year that assessed physician responses to unsolicited patient e-mail requests for medical advice; it showed that the physicians studied were frequently reluctant and ambivalent about how to respond to a fictitious inquiry despite its clearly urgent, emergency medical nature (Eysenbach & Diepgen, 1998a). The study suggested that some of the reasons physicians were unsure about responding to patient e-mail inquiries was potential volume of e-mail inquiries and a subsequent increased workload, fear of liability for incorrect diagnosis, and worries about confidentiality and security issues. Although guidelines have recently been suggested for physician-patient e-mail correspondence, they have yet to make provision for inquiries outside the traditional patient-physician relationship (Kane & Sands, 1998).

Although physicians may hesitate to interact with their patients by e-mail, the same does not hold true for the patients. A study on patient and family requests for advice from health care providers publishing over the Web found patients eager to consult providers by e-mail to solicit second opinions on medical advice or to ask for a referral (Wideman & Tong, 1997). The study also indicated that patients could make appropriate decisions about whom to ask for information. As both health providers and patients become more familiar with e-mail and as more guidelines are set and adopted to govern questions of e-mail legitimacy and liability, access to providers and other clinical staff by e-mail will eventually evolve into a consumer demand that will drive the market.

The ability for physicians, nurse practitioners, and patients to use e-mail to interact with one another may soon be seen as an enhancement to practice, allowing them to communicate with their patients at greater convenience to all, adding electronic communication with their patients directly into the medical record, making some office visits obsolete, and generally improving the provider-patient relationship.

Mail Lists and Listserves

Mail lists and listserves are communication exchanges that occur via an e-mail medium among many people with a common interest. Mail lists are available for almost every imaginable health and medicine related subject or specialty. For example, PatEdNet, a restricted mail list for professional patient educators, is available by inquiry at *patednet@hsc.utah. edu.* Online subscription to 16 mail lists or online bulletin boards especially focused on the needs of Nurse Practitioners is available from NP Central (*http: //www.nurse.net*).

Mail lists foster a sense of community for patients and broaden their networks for self-help and support. Mail lists allow people to participate in person-to-person conversation with various people, providing a wide spectrum of perspectives and information on topics that relate to their particular health care issue or interest. Patients can frequently ask questions, share confidences, or solicit and receive caring support in a way that may not always be available from family, friends, or their personal health providers. Mail lists represent dialogue that is frequently intimate, but not personal to the degree of a direct post to an individual mailbox.

These lists encourage the breakdown of barriers between patients and health providers. Physicians who would not respond to their own patients via e-mail will advise in a more general, consulting capacity, to a group of subscribers on a listserve. Likewise, informed patients, who feel intimidated sharing concerns and doubts about treatment with their personal physicians, will not hesitate to engage a physician online with direct and pointed questions. This community of patients and clinicians, bonded together by shared experiences, provides unique opportunities for sharing specific and personal information. Also, this community is an outlet for expressions of grief, suffering, concern, and compassion. Two

of the most well known compilations of mail lists are Tile Net (*http: //www.tile.net*) and Liszt (*http: //www.listz.com*), which provide information on more than 66,000 lists.

Newsgroups

The biggest difference between a mail list and a newsgroup is that messages are not automatically sent to individual members' e-mail addresses daily; thus, they have the advantage of not requiring personal management of the sometime large quantity of postings that are submitted to the mail lists. One of the longest established and complete database of newsgroups can be found at Deja.com (*http://www. deja. com/usenet*).

Newsgroups, because of their broader distribution, lack some of the intimacy of mail lists. However, they remain a unique source for information. They are perhaps most useful for the value in providing a forum for grassroots opinions. For example, you could find a general discussion by well-informed consumers on the merits of a particular breakthrough in medical research or a recent healthcare bill in Congress on a newsgroup. A newsgroup would be the place to visit to get a wide variety of opinions and to post your own. The broader range of input from a more diverse population is possible in a newsgroup, which, unlike listserves, does not require subscription before posting. In 1995, one researcher took advantage of the ability of newsgroups to reach, easily and inexpensively, a vast population around the globe by piloting a medical research study using two Usenet newsgroups (Engstrom, 1997). Although the data collected admittedly reflected a bias in the study group, it had the advantage not only of reaching a large and yet selective study population, but also enabled data to be collected and results published in 2 months.

Internet Relay Chat (Chat or Chat Rooms)

One of the most popular forms of Internet synchronous communication is Internet Relay Chat (IRC), more universally known as *chat* or *chat rooms*. Because conversations are live, it is much easier to accomplish a conversational dialogue with another user than it is via e-mail or newsreaders. This medium also has the advantage of promoting intimacy and anonymity. Scheduled chats (as opposed to channels that are open to a casual lurker) in which a group of people gather at a specific time to simultaneously discuss a particular issue, can offer a unique opportunity for animated and informative discussions.

Chat is becoming more acceptable as an adjunct to other types of educational formats for teachers, presenters, or authors to be available for specific times to lead or facilitate groups in chat discussions. The primary disadvantage to this communication medium is that the discussion is not monitored and is prone to conversations that can be off-topic, monopolizing, or even distracting.

Web Videoconferencing

A relative newcomer to synchronous communication is Web videoconferencing. Special cameras and software allow a user on one computer to receive a live sound and video broadcast from another computer simultaneously. Online whiteboards allow the users to share documents and collaborate directly on materials while maintaining the online connection. Videoconferencing applications in the future will hold the potential not only for tele-education over distance between patient and educator, but for telehealth between a provider and a remote patient.

Information Tools

The unique capabilities of hypertext markup language (HTML) or hypertext links for information dispersal via the easy-to-use graphical interface of the World Wide Web, provide a mixed blessing for information searchers. Because publication to the Web is both easy and fast, the amount of information is increasing by thousands of Web pages daily, creating potentially better access for patients to more current and in-depth information. Simultaneously, this proliferation of information on the Internet can be difficult for searchers who must filter and evaluate more material in the quest for accurate and relevant information on a specific topic.

Two of the primary types of organizational tools designed to help users with the explosion of information on the World Wide Web are:

1. **Subject directories.** These directories are sometimes referred to as indexes or libraries. These also are reviewed (or rated) subject directories.
2. **Search engines** and the subcategory metasearch engines

The primary difference between subject directories and search engines can be described in terms of recall versus relevancy. *Recall* is the process of gathering the total number of documents on a particular topic. *Relevancy* is the process of gathering relevant documents on a particular topic. The index of a search engine is created mechanically and therefore tends to provide more recall than relevancy. Subject directory indexes are created by humans, and therefore tend to provide more relevancy in their retrieval than do search engines. Previously, it was easier to determine the difference between search engines and subject directories. Currently a marriage between the two exists, and most indexing sites have both. Still, it is useful to know the difference to assess and evaluate the results of search retrieval (Fig. 11-1).

Search Engines

Search engines use mechanical software programs that visit Web pages on a routine basis. These programs collect data for each page in a huge database, break down the content into an index organized by keywords, move on to follow links attached to the page, and then initiate the process again.

The success of a search depends on three factors: creating exact matches between terms searched and terms used in the documents you want to find; the size and contents of the database; and its features for searching its contents successfully.

A complex search, with highly specific terms and multiple concepts, requires a search engine. Determining which search engine to use varies according to the nature of the question and the specific features needed to refine or

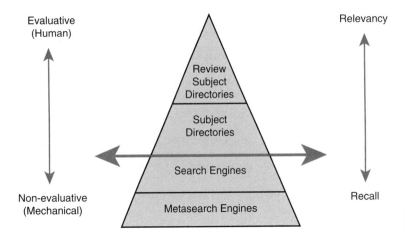

FIGURE 11-1. The search tool structure for the World Wide Web.

focus your search. Every search engine is different and varies according to size of the database, currency of database, search features, and indexing components. To ensure a greater degree of reliability in search results, it is recommended that users become familiar with at least three general search engines with varying capacities and features, and replicate their searches in each of them.

Metasearch Engines

Metasearch engines allow a single query string to be sent to several search engine databases simultaneously, retrieving a listing of top-ranked listings from each source. Metasearch engines, because they search multiple databases, are generally limited to simple and straightforward searches. They are most useful for finding "needles in haystacks" (ie, information that can be described by a distinctive word or name, but also unlikely to be found in many resources). Metasearch engines can give a quick overview of the kind of retrieval likely to be found in several sources and can lead to the places most likely to provide you with hard-to-locate information (Table 11-2).

Subject Directories

Subject directories, indexes, or electronic libraries represent a human effort to organize Web sites into categories by subject content.

Although subject directories may begin with mechanical retrieval from a Web search engine, they usually require some further filtering according to specific indexing schemes.

Although a comprehensive search requires a search engine, the smaller size of a subject directory, generally sorted to eliminate sites that refer to the subject in only a limited way, can provide quick and easy access to primary, well-known sites on a particular topic. Many health and medical related subject directories provide general overviews of health information and are good starting points to look for in-depth information. Many of these sites list links to medical information or handouts that are geared to the understanding of patients and health consumers.

Review Subject Directories

A review subject directory further filters and refines a subject directory. Not only are listings on these websites indexed and displayed by subject, but they are frequently evaluated by specific criteria. For example, a review subject directory may rank sites according to the criteria of clinical applicability or appropriateness for use by a particular population of health providers or patients.

If your question is *What is the best information on this topic?* then a review subject directory of sites selected by a recognized authority on the given topic is recommended.

TABLE 11-2. Metasearch Engines

NAME	ADDRESS (URL)
All-in-one-Search	www.allonesearch.com
Ask Jeeves	www.askjeeves.com
Dogpile	www.dogpile.com
Highway 61	www.highway61.com
Inference Find	www.inferencefind.com/infind
Internet Sleuth	www.isleuth.com
Mama	www.mama.com
Metacrawler	www.metacrawler.com
Profusion	www.profusion.com
SavvySearch	www.savvysearch.com

A review of each of these metasearch engines is provided by Cnet's SearchEngine Shootout at: *http://home.cnet.com/category/topic/0,10000,0-3817-7-276933,00.html*

Directing a patient to a medical review subject directory is probably the most reliable method of assuring quality Internet information content on a general topic, because the reviewers of these sites pay particular attention to identifying and verifying the accuracy of these sources of information (Table 11-3).

Portal Sites

Portal sites are newer types of Internet search tools. They represent a marriage of subject directory, search engine, newsreader, bulletin board, chat room, and even e-mail. Some of the best know portal sites are Yahoo!'s *My Yahoo* and Netscape's *My Netscape*. *My Health-AtoZ* is a recently developed healthcare-based portal site.

Proprietary Health Information Databases

Many resources provide access to proprietary content information, or databases. Although not technically part of the Internet or the Web, they are accessible from a graphical Web browser and server. These databases have a customer-friendly Web browser interface, but their information is self-contained and is accessible only by use of an internal searching program or mechanism. These databases are not accessible by general Web search engines, and they use retrieval programs specific to their database. These databases are generally restricted for use by authorized subscribers who may or may not pay a fee for access.

Because each searching tool retrieves and

TABLE 11-3. Health/Medical Subject & Review Directories

NAME	ADDRESS (URL)	DESCRIPTION
CliniWeb	www.ohsu.edu/cliniweb	Searches in 5 languages and by MeSH headings. Retrieves information found in PubMed.
Harden Meta Directory	www.arcade.uiowa.edu/hardin/med.htm	Large listing of health sites selected for consistent connectivity.
Health A–Z	www.healthAtoZ.com	Consumer health site maintained by health professionals.
HealthFinder	www.healthfinder.org	Produced by U.S. government—organized using lay language.
Healthwise Knowledge base	www.betterhealth.com	More than 30,000 listings. Provides expert advice from physicians and nurses.
Medhunt	www.hon.ch	Sponsored by Health on the Net Foundation; targets information for patients, professionals, physicians.
Medical Matrix	www.medmatrix.org	Sponsored by the AMIA; sites selected for clinical applicability.
Medical World Search	www.mwsearch.com	Designed primarily for medical field. Uses MeSH headings.
MedicineNet	www.medicinenet.com	Doctor-produced consumer health information.
Omni	www.omni.ac.uk/	Highly edited resources indexing medical information from the United Kingdom.
Oncolink	www.oncolink.com	Produced by the University of Pennsylvania Cancer Center. Comprehensive listing of resources on cancer.
Six Senses Review	www.sixsenses.com/	Reviews directory of rated sites designed for medical professionals.
Yahoo Health	health.yahoo.com	Popular listing of sites, plus chats and "ask an expert".

TABLE 11-4. Guide to Selecting Search Tools	
INFORMATION NEED	**INFORMATION TOOL**
I want a broad overview of a topic.	Subject directory
I don't know where to begin to look for an obscure topic.	Metasearch engine
I have a complex search question that requires linking a number of concepts.	WWW Search engines that permit Boolean searching.
I want to meet/talk with people online.	Internet relay chat
I want to read discussions on current events.	News reader
I want a few relevant resources from sources I can trust.	Review subject directory
I want to find the e-mail address of a friend.	Database of people
I want to find information that occurred on a specific date.	WWW Search engine that limits by date.
I want to discuss professional issues with a small group of people in my field.	Monitored listserve
I want to locate information in another language.	WWW Search engine that limits by language.

displays data in a different manner, each tool is useful for locating different types of information. The type of question to be answered should determine the type of site selected for finding information. Table 11-4 lists the types of information needs that can best be met by a particular resource.

Searching for Internet Information Resources: Knowing How to Retrieve Information

The second step in the information retrieval process is to use the selected search tool effectively. One must identify the nature and scope of the information question, and specific techniques for retrieving information from each of the tools.

Equipped with an understanding of the types of information resources available on the Internet, and a general knowledge of which search tool can be used with each type of resource, the informed searcher is ready to define a process for extracting the particular information needed. The biggest barrier to effective information retrieval by the inexperienced searcher is not the quantity or organization of information, but it is the failure to adequately plan a searching strategy. One needs to spend time thinking about the specific information needs of the individual patient and the most likely method to pursue answers. To maximize time and effectiveness of searching it is necessary to take some time initially to query the patient, determine the type and format of information needed, and to plan and develop a strategy for searching.

A 10-step information retrieval process can bring a searcher more satisfactory results in a more timely manner (Fig. 11-2). Although this process is applicable to most queries on an Internet-based searching tool, it is easiest to understand this process in relation to searches conducted on a general Web search engine. For that reason, the 10-step process is presented as it applies to a general purpose search engine. The clinical scenarios at the end of the chapter are illustrative of a search in that type of tool.

Step 1—Define the Problem Statement

The information retrieval process always begins with an information need, in response to an information problem, which is stated in the form of a single question. Although this may state the obvious, few people consciously and specifically define what it is they hope to discover on the Internet. Many people begin a search without realizing that they are looking for answers to many interrelated questions,

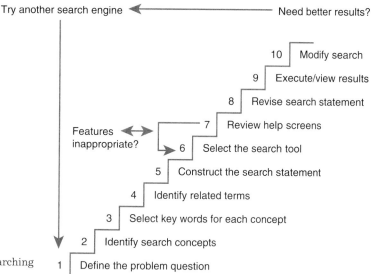

10 Steps to Effective Searching

Try another search engine ◄──────────── Need better results?

10	Modify search
9	Execute/view results
8	Revise search statement
7	Review help screens

Features ◄──► inappropriate?

6	Select the search tool
5	Construct the search statement
4	Identify related terms
3	Select key words for each concept
2	Identify search concepts
1	Define the problem question

FIGURE 11-2. Ten steps to effective searching on the Internet.

some of which are better answered by one source than another and some of which have answers that build upon or redirect other questions. For example, a patient may ask a nurse for information that would help him or her understand a diabetes diagnosis better. Rather than searching on the single word *diabetes,* the nurse would query the patient further about his or her information needs and add more details to the search statement based on the need to know about treatment, prognosis, genetic origins, or factors related to the patient's age, gender, or race.

Developing a good searching statement that translates into an effective machine-readable query involves defining these generalized information needs into a series of single, clear, and unambiguous statements.

Step 2—Identify Search Concepts

Once a single problem statement has been defined, it should be further refined into discreet concepts. Clarify any ambiguity that may exist in each concept. For example, if one seeks information on acquired immunodeficiency syndrome (AIDS), would additional words or con-

cepts in a problem statement help distinguish between the effects of human immunodeficiency virus (HIV), teaching aids, hearing aids, or nursing aids? Would a query be better served using "drug therapy" as a single concept or by combining the two individual concepts "drug" and "therapy"? Because word order may be significant in the interpretation of concepts, be sure to list concepts in order of their importance when defining the overall search statement.

Step 3—Select Key Words for Each Concept

After determining the concepts that define the search statement, and placing them in order of importance, specific key words or phrases for each concept should be defined. A key word is a term that would most likely be used to identify a particular concept in an index. When trying to identify a site that would discuss "childhood diseases" that occur "between birth and 6 years" should we select the key word child? Children? What about infant? Baby? Newborn? Preschooler? What about pediatric or pediatrics? Although some health and medical sites will provide a browsable cross-referenced thesaurus of index terms (for example, Clini-Web — *http://www.ohsu.edu/cliniweb* — uses National Library of Medicine (NLM) Medical Subject Headings), it may be difficult to determine exactly which terms will be selected for use by most sites in their texts or by most subject directories in their indexes. When in doubt about which key words to use, repeated efforts may be needed to locate the search terms most likely to return relevant results. To plan for the need to select alternative words, complete the fourth step in this process.

Step 4 — Identify Related Terms

After selecting the best key words to define each search concept, evaluate each term to determine if synonyms or related terms exist that may be used by some search tools to define the concept. If initial attempts to apply the primary key words fail to render quality results, a searcher may substitute one or more synonyms or related terms into their search string with perhaps better results. Many search tools allow truncation or wildcard symbols (see Step 7) to be used to retrieve many words with a common root stem or words for which spelling is uncertain.

Step 5 — Construct the Search Statement

Once key words and related words have been selected, construct a search statement that can be placed in a search window as a search string. Constructing the search statement consists of:

1. Selecting the key words (eg, *diabetes, adolescence, drug therapy*)
2. Ranking the key words according to priority and degree of relevance (eg, 1. *diabetes*, 2. *drug therapy*, 3. *adolescence*)
3. Grouping the key words systematically according to the principles of the logic applied to the search mechanism (eg, using Boolean logic: *diabetes* AND *drug therapy* AND *adolescence*)

The traditional information retrieval algorithm used by search engines has been Boolean

logic. Boolean logic uses the operators *AND, OR,* and *NOT* to combine terms and establish a relationship between terms. This system functions effectively in a database (eg, *Medline*) when it is used within a limited data set that is indexed using a controlled vocabulary. One of the difficulties of understanding Boolean operators is that they are counterintuitive to the manner in which we usually use these terms. In general usage, the word *OR* is an excluder and the word *AND* is an excluder (Fig. 11-3).

Step 6 — Select the Search Tool

If a search statement has been defined carefully, it is relatively easy to discern what type of Internet tool should be queried to deliver the appropriate response to the query.

If the statement is simple and comprised of one or two general keywords, a subject directory is the best place to begin a search. There are many health and medical subject directories to begin collecting information for patient education. Many of these subject listings also have search engines, which allow the searcher to retrieve sites collected on the site directory based on key word searching. If a search is complex, requiring linking of multiple synonyms or concepts, a search engine would be required. Well-known and effective search engines include Hotbot.Lycos, Altavista, and Infoseek.

Step 7 — Review the Help or Tips Screens

A common mistake of novice searchers is to immediately apply the search statement they have created in Step 4 to the search engine they selected in Step 5 without reviewing the *Help* or *Tips* screen. Even the experienced searcher should review the Help screens frequently, because database search tools evolve rapidly. Help screens give tips and strategies accompanied by examples that can provide clues to searching characteristics or capabilities that are unique to the specific search tool. Although subject directories and proprietary databases generally have their own unique searching syn-

Boolean Operators

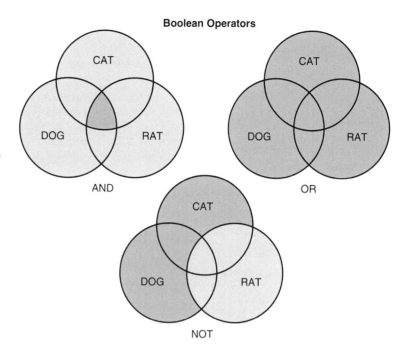

FIGURE 11-3. Boolean logic used for Internet search strings. The Boolean *OR* means one wants to retrieve *anything* on *either* cats OR dogs OR rats. In other words, a retrieval of *all* sites which contain *any* of those words. Boolean *AND* is not, as in natural language, an inclusive term. In Boolean logic the *AND* is an excluder. It requires that *only* those sites, which contain *all* of the terms (cats, dogs, and rats), should be in the retrieval. The Boolean operator *NOT* is a more selective excluder. It means those sites which include the specific search term should be eliminated from the retrieval. In other words, retrieval would be the set of all sites that include discussions of both cats and dogs, but not sites that also discussed rats.

tax, some elements are common to most of the primary Web search engines (Box 11-1).

Step 8 — Revise the Search Statement

A key to effective searching is to apply and execute the features and syntax rules that are specific to the individual search engine design. Having reviewed the help screens of the search tool selected for your query (and having noted particular features it uses to retrieve data sets), return to the search statement created in Step 4 and revise it appropriately. It may even be appropriate, based upon the nature of your search and the features provided by the search engine help screens, to return to Step 5 and select a different search engine.

Step 9 — Execute Search and Review Results

Once the search has been executed, review the results. Some worthwhile hits should occur within the first 10 sites listed in the retrieval.

If this is not the case, return to Step 6, review the searching tips again, revise the search statement, and execute the search again. If the search fails again to retrieve the desired results, return to Step 5 and follow the process through the remaining steps with another search engine.

Step 10 — Modify Search or Execute Search in Another Database

Because of the differences in search mechanics, in which sites they have indexed in their database, and in the currency of the indexing, no two search engines will ever retrieve identical data sets. If first efforts do not provide the desired answer, or if a need exists for more comprehensiveness in the search results, return to Step 5 and replicate the search in another search engine. A good rule of thumb: Learn the features and syntax commands of three search engines well and use these first for your search. Expand to other search engines after you become familiar and can monitor the changes of the original three.

BOX 11-1.   Common Search Engine Syntax Strategies

Use quotation marks around phrases or proper names of more than one word. Many search engines default to a Boolean OR. That means that if you simply key in "breast cancer," the search engine will interpret the statement as breast OR cancer, retrieving all of the sites that contain the word breast and include them with all the sites that contain the word cancer—regardless of what type or in what context. Placing quotation marks around the terms cues the search engine to search just for the occurrence of "breast cancer" as a phrase, with the terms taken together as a single concept.

Select search terms carefully and use the most uncommon and specific terms that will describe your topic. Common words produce far to many results. For example, if you were looking for information on how to prevent heart disease, instead of searching on the terms *heart* and *disease* and *prevention* better results might be retrieved by searching for the phrase *low-cholesterol diets.* The more terms you can combine to describe the topic, the more restricted the search results will be.

Substitute a plus sign (+) for the Boolean operator AND and a minus sign (−) for the

Boolean AND NOT. Many search engines either use these characters as substitutes for the Boolean operators or allow them to be included as alternatives to require that the word appear (+) or not appear (−) in the retrieval.

Use nesting when using multiple Boolean operators. Search engines that permit long Boolean strings sometimes permit the use of ( ) parenthesis to indicate "nesting" which instructs the search engine to conduct certain Boolean operations before others.

Use capitalization as necessary. Most words should be capitalized if they would normally occur in that matter in most written texts.

Truncation and Wildcards. Most search engines allow the use of a special character (usually an asterisk *) to permit searching for words that have the same prefix. For example, by typing in "inform,*" you can call up pages containing the word "informatics," "information," etc. Questions about correct spellings of words can sometimes be resolved by placing wildcard characters (such as a # or ? sign) in the center of word to retrieve all possible spellings. For example, searching for a proper name G###er would retrieve Gunter, Garner, Grover, etc.

Evaluating Internet Resources: Knowing What Information Is Appropriate

Equipped with an understanding of Internet search tools and how to plan a search strategy that ensures those tools are used effectively, it should be possible to generate a listing of Internet resources that will be potentially useful in answering a specific query. Many of these resources are reliable and authoritative. Others are biased, inaccurate, and may even be deliberately misleading. This bias could provide the opportunity for misinformation, po-tentially causing harm to those who are using the Internet to locate health and medical information. It is essential that all Internet users become adept at critically evaluating the quality of information retrieved from this new resource. How does a discriminating information searcher know the difference?

Many groups (eg, Consumer and Health Evaluation Informatics Working Group of the American Medical Informatics Association) are committed to help both health providers and consumers determine the quality of Internet information. One of these efforts, sponsored in part by grant funding from the Agency for

Health Care Policy and Research, was the convening of a Health Summit Working Group comprised of healthcare providers, librarians, Website developers from health-related organizations, and the general public (Health Summit Working Group, 1997). Three Health Summit Meetings were held at the Health Information Technology Institute of Mitretek Systems, Inc. (McLean, VA) between 1996 and 1998 to develop a set of criteria for assessing the quality of information delivered over the Internet. With their ultimate goal the creation of an Internet tool to assist the general public in assessing the quality of Internet resources, the group developed a consensus on seven criteria necessary for assessing the quality of health information. Although creation and testing of this tool has not been completed, the criteria developed by the group for evaluating Internet Health Information provides an excellent blueprint for discussing the elements that determine quality on the Internet.

Criteria for Evaluation

Credibility

Given the lack of prepublication filters, determining the credibility of sources of medical information on the Internet is the most important factor in evaluating the quality of the information. To determine the quality of the source of information the user must ask: Who is publishing the information? What are the credentials for publishing the information? Are they providing information or advice that is beyond the scope of their expertise? What person(s) or organization is sponsoring the information? How well are they reviewing the material?

A quality Web site displays the name and biographical information of all authors. It also includes the names and qualifications of the sponsoring organization and criteria for publication. There should be disclosure of the relationship of the author(s) to the sponsoring organization to help the user determine motivation of sponsors and potential conflicts of interest.

Currency is another determiner of the cred-ibility of the source: When was the information originally published? When was it last updated? How relevant is the currency of the material to the topic being discussed? Because of advancements in the pharmaceutical industry, drug information should be current; currency is much less important on sites of more enduring natures (eg, those displaying anatomy information).

Content

Determining the accuracy of content on the Internet is often difficult to do and frequently requires the user to comparison search to validate accuracy. The user must ask:

How accurate is the information on the site? Is it replicated in other resources in other mediums? Can the facts be checked for accuracy and does the site provide links or descriptions of these resources? Are clear distinctions made between clinical or scientific evidence and conjecture or personal testimonials? What coverage of the topic does the site provide? Does it indeed provide what it purports to provide? Does it claim to provide comprehensive coverage of a subject but then fail to do so? Does the site provide a disclaimer that describes the limitations of information on the site?

All quality medical sites should provide a disclaimer that the material provided is for general information only, and that advice of a physician should be sought for authoritative information that relates to their specific issue.

Disclosure

The ability to easily determine the purpose of a site is a key to its quality.

Is the mission and purpose of the site clearly stated? Who is the intended audience of the site? Is the work written in a style that is not too simple or too complicated for the intended audience? Is the material free from bias? Does it promote a particular position that casts doubt on the objectivity of the material? If a site requires registration or other forms of collecting personal data about the site visitor, are the purposes for that information disclosed? Do statements attest to the confidentiality of information gathered in this fashion or does the site designate the manner in which the data will be used?

Links

Links are extensions of the original site, and therefore should be analyzed for their value in supporting the viewpoint demonstrated on the original sites. Do the links relate to the purpose and content of the site? Are criteria for links established and clear, supporting the content of the site? Is the person or persons responsible for link selection identified and are methods of contacting them provided? Are links clearly labeled within the context of the displaying site and is it easy to navigate back and forth between links? Are links described or annotated so viewers will have some idea of the nature of the linked site before following the link? Are site links maintained without a lot of dead links or links to outdated resources?

Design

The arrangement of information on an Internet site is often more important to the user's ability to access the information than it is in more traditional resources. Although the design and layout of the site do not determine the quality of the content, they affect the ability to access the information. Users should ask: Does the design facilitate the delivery of content and not distract from it? Does the page load quickly? Is it easy to navigate? Do all pages within the site refer to the primary pages so users can clearly identify the source of information? Is the site organized effectively for the intended audience and does it reflect a logical structure? Has the site been created to meet the technical and equipment needs of most intended users? Does the overall design contribute to the purpose of the site in terms of balance in graphics, text, and multimedia elements? If the site has extensive content, does it provide a mechanism for internal searching? Is there an internal search engine to help users locate selected information without browsing through many pages? Are links off of the page described or annotated?

Interactivity

Many sites have interactive features that contribute to their authority, accessibility, and scope. Are provisions made for contacting site content and/or developers by e-mail to offer comments or ask questions? Do sites provide mechanisms that allow for interactivity, or an exchange of information between site viewers (eg, discussion groups, forums, or chat rooms)? Can users customize the content or features they review, and if so, are methods used to profile the person clearly delineated? Are there options for use by people with hearing or seeing disabilities, viewers with low literacy levels, or foreign language users?

Evaluation at a Glance

A quick review of three components of every Web page—the header, body, and footer—can help the user evaluate the quality of the site. The *header* usually provides the logo or link to the institution creating the information and to any sponsoring organization. Opportunities for interactivity also should be clearly visible somewhere near the top of the document through e-mail, chat, or discussion links, as would any search engine, if available. The *footer* of the document generally provides information on the content author, the contact person for questions, the Website designer, and date of creation or revision of the document, and any disclaimer for the scope of the material. A cursory review of the *body* of the document should clearly identify its intended audience and the purpose of the site, and testify to the balance and appeal of its layout, organizational quality, and navigability.

Another quick check for quality is to use the *IQ: the Health Information Quality Assessment Tool* (*http: //hitiweb.mitretek.org/ iq/default.asp*). This Web-based, interactive tool was developed by the Health Summit Working Group to electronically assess any page to which it is directed.

Evaluating Materials for Patient Populations

Although the factors discussed may help evaluate the quality of the information presented in an Internet resource, determining that the information has been produced by a reputable authority and is both accurate and current still may not render it suitable for patient education purposes. The information also must be appropriate to meet the needs of the specific patient. Many sites maintain patient information handouts in a ready-to-print format (Table 11-5). But these must be further analyzed to determine if the individual patient can understand them. This is particularly important for patients with low literacy levels, patients with physical or mental disabilities, or patients from other cultural or ethnic backgrounds.

A great tool for quickly assessing the appropriateness of materials for a specific population is SAM—a suitability of materials instrument (Fig. 11-4) (Doak, Doak, & Root,

TABLE 11-5. Sites for Patient Education Information

NAME	ADDRESS (URL)	DESCRIPTION
ADAM	www.adam.com	Full color medical artwork. Illustrates 45+ surgeries.
AAFP - Health information for patients	www.aafp.org/family/patient.html	Includes self-care flowcharts, and education resources by topic.
AltaVista translation service	http://babelfish.altavista.com/cgibin/translate?	Translates documents into six languages.
Drug reference center	www.nursespdr.com/members/databse/content.html	Complete monographs on drugs.
Family health radio	www.fhradio.com	2 ½ minute audio presentations on health topics.
Health A–Z	www.healthAtoZ.com	Consumer health site maintained by health professionals.
Health answers	www.healthanswers.com	Sponsored by several healthcare associations. Newsletters, streaming video.
HealthFinder	www.healthfinder.org	Produced by U.S. government—offers reference service to the public. Fact sheets.
HealthTouch	www.healthtouch.com	Single-page patient education documents from professional organizations.
HealthWeb	www.uic.edu/depts/lib/health/hw/consumer	Strong emphasis on full text educational materials.
Healthwise Knowledgebase	www.betterhealth.com	More than 30,000 listings. Provides expert advice from physicians and nurses.
Intelehealth	www.intelihealth.com/IH/	Topical information by experts at Johns Hopkins.
Mayo Clinic health watch	www.mayohealth.org	Topical new items, experts.
MedicineNet	www.medicinenet.com	Doctor-produced consumer health information.
Medline plus	www.nlm.nih.gov/medlineplus/	Produced by NLM. Links to medical dictionaries, full-text resources.
Merck manual online	www.merck.com/pubs/mmanual/sections.htm	Full-text of the 1992 manual online.
NIDDK Digestive and diabetes disease briefs	www.niddk.nih.gov/health/health.htm	High quality fact sheets produced by National Institutes of Health.
OSU patient education materials	www.osu.edu/units/osuhosp/disclaim2.htm	Well formatted teaching guides.
Netwellness	www.netwellness.com	Links to clinical trials, physician referrals, and online textbooks.
NOAH	www.noah.cuny.edu	Material in Spanish. Strong mental health focus.
Peoples Book of Medical Tests	www.thriveonline.com/health/library/lookitup.html	Consumer information on test preparation, risks, results. Requires registration.
ThriveOnline	www.thriveonline.com	Interactive programs, fact sheets, article summaries, MDX health Digest, Consumer reports.

SAM (Suitability Assessment of Materials)

	Superior	Adequate	Not Suitable
CONTENT			
Content focused on a specific patient issue			
Scope limited to what can be absorbed			
Directed towards behaviors - not information			
Keypoints are reiterated and summarized			
LITERACY LEVEL			
Appropriate reading level (9th grade or below)			
Conversational writing style using active voice			
Common word vocabulary, no jargon			
Advanced Organizers (topic statements) precede new content			
GRAPHICS and MULTIMEDIA			
Illustrations and multimedia presentations are simple and relate to content			
No distracting elements are present			
All graphics and multimedia elements are explained by text			
Audio tones are of appropriate pitch and quality			
Video is of appropriate resolution and clarity			
Audio/video elements are brief and realistic			
LAYOUT			
Illustrations are adjacent to text			
Limited scrolling (two pages) occurs			
Layout compliments and does not distract from text			
White space is prevalent			
Hypertext is limited if used at all			
Type size is suitable for easy viewing			
Type is sufficiently varied to divide information into small, discrete sections			
LEARNING STIMULATION and MOTIVATION			
Opportunities for interaction are included			
Behavioral activities are modeled and subdivided into small "doable" segments			
CULTURAL APPROPRIATENESS			
Logic, language, experience present match patient			
Realistic portrayal of cultural images			
TOTALS			
SAM PERCENTAGE RATINGS			
35 to 50 points (70% - 100%)	X		
20 to 34 points (40% - 69%)		X	
0 to 19 points (0% - 39%)			X

Adapted from SAM, Suitability of Materials by C. Doak, L. Doak, and J. Root, (1996)
Teaching patients with low literacy skills. Philadelphia: Lippincott.

FIGURE 11-4. Suitability assessment of materials (SAM) tool. Each Internet or web page document is evaluated according to 25 factors. A value from 1 to 3 is recorded for each item, based upon a scale from 0 to 2, in which a rating of *Superior* receives two points; a rating of *Adequate,* one point; and a rating of *Not Suitable,* zero points. By this accounting, a perfect score of 50 points would equal an overall value of one hundred percent. Items on the rating scale that are not applicable receive a rating of N/A and the total possible number of points should be reduced by two for each N/A tabulated and percentages calculated accordingly.

1996). Developed from a Johns Hopkins School of Medicine project, SAM was originally designed to apply a numeric rating system to patient education text and illustrations. However, it also can be easily revised and adapted for multimedia and Internet-based resources.

The SAM scale should be used to determine the suitability of the material for a specific patient. For example, although patient education material may be written at a sixth-grade reading level, and thus suitable in that category for the average patient, it would still not be suitable for a patient who could not read at all. Another patient education material may be written in 12-point typeface and be acceptable for most patients. However, a patient with visual impairment may need at least a 16-point typeface. Video or audio clips that might enhance the education of the average patient, might be a hindrance to older patients or patients who need to digest information at a much slower pace.

USING THE INFORMATION RETRIEVAL PROCESS TO MEET YOUR PATIENT'S NEEDS

Patient educators should complete the following three techniques that can be applied to a specific patient's care:

1. Develop a general road map of the Internet so they can locate resources on a specific topic.
2. Become sufficiently familiar with the 10-step searching plan and techniques for narrowing down resources to specific, relevant educational materials.
3. Integrate a system of evaluation into materials review that will help assess the quality of the resource in terms that are specific to the patient's educational need.

Patient educators can use the Internet and the Information Retrieval Process to expand their knowledge about a particular condition or treatment that affects a patient; to retrieve materials they can integrate into their teaching; or to assist a patient with direct self-education.

Although the primary thrust of discussion in this chapter has been directed at patient educators who want to integrate the wealth of Internet information into the materials they develop for teaching, the Internet can also be used as a medium for direct patient education. For patients who are physically and mentally able to use computers, the Internet is a medium that can enhance educational motivation and provide a participative learning environment that can promote effective teaching strategies. The computer and an Internet connection can help patients meet learning objectives regardless of which area of learning outcomes are defined: knowledge, skills, attitudes or practices (KSAP) (Chatham, Hoffler, & Knapp, 1982). For example, occasionally a patient will need some additional information, facts, or concepts that can broaden an understanding of his or her health situation and contribute to a change in behavior. Many Internet sites contain brief, easy to read or print, factual information that describes, in language appropriate to the patient, particular concepts related to symptoms, disorder, or treatment.

The Internet can also enhance a patient's ability to perform a specific skill related to improving health outcomes or activities of daily living. By following a simple step-by-step illustration on the Internet (which may be accompanied by an audio description), patients can see a demonstration of the skill they need to imitate. As video becomes more common on the Internet, patients can see with even greater clarity how to accomplish a given skill. Because Internet material can be accessed repeatedly, the patient can use the materials as frequently as needed to reinforce skill development.

Attitudes are learned responses that are shaped through a lifetime by the cumulative effect of daily encounters with other people and events. The Internet can help patients shape healthy attitudes toward their illness or treatment by allowing them to engage in Internet discussion or chat groups with persons who have similar health problems. These resources can help patients and their families cope with the changes brought on by illness and reinforce desired belief systems. Once a patient has developed sufficient knowledge, skill, and a positive attitude about his or her illness, the Internet can continue to help establish positive health practices by involving the patient on an ongoing basis as a participant in activities that promote integrated changes in health behavior and lifestyle (Box 11-2).

How the Internet is used in the patient education process and the degree to which patients are themselves encouraged to use the Internet will be largely determined by three factors:

1. **Technological access factors.** These factors include the degree to which a computer with sufficient access to the Internet is available. This includes not only the features and location of the computer and the quality and stability of the Internet connection, but also the amount of time the instructor or patient can use the equipment.
2. **Technological competency factors.** These factors include the computer and Internet literacy level of both instructor and patient, and the comfort level each has using the Internet as a teaching methodology.
3. **Physical and emotional factors.** These factors include both physical limitations (eg, pain and fatigue; visual, audio, neurological, and motion deficiencies that would prevent a patient from using a computer) and emotional limitations (eg, depression, anxiety). See Chapters 4, 8, and 9 for discussions on patient readiness to learn, interests, and motivation.

BOX 11-2. Using the Internet to Reach KSAP Education Objectives

- **Knowledge**—fact sheets, articles
- **Skill**—illustrations, animations, video demonstrations
- **Attitudes**—Discussion groups, listserves
- **Practices**—ongoing participative activities for health promotion

---

Many of the technological barriers to Internet use can be overcome with a little effort and perseverance, and competency can be improved by using online Internet tutorials. Many of the physical problems associated with computer use can be overcome by adjusting audio sound or configuring browsers to display in larger font texts. This is an especially appropriate medium for older patients who may have difficulty seeing or hearing other mediums of instruction. Text on computers can be configured to up to 72-point typeface to allow for reading by people with vision problems, and head phones can be attached and allow audio files can be adjusted to ranges that would be picked up by patients with hearing problems. It takes little dexterity (and only a little practice) to move a mouse or to type on a keyboard, and with time and patience, these skills can be achieved by most patients. The computer and an Internet connection can sometimes be just the thing to distract a depressed or anxious patient from concerns about his or her illness, granting a new and interesting device that can help one cope with illness in a proactive and positive manner.

If the patient cannot access the Internet directly, the nurse can always download relevant information and provide it in printed form to the patient. Caution should always be exercised when downloading or printing information off the Internet that copyright restrictions, which apply to Web site material as they do to other intellectual property are not violated. For additional information on electronic copyright, see the Library of Congress Copyright Office site at *http: //lc.web.loc.gov/copyright*.

The Internet can be used many ways in the patient education process. The following three clinical scenarios suggest ways in which the information retrieval process can be applied to actual situations.

Clinical Scenario 1: Self-Directed Learning

A 45-year-old woman has been taking Prozac for 6 months to alleviate the symptoms of depression. She has experienced some mild side effects from the drug. She has been told by friends that St. John's Wort is an effective, natural alternative treatment for mild depression. After the patient consults her physician, she asks the nurse educator for help to learn more about St. John's Wort.

The nurse uses the Internet to learn more about St. John's Wort. The patient says she wants to 1) talk to other people who used the product and see what kind of reaction they have had, 2) determine if any studies (preferably clinical trials) have been conducted on St. John's Wort, and 3) determine if any general information available on the Internet compares the effectiveness of Prozac and St. John's Wort.

Strategies

What can the nurse do?

Strategy 1. The nurse determines that the information for query 1 is most likely in discussion groups, listserves, and newsgroups. A search of the Deja News site (*http://www.deja. com*) reveals 16 newsgroups on depression (eg, *soc.support.depression.treatment, misc.health. alternative*). The nurse asks the patient to read some of the discussions on those newsgroups and to post her questions there. The nurse also suggests that the patient start her own community at that site to make connections with others who currently use St. John's Wort.

Strategy 2. The nurse determines that the information for query 2 is most likely in an authoritative proprietary database of peer-reviewed medical journals (eg, Medline). The nurse has two premier medical sites already bookmarked—Medical Matrix and the National Library of Medicine—so established access to Medline through various search engine interfaces already exists. The nurse selects the National Library of Medicine's PubMed, because it is highly ranked by Medical Matrix and it is free. The nurse visits the PubMed site and reads instructions about using search terms. (PubMed basic search uses natural language queries). The nurse types in St. John's Wort clinical trials and retrieves 87 articles that match this topic. The nurse browses several abstracts and discovers that there was a randomized controlled clinical trial conducted in 1998 to test the efficacy of St. John's Wort for depression.

Strategy 3. The nurse uses the 10-step plan to search the Internet for information that compares the effectiveness of Prozac and St. John's Wort for depression. (Remember: There are no gold standards for Internet searching. The strategy outlined below is just one of many possibilities.)

Step 1. Are there any studies that compare the effectiveness of St. John's Wort and Prozac as a treatment for depression?

Step 2. Depression, St. John's Wort, Prozac. Comparison, effectiveness, treatment.

Step 3. Because the words *comparison* and *effectiveness* are likely to generate many irrelevant hits, it would be better to restrict the keywords to *depression*, St. John's Wort, Prozac and *treatment* and add the other terms only if needed and only if conducting the search in a database which uses subsearching.

Step 4. Begin by asking if there are generic words for Prozac or medical terms for St. John's Wort? If not, are there additional terms that could be used for depression (eg, major depression, depressive disorder, bipolar)? Would it be better to search for the concept "drug therapy" rather than treatment? Do you need to account for possible alternative spellings, such as *Saint* for *St.*? Should you use a truncation symbol on the term *treatment* (ie, *treatmen**) to retrieve the singular and plural forms of the word?

Step 5. Because many concepts will require combining, it might be useful to use a complex Boolean operation algorithm to ensure the proper relationship of terms. For example, a search statement that captures most of the elements in Step 5 may look like:

Depression AND Prozac AND ("St. John's Wort" OR "Saint John's Wort") AND ("drug therapy" OR treatmen*)

Step 6. Because this is a complex Boolean search, the first attempt in the search should probably be in Altavista Advanced Search. Altavista also allows you to limit the search by a date range; given that St. John's Wort has received a lot of news coverage recently, this could be a helpful feature. Altavista also provides ranking of results by selected keywords; the nurse may want to select the term *Prozac* as the most unique identifier and have those results ranked first.

Step 7. After reading the advanced tips screen on the Altavista page, the nurse notes that all of the parameters used in the search, Boolean operators, phrase searching, and nesting are available, although you see no mention of truncation. The Help screens also tell you how to enter the date range.

Step 8. Our search appears to be formulated correctly according to the help screens, so we need not reuse the search strategy for this example.

Step 9. The nurse executes the search and gets results, but Altavista asks if the nurse meant *treatment* for *treatmen** so the nurse eliminates the truncation symbol and reruns the search. The nurse retrieves 490 items.

Step 10. The nurse knows that the Infoseek search engine allows subsearching, permitting the nurse to refine the sets one word at a time, which may work better given the complexity of the search. The nurse accesses the database and returns to Step 6 to review the Infoseek help screens.

Clinical Scenario 2: Working With Children and Adolescents

A nurse is working with a 12-year-old boy who has recently been diagnosed with type I diabetes. He is active in sports and is the captain of his soccer team. He generally feels good, so it is difficult for him to take his illness seriously. He admits to skipping his medication sometimes, and he admits to not being careful about his diet. The nurse's goals for the boy are that he take more interest and responsibility for monitoring his illness. The nurse knows that the boy has a computer in his bedroom, which he uses to play games and to chat with a group of his close friends.

Strategies

What can the nurse do?

The Internet is an especially valuable tool for educating children and adolescents because of its multimedia components and interactivity. By making learning fun and interesting, educators can frequently get children and adolescents to overcome anxieties about a health issue and cooperate more fully in their own health care. With this patient the nurse can:

1. Develop an Internet searching strategy to retrieve information on children and diabetes.
2. Discover a site titled "Children with Diabetes" and begin to explore related links.
3. By clicking on a hypertext link titled *food links* on the main page, discover an animated food pyramid that can help the patient learn more about the kinds and amounts of food he should eat. He can even download a full color food pyramid that he can hang on his wall to help him remember food groups.
4. Explore some links to software, read the reviews, and determine if any free shareware computer programs can help with tracking medication and food. The patient finds one he can download and install. He is excited at the thought of using software to monitor the changes in his glucose level and is eager to try it out.
5. Explore additional links and learn about many diabetes summer camps where he can go and learn more about his illness. The patient seems both surprised and eager to visit a camp outside his home state.
6. Discover an online chat room. The nurse and patient find that entertainer Alan Thicke, father of a child with diabetes, is currently online discussing diabetes.
7. Discover a link to the American Association of Diabetic Educators. The nurse finds some interesting audiovisual materials to order that will help the patient and other young patients with diabetes take more control of their illness.

Clinical Scenario 3: Working With Families

A nurse enters the room of a young woman who has recently undergone a radical mastectomy for breast cancer. The woman is single, and her closest relative and primary caretaker is her younger sister. Although the patient is sleeping comfortably, the nurse finds the sister crying by the patient's bedside. The nurse asks if she can get her anything, and she seems eager to talk. The sister confesses that although she feels comfortable about the clinical decisions and quality of care her sister is getting, she is worried about her own ability to adequately care for the patient during her illness. The patient will be living with the sister during chemotherapy, and the sister is not sure how to respond to the needs of the patient or how to help her own family (she has two young children) understand what is happening to their aunt. The sister also expresses some concern about her own potential risk of developing breast cancer.

Strategies

What can the nurse do?

1. The nurse has already assembled a list of resources on major medical topics. This list has been reviewed and evaluated according to the seven criteria of quality. The nurse opens her bookmark listings under *cancer* and clicks on *Oncolink* (*http://www.oncolink.upenn.edu/*). Oncolink is a major resource for cancer topics, has been a longstanding site of good reputation, and is sponsored by the University of Pennsylvania Cancer Center.
2. The nurse notices immediately a hypertext link titled "Psychosocial Support and Personal Experiences," which leads to another page of resources titled "Information for Caregivers."
3. The nurse clicks on a link that allows her to subscribe the patient's sister to a discussion group called "Caregivers" for family members of cancer patients.
4. Also, a link to a "Caregiver Education Course," allows the nurse to print step-by-step written instructions related to caring for a cancer patient. Three modules comprise the course and they are titled "Common Issues and Problems, Signs of Distress, and Issues of Caregiving."
5. On the same general page, the nurse discovers a link to several multimedia video presentations for "Giving Care to the Patient at Home." The nurse makes a note of two, ("Giving Physical Care" which deals with issues of transfer, bathing, repositioning and "Living and Laughing with Cancer"). The nurse plans to let the sister view these at a later date.
6. Another link from the "Psychosocial Support and Personal Experiences" page links to a page titled "Information for Patients and Families." The nurse finds a link to an online book titled *Kemo Shark*, which provides full-color story book pages of the Kemo Shark that attacks cancer cells and provides an excellent and entertaining handbook for informing children what to expect from a person who is undergoing chemotherapy.
7. The nurse follows a link to an external site at the National Cancer Institute (*http://www.nci.nih.gov/*) that delineates the risk factors and screening procedures for estimating the likelihood of breast cancer. At this site you can sign up and order a free computer program, Breast Cancer Risk Assessment Tool, which can help the patient's sister understand her risk for breast cancer.

SUMMARY

The Internet is a vast publishing medium that provides a unique opportunity for communication, information dispersal, and education. Its continued global growth both in total numbers of users and frequency of use has ensured continued commercial development for some time to come. As technologies develop that will enable computer equipment to increase in performance and decrease in cost, access to the Internet will increase as will accessibility to much relevant and customized information. A primary target for Internet development is the professional health provider and the consumer health markets. As security systems are enhanced and computerized patient records become more commonplace, data and order entry will increasingly be delivered electronically at the point of care. Patient records will be integrated with links to the medical literature, pharmaceutical information, clinical decision-making tools, patient education handouts, and brief continuing education opportunities for a provider who needs to be updated to the most recent information related to his or her patient's disease, treatment, or procedure.

Patient information will increase both in quantity and formats, with a particular emphasis on multimedia delivery. It will become easier to customize information and accommodate the learning styles and educational assessment profile of each person. New hardware and software development will enhance and increase the opportunities for self-directed learning by both provider and patient, ultimately resulting in improved health outcomes. To prepare for the acceleration of technology-based and Internet-accessible learning, the nurse educator or student nurse must develop skills that integrate information technology into daily practice routines. They must adopt an attitude toward computerized educational technology that is open, flexible, and adaptable. Keeping pace with rapidly changing and developing modalities for patient education will require that current nurse educators become discriminating information searchers, qualified information intermediaries—dedicated professionals who are personally committed to lifelong learning into the next millennium.

STRATEGIES FOR CRITICAL ANALYSIS AND APPLICATION

1. Discuss when the Internet is an appropriate vehicle for answering health-related questions and discuss when it is not.
2. Develop a searching strategy for locating and compiling a reference list of complementary and alternative medicine therapies on the Web.
3. Outline and develop a plan for using the Internet to help a French-speaking mother understand the health issues of her child who has been diagnosed with sickle cell anemia and how she can be involved with the child's care.
4. A young patient suffering from partial

paralysis from stroke is confined to a wheelchair. The patient has sufficient dexterity to manage a computer keyboard and wants to communicate with other patients who have had strokes. Develop a plan for helping him or her access support groups, listserves, and Usenet resources.
5. Apply the 10-step search planning and implementation process to locate educational and self-help resources for non-English speaking patients.

REFERENCES

About Health Commons Institute. (1999). Available: http://www.maine.com/hci/links/abouthco.html. Accessed June 6, 1999.

Chatham, M., Hofler, A. & Knapp, B. (1982). *Patient education handbook.* Bowie, MD: Robert J. Brady, Co.

Criteria for assessing the quality of health information on the Internet—a policy paper. (1999). Prepared by the Health Summit Working Group. Available: http://hitiweb.mitretek.org/docs/policy.html. Accessed June 25, 1999.

CyberAtlas. *Doctors' net use keeps increasing.* (1999). Available: http://www.cyberatlas.com/market/professional/physician.html. Accessed June 26, 1999.

Cyber Dialogue Study. Available: http://www.cyberdialogue.com/pdts/whitepages/intel.pdf. Assessed July 1998.

Dearlove, O., Sharples, A. & Stone, C. (1997). Internet is useful for information on rare conditions. *British Medical Journal, 315* (7106), 491.

Deja.com (2000). Deja.com's usenet discussion service. Available: http://www.deja.com/usenet. Accessed October 3, 2000.

Doak, C., Doak, L., & Root, J. (1996). *Teaching patients with low literacy skills* (2nd ed.). Philadelphia: Lippincott.

Engstrom, P. (1997). How a scientist tapped Usenet for clues to an inexplicable disease. *Medicine on the Net, 2*(3), 1–4.

Eysenbach, G., & Diepgen, T. (1998a). Responses to unsolicited patient e-mail requests for medical advice on the World Wide Web. *JAMA, 280*(15), 1333–1335.

Ferguson, T. (1996). A guided tour of self-help cyberspace. *DocTom's online Self-Care*

Journal. Available: http://www.healthy.net/home/tomonline/tomstour.html. Accessed July 17, 1999.

Health Summit Working Group. (1999). *IQ: Health informaton quality assessment tool.* Available: http://www.hitiweb.mitretek.org/iq/default.asp. Accessed June 27,1999.

How many online? (1999) NUA Internet surveys. Available: http://www.mua.ie/surveys/how_many_online/world.html. Assessed June 27, 1999.

Howe, W. (1999). *A brief history of the Internet.* Available: http://www.delphi.com/navnet/faq/history.html/, July 27, 1999

Impicciatore, P., Pandolfini, C., Casella, N., Bonati, M. (1997). Reliability of health information for the public on the World Wide Web: systematic survey of advice on managing fever in children at home. *British Medical Journal, 314*(7098), 1875–1884.

Jadad, A. & Gagliand, A. (1998). Rating health information on the Internet: navigating to knowledge or to babel? *JAMA, 279*(8), 611–614.

Kane, B., & Sands, D. (1998). Guidelines for the clinical use of electronic mail with patients. The AMIA Internet Working Group, Task Force on Guidelines for the Use of Clinic-Patient Electronic Mail. *Journal of the American Medical Informatics Association, 5*(1), 104–111.

Kassirer, J. (1995). The next transformation in the delivery of health care. *New England Journal of Medicine, 332*(1), 52–54.

Lawrence, S. (1999). *Online Health.* Available: http://iconocast.com/iconoarchive/icono.070899.html. Available: August 16, 1999.

Miller, T. & Reents, S. (1998). *The health care industry in transition: the online mandate to change.* Cyber Dialogue. Available: http://www.cyberdialogue.com/pdfs/whitepapers/intel.pdf. Accessed July 27, 1998.

McClung, H., Murray, R., & Heitlinger, L., (1998) The Internet as a source for current patient information. *Pediatrics, 101*(6)e2. Available: http://www.pediatrics.org/cgi/content/full/101/6/e2. Accessed June 17, 1999.

Netcraft Web Server Surveys. (1999). Available: http://netcraft.com/survey. Accessed June 25, 1999.

Nurse Practitioner Support Services. (1999). *NP Central* Available: http://www.nurse.net. Accessed July 27, 1999.

Office of Patient Education, University of Utah Hospitals and Clinics (1999). *Patient Education Network*. Available: http://www.med.utah.edu/pated/patednet. Accessed July 27, 1999.

Silberg, W., Lundberg, G. & Musacchio, R. (1997). Assessing, controlling and assuring the quality of medical information on the Internet: caveat lector et viewer-let the reader and viewer beware. *JAMA, 277*(15), 1244–1245.

Sonnenberg, F. (1997). Health information on the Internet: opportunities and pitfalls. *Archives of Internal Medicine, 157*(2), 151–152.

The numbers behind the e-mail. (1999). CyberAtlas. Available: http://cyberatlas.internet.com/big_picture/article/0,1323,5931_151911,00/html. Accessed September 6, 1999.

University of Pennsylvania Cancer Center (1999). *Oncolink*. Available: http://www.oncolink. upenn.edu. Accessed July 27, 1999.

Wideman, L., & Tong, D. (1997). Requests for medical advice from patients and families to health care providers who publish on the World Wide Web. *Archives of Internal Medicine, 157*(2), 209–212.

Weisbord, S., Soule, J., & Kimmel, P. (1997). Brief report: poison online—acute renal failure caused by oil of wormwood purchased through the Internet. *New England Journal of Medicine, 337*(12), 825–827.

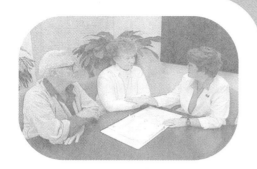

Evaluating Patient
Education Outcomes

LEARNING OBJECTIVES

After reading this chapter, the nurse or student nurse should be able to:

1. Describe how evaluation and documentation of learning can be integrated into basic nursing care, including medication administration, dressing changes, and bathing.

2. Identify four levels of evaluation and provide examples of patient learning outcomes that can be identified in each level.

3. Discuss how the problem-oriented record (POR) can be used to encourage interdisciplinary collaboration.

4. List 10 common mistakes that can have a negative impact on patient education outcomes.

5. Discuss how evaluation relates to assessment in the nursing process.

INTRODUCTION: ASSESSING OUTCOMES

Patient education is an appealing concept, and the instructed patient fares better than the uninstructed one. However, nurses find it challenging to concretely evaluate patient education outcomes. Evaluation, an essential component of the nursing process, is often neglected and misunderstood. Why are nurses frequently unable to find time to evaluate patient education or to document learning? Why does the word *evaluation* cause unease and uncertainty?

To evaluate is "to determine the significance or worth of by careful appraisal or study." Both nurses and patients may feel threatened by the thought of evaluation. Some may worry about being personally devalued or about judged unworthy. Some may recall humiliation when one failed a test and may not want to feel that way again. Some may fear that if they fail to achieve what others expect of them, they will lose love, support, assistance, esteem, and credibility.

Evaluation is not intended to place a value or a worth on patients or nurses. Its purposes are to measure the results of care, to define specific outcomes, and to redirect patient care. Outcomes measurement is central to assessment of the cost, quality, and effectiveness of care and organizational performance (Jennings, Staggers, & Brosch, 1999). Evaluation of patient education involves collecting specific and descriptive data related to behaviors targeted as patient learning objectives. Through evaluation, the nurse and the patient determine the value of the nursing interventions that help the patient perform desired behaviors (Oermann & Huber, 1999). The nurse must also determine the likelihood that the patient can be safely discharged from care based on the ability for self-management and the resources needed for continuing care (JCAHO, 1998).

Many nurses underestimate the importance of evaluation in patient education. Many nurses once thought patient education simply involved giving information. Nurses have not always considered patient education a valid nursing intervention for response to specific client needs or problems. As the nursing process increasingly directs the delivery of patient education, evaluation is recognized as a component of the nursing process that deserves attention (Fig. 12-1).

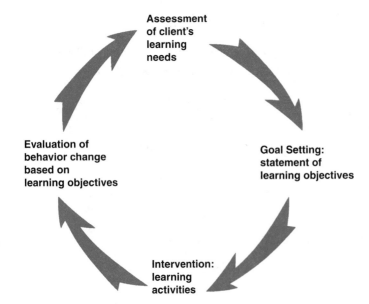

FIGURE 12-1. Evaluation is part of a continuous process in patient education.

This chapter offers a better understanding of evaluation, addresses methods of data collection, and discusses how to use the information from the evaluation process to reinforce learning and to plan future learning opportunities for patients. The examples offered in this chapter focus on education of individual patients and their families. Strategies for evaluating organizational approaches and community programs for patient education are discussed in Chapter 14.

Although evaluation is the fourth step in patient education, it is not an end point. As illustrated in Figures 8-1 and 12-1, evaluation links to assessment, and the nursing process continues. Not only does the nurse determine if the patient met the goal, but why or why not. The barriers that prevented the targeted outcomes must be confronted as the nurse-patient relationship continues.

A staff nurse from an outpatient clinic in the Boston area shared this experience:

There are numerous barriers when educating a client with HIV/AIDS. One of the more pronounced barriers I have encountered in my career is when the nurse recognizes the need for a client to change behaviors, but the client does not agree to this goal. A person with HIV/AIDS has a great responsibility to society to slow the rate of transmission of this virus. The nurse can facilitate education, provide information, and make recommendations for a healthy lifestyle, but the ultimate responsibility is the client's. The educator is further challenged when the client is an active injection drug user, or when the client has expressed a loss of hope for the future. Instilling that hope and setting individualized goals with clients is the first step in overcoming barriers to patient education and ultimately changing behaviors.

We also address documentation of learning in this chapter. The patient's record should reflect what the patient knows, understands, or performs; it emphasizes patient outcomes. Components of nursing documentation systems are reviewed and discussed as they relate to patient education.

SCOPE OF EVALUATION

Evaluation is closely related to assessment. Both involve formulating criteria or questions, gathering and categorizing data, and writing a summary statement. These findings are used in patient care planning. Assessment usually refers to building a database that includes nursing diagnoses and outlines the patient's needs or problems. Evaluation is essentially the follow-up assessment that is continuously conducted as nursing interventions are performed. Therefore, evaluation occurs throughout the learning activities and is used to assess the patient's progress toward meeting learning objectives.

Evaluation is conducted using the behavioral objectives discussed in Chapter 9. If the patient objectives are clearly defined, evaluation is straightforward. Measurement is based on the stated behaviors (Mager, 1997a; Mager, 1997d). The patient and family should be active participants in evaluating learning. Through self-evaluation, based on his or her own learning objectives, a patient can define what is expected of him or her, can plan and participate in learning activities, and can seek feedback to direct his or her performance. Evaluation becomes a learning experience that can increase the patient's self-esteem as the patient recognizes his or her own accomplishments and gains positive feedback and support from others.

Evaluation is also a learning opportunity for the teacher. The feedback the nurse receives from the patient's progress or lack of progress helps the nurse modify the approach and consider alternate teaching strategies (eg, providing more review, clarifying learning objectives, and changing teaching methods or media).

Using the evaluation process, both the nurse and the patient benefit from feedback that reinforces successes and readdresses problems. At times evaluation is conducted in a formal manner, using written documentation and oral feedback. This documentation usually occurs at the end of a nursing shift, after classes or skills training, and before a patient's discharge from the hospital or outpatient office. Just as the assessment process involves asking questions to gather specific information, so does the evaluation process. The evaluation process should include:

1. Measuring the extent to which the patient has met the learning objectives: What are the outcomes of patient education?
2. Indicating when there is a need to clarify, correct, or review information
3. Noting learning objectives that are unclear to the patient, family, or health care providers
4. Pointing out shortcomings in the patient teaching interventions, specifically addressing content, format, activities, and media
5. Identifying barriers that prevented learning

In patient education, it is the teacher's responsibility to initiate the evaluation, summarize the findings, document findings in the patient record, give constructive feedback to the patient and family, plan future experiences to reinforce learning, and design learning opportunities to foster behaviors that were not initially accomplished.

The teacher must be prepared by knowing what questions to ask and by understanding each component of the patient education process. In addition to measuring behavior, the nurse looks critically at nursing care and identifies problems that have prevented learning.

THE FOUR LEVELS OF PATIENT LEARNING OUTCOMES

Evidence of patient learning outcomes is emphasized in the guidelines of the Joint Commission on the Accreditation of Healthcare Organizations (JCAHO) (1998). Nurses express concern that with shorter inpatient stays, they are expected to produce unrealistic learning outcomes. Chapter 5 outlines the JCAHO patient education standards, emphasizing that teaching should be appropriate to length of stay and understandable to the patient.

Learning outcomes can be accomplished in any setting, even if the patient is there only a matter of minutes. Four levels of learning outcomes address different increments of learning (Fig. 12-2). The nurse should evaluate a patient's learning in one or more levels.

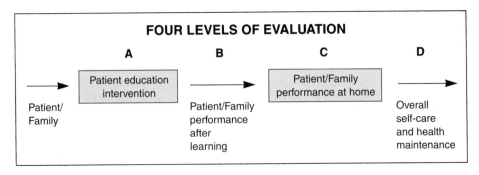

FIGURE 12-2. *Note.* From *"The four levels of evaluation,"* by Brethower, K. S., and Rummler, G. A. (1979). *Training and Development Journal, 79*(5), 12–20. Adapted with permission.

Level A: Patient and Family Involvement During Interventions

We surveyed our patients before and after implementation of our new patient care map, which includes patient education. The entire health care team [narrowed] and prioritized patient education interventions. We surveyed patients about their preparation for discharge and their satisfaction with the information they had been given. We were pleased to find significant increases on all 15 variables.

L.P. (STALLINGS, 1996)

The teacher assesses the level of involvement of the learners. Was education provided for the patient and family? Was a standardized approach or teaching plan followed in accordance with the policies of the agency and expectation of third parties (eg, health plans)? Was the learner present (ie, physical presence at a class or alert presence for individual teaching)? Does the patient ask questions? Does the patient seem alert and interested? Does the patient comprehend instructions? Is the patient willing to assume responsibility for learning? Are learning experiences relevant to the patient's unique situation? Are culture and beliefs accounted for during the teaching? Does the patient participate in discussion, demonstrations, and problem solving? Were concepts too basic? Or did the patient feel overloaded and overwhelmed by the amount of instruction and information? Were learning objectives and desired outcomes clear to the learner (ie, did the patient know what he or she was expected to do)? In what ways did family members participate?

Evaluation of the patient's readiness to learn should not be overlooked. Counseling patients during the initial shock of an illness or disability, helping them accept it, and encouraging them to focus on how they will live their lives in the future are great challenges nurses

face. Interventions and evaluation related to this counseling and the patient's responses are seldom documented.

JCAHO (1998) identifies the following outcomes in accreditation standards:

- That the patient and family understand the patient's current health problem or reason for admission
- That the patient receives informed consent
- That the patient and family understand the treatment plan and the role they will play
- That the patient has an overview of the survival skills needed for safe discharge

Level B: Patient Performance Immediately After Learning Experience

One of the biggest successes from our patient education classes has been the ability of patients to recall their medications. We've ensured this by outlining specific objectives at the beginning of the class and then evaluating learning at discharge or shortly thereafter. We know that if individuals are discharged and don't take their medications accurately, they will relapse. We ask the patients to name their medication, tell us the reason they are taking it, tell us when they will take it.

A.C. (STALLINGS, 1996)

When evaluating patient performance after a learning experience, the nurse should ask: Could the patient meet performance standards (ie, objectives) as a result of the learning experience? To what extent did the patient meet objectives? The nurse should describe the *patient's* performance rather than what the nurse did. How should future teaching be conducted? Outcomes should reflect knowledge and survival skills to participate in self-care.

Individual needs, patient readiness, and patient learning abilities should be assessed.

JCAHO is particularly interested in the following areas of teaching:

- Safe and effective use of medications and medical equipment
- Potential food-drug interactions
- Rehabilitation techniques
- Community resources
- How to obtain further treatment
- Ongoing health care needs

Level C: Patient Performance at Home

In providing discharge instructions, I always try to include the patient's family so they can remind the patient of some of the things they did in the hospital that they need to continue to do at home. An example is abdominal splinting. The patient with an abdominal incision is likely to be uncomfortable. The family member can keep a blanket or towel at the bedside and encourage the patient to mobilize by reminding them, "here, use this to take away some of the discomfort." We find that this helps the patient extend more and it also helps the family in the caregiver role."

N.B. (STALLINGS, 1996)

When evaluating the patient's performance at home, the nurse should ask: Was the patient given written discharge instructions that were understandable? Did patient and family perform the desired behaviors at home? To what extent did they follow the recommended plan? If they had difficulty, was this a result of not remembering, inability to perform the skill, or misunderstanding instructions? Did they change their minds about willingness to perform the behaviors? Did physical limitations or financial barriers prevent them from self-care?

Was a continuing care provider identified and given instructions to promote continuity of care?

Level D: Patient's Overall Self-Care and Health Management

If a patient is readmitted, especially if they relapse, we look at what caused that to happen, and then we try to put that into a discharge plan right on admission. A common reason is noncompliance with medications. We look at how this can be corrected. Often, patients cannot afford the medication or cannot remember to take it."

A.C. (STALLINGS, 1996)

When evaluating the patient's overall self-care and management, the nurse should ask: was overall management successful in preventing or controlling health problems? Did physiologic data (blood pressure, blood glucose level, handling emergencies, readmission rates) reflect successful self-care? What were long-term results 6 months to 12 months after teaching was initiated?

Patients with a chronic disease may have side effects from their treatment, may be depressed, or may have problems in the workplace, all of which affect their continued health. Outpatient rehabilitation programs to assist cardiovascular patients with exercise, smoking cessation, and emotional aspects of recovery are often key to long-term, successful behavioral change (Carter, 1999).

Which Level of Evaluation Is Best?

Summary: Comparing Four Levels of Evaluation

Data from a combination of evaluation sources should be assimilated and the results should be summarized. This procedure is similar to that of categorization of information and writing a summary statement in assessment.

When summarizing results, the nurse should ask: *To what extent were the learning objectives accomplished?* The answer to this initial question leads to more questions:

- If the behavior was successfully performed, how can it be reinforced?
- If the behavioral objective was *not* met, could the patient perform the behavior in the past?
- If he could perform it in the past, why has he failed to perform it now?

Evaluation does not simply provide nurses with a single *Yes* or *No* answer. Instead, evaluation becomes another starting point in the continuous nursing process. Data is gathered, feedback is offered about the learning experience from the patient, the family, the health care team, and the institution. The nurse looks to others for feedback about the quality of the nursing interventions. Feedback is a learning tool that can be powerful in guiding behavior when used positively. Tips on giving feedback are offered later in this chapter.

Conclusions drawn from evaluation should be carefully considered. Often data are limited or absent at one level of evaluation. In this case, conclusions at a higher level may be inaccurate.

For example, if information is collected at level D (overall self-care) to reflect that blood pressure has not declined, it is inaccurate to assume that the patient did not know how to follow the regimen (level B) or that he or she did not follow the treatment plan at home (level C) unless evaluation was conducted at all levels. Ideally, evaluation occurs at each level and modifications are made to the teaching plan to build success at each level.

Ideally, the nurse can assess evidence of patient learning in each evaluation level. However, evaluation has limits if the nurse cannot follow the patient's entire course along the continuum of care. Regardless, all levels of evaluation provide important evidence. For example, if a patient does not perform a skill at home,

such as insulin administration or blood glucose testing, we must know whether he or she was provided and received instruction. Otherwise, it is difficult to learn why the skill was not learned and to improve the intervention. Valuable time may be lost recreating the assessment of potential barriers to learning. All patient education outcomes can be documented at some level, including daily documentation in the patient's record or when a nursing visit is made.

The authors frequently hear nurses say, "I'd love to do patient education, but I don't have the time to teach and document it with all the paperwork and other demands." Opportunities for patient education are lost during the typical day in all settings. For example, bath time can be used for teaching the patient with diabetes about good skin and foot care, the surgical patient about dressing or cast care, the patient with chronic obstructive lung disease about breathing exercises, and so on. Medication time can be used to teach the patient with congestive heart failure how to take his or her pulse before self-administering medication or to teach the patient with rheumatoid arthritis to safely taper off steroids. Every patient encounter is an opportunity for patient teaching. The astute nurse who capitalizes on these moments should always document the teaching in the patient's chart.

EVALUATING PATIENT EDUCATION INTERVENTIONS

This step in evaluation considers the performance of both the teacher and the learner. The nurse needs to know if the teaching environment was set for the patient to be a colleague and the nurse to be a consultant. The nurse must determine if the teaching-learning process was interesting, clear, and stimulating to the learner. The nurse especially wants to know if the patient and family understood the learning objectives and desired outcomes for learning (Weinrich, 1999). Data gathered in this step are used to modify the climate or patient education interventions. Data are gathered by interview, questionnaire, and observation.

We suggest that nurses formulate a series of questions to provide direction in the evaluation of the patient education process (Box 12-1).

The nurse looks critically at the teaching interventions that were designed to help the patient achieve his or her goals and gain knowledge, attitudes, and skills. The following questions help determine effective interventions and areas of nursing care that need improvement.

Evaluating format and content. Was the patient taught by self-study, individual instruction, or group instruction? Was the format compatible with the learning objectives and with the patient's condition and learning style? Did the patient receive the necessary facts and training to learn the desired behaviors?

BOX 12-1. Evaluation Checklist for Patient Education

Questions

✔ Did the objectives clearly state observable patient behaviors? ‡
✔ Were the objectives realistic for the client? † ‡
✔ Was the original assessment complete? †
✔ Did the client perceive the identified problem as important? Did he or she want to change? * † ‡
✔ Did new problems pose obstacles to behavioral change? †
✔ Did the client participate in goal setting? * ‡
✔ Were the interventions tailored to meet the objectives? §
✔ Was behavioral change measured and documented accurately? //
✔ Is there a skill deficiency? Should there be changes in the nursing interventions? § //

---

* See Chapter 4
† See Chapters 8, 9, 10
‡ See Chapter 9
§ See Chapters 10, 12
// See Chapter 1

Evaluating teaching activities and media. Was the patient given an opportunity to actively participate, ask questions, and practice? Were the patient's past experiences used as resources for learning? Were the patient's social roles and developmental tasks acknowledged? Was learning practical and problem centered? Was there an opportunity for immediate application by the learner? Were the learning methods and media appropriate for the types of learning objectives? Could the media deliver the message in a manner that the patient and family could understand?

Evaluating patient and family satisfaction. Do the patient and the family have suggestions for improving the patient education experience? Which activities did they find most helpful and which did they find least helpful? Did they feel supported in the learning environment? Were their concerns addressed? Did they feel confident with the staff's preparation to teach? Was the content understandable and practical?

Evaluating the resources and staff recommendations. Were staff and facility resources adequate for teaching? If not, which unmet staff needs posed barriers to patient learning? Do nurses and other members of the health care team have suggestions? How do they assess the quality of the patient learning experience? Were the contributions of staff members in teaching the patient and family coordinated? Did they feel prepared to teach? If not, what training should be offered to the staff? (Refer to Chapter 5).

Evaluating Patient and Family Performance

Learning objectives are a yardstick to measure the patient's ability to assume self-care. Learning objectives are the behaviors the patient *will perform* to show that he or she has mastered knowledge, attitudes, and skills. They are tailored to the patient's individual goals.

Recall that a learning objective has three components: performance, conditions, and criteria (Mager, 1997a). See Chapter 9 for detailed definitions of these components. To evaluate patient education, the teacher uses performance, conditions, and criteria to measure the patient's progress. The measurements should be collected accurately and should reflect qualitative and quantitative data (Mager 1997b; Mager 1997c).

In Chapter 9 the following learning objective was offered as an example: The patient will draw up and administer 22 units of insulin using sterile technique at 7:00 AM on 3 consecutive days.

Qualitative data might include the following statement: "The patient could perform sterile technique in preparing the injection but could not accurately measure the units of insulin." Quantitative data might include this statement: "The patient could perform sterile technique correctly only once. In the other two efforts, he or she contaminated the needle by placing it on the table uncapped." Specific data help the nurse and the patient to focus on problem areas and to acknowledge progress that is made toward meeting the objective.

Evaluating Performance in the Home

Evaluating performance in the home is often difficult because continuous care is not always possible from the hospital, clinic, or school setting. Outpatient follow-up may be difficult because the patient is discharged to a different city, follow-up appointments are infrequent, home health services may not be available, or there is little communication about patient teaching between agencies.

The nurse needs to know how a patient is doing at home. Does the patient feel competent to manage self-care? Does the home environment present any barriers to self-care? Is the regimen flexible enough? Can the patient handle problems or temporary relapses constructively? If emergencies have occurred, did the patient or family respond appropriately? Does the patient still assume responsibility for self-care?

Unfortunately, nurses often don't learn about patient difficulties until a crisis (eg, hospital readmission or ER visit) occurs. Interventions (eg, telephone follow up, postcards, home

visits by students, and better communication between the hospital and outpatient clinic) can improve evaluation of the patient and family performance.

 A growing role for advanced practice nurses exists in the home health care setting, particularly for geriatric care. The potential to improve outcomes and reduce costs is especially demonstrated with patients who have dementia and cannot cope well with changes, and with patients and families who need case management, education, and advocacy (Pierson, 1999).

One of the most important things a home health nurse does is to continue patient education. A home health nurse offers the following advice:

> *You've [must] be a good listener, a teacher, and an observer. The patient and family may tell you one thing, and you observe another. You can't assume anything. They have to demonstrate back to me. Are they living it? You can't force them to change their lifestyle. It's not like the hospital where if you don't want them to have sweets or salt, you simply refuse them. This is the real world where they have a salt shaker on the counter and a daughter who brings in doughnuts. We're there to teach and encourage, not boss and demand.*

(BOVENDER, 1994)

Evaluating Self-Care and Health Maintenance

This level of evaluation takes a broad look at the patient's course of care before and after the learning of new behaviors. Information is collected about absences from work or school, hospitalizations, episodes of acute complications, and daily management. Research data are usually gathered to measure the long-term value of patient education interventions. In addition, the data may be used to substantiate requests for third-party reimbursement of patient teaching and negotiated managed-care contracts.

For patients managing type 1 and type 2 diabetes, treatment goals (eg, medication, nutrition, and exercise outcomes) are continually evaluated (Magoon, 1999). Clinical and financial outcomes targeted for evaluation of a population of patients with diabetes includes decreased drug spending, decreased hospitalization, decreased emergency department visits, and decreased outpatient visits for acute episodes (Ziegler, 1996).

Methods of Measurement

Several methods exist to gather information to evaluate learning. In general, nurses should remember that adults learn best with immediate application of knowledge, attitudes, and skills. Evaluation becomes a learning experience when it is prompt and when it is an exercise shared with the learner. The feedback reinforces positive behaviors and guides the correction of misunderstandings and performance problems. Because evaluation is a problem-solving process, the learner gains skill in managing problems by working with the teacher.

The following seven methods (direct observation, patient records, reports, tests, interviews, critical incidents, length of stay) are commonly used by nurses to evaluate patient learning.

Direct Observation

Watching the patient perform a skill or having him or her role-play a situation offers two valuable opportunities. First, accurate, descriptive data can be collected. Second, the learner receives immediate feedback and guidance. Use direct observation whenever possible (as opposed to relying on reports and assumptions). Patients should be encouraged to demonstrate self-care activities and should be given professional guidance to reinforce learning. Examples of opportunities for direct observation are when the patient changes dressings, administers medication, performs breast self-examination, or selects foods according to a prescribed diet.

Preventive education for children also can be evaluated through return demonstration. Age-specific teaching for burn prevention by a pediatric nurse practitioner helps young children create an escape plan and has them demonstrate "stop, drop, and roll." Second and third graders crawl through a simulated smoke tunnel, and older children learn about burn staging and skin grafting through simulations (Gregory, 2000).

Patient Records

A nurse must often rely on patients to keep records of their performance. Although teaching begins in the company of health care professionals, much of the actual learning occurs in the home when the patient and family assume total responsibility. Although reinforcement of positive behavior is essential to the continuance of learning, it is not easily provided when opportunities for observation are lacking.

Ask the patient to keep specific records and to present them to the nurse at a later time; this reinforces the patient's responsibility, reinforces positive behaviors, helps the patient evaluate his own progress, and provides the nurse with data for evaluation. This method has worked well in evaluating compliance with medical regimens, diet modification, stress management, and treatments carried out at home. When possible, supplement the patient records with direct observation, which will increase objectivity.

Reports

Patient and family reports are used as sources of data although their objectivity is often questioned. Measurements (eg, pill counts, weight, and blood tests) can accompany reports.

Reporting should be solicited from the patient and family through carefully constructed questions. For example, the nurse will get more specific and descriptive data by asking, *What medications did you take today and at what times did you take them?* than by asking, *Are you taking your medication as you were instructed?* Patients can be taught to be good reporters if they are given specific directions about collecting and recording significant information and if they are told how they are expected to contribute to the evaluation process.

Tests

Oral and written tests can be used before learning activities and repeated at intervals following instruction. Tests can measure the patient's progress toward meeting cognitive objectives, and they offer objective data about learning retention. Tests require the patient to be an active participant in defining learning needs and in recognizing positive change. Tests are often used to teach and evaluate daily management decisions made by patients and their families dealing with chronic illness.

Tests used when patients with asthma come to the hospital emergency room can help nurses identify critical learning outcomes needed by their patients. For example, through questioning, the staff can discover that some patients do not understand their disease, the triggers of their asthmatic episodes, and how to use their special medications to prevent asthmatic episodes. Some patients did not have a peak flow meter or did not know how to use it (Finerty, 2000).

Tests used for evaluation should present problems in a sequence, from simple to complex, and the tool should be appropriate for the patient's literacy level.

Interviews and Questionnaires

With Patients and Family

Patients and their families may be interviewed or given written questionnaires to assess their expectations, opinions, degree of confidence in new knowledge, and self-efficacy (Redman, 1998). In these interviews and questionnaires, patients may evaluate their own progress, define their learning needs, and offer suggestions for future training.

The authors have used questionnaires to evaluate prenatal classes, newborn care instruction, and stress management classes. Ask specific questions that do not require long, general responses and to phrase the questions so that the learner can understand them. Questionnaires are inappropriate for illiterate patients and family members. A nurse may want to ask a patient to write a letter describing the birth experience or a surgical experience and explain how prepared he or she felt for it. The patient can offer suggestions for how to best prepare others based on his or her experience.

With Staff

Staff members involved in the patient's care offer important information about a patient's progress. Although one nurse coordinates the patient's care, many health professionals, including those from other disciplines, gather evaluative data. These health care professionals should be asked to contribute these important measurements. Brief, carefully worded questions can be used in interviews and surveys for staff. The questions should focus on specific, measurable behaviors. Data are also found in their notes in the medical record.

Critical Incidents

Research can be used to follow-up with patients for a predetermined time to look for critical incidents, such as readmission, complications, and mortality. Emergency room (ER) visits for acute asthma episodes often reflect patient learning and self-efficacy.

Length of Stay

Patient education can reduce length of stay by enabling the patient to better participate in recovery and preparation for discharge. Teaching must be updated and streamlined to accommodate shorter hospital stays. When determining goals for patient teaching, estimated length of stay associated with the diagnosis-related group (DRG) or the case type will guide the nurse in keeping the teaching plans realistic. The nurse should be familiar with

DRGs frequently seen on her unit and the associated length of stay.

Nurses and administrators may evaluate a patient education program by averaging the lengths of stay for a patient population that has participated in a patient education intervention (usually for the purpose of making a case for the program's impact). Consider the following advice:

 The median is the same as the 50th percentile rank, the score in a distribution of scores above and below which one-half of the scores fall. It is the middle score, if all scores are laid out in numerical order. The median is less sensitive to outlier scores than in the arithmetic mean (the average of all scores). Therefore, the median is a better statistic to use when evaluating impact on length of stay, particularly when outliers can reduce the appearance of a program's success for most patients. ■

Identifying Needs and Performance Problems

The behavioral objectives in the learning process (see Figure 9-1) guides the nurse in the evaluation process.

If the desired behavior is accomplished, the nurse provides opportunities for reinforcing the positive behavior. Clinic visits, home visits, telephone calls, and community resources offer such opportunities. The patient and the family can demonstrate the knowledge and skills they have retained and ask for the review or guidance that they need. The health care team should encourage clients to take advantage of these learning resources.

When learning behaviors are not accomplished, or are only partially accomplished, the patient educator must reassess and readdress barriers to behavioral change. Pipe and Mager (1997) provide a model for problem solving to determine client learning needs (Fig. 12-3). The nurse must reconsider whether the particular behavior is important and necessary if a skill deficiency is present. If the patient has never been able to perform the skill, the teacher should provide additional training. If the skill will be used infrequently, feedback and practice should be arranged. For example, insulin injection is often learned with some initial difficulty, but the skill is used so often that it is retained and reinforced. Breast self-examination is performed less often, so

---

WHEN CLIENTS FAIL TO MEET LEARNING OBJECTIVES: IS THERE A SKILL DEFICIENCY?

Yes	No
1. Has the client ever demonstrated the ability to perform the skill? If not, *formal training* is required.	1. Is the performance of the skill punishing? If so, *remove punishment.*
2. Is the skill used often? If not, *arrange practice.* If so, *arrange feedback.*	2. Is nonperformance rewarding? If so, *arrange a positive consequence.*
	3. Does the client feel that it doesn't matter if he performs the behavior? If so, *arrange a consequence.*
	4. Are there obstacles to performing the behavior? If so, *remove obstacles.*

FIGURE 12-3. *Note.* From *"Analyzing Performance Problems,"* by Pipe P., & Mager R. (1970, 1997). Atlanta: Center for Effective Performance. Adapted with permission.

this technique and the importance of its performance may need more reinforcement.

If the patient has demonstrated the ability to perform the skill but has not continued to perform it, four additional questions direct the teacher's problem-solving. Mager and Pipe suggest that if performing the skill somehow "punishes" the patient, the nurse must identify the source of punishment and remove it.

1. **Why does the patient feel punished?** For example, patients who are on special diets often complain that they cannot follow their diet while socializing with friends. Locating other sources of support, such as support groups of dieters, may remove the feeling of being different or punished.
2. **Does the patient see the performance as unrewarding?** If so, the teacher can arrange positive consequences by offering additional support and more frequent follow-up visits and reporting mechanisms, so that the patient will see his improvement more clearly.
3. **Does the patient think that it doesn't matter whether he or she performs the behavior?** If this is the case, as with patients who have hypertension and who fail to take their medications regularly, more frequent blood pressure checks can reinforce the patient's awareness of the seriousness of omitting the medication.
4. **Do obstacles prevent the patient from performing the behavior?** If so, the teacher will want to review these obstacles and help the patient deal with them. For example, the snack machine at work, which contains only candy and chips, may be less of a temptation if the patient brings a nutritious snack to work in the morning. If a mill worker feels self-conscious about wearing a protective mask on the job, because "nobody else wears one," the company manager and employee health nurse may insist that all employees wear the recommended masks.

The nurse must become a detective to help patients overcome stumbling blocks in the learning process. This requires the skills of making astute observations, using active listening, and approaching individual situations creatively.

The continuous cycle of teaching and learning brings us back to formulating objectives. The nurse, the patient, and the patient's family must once again discuss their mutual goals: Where does the patient want to be in terms of his or her behaviors? What can the nurse offer to assist him or her in carrying out these new behaviors? Just as negotiation and the formulation of a learning contract were emphasized in Chapter 9, they are also priorities in evaluation. The original learning contract should be modified according to the oral agreement between the nurse and the patient.

Feedback

Feedback is a communication process that involves sharing perceptions. The patient and family can be supported and guided in learning when they are given constructive feedback. They can be directed toward meeting their goals. Nurses often comment that they wish patients, families, and staff would give them more positive feedback about the nursing care they provide. Health care institutions ask for feedback from the public about how they are meeting community health care needs.

Feedback is seen as a valuable commodity. People generally refer to two types of feedback: positive and negative. *Positive feedback* compliments a person's behavior. *Negative feedback* communicates displeasure or disappointment with a person's behavior. Most people describe positive feedback as being of great importance to them. It means more when it comes from someone we respect, from someone who values us, and from someone who understands our situation. Feedback is provided in the home, workplace, and health care settings. In patient learning, patients and their family members expect to receive feedback from nurses and other team members.

Feedback guidelines can increase the likelihood that the feedback given by professionals to clients will be constructive and helpful. Rather than focusing on positive versus negative feedback, consider how the evaluation process can offer opportunities for useful feedback. Box 12-2 describes the characteristics of constructive feedback and includes tips for giving feedback to the patient and family in a manner they can understand.

DOCUMENTATION OF PATIENT EDUCATION

Written documentation of all aspects of patient care, including patient education, is essential. Documentation is critical for communication among team members, to provide a legal record, to support quality assurance efforts, to meet JCAHO standards, to promote continuity of care, and to promote reimbursement. Documentation should reflect the following elements of patient care and patient education:

- Initial assessments and reassessments
- Nursing diagnoses and patient needs, priorities
- Interventions planned
- Interventions provided
- Patient's response, outcomes of care
- Patient and family ability to manage needs after discharge

Documentation is time consuming, especially in light of increasing patient acuity, complex care, and expanding clinical responsibilities. However, nurses must provide timely, accurate documentation that shows the basis of their clinical judgments and evidence of nursing interventions provided to the patient.

We believe that nurses should make every

BOX 12-2. Guidelines for Obtaining and Giving Constructive Feedback

Characteristics of Constructive Feedback
- Descriptive rather than judgmental, it offers objective data and suggestions for improvement.
- Specific rather than general, it does not include absolute words such as *always* or *never*. It is concerned with the here and now.
- Focused on the person's *behavior* rather than on the person.
- Given at the earliest opportunity after the behavior is performed; it is timely.
- Considers the needs of the learner. It is given to help, not to hurt.
- Directed toward a behavior about which the learner can do something. The person will only become frustrated and discouraged when he or she is unable to control a situation.
- Involves sharing information and offering guided choices rather than giving advice such as "You should. . . ."
- Considers the amount of information that the learner can handle. It does not overload the person.

Tips for Giving and Soliciting Feedback
- Ask whether feedback is wanted. It is most useful when it is solicited rather than imposed.
- Be prepared to listen.
- Give positive feedback first. Reinforce positive behaviors, then discuss weaknesses.
- Don't argue or push. Present alternatives.
- Ensure that your feedback is interpreted correctly.
- When requesting feedback from others, tell them what kinds of specific information you want. Offer them structured questions, but encourage them to use open-ended responses.
- When you want feedback from others, be open to it. Observe patients' expressions or comments. Listen for the intended message.

effort to improve documentation systems by designing all components to fit together. Documentation can be streamlined to avoid duplication of charting and to accurately reflect the nursing process in which nursing diagnoses either are resolved or referred. To demonstrate quality care, nurses must integrate all clinical data, including those gathered by other health care team members. This approach necessitates a single, integrated, patient-centered database (Eggland & Heinemann, 1994; Mowry, 1992; Darby, 1999).

We have witnessed increasing use of computerized documentation systems, with data entry at a bedside terminal. Research on the use of bedside computers shows that automation enhances the amount and accuracy of information documented by nurses (Eggland & Heinemann, 1994) and increased focus on recording patient outcomes data (Patient Education Management, 1999).

A documentation system should be concise, organized, and focused on patient outcomes. When charting patient education, the mastery of learning objectives is highlighted and a snapshot of what the patient knows and can do is included. Statements in the charts such as "patient teaching done" describe the nurse's behavior rather than the patient's behavior and in such general terms that evaluation is meaningless.

Although documentation systems look different from one setting to another (and even among units in the same agency), they have common components (Montemuro, 1988; Eggland & Heinemann 1994). Successful documentation for outpatient settings is streamlined to reflect the length and scope of the visit, but is just as vital to communication. Duplication of charting should be avoided and timesaving methods encouraged. One of the biggest problems with traditional narrative charting has been the quality of data nurses documented and the ability to reflect both the nurse's clinical decision-making and the patient's outcomes.

Nurses often ask: *Is a special form needed for documenting patient education? Would documentation improve if we had a better check-list or flow sheet specifically for patient teaching?* No universal answer to these questions exist for every situation and setting. The nurse should ask: Where is patient education currently documented and is it working? Staff often have no clear understanding or mandate for the use of progress notes and how to chart patient education outcomes as an integral part of care. Creating new forms often leads to fragmented communication, the perception that patient education is separate from routine care, and the belief that patient teaching requires extra work that is unrealistic. A rule of thumb: If you create a new form, one or more existing forms should be eliminated.

Critical pathways (Chapter 13), which identify key learning outcomes and related variances, should be a focus of interdisciplinary teaching. To promote documentation by all staff, share information gleaned from chart audits, include staff in the development of new forms, make sure staff understand how to use the forms correctly, and incorporate documentation of patient education into employee appraisals (Patient Education Management, 1996).

A review of the common components of a documentation system allows nurses to consider how they can integrate the documentation of patient education into the patient record. The components are:

Nursing admission assessment (data base)
Problem list
Care plan or critical path
Flow sheets (optional)
Progress notes
Discharge summary

Nursing Admission Assessment

Client profile and history are completed by the nurse on admission. Functional assessment is highlighted to aid the formulation of nursing diagnoses. Patient assessment forms are designed to complement whatever assessment guide the nurse uses. Forms vary according to setting and patient needs. Assessment is described in Chapter 8 and emphasizes the identification of barriers to learning (eg, lack of readiness, culture, language, physical problems). Assessment forms may be designed strictly for patient teaching purposes to pinpoint potential problems or barriers that high-risk patients may face following medication regimens, for example (Gibson, 1989).

Problem List

A list of actual and potential health problems identified by health care providers, individually or collaboratively, is placed at the front of the chart. Nursing diagnoses are added to this list and numbered as they are identified (not necessarily in order of priority or intensity). A date is entered next to each problem as it is identified, and another date is recorded to reflect when the problem is resolved. The problem list is used as an index. Problem numbers are used throughout the record to streamline documentation, whether manual or computerized. Nurses in many agencies use standardized care plans that are generated based on DRGs and nursing diagnoses.

Care Plan or Critical Pathway

An individualized care plan for each patient accounts for nursing diagnoses, patient goals or outcomes (including learning goals), interventions (including patient education and discharge planning), and actual outcomes.

Flow Sheets

Routine or repetitious actions can be systematically documented with flow sheets. Flow sheets can be kept at the bedside to record vital signs, medication, positioning, and so forth. Paperless flow sheets can be used at bedside computer terminals. Flow sheets list observations in a clear, concise check-off format to encourage rapid and immediate documentation; abnormal findings or patient responses must be recorded in narrative notes. This method of charting assumes that all abnormal findings, or variances, are charted; this is referred to as "charting by exception" (Eggland & Heinemann, 1994). If flow sheets are used to

record patient teaching, they should be organized by patient response, not by "what the nurse did" to teach the patient.

Progress Notes

Narrative notes show the patient's progress as viewed by all health care professionals involved in the patient's care. Evaluation of the patient's responses to nursing interventions should be evident. Each problem is referenced with a number corresponding to the problem list.

Patient education is ideally documented in the progress notes section of the medical record. Because patient education is a problem-solving process, documentation includes a clear statement of needs or problems, significant data contributing to these nursing diagnoses, and the plan for nursing care. The evaluations of the outcomes of care are essential ingredients in the care plan. Narrative notes also encourage the charting of the patient's own words to illustrate outcomes of patient education and evidence of individualized care.

POR and SOAP

Dr. Lawrence Weed (1971) developed the problem-oriented record (POR), a systematic tool for communication and problem-solving. All team members (physicians, nurses, physical therapists, dietitians, pharmacists, and social workers) contribute to the one problem list that focuses on *patient* problems rather than on *provider* problems. Team members write narrative and discharge notes using the SOAP format to document subjective and objective data, assessment (or identification) of problems and the planned course of intervention. The SOAP note was later modified to include intervention, evaluation, and revision, and referred to as SOAPIER. This method increases awareness of the contributions of others and encourages the members to function as a team. There are no divisions of nurses' notes, physicians' notes, and so forth. All health care professionals document information on the patient's progress notes. The patient is clearly the center of the team and the focus of care.

We recommend this method, and in our own experiences in patient education, it has increased communication and collaboration. It helps team members to know what has been taught by others and facilitates reinforcement of learned behaviors.

The POR highlights the use of the nursing process, which is based on problem-solving. Narrative notes begin by naming the problem, and they then offer subjective and objective data, the assessment, and the plan, as detailed in Box 12-3.

Many formats exist for progress notes, all of which can promote interdisciplinary coordination, a focus on the patient's functional health problems, and a record of the patient's learning outcomes as an integral part of documenting care. Regardless of the type of progress note, the nurse should shift the focus of care from the medical diagnosis to the individual patient's response to it (ie, the functional problems). This can be encouraged throughout the course of patient care by asking, *How does this diagnosis affect this patient?* Nurses' responses to this question help us to keep patient care centered on the patient.

Discharge Summary

Summaries or reports written at the time of discharge or transfer communicate to other health care providers the patient's needs for reinforcement and continued learning. This documentation is important because learning is a continuous process. It often begins in the hospital, but it must be resumed in the clinic or home. Nurses are encouraged to use written and telephone consultations in planning to meet the patient's learning needs.

A significant amount of patient learning occurs after patients leave the sheltered hospital environment, and most of them need continuous patient teaching to responsibly and capably manage their daily care. Suggestions for patient-centered one-page discharge instructions are offered in Chapter 10. Many agencies require that discharge instructions be developed in triplicate; the patient and family sign a copy for the patient's record indicating instructions were received, a copy is given to the patient, and a copy is provided to the individual or agency responsible for continuing care.

Patient Contracts

Patient contracts may also be entered as a permanent part of the patient record (see Chapter 9).

CLINICAL APPLICATION OF EVALUATING PATIENT EDUCATION OUTCOMES: CASE STUDIES

In Chapter 8, the reader was introduced to Mrs. Dawe, who is struggling with her daily management of diabetes and hypertension. Her case has been followed in Chapters 9 and 10.

BOX 12-3. The SOAP Format for Notes in Problem-Oriented Records

— —:Problem
S: Subjective data—what the patient reports
O: Objective data—what is observed through the senses and diagnostic tests
A: Assessment—the nursing diagnosis based on categorization and interpretation of data; patient responses to health problems
P: Plan—includes diagnostic, therapeutic, and patient education interventions and reflects immediate and future actions and the evaluation of these actions
For a SOAPIER note, add:
I: Intervention
E: Evaluation
R: Revision

C A S E   S T U D Y   1

EVALUATION OF MRS. DAWE'S BEHAVIORAL CHANGE

After the home visit for Mrs. Dawe, the nursing students offered a summary of patient learning outcomes. Reassessment of patient needs and modifications to the teaching plan are also noted.

Problem 3: Altered Nutrition. Mrs. Dawe correctly outlined food exchanges for breakfast, lunch, and dinner using her American Diabetes Association meal plan. She wrote three sample menus for each meal. She included one-half cup of ice cream in one of these meals and substituted accurately. She returns to the clinic for her first weekly visit with 2 days of food intake recorded in her notebook. Both days she had followed her diet plan. She reports that on the last 5 days she "cheated" on her diet and ate several desserts, failing to record what she ate. She states that she feels guilty not following the diet and explains that she knows weight control is important for her diabetes management.

Her weight at the clinic visit is unchanged from her last clinic visit. The nurses review her goals and learning objectives. Mrs. Dawe states that she is still interested in following her diet and wants a nurse's help in doing so.

The nurses reinforce Mrs. Dawe's knowledge about her diet and her understanding of the importance of weight control for her condition. The nurses stress that she must take responsibility for changing her habits but that the nurses will help her come up with strategies to confront problems. She states that she would like to resume her diet plan today and come back to the clinic next week. The nurses agree and give positive reinforcement to the fact that she had 2 days of success with her plan.

Problem 4: Altered Tissue Perfusion. Mrs. Dawe reported that she took her medications and showed the nurses the record of medication in her notebook. She reports that she omitted salt in cooking during the week and that she did not use any canned foods except for water-packed fruits. She recalls ten high-sodium foods when asked to do so.

Her blood pressure at the clinic visit is 188/96 mmHg.

Mrs. Dawe reports that it was less difficult than she thought to avoid high-sodium foods and that Mr. Dawe had encouraged her to do so. In fact, when she was about to use canned tomato sauce in cooking, Mr. Dawe reminded her of its high sodium content. The nurses commend the Dawes on their positive behaviors and show them how the blood pressure measurement highlights their success.

Boxes 12-4 and 12-5 illustrate SOAP notes written by the nursing students to document Mrs. Dawe's care.

BOX 12-4. 3/31/00 Home Visit of Mrs. Dawe

Nursing Note

Altered Nutrition

S: "I want help with my weight problem. I know I'm too heavy and it's making my diabetes difficult to manage. My diet is too limited. I just can't follow it."

O: 5'3" tall, weight 170 lb. at last visit. 45 lb. above prescribed weight. Unable to follow American Diabetes Association meal plan. Gets little exercise except for housework.

P: Negotiate weight loss goals. Change diet to updated ADA low-fat meal planning. Outline menus with Mrs. Dawe and make referral to the dietician to build variety into her meal plan. Discuss importance of weight loss in management of diabetes. Refer to diabetic luncheon. Schedule clinic visit for 1 week from now.

Altered Tissue Perfusion

S: "I know I need to cut down on salt and lose weight to get my pressure down."

O: Blood pressure 220/190 today. Reports taking medication.

A: Blood pressure poorly controlled. Food intake recall reveals salt used in cooking and at the table, with canned foods frequently included.

P: Continue medication as ordered. Patient to keep written records. Follow weight-reduction diet as ordered. Omit salt in cooking and avoid canned foods. Mrs. Dawe agrees with the plan. We discussed high-sodium foods to be avoided. Return to clinic in 1 week for blood pressure check.

BOX 12-5. 4/7/00 Clinic Visit of Mrs. Dawe

Nursing Note

Altered Nutrition

S: "I followed my meal plan the first 2 days, but cheated after that. I just couldn't pass up desserts when I thought about having them. I didn't keep records of what I ate, because I was embarrassed. I really do want to lose weight and wish you would help me to do it."

O: Weight 170 lb. (unchanged from last visit). The 2 days of recorded meals indicated Mrs. Dawe followed diet plan.

A: Poor cooperation with meal plan. Understands meal spacing and can select menus. Understands importance of weight control but does not

perform necessary behavior modifications.

P: Review goals. Stress Mrs. Dawe's responsibility. Offer assistance for problem-solving and role-playing. Reinforce 2 days of positive behavior. Return visit in 1 week.

Altered Tissue Perfusion

S: Reports taking medication. Reports omitting salt in cooking.

O: Blood pressure 188/96 today.

A: Blood pressure lower. Good cooperation with reducing sodium intake. Knows name and dosage of medication. Identifies high-sodium foods to avoid.

P: Reinforce progress. Continue weekly blood pressure checks.

MR. STRAMINSKY'S AMBULATORY SURGERY

Mr. Straminsky is 73 years old. His wife, Alice, is 70 years old. They live in the suburbs, 30 miles from a large teaching hospital where Mr. Straminsky is to have a bladder biopsy in ambulatory surgery. He was a patient in the same hospital 3 years before when he had a coronary artery bypass graft.

Nurses in the ambulatory surgery unit recognize that all patients have some degree of anxiety before the procedure. During the preoperative assessment, the nurses ask about concerns the patient and family have. Patients usually come to the ambulatory surgery center 2 days to 4 days before surgery. Before beginning patient teaching, the nurse tries to determine the following factors:

The patient's knowledge about the expected surgery or procedure
The patient's previous surgical experiences or hospitalizations
Other illnesses the patient may have
The patient's support systems
The patient's concerns about his or her occupational or related issues (eg, when work or activity can be resumed)
Effective ways of coping with pain

Unfortunately, nurses at the center find that they usually have about 15 minutes to complete the assessment, and often patients do not share their concerns in depth with the nurse. This is particularly true of older patients (Kempe, 1987; Leyder & Pieper, 1986).

Patient teaching preoperatively for Mr. Straminsky addressed what to expect in the surgical procedure and instructions for discharge (Connaway & Blackledge, 1986). The patient and his wife seemed to understand the instructions, although Mrs. Straminsky made a comment about how they had seen so many doctors, specialists, residents, and medical students, and they were overwhelmed with instructions. They were given a pamphlet explaining the ambulatory surgery unit and told the logistics of arriving the next morning for the surgical procedure.

The nursing diagnoses identified for most patients in this unit are appropriate for Mr. Straminsky:

1. Knowledge deficit related to the ambulatory surgery unit and the surgical procedure
2. Anxiety related to surgical procedure and discharge from unit

The short teaching session with the Straminskys seems to go well. The Straminskys ask questions about the procedure and repeat what they should do after discharge. They seem interested and capable.

When they return for the husband's bladder biopsy, the admissions nurse greets them. They were asked to report at 6:30 AM, and they arrive early, at about 6:00 AM. Mr. Straminsky is assigned a bed and his wife waits for a few minutes before joining him. Throughout the morning, Mrs. Straminsky seems anxious. Despite the procedure, which according to the health care team goes well, Mrs. Straminsky seems distracted and unsettled. She tells the nurse assigned to recovery that she was not well prepared for this "ordeal."

The nurse gives Mrs. Straminsky a form and asks her to describe her concerns in writing, reviewing her experience. This evaluation method helps the patient (or in this case the spouse) verbalize her feelings, and it can also be used to better teach other patients. Mrs. Straminsky agrees and begins making notes. Three days later, her "surgical experience" is delivered by mail to the nurse.

My Husband's Bladder Biopsy

The various physicians who have sent my husband and me for the many outpatient procedures are intelligent, caring, and extremely busy people. They certainly never indicated that they were sending us to the Ritz, but neither did they prepare us specifically for conditions in a large suburban outpatient facility.

In the preliminary visit, more discussion, or a videocassette, would all have been helpful. Some of these things could certainly be the responsibility of the hospital.

The first shock to me was the size of the tiny cubicles to which a patient is assigned. The only similar situation I have seen was an emergency room 25 years earlier. My sister had been taken there after an accident. I accepted the lack of privacy because of the need for immediate attention in that case.

This time we were scheduled and asked to report at the usual crack of dawn. One lonely nurse was on duty and she got my husband into bed. I was allowed to sit in a straight chair by his side as many other patients joined us, each in his curtained rectangle, each giving his history, giving blood, giving urine, and surrendering all thought that some items might be personal and private. There was no way to avoid hearing the details of others' dilemmas.

When my husband was finally wheeled away to surgery, it was a relief for both of us. I escaped first to the cafeteria, then to a waiting room near surgery. After the surgeon spoke to me about my husband, I was allowed into a recovery room where he was blessedly alone with a nurse in attendance.

"Good," I thought, "He'll be here in peace and quiet for a while."

It was a short time. Responsive but groggy, he was wheeled back to the outpatient area, now a bustling place. We were informed that as soon as he could urinate on his own, my husband would be discharged. There were many disappointing trips to the lavatory, and often other patients were waiting to use the facility. We waited about 8 hours before he was discharged. I believe it was that time that I inquired about whether it would have been better if he were admitted to the hospital. We were advised that neither Medicare nor our insurance would cover the cost, and the nurse advised against it. Evidently patients do best spending as little time as possible in hospitals!

"You don't want him to be in the hospital; terrible things happen in hospitals," were the exact words from the spouse of another patient. At least in the outpatient facility I could sit with my husband and watch for those terrible things.

The nursing staff was wonderful. Competent, professional nurses stayed aware of all that was going on. I imagine that they too wish for a better environment for themselves and their patients.

This experience (which bothered me much more than it did my spouse) could have been alleviated by some preparation such as the ones suggested at the beginning of this account. In addition, a waiting area adjacent to the patient holding area could be provided with video or slide viewers to help explain what is happening.

After reading Mrs. Straminsky's letter, the nurse realizes that more explanation of the physical layout of the unit is needed in the preadmission program. She also knew that patients and families experience more anxiety than they expect to feel because of the loss of control on the morning of surgery. The nurse decides to convene a group of patients and family members who had surgical procedures on the unit and ask them to share questions or concerns that they each had before, during, or after the procedure.

A 15-minute videotape is added to the pread-mission program, showing what the facilities looked like and following-up on a patient through the surgical procedure. It could also be shown the morning of surgery. The video-tape features a spouse who described how she handled such things as waiting, getting infor-mation about her husband's status, and so forth. This videotape is shown to groups of pa-tients the day before the surgery, and a nurse is available to answer questions after the film. She finds that patients and family members learn from each other and also get support from each other, which may continue through the surgical experience on the unit.

Commentary on the Straminsky Case

Research indicates that preoperative infor-mation alleviates anxiety and aids in postop-erative recuperation. However, preoperative instruction for the family has been largely overlooked. Studies have indicated that by al-leviating a family member's fear and anxiety, he or she can be a better source of support for the patient. Fear and anxiety have different characteristics and are subjective experiences. We know through the case study of the Straminskys that sensory experiences of the spouse can be a source of anxiety caused by lack of preparation. Particularly with older patients, nurses should use patient education to decrease anxiety related to the ambulatory surgery environment. Evaluation should con-tinue to be done to see how the patient and family perceive the adequacy of preoperative instruction. Although the results of preopera-tive patient teaching are well documented, this has not been true for family member teaching. One extensive review of the litera-ture shows a lack of:

- Studies that examine the impact of preoperative instruction on significant family members
- Studies that measure fear and anxiety in family members
- Tools to measure family members' psychological reactions to surgery

- Studies to determine potential positive impact of preoperative teaching interventions with significant family members and the patient (Moss, 1986).

CASE STUDY 3

MR. HORTON IN THE CORONARY CARE UNIT

Mr. Horton is the 67-year-old owner of a large retail store. He is admitted to the coronary care unit (CCU) with symptoms of coronary artery disease. Like most patients in this situation, he is anxious, depressed, and angry.

The nurses in the CCU are using patient-nurse contracts to help patients who are physiologically stable regain a feeling of control. They recognize that the routines and sensory experiences of the CCU are depersonalizing and that unit procedures and policies (eg, restricting visitors, telephones, and newspapers) make matters worse. They also know that research studies indicate that stress reduction measures to counteract environmental stressors positively affect patient attitudes and the return of functioning.

Commentary on Mr. Horton's CCU Experience and Nurse-Patient Contracts
Mr. Horton was oriented by audiotape to patient-nurse contracting, and then a nurse worked with him to offer choices about visiting privileges, hygiene time, room arrangements, teaching preferences, activity, and other areas of patient concern. The contract was shared with the nursing staff, who honored the terms of the contract whenever possible. Through this process, he was taught about how and why to manage aspects of his own care. Mr. Horton's anxiety decreases when measured 24 hours after contracting with his primary nurse.

(case study continues on page 345)

The CCU nurses in the case study on Mr. Horton evaluated the effectiveness of this intervention by studying control and experimental group outcomes. They use two questionnaires and a checklist designed to measure anxiety, depression, and hostility. The results of the study are rewarding. Although baseline data indicate no statistical difference between the two groups, significant differences were found when overall scores for both groups continued to change in opposite directions during time. The contract worked as an intervention to decrease anxiety.

Patients in the experimental groups were most interested in controlling the number and length of family visits, highlighting the support of family as a means to decrease stress. Overall, male patients in both control and experimental groups reported higher levels of stress than did female patients.

Nurse researchers (Ziemann & Dracup, 1989) in this study have made an important contribution to patient education efforts in the CCU by presenting a model for patient contracts in this setting. When teaching attempts are hampered by the patient's anxiety and depression, CCU nurses can use patient contracting as a powerful intervention that gets results.

SUMMARY

Evaluation occurs at different points of the teaching and learning process and uses different methods to gather the types of information needed. The nurse uses evaluation to measure the degree to which patient learning goals have been met and also uses findings to improve or redirect patient care. Documentation of the results of patient education focuses on patient outcomes: knowledge, skill, and health behaviors. Good documentation improves continuity of care, satisfies legal responsibilities for charting patient care, and provides evidence that standards for accredi-

tation are met. Understanding patient expectations and improving patient satisfaction are key to providing consumer centered care (Jennings & Staggers, 1999).

Through evaluation we learn valuable lessons from our patients and their families about teaching priorities, who needs to be taught, how to share responsibility for learning with the patient and family, and how difficult long-term change can be.

Despite good intentions, new knowledge and skills and behavior modification strategies, patients may only partially achieve the health outcomes nurses desire. Obstacles to change are often less tangible than, for example, exposure to party foods or pressure from family and peers. Obstacles are closely related to self-esteem, the patient's view of himself as a whole person. The feedback and counseling offered to patients in the health care setting may help them to place greater value on themselves and their health. This often takes time to develop, and many patients have difficulty accepting their own responsibilities in daily health management.

The provider-patient relationship offers an opportunity to help the patient grow in assuming his or her role as a member of the health care team. It is important to communicate confidence in the patient's ability to choose responsibly. It is also important to offer encouragement and guidance for change. Evaluation is a tool used to strengthen the provider-patient relationship and to continue patient-centered care through the nursing process. Documentation that includes evaluation of patient learning outcomes provides critical evidence of such patient-centered care.

In addition to meeting agency mandates for evaluating and documenting patient learning outcomes, nurses gain important personal and professional rewards by engaging in the process. In acute care settings, teaching can make the critical difference in helping a patient survive through an illness or injury. Nurses on a neurosurgery service described the importance their patient education made during an awake craniotomy. They stated that throughout surgery they showed the patient pictures, answered her questions honestly, provided comfort measures, and cared for her emotionally. "We helped maintain the patient's low anxiety level and received excellent feedback and cooperation" (Fuchs, Porter, & Clark, 1994).

In rehabilitation settings, nurses describe the rewards of patient teaching in different ways: "It makes you feel really good to see your teaching help a patient master self-care activities and to see these regained skills restore self-esteem, a positive outlook on life, and in many cases, independence. Nursing empowers patients to make decisions independently and improve the quality of their life" (McDonald, 1994).

STRATEGIES FOR CRITICAL ANALYSIS

1. Consider nursing care provided in the following settings: preoperative visit in day surgery, prenatal outpatient visit, recovery room, medical-surgical orthopedic unit, pediatric office, home health, long-term care, elementary school, and occupational health. Identify what types of patient learning outcomes are realistic, in which level they belong (Level A, B, C, or D), and how you would document them in the patient record.
2. Describe two strategies a nurse can use to help patients and families become involved in evaluating patient education efforts and offering suggestions for improving patient education services.
3. Describe two ways that members of the health care team could become more involved in evaluating patient education efforts and offering suggestions for improving patient education services.
4. How would you assess whether a new form is needed for documenting patient education in your agency? What are the pros and cons of creating a new form? Which existing form or forms could be eliminated? How can the health care team provide input in the decision?

REFERENCES

(1996). Documentation proves tough issue for educators. *Patient Education Management,* 3(12), 135.
(1999). Automate patient documentation with pop-up menus and mouses. *Patient Education Management,* 6(4), 37–39.
Bovender, N. (1994). Home care: nurses discover the rewards and challenges of this growing frontier. *North Carolina Nursing Matters,* 4(11), 6–7.
Brethower, K. S., & Rummler, G. A. (1979). Evaluating training. *Training and Development Journal,* 79(5), 12–20.
Connaway, C., & Blackledge, D. (1986). Preoperative testing center. *AORN Journal,* 43(3), 666–670.
Carter, B. (1999) Compliance and cardiac disease. *American Journal of Nursing,* 99(11), 24c.
Darby, M. (1999). Coordinating care in an integrated delivery system. *The Quality Letter,* 11(7), 1–5.
Eggland, E., & Heinemann, D. (1994). *Nursing documentation: Charting, recording, and reporting.* Philadelphia: J. B. Lippincott.
Finerty, P. (2000). Filling educational gaps. *Patient Education Management,* 7(1), 3–4.
Fuchs, K., Porter, M., & Clark, M. (1994). Caring for a patient during an awake craniotomy. *North Carolina Nursing Matters,* 4(8), 5.
Gibson J. (1989). A new approach to better medication compliance. *Nursing,* 19(4) 49–51.
Gregory, C. (2000). Age-specific education targets burn prevention. *Patient Education Management,* 7(1), 2.
Jennings, B., Staggers, N., & Brosch, L. (1999). A classification scheme for outcome indicators. *Image—The Journal of Nursing Scholarship,* 31(4), 381–388.
Joint Commission on the Accreditation of Healthcare Organizations. (1998). *1998 Comprehensive accreditation manual for hospitals.* Chicago: Author.
Kempe, A. (1987). Patient education for the ambulatory surgery patient. *AORN Journal,* 45(2), 500–507.
Leyder, B., & Pieper, B. (1986). Identifying discharge concerns. *AORN Journal,* 43(6), 1298–1302.
Mager, R. (1997a). *Preparing instructional objectives* (3rd ed.). Atlanta, GA: Center for Effective Performance, Inc.
Mager, R. (1997b). *Goal analysis: How to clarify your goals so you can actually achieve them*

(3rd ed.). Atlanta, GA: Center for Effective Performance.

Mager, R. (1997c). *Preparing instructional objectives: A critical tool in the development of effective instruction* (3rd ed.). Atlanta: Center for Effective Performance.

Mager, R. (1997d). *Measuring instructional results* (3rd ed.). Atlanta: Center for Effective Performance.

Magoon, L. (1999). The diabetes project. *American Journal of Nursing, 99*(10), 24c–24f.

McDonald, K. (1994). Rehab nursing: Helping patients be all they can be. *North Carolina Nursing Matters, 4*(8), 6–7.

Montemuro, M. (1988). CORE documentation: A complete system for charting nursing care. *Nursing Management, 19*(8), 28–32.

Moss, R. (1986). Overcoming fear. *AORN Journal, 43*(5), 1107–1114.

Mowry, M. Computerized and quality. In Johnson, M. (Ed.). *The delivery of quality healthcare.* St. Louis: Mosby-Year Book.

Oermann, M., & Huber, D. (1999). Patient outcomes: a measure of nursing's value. *American Journal of Nursing, 99*(9), 40–47.

Pierson, C. (1999). APNs in home care. *American Journal of Nursing, 99*(10), 22–23.

Pipe, P.. & Mager, R. (1970). *Analyzing performance problems.* Atlanta: Center for Effective Performance.

Pipe, P., & Mager, R. (1997). *Analyzing performance problems: Or you really oughta wanna* (3rd ed.). Atlanta: Center for Effective Performance.

Redman, B. (1998). *Measurement Tools in Patient Education.* New York: Springer Publishing Co.

Stallings, K. (1996). *Integrating patient education in your nursing practice.* [Video]. Reproduced with permission of GlaxoWellcome, Inc. (Produced by Horizon Video Productions, 4222 Emperor Boulevard, Durham, NC 27703.)

Weed, L. (1971). *Medical record, medical education, and patient care.* Cleveland: Press of Case Western University.

Weinrich, S. (1999). The high risk of low literacy. *Reflections, 25*(4), 22–24.

Ziegler, J. (1996). Improving diabetes management through employer/provider partnerships. *Business and Health, special report, 14*(1), (Suppl. A), 25–30.

Ziemann, K., & Dracup, K. (1989). How well do CCU patient-nurse contracts work? *American Journal of Nursing, 89*(5), 691–693.

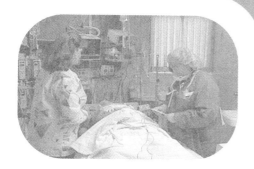

Case Management
and Patient Education

LEARNING OBJECTIVES

After reading this chapter, the nurse or student nurse should be able to:

1. Explain why the evolution of case management systems, with the goals of controlling health care costs and improving the quality of care, emphasizes the need for patient and family education.

2. Describe how patient learning outcomes are integrated in critical pathways and patient care maps.

3. Describe two ways staff nurses can provide leadership in promoting patient education as an integral part of case management.

4. Identify the philosophical differences of traditional and progressive health care providers that can challenge unification of patient education efforts.

5. Discuss the types and sources of power that nurses can use to promote patient education and to secure needed resources.

INTRODUCTION

Case Management: Controlling Costs and Improving the Quality of Care

Case management has been used for more than 25 years to allocate health care resources across various settings to meet individual client needs. The term *case management* typically described the model used by social workers in welfare settings (Kovner, Hendrikson, Knickman, & Finkler, 1993).

Case management has been adapted to inpatient, acute care settings and various outpatient settings in which nurses recognize the shift to outcome-oriented and fiscally responsible care (Powell, 2000). Health care delivery has shifted from fee-for-service plans to managed care or capitation plans. Managed care is a process in which all components of health services for a particular population of patients are brought together in a coordinated and accountable way (McEachern, Curley, & Neuhauser, 1995). In response, nurses have developed new professional practice models that incorporate principles of managed care. The models encompass clinical and financial outcomes, nurse as case manager, nurse-physician collaborative practice, and increased patient and family participation.

Patient education is an integral part of case management because it enables patients and families to participate in care and to gain survival skills needed to promote decreased length of stay and safe discharge (Powell, 2000; Oermann & Huber, 1999; Zander, 1988-1998).

Integrating Patient Education Into Case Management Models: Product and Process

Nurses provide important leadership in the practice innovations associated with case management models. They fulfill various roles and job descriptions (Powell, 2000). It is essential for staff nurses, who provide direct patient care, to understand the approaches and tools of case management. Interdisciplinary collaboration and communication and streamlining patient education approaches also are critical to assuring that patients have the right information at the right time (Darby, 1999). To address these issues, the first section of this chapter discusses the *products of case management* and suggestions for designing realistic patient education interventions.

Nurses may be managed care coordinators, case managers, clinical specialists, or patient education coordinators. In these positions, nurses fulfill the important roles of manager, consultant, liaison, advocate, facilitator, gatekeeper, negotiator, educator, and researcher (Tahan, 1999). If they do not directly deliver patient education, they are instrumental in coordinating case management system development. They also must promote innovative, interdisciplinary patient education interventions as part of patient care, design ways of evaluating complex patient needs and responses, and assess nursing staff knowledge and skill to teach patients (Wayman, 1999; Powell, 2000). These roles increase the nurse's power to improve patient education, yet simultaneously challenge him or her to appear neutral in the eyes of the interdisciplinary team and to gain the trust and respect of clinicians and administrators.

Process issues, including assessing and using power, dealing with politics in the organization, and promoting constructive change are key to successfully leading case management efforts (Kortbawi, 1993; Cahill, 1995; Lachman, 1999). The development process for critical paths (a tool used in case management) involves eight primary stages, which take place during 2 years for the creation of a single path (Hofmann, 1993):

1. Literature search
2. Steering group
3. Targeting diagnoses
4. Designing paperwork
5. Gaining consensus
6. Implementing trial program
7. Refining program
8. Full implementation

Gaining consensus of many caregivers is the most challenging task of nurses in leadership roles (Marquis & Huston, 1998), and it is an issue at all stages of group work. The nurse leader must address nurses and other caregivers who do not understand or who do not trust case management and think it is merely an administrative, money-saving strategy (Hofmann, 1993; Freed, 1998; Lachman, 1999). Turf battles (eg, how to implement patient education, how to standardize patient education materials, and how to integrate prevention approaches in the acute care setting) must also be addressed. These process issues and the use of power and politics are covered in the second section of this chapter.

PRODUCTS OF CASE MANAGEMENT

Key Elements of Case Management Models

One of the first models of nursing case management was developed by The Center for Nursing Case Management at Boston's New England Medical Center. It adapted the case management concept to the acute care setting with the nurse caregiver as case manager. This model has four essential elements:

1. Achievement of clinical outcomes within a prescribed time frame
2. Caregiver as case manager
3. Episode-based nurse/physician practices that transcend units
4. Patient and family participation in goal setting

Patient education is an integral part of case management efforts (Zander, 1988–1998).

Critical Pathways and Care Maps

Managing care is routinely accomplished by using an overall, standardized plan for a patient, which includes specific outcomes and time frames, and that is based on a diagnosis-related group (DRG) or case type. *Case type* refers to the medical diagnosis and is used for reimbursement purposes similar to DRGs (Bower, 1988). *Critical pathways,* one-page summaries of case management plans, plot the course of a patient's hospitalization (Leininger, 1997).

The critical path method, an industrial model from the mid-1950s, has been adapted to the delivery of patient care in the following way. A *critical path* outlines key incidents that typically occur at predictable times during a patient's hospital stay and according to the patient's case type. A one-page time line accompanies the critical pathway to help nurses and other professionals see how key incidents are managed in patient care (Zander, 1997). The one-page time line describes what is done each day for the patient according to the diagnosis and the milestones should be met by the typical patient of this case type. If the patient's clinical course deviates from the goal, the plan is revised.

For high-volume case types with predictable care patterns (eg, cardiac bypass patients), critical pathways are condensed into user-friendly documents called *care maps,* which can be used by the nurse to replace the patient care plan. Care maps are shared with the patient in the form of a patient care map, so the patient can anticipate discharge and track his or her own progress.

Critical pathways are developed collaboratively by nurses, physicians, and other health professionals involved in patient care. The goal is to incorporate an interdisciplinary perspective, identify expectations and events that are critical to achieving a desired length of stay, and implement strategies that improve the quality and cost effectiveness of care. The critical pathway does not take the place of physician orders. Patient education is one of the key activities sequenced in the care map; other activities include consultation, diagnostic testing, discharge planning, patient teaching, activity, diet, and medication. Timing and content for effective patient teaching are emphasized.

Nursing assessment and documentation reflect the progress or lack of progress made according to the critical pathway.

An example of a patient care map for open-heart surgery patients at High Point Regional

Hospital in North Carolina is shown in Figs. 13-1 and 13-2. It is designed for DRG #106 (coronary artery bypass graft with catherization) based on a length of stay of 4 to 5 days. The cardiovascular clinical care coordinator incorporated patient focus groups in the design of the patient care map. Based on patient input, the care coordinator collaborates with physicians, home health, and cardiac rehabilitation to develop a second care map (patient plan), which addresses the patient's course during the first 2 weeks after discharge. The care map is designed as a picture plan to aid the teaching of patients with limited reading skills. It also explains in narrative the expected events during the patient's recovery.

Most hospitals have adopted some form of critical path and care map system for patient care. Similar efforts to coordinate and standardize clinical care may be referred to by different names, including *clinical paths, practice guidelines,* and *coordinated care plans.* Time lines for critical paths can occur by visit (home health), by month (extended care), by week (rehabilitation units), by day (medical-surgical unit), or by minute (emergency department).

Patient Case Management and Variances

The term *patient case management* is often used to describe the close tracking and specialized individual intervention along the continuum of care that are needed to manage high-risk, high-cost patient cases. Although all patients benefit from nurse-managed care, case management frequently targets patients vulnerable to readmissions and an unpredictable course of care, including the following:

- Low birth weight infants
- Pediatric patients with special needs
- High-risk obstetric patients
- Patients with terminal illness
- Patients with multiple trauma
- Patients with human immunodeficiency virus (HIV)/acquired immunodeficiency syndrome (AIDS)
- Patients with radical surgeries (eg, amputation)
- Patients on long-term ventilation

Variances, which prevent the patient from staying on the expected course, are identified (Zander, 1997). A *variance* is a deviation from the projected critical path. For example, new nursing diagnoses may be identified, and the plan of care is revised. Quality improvement monitoring involves tracking variances; if patient outcomes vary from those expected, the nurse or other health care team member documents the variance and its reason (Leininger, 1997). Common reasons for variances may reflect patient, family, and provider outcomes, as detailed in Box 13-1.

Although exceptions are expected as plans are individualized, the targeted length of inpatient stay remains unless it can be justified by the variance. Variances can lead to a shortened length of stay or an extended length of stay (because patients may progress more quickly than expected). All variances are noted, with efforts to resolve negative variances as priorities in care planning and to examine positive variances that may lead to decreasing lengths of stay.

Documentation of Case Management

Documentation that supports case management continues to evolve. The trend toward computerized systems, often called *decision support systems,* integrates many facets of tracking, communication, and quality improvement (Patient Education Management, 1999b). It is also possible to automate the development of critical paths and patient education paths, similar to the development of standardized care plans with which most nurses are familiar. Software programs are capable of developing reports for physicians, nurses, and other staff, which reflect actual length of stay, patient and procedure variances (including those related to patient education outcomes), and actual outcomes of care. A charting-by-exception format is commonly used with bedside computer terminals.

Nursing Responsibilities in Case Management

Benefits of Nursing Case Management

The New England Medical Center model of nursing case management illustrates the

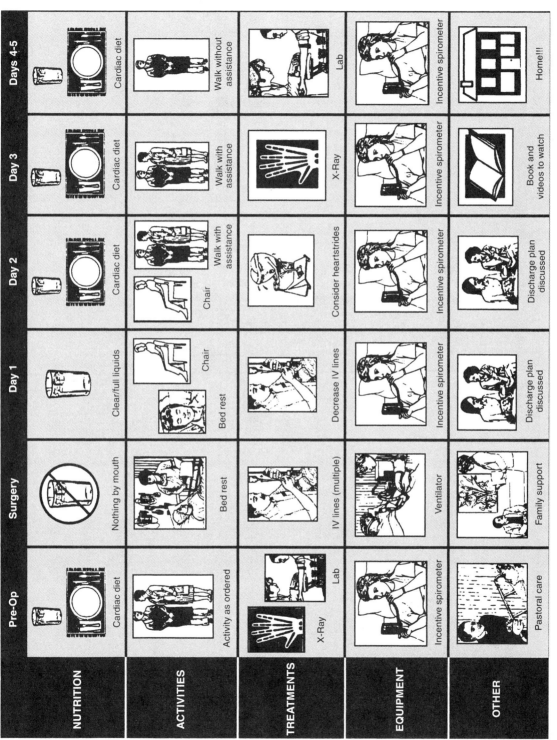

FIGURE 13-1. High Point Regional Hospital open heart surgery patient plan (picture path).

Open Heart Surgery Plan

Welcome to High Point Regional Hospital. This plan is to share with you and your family a picture of what to expect during your hospital stay, one day at a time. If you have questions or concerns, please ask your doctor, nurse, or members of our health care team.

Before Surgery: This is a busy day for you, but you can still enjoy your cardiac diet/food until midnight. You can also do the same activities the doctor has ordered for you until surgery. You will have a chest x-ray and blood and urine tests done. Teaching by your health care team members will also be done today. This will include: coughing, breathing exercises, ankle exercises, the equipment used to watch you during and after surgery, and about the surgery itself. A visit from Pastoral Care is also available.

Surgery: The events of the day of surgery begin at an early hour. Medicine will be given to you that makes you sleepy and relaxed. Your only activity will be bed rest. Before surgery, please do not get up after taking your medicine. After surgery, you will wake up in the Surgical Intensive Care Unit (SICU) with a breathing tube in your mouth, which is connected to a ventilator (breathing machine). You will not be able to talk until the tube is taken out, but the nurses will ask you yes/no questions so you can let the nurses know what you need. The nurse will explain things to you. Your family may visit you in the SICU at pre-set times, since it is a good idea for them to get some rest, like you, after you return from surgery. The doctors and nurses will also explain to them what is happening and why.

Day One After Surgery: By morning, the breathing tube is usually removed and you can talk again and start taking sips of clear liquid (apple juice, jello). You will wear an oxygen mask and will work on your deep breathing and coughing. An IV will be kept in place, but all the other equipment will be removed, if not needed. Usually you will be transferred to the Cardiac Telemetry Unit (CTU) where you continue your progress towards going home. Your activity will gradually increase during the day and you may get up in the chair. Your emphasis is to stay comfortable and rest.

Day Two After Surgery: Your diet will return to a cardiac diet. Your activity will increase and you will get in the chair several times. Teaching for going home will be continued.

Day Three After Surgery: You will continue with the cardiac diet throughout your stay. Your activities will increase each day. You will have an x-ray. You might feel sore, so please take your pain medicine to keep you comfortable. The most important activities for you to do are coughing and deep breathing. You and your family or care person will watch videos and learn discharge activities daily to help get you ready to go home. Your discharge plans will be reviewed and finalized.

Day Four or Five After Surgery: You will be walking and doing your coughing and deep breathing exercises by yourself. You will have blood tests. You will be ready to go home.

Remember, each person is special and may progress at a different rate. The plan is adapted to meet the needs of all our patients. It will allow you to set goals for yourself and keep you on course to go home. All your needs are taken into consideration as we work with you to return home. For more information, please read your books: *Going for Heart Surgery, What You Need To Know,* and *Moving Right Along After Open Heart Surgery.*

FIGURE 13-2. High Point Regional Hospital open heart surgery plan (text).

BOX 13-1. Common Reasons
for Variance

- Patient condition, complication
- Patient pain, fatigue
- Patient decision
- Patient's limited mental status
- Medication or treatment not administered
- Additional tests needed
- Care map modified because of admitting diagnosis or pre-existing condition
- Family decision or unavailability
- Equipment, medication, referral, transfer bed not available

---

responsibility nurses have assumed in managing patient care, which is goal directed and cost effective. New England Medical Center nursing staff (Bower, 1988) identified the following benefits that can be demonstrated with case management:

1. Patients are more aware of their progress, have more insight into their care, anticipate their discharge, and participate more in their care.
2. Nursing assessments are more outcomes oriented and address variances that influence length of stay.
3. Length of stay is controlled and often reduced.
4. Staff nurses think they have more control over patient care and feel more satisfied.
5. Orientation of new staff is more effective: new staff learn about case types and the goals and standards of care.
6. Shift report is more meaningful: Nurses share information about estimated length of stay, critical events anticipated for that day, and difficulties in achieving outcomes.
7. Documentation reflects patient progress toward goals.
8. Consultation, collaboration, and continuity of care are increased.

Case Management in Various Settings

Case management is not restricted to acute care; it also can be practiced in outpatient settings with many of the same successes (Marrelli & Hillard, 1996; Huggind & Phillips, 1998). These programs are often referred to as care management, and implying a continuum of care involving multiple settings and providers. Nurses are a link to health promotion, reduction of acute episodes, better utilization of resources, and often reduced costs.

For example, nurse case managers have successfully managed the care of older people who live in the community. The nurse works as a liaison to coordinate services for the older client and as an advocate when the client needs additional assistance. A plan of care and goals for rehabilitation are established for the client in a fashion similar to the critical pathways mechanism, and this plan is shared with the client and family members.

Another example of nursing case management concerns AIDS patients in the San Francisco Bay Area. The same case management process has been used to manage health care services for these clients. Case management goals in the community may differ from those in the acute care setting; however, managed care is still critical for the quality of life of these patients. Care management programs frequently target patients with asthma, breast cancer, CHF, diabetes, mental illness, and other chronic health problems (Brass-Mynderse, 1996).

Discharge Creep and Issues of Timing: Implications for Patient Education

Providing patient education as a critical facet of case management requires indentifying when to initiate patient teaching. Involving the patient throughout the case management process requires a commitment to openness and sharing with the patient and family, and respect for patient readiness. The nurse case manager is in a unique position to improve patient outcomes and control health care costs by addressing the need for innovative, product-line approaches to patient education (Powell, 2000). Nurses recognize that rising health care costs create financial incentives for early discharge and promote shortened lengths of stay.

 As inpatient length of stay decreases, critical paths must be redrawn to reflect a new time line for the delivery of procedures, tests, treatments, and patient teaching. For example, nurses must acknowledge and advocate that a 7-day patient education program cannot be automatically condensed into 4 days with the same patient learning outcomes achieved. Also, all days are not equal: the patient's physical and psychological ability and the need for reinforcement of learning must be considered when allocating teaching responsibilities to the path. Planning integrated patient education approaches that cross service areas is needed to increase patient safety and to provide continuity of care. ■

Carondelet Nurse Case Management Program

A model of *internal case managers* (ie, nurses who specialize in high-risk, high-volume cases) and community-based nursing case managers, comprises the system implemented by the Carondelet Health Care System in Tucson, Arizona. For example, at this health care system, the program for heart surgery patients includes well-managed teaching and care management in preadmission, intensive care unit (ICU), stepdown unit, telephone follow-up, and home visits.

By managing the entire service-line care experience rather than only the acute care experience, the Carondelet Nurse Case Management Program documented a 30% reduction in length of stay, a more than 10% reduction of costs, and a 58% reduction in adverse outcomes (Mahn, 1993). The managed care movement also has been the catalyst for nursing leaders to develop new models of theory based nursing practice (Tritsch, 1998).

Patient Input to Streamline Patient Education

Chapters 8 through 12 offer various approaches that can be used to streamline teaching in light of the trend for decreased length of inpatient stay. Repeated throughout the text is the advice: Choose no more than three or four critical learning objectives, observe patient performance, and document. Nurses are often stymied at the prospects of teaching less content in favor of survival skills because they worry that patients will be undereducated. The reality of short stays is that teaching too much can mean that the patient learns less, feels overwhelmed and frustrated, and fails to perform the most essential self-care responsibilities.

An innovative product-line model for educating cardiac rehabilitation patients (Hanisch, 1993) was implemented in South Dakota (Royal C. Johnson V.A. Hospital, Sioux Falls). It provides incentive for using patient input to streamline patient education that is useful and that promotes safety. The model can be applied to other patient populations in which patients are discharged quickly and cared for across multiple settings, such as in obstetrics and orthopedic surgery (Patient Education Management, 1998; Darby, 1999).

A cardiac rehabilitation coordinator in this South Dakota institution believed that to accomplish effective patient education, nurses must understand the perceived educational needs of cardiac rehabilitation patients and then develop a program that meets both the needs of the patient and the most effective time for learning (Hanisch, 1993).

The rehabilitation coordinator studied the topics taught by the interdisciplinary cardiac team (physician, nurse, physical therapist, social worker, pharmacist, dietitian, and chaplain) during the cardiac rehabilitation period (6 weeks to 6 months) after hospital discharge. She then constructed a questionnaire that was given to cardiac patients and their spouses. In addition to demographic data, the questionnaire asked patients to rate 30 topics believed by health care practitioners to be essential in cardiac patient education.

Respondents were first asked to rate (using a 7-point Likert-type scale) how important learning about the item was, and then to indicate the time during which it would have been most helpful. The four choices for time interval were: preoperative, intensive care unit (ICU), before discharge (stepdown unit), or posthospitalization. More than 75% (32 of 41 of respondents) indicated that four items were extremely important during all phases of recovery:

1. Specific instructions on type and amount of activity or restrictions
2. What is physically and psychologically normal and to be expected after cardiac event
3. Medication (names, dosages, side effects, scheduling)
4. Signs and symptoms of complications that need medical attention

These four items could be considered safety needs. Also, patients rated the following items as important to learn during the preoperative period: cardiac risk factors, anatomy and physiology of coronary artery disease, and explanation of the surgical procedure. In the ICU, the priority learning need was about ICU policies and procedures. In the stepdown unit, patient priorities were how to manage incisional pain and receiving written instructions for discharge, including diet. After hospitalization, patients placed priority on a follow-up telephone call, advice on resuming sexual activity, and managing decreased energy levels (Hanisch, 1993).

Table 13-1 presents the informational needs of cardiac rehabilitation patients. Note the growing use of telephone advice, e-mail, and tailored mailings (eg, newsletter to support patients after hospital discharge) to prevent unnecessary hospital admissions and costly office visits (New, 1998; Green, 1996; Wright & Arthur, 1996; Patient Education Management, 1998, 1999b, 1999c).

Although patients and spouses in this study perceived all 30 items as important, they offered valuable insights to nurses to redesign and streamline patient teaching for product-line or critical path models. They cited the four critical learning objectives targeted for every patient that can be reinforced in every setting, by every member of the health care team, and reflected in documentation. They also pointed

to scant learning needs that were specific to each of the four settings, thus enabling nurses to provide information at a teachable moment for the patient, when he or she is most motivated to learn it.

This study should inspire nurses to resist the urge to teach a 30-item list from top to bottom. Rather, patient input helps streamline the list and the process in ways that promote teaching smarter and achieving critical learning outcomes. Health care providers, especially nurses, should eagerly abandon outdated patient education approaches and design innovative interdisciplinary models such as the one described.

The remainder of this chapter addresses the process issues, which, unless skillfully dealt with, can prevent needed innovation.

PROCESS ISSUES IN CASE MANAGEMENT

Philosophical and Power Issues: Implications for Case Management and Patient Education

When care coordinators, case managers, nurse managers, and staff nurses involved in creating critical paths are interviewed, they invariably mention philosophical issues and power (or political) issues. Confronting these issues is essential to successfully streamline and integrate patient education into innovative case management efforts, including the development of critical paths and expert patient teachers (Benner, Tanner, & Chesla, 1996; Powell, 2000).

Despite evidence indicating that patient education improves the quality of care and reduces costs, nurses who promote patient education efforts must compete with other departments in their institutions for budgets and organizational influence (Bartlett, 1986). With the focus of patient education on interdisciplinary planning and coordination involving many providers, and frequently crossing divisional lines in the institution, a political

TABLE 13-1. Informational Needs and Preferred Time to Receive Information for Phase II Cardiac Rehabilitation Patients

	TABLE 1A								TABLE 1B			
LIKERT-TYPE SCALE **(NOT IMPORTANT) (VERY IMPORTANT)**									**TIME**			
1	2	3	4	5	6	7	**INFORMATIONAL ITEM**	PRE OP	ICU	POST EVENT	POST HOSP
			3	3	5	30	1. Cardiac Risk factors	23	4	11	2
2	2		3	5	7	21	2. Anatomy-physiology of heart	18	1	12	5
	1		2	6	4	27	3. Atherosclerosis/coronary artery disease	19	2	11	6
			3	1	1	26	4. Explanation of surgical procedure (bypass only)	29		2	
				2	6	25	5. Myocardial infarction	14	7	11	1
	3	2	4	5	4	23	6. ICU/CCU policies & procedures	17	18	4	
1		3	3	3	5	26	7. Effects of cardiac event on body functions	10	5	19	6
4	1		7	4	4	19	8. Effects of cardiac event on sexuality and sexual functioning	8		19	10
1	1		5	5	8	21	9. Possible emotional reactions to cardiac disease/event	11	3	18	8
1		1	2	8	4	24	10. How to communicate special needs to health professionals	13		19	7
	1		1	4	7	27	11. Involvement of partner or family in teaching program	12		13	14
1		1	1	5	10	21	12. How to communicate feelings and concerns to partner/family	8	2	20	9
		2	6	3	8	22	13. Available resources for assistance at home	2		20	18
		1			8	32	14. Specific instructions on type and amount of activity/restrictions	2	1	27	10
1			1	5	11	23	15. Specific time for resuming work and/or leisure activities	2		19	18
2	2		6	10	4	15	16. Suggestions on how to resume sexual activity	2		17	17
					9	32	17. What is normal and to be expected after cardiac event	7	2	21	9
			2	3	8	28	18. Dietary modifications	4		27	9
			2	2	5	32	19. Medications	4	2	28	6
			4	10	6	20	20. Time required for hospitalization and recovery	14	4	17	2
2	1	1	7	7	5	17	21. Follow-up phone call by health professional	2		14	22
	1			5	4	31	22. What will be experienced before, during, and after surgery/heart attack	25	5	6	2
				6	2	17	23. Removal of stitches and care of incision (bypass only)	2	5	16	3
			2	5	9	23	24. How to manage incisional pain and/or anginal discomfort	4	6	26	1
	1		2	8	6	24	25. Pulse taking	4	3	23	10
				2	7	32	26. Signs and symptoms of complications that need medical attention	5	3	23	7
		1	1	2	7	30	27. Common symptoms that occur during recovery	7	5	20	7
	2			8	5	24	28. How to manage decreased energy level	4		18	16
1			1	5	5	27	29. How to care for self after return home	2		19	15
		1	3	4	7	24	30. Written information about cardiac disease	8		15	14

Table 1A shows the rating of information. Table 1B shows preferred time to receive information. The numbers in the columns indicate the number of respondents selecting each informational item and time period. Not all respondents answered every question.

From Hanisch, P. (1993). Informational needs and preferred time to receive information for phase II cardiac rehabilitation patients: What CE instructors need to know, *Journal of Continuing Education in Nursing, 24*(2), 86.

coalition is necessary to support patient education services (Redman & Levine, 1987). In attempting to build coalitions, nurses encounter philosophical and political issues.

Philosophical issues concern one's approach to patients and basic beliefs about how patient education should be implemented. These issues tend to vary with educational background: nurses or other health care professionals tend to practice patient education in a manner consistent with their own educational preparation. Power and political issues usually concern control—who teaches what, to whom, and when.

This chapter presents skills that will enhance the effectiveness of the practicing nurse who confronts philosophical, power, and political issues in promoting patient education. These skills will also help prepare the student nurse to become an agent for change. We also explore the impacts that different professional roles and institutions exert on the delivery of patient education, criteria to help a practicing nurse determine who has power in a given setting and gain power herself to improve patient education, methods used to bring about planned change, such as change-agentry skills, and practical suggestions for managing philosophical and political issues.

Traditional Versus Progressive Health Professionals

Through years of nursing practice, we have noticed that, in general, two types of health care professionals exist: *traditional* or *progressive*. Although we speak of health care professionals as the entire health care team, the following discussion focuses on physicians and nurses.

The traditional health care professional is accustomed to a hierarchical approach to medical care, in which the physician is the dominant decision-maker and the focus of patient care activities. Those who subscribe to this model view the physician as totally responsible for all aspects of the patient's care and tend to regard the patient as belonging to the physician. The physician operates from a position of centralized power. These traditional models assume that the physician always

knows what is best for the patient and that the patient concurs with this attitude. The patient exhibits this concurrence by responding without question to the medical regimen.

Physicians practicing in medical and surgery specialties are often described as "traditional" in their approach to patient education. They are among those with a high risk of medical malpractice suits. This risk may account for this group's less than enthusiastic acceptance of nurse-sponsored patient education. Implications for nursing are that this group of physicians must be persuaded that patient education can actually reduce litigation. Accurate and concise documentation will establish a channel of communication, keeping the physician aware of all information given to his or her patients.

A traditional nursing orientation to patient education is most likely associated with nursing education prior to 1970, when nurses were taught in a medical model, often with physician instructors. The current approach to nursing education in both degree programs and continuing education, which uses the nursing process, has resulted in a more eclectic, holistic appreciation of humankind that does not depend on one particular approach or model.

The progressive health care professional may be younger, more accustomed to a team approach with the patient as the focus, and less likely to view the physician as the dominant or sole decision-maker. The progressive health care professional eschews centralized power in favor of decentralization, so that all team members have authority in their specialty areas.

We emphasize that both traditional and progressive approaches are appropriate; in some cases, the traditional approach may be better suited to some situations than the progressive approach. However, as readers can probably tell, our bias is in favor of the progressive health care professional.

Examination of the Issues

Philosophical Issues
Self-Care Approach
Self-care is a term coined by Dorothea Orem. As a conceptual basis for nursing practice, it

is "the production of actions directed to self or to the environment to regulate one's functioning in the interests of one's life, integrated functioning, and well being" (Orem, 1985). The nurse's function is to help the client achieve a level of wellness consistent with the client's own lifestyle and value system (but not necessarily with the value system maintained by the health care purveyors). In self-care, the client controls his or her medical regimen and makes choices regarding medical management. In the United States, the traditional health care system emphasizes acute management, which leaves the physician little opportunity to assist the patient in accomplishing self-care activities and skills.

Patient education is an integral part of self-care practice, because most patients lack the requisite knowledge to promote health or to manage problems related to disease.

Ideally, patient education reduces a patient's dependency on the health care system (it does not increase his or her need for services). Self-care activities promoted by the nurse attempt to make the system conform to the client's needs. Patient education activities encourage self-care and greater independence from the traditional health care system. Wellness and prevention are also promoted when health care professionals interact with patients and families.

We believe that traditional health care professionals are changing their attitude toward the self-care approach, partly because of consumer desires and pressures and partly because of a changing philosophy in many nursing and medical schools. Also, the standards of the Joint Commission on the Accreditation of Healthcare Organizations (JCAHO) support empowering the patient for self-care and wellness (JCAHO, 1998).

Patient Education Model
Progressive and traditional health care professionals adhere to different models of patient education. In our experience, traditional health care professionals tend to approach patient education from the perspective of the medical model: diagnosis, prognosis, and therapy. Teaching is oriented toward imparting knowledge about these three entities. Although most medical students receive this type of education, nursing students (especially recent graduates) usually receive instruction in teaching and learning theories, which assert that although information is imparted, there is no guarantee it is learned.

Nursing students are required to put teaching and learning theories into practice, and almost all recent nursing graduates can remember being evaluated on a patient education project. But as these theories assert, all students do not learn and practice the precepts as comprehensively as they should. A recently evaluated baccalaureate nursing student in a patient education setting said to a patient, "Because you've had a heart attack before, I know you understand what it's all about. I'll leave you a handout that will give you more information." The student made no effort to assess the patient's level of understanding or his or her possible misconceptions about the previous myocardial infarction. This student wrongly assumed that delivering information constituted patient education. (For more information on assessment in patient education settings, see Chapter 8.)

The progressive health care professional views patient education as a process with discrete steps, whereas the traditionalist frequently views patient education as the imparting of information. Progressive health care professionals also understand the value of tailoring teaching to individual patient needs and beliefs.

Information Sharing
Another philosophical issue is sharing information. Progressive health care providers are generally more willing to share information with patients. One nurse related an incident that occurred in a hospital where she worked, in which several physicians did not want their patients told about the potential side effects of a particular medication. In another example, a nursing student was forbidden to make home visits to an oncology patient because the physician did not want the student to tell the patient the possible side effects of chemotherapeutic agents. When a physician forbids a nurse to

give information to a patient, issues of power and control are definitely at stake (Benner & Tanner, 1996).

Obviously, instances occur when nurses impart incorrect information or choose the wrong time to attempt patient teaching. A nurse may completely overwhelm a presurgical coronary bypass patient with teaching, such that the patient approaches surgery with an unhealthy level of anxiety. It is the nurse's responsibility to ensure that his or her information is correct and that he or she properly assessed the patient's ability to learn. It is the physician's responsibility, in keeping with the patient's right to know, to impart all pertinent information to the patient in such a manner that the patient can understand the information.

One of the best ways to get physicians to support patient education is to show how it benefits them. Find out what physicians repeat to their patients, or what patients repeatedly phone the physician about during or after office hours (eg, pain or constipation). Create a handout to remind patients of what they were taught. An orthopedic surgeon may sit down with a patient and review exercises that the patient is to perform after surgery. The nurse can create a teaching sheet to reinforce the instruction and use it for follow-up by the nurse. It can also include information on how to deal with pain. Nurses find that resistant physicians appreciate the nurses' skills as patient educators when patients remember and follow instructions better (Patient Education Management, 1999a).

Holism

The *holistic concept of man* implies that we view a person as a total, nonfragmented human being, who is a sum of all his or her parts (Menke, 1985); this concept has an impact on patient education. When we assume the holistic approach, we are interested in the total person, not just his or her diseased or dysfunctional part. The medical model, which the nursing profession endorsed in the past, separates mind from body from spirit. This model presumes a nonholistic approach, one looks at the child's broken leg, diagnoses it through the use of x-ray films, casts it, and prescribes an analgesic.

According to the medical model, the fractured femur is the dysfunctional part, the part that is treated. A holistic approach expands the focus on the child with the broken bone to include assessing the parents' need to be taught childhood safety. When the holistic approach is applied to patient education, it is evident that patient education should include more than just teaching about a single dysfunction or problem.

Another example of holism and its effect on patient teaching involves a 44-year-old man with gastric carcinoma. A nursing student who had cared for the patient in the hospital made a home visit to evaluate his status and do any necessary teaching. She found that the patient's family had learned the necessary skills of dressing changes and tube feedings and that they were doing much better with the physical care than had been expected. However, she noted that the teenage son exhibited inappropriate behavior by ignoring his father. During discussions with the mother and son she learned that the son feared a bloody, gruesome death scene. The nursing student could clarify the misconceptions and alleviate a great deal of the adolescent's anxiety. Her holistic approach also included a referral to a local hospice group.

In the past, most nursing education paralleled medical education, and nurses were instructed according to the medical model. Some nurses still subscribe to the medical model but, as nursing education has progressed, many nurses abandoned the old model in favor of a view of the patient as a unified whole. There is also a growing trend among physicians to ascribe to a holistic concept, and it is not unrealistic to hope for a unified nursing-medical approach in the future.

Education for the Chronically Ill

Viewpoints about educating chronically ill patients differ between traditional and progressive health care professionals. Most progressive professionals believe that patients with chronic illnesses need more in-depth education than is ordinarily offered by the medical regimen (ie, more information than indicating on a chart when medications should be taken). Nurses and other progressive health care professionals undertake teaching about chronic illness in an effort to assist the client in attaining the highest level of wellness possible.

Ruth Wu states in her book *Behavior and Illness* that the chronically ill person maintains a secondary role, the chronic-illness role, on a permanent basis or until he or she becomes acutely ill, at which point he or she reverts to the sick role (Wu, 1973). The chronic-illness role requires greater patient adaptation in most situations than does the more acute-sick role. Social expectations are vague for the patient in the chronic-illness role. He learns that the condition, unlike acute illness (the sick role), is not reversible; this awareness greatly influences the informational needs of the patient.

For example, a nurse spent 3 hours with a 12-year-old girl who had insulin-dependent diabetes and her parents, attempting to educate them about the intricacies of diabetes management. This preadolescent girl and her family not only had to learn about insulin administration, diet, exercise, blood glucose monitoring, and the signs and symptoms of hypo- and hyperglycemia, but they also had to learn how to work this regimen into the lifestyle of a 12-year-old. The patient and her parents needed to actively set goals for her own care (Jacobson, 1996). At one point they realized that they had to weigh the option of less strict control against the possible dangers of later complications and even premature death.

When an adolescent is diagnosed with type 2 diabetes, it is likely that other family members also have diabetes or are glucose impaired. Obesity, high-fat, low-fiber diets and lack of physical exercise are also a common family pattern. Nurses should review the entire family dynamic and help the family make healthy lifestyle choices (Diabetes Management, 1999). Imparting all information to the chronically ill patient and his or her family is especially important. Long-term plans must be made and long-term goals defined by the family and the nurse.

The AIDS epidemic and consideration of cancer as a chronic, terminal illness have resulted in additional efforts to increase the quality of life for these patients through effective patient education (Pollock, 1987; Adinolfi,

1996). The growth of support groups among the gay community in San Francisco demonstrates the importance of self-help, but also the failure of the established health care community to effectively share information on pharmaceutical agents, treatments, and other issues of utmost importance to the community most at risk for developing AIDS. The necessity of increasing quality of life for those living with AIDS is imperative. Quality of life can be enhanced through the immediate sharing of information and through agencies (eg, hospice) that offer emotional and instrumental support.

Quality of life for cancer patients has been improved by the research of nurses that has been shared and put to practice. For example, Weekes & Savedra (1988) studied the coping strategies used by adolescents responding to chemotherapy or bone marrow treatments. The implementation of their findings will assist chronically ill adolescent cancer patients to improve their quality of life through patient education.

A nurse who is educating a patient and family about chronic illness is responsible for covering the details of the medical regimen. If, however, the nurse does not discuss the regimen in the context of the patient's lifestyle (including educational background, socioeconomic status, marital and family status, belief system, and occupation), then the teaching is virtually useless (Patterson, Thorne, & Dewis, 1998).

Power and Political Issues
Compliance
An important topic in any discussion of patient education is compliance. Many traditional health care professionals claim that the goal of patient education is compliance and that patient education is worthless if we cannot prove that it increases compliance.

The authors believe that compliance with a medical regimen is an important, but not the only, goal of patient education. A significant process occurs between education and compliance, in which the client internalizes the teaching and then makes informed choices about applying the teaching to his or her life.

It is the coercive aspect of compliance that relates this issue to power and control. Who has power in a patient education situation, the health care provider or the patient? Obviously, the patient should have the control, but too often patient educators try to control the situation for the patient, subtly threatening removal of support or services if instructions are not followed.

Health care providers, especially physicians, have usually been viewed as authority figures whose will must be obeyed. As consumers demand greater accountability of health care professionals, many providers have dropped the traditional, paternalistic roles. We hope that all health care professionals will eventually view compliance as only one part of the provider-client relationship, instead of as an end in itself.

Responsibility for Teaching

Determining who should teach is another power and political issue on which progressive and traditional providers frequently disagree. Nurses have a legal responsibility to provide health teaching for their patients (see Chapter 6). Yet nurses still encounter some physicians who believe that nurses should not perform health teaching. In some hospitals, physicians require nurses to wait for an order before their patients may be shown hospital-approved videos or literature. Although in some cases a physician's order is required to facilitate third-party payment for patient teaching activities, in many situations the requirement of a physician's order for patient education is an issue of power and control.

A physician's reluctance to allow nurses to perform this as an independent function may be related to incidents they have seen involving novice nurses who were clinically unprepared to teach (Benner & Tanner, 1996). Licensed practical nurses (LPNs) are not prepared in their educational programs to assess and plan for patient education. This is not to say that few LPN patient educators carry out effective patient teaching, but it is unrealistic to expect all of them to be as well prepared, without staff development and continuing education,

as the baccalaureate registered nurse (Balik, 1998). Granted, some professional registered nurses (RNs) are ineffective as patient teachers because of either personality factors or lack of preparation. A few experiences with these nurses tend to dampen the enthusiasm of even the most strongly patient education-oriented physician. However, nurses who have been rebuffed in their patient education efforts by physicians, are inclined to lose some of their enthusiasm. Patient education must be a team effort.

Most nurses are not interested in appropriating the physician's role in discussing the diagnosis, prognosis, and therapy with the patient. Instead, they interpret their role in patient education as that of making themselves available for clarification and discussion of daily management of the problem. This role seems appropriate for the nurse if we accept the goal of nursing as the promotion and maintenance of health in individuals, families, groups, and the community (Weaver, 1985; Roy, 1984; American Nurses Association, 1980). Again, collaboration is a key to effective patient education. It is often necessary to spend time one-on-one with physicians to garner trust and to gain support for patient education programs (Patient Education Management, 1999a).

Patient Education Referrals

The third political issue is the willingness to refer patients to other patient education resources, especially self-help groups. It is frequently appropriate to refer patients to extramural resources so that they can receive ongoing support (and ongoing teaching) from like-affected people, as in the cases of patients with Alzheimers disease, their families, and patients with substance abuse problems.

Nurses and physicians frequently do not know about groups and online computer resources to which patients could be referred. Part of this lack of awareness is undoubtedly caused by the proliferation of information with which health professionals must be familiar. Also, it represents a lack of concern regarding the development of patients' coping and adaptive resources.

A more disturbing attitude, however, is the paternalism found among traditional health care professionals who are reluctant to suggest community resources unless they can vouch for their value. The idea of ownership of patients is not a viewpoint congruent with the prevailing belief that adults are responsible, autonomous human beings who make their own choices about health care. If a physician or nurse refuses or neglects to give a patient information about self-help groups, the health care professional has single-handedly decided that the patient cannot judge whether such a self-help group might be useful. This type of attitude effectively places the power for decision-making in the physician's or nurse's hands instead of in the patient's, where it rightfully belongs.

All physicians and nurses should acquaint themselves with self-help and support groups that may aid their patients. The health care consumer recognizes the need for self-help resources and is becoming more aware that the traditional social and medical institutions cannot provide complete support for the handicapped, the needy, the deviant, or the socially isolated. Health professionals cannot be all things to all people; we must give some of our power to self-care and avenues for self-help support resources if the client desires it.

Power in the Patient Education Setting

Stephen Robbins defines power as the influence a person or a group has on the decision-making process (Robbins, 1980). John Wax's definition supplements Robbins, stating that power is "the control of resources essential to the functioning or survival of individuals and the organization" (Wax, 1971). Nurses have begun to recognize power as a legitimate function in nursing, and nurse educators promote its use.

Recognizing Types and Sources of Power

Power is a quality that is developed over time with a great deal of hard work. The clues to recognizing power and influence in others are subtle. To implement patient education, first recognize where power resides by asking the questions in Box 13-2. Because power includes decision-making and control of resources, nurses should learn to answer these questions correctly and to approach the power source or sources.

Power emanates from various sources, which in turn strengthen or lessen the power. The following typology of power outlines its sources, starting with the most and ending with the least influential:

1. Expert power
2. Positional power
3. Personality, or charismatic, power
4. Social power

Expert power is the most effective type of power. The person with expert power knows what he or she is talking about, and people respect what he or she has to say. This person may or may not possess positional power. A nurse who attempts to coordinate or initiate a patient education program on pain management must

---

BOX 13-2. Questions to Determine Who Has the Power Regarding Patient Education in an Institution

- Who decides if this patient is to receive teaching?
- Who assesses the value of a teaching program and mandates its operation in the hospital?
- Whom do I approach for obtaining necessary funding for audiovisual equipment to enhance patient education?
- Who knows what is really going on in this institution?
- Who seems to be "in control" at meetings on patient education?

have expert power if his or her efforts are to succeed. He or she provides pertinent information in a logical, concise manner, citing accepted guidelines for analgesics (Collins, Sparger, Richardson, Schriver, & Bergenstock, 1999).

Expert power may be a type of formal power (eg, in a nurse clinical specialist) or it may be informal power (eg, the staff nurse everyone turns to when a patient needs teaching). Formal education or on-the-job training can develop expert power, but expert knowledge makes this person credible. Being an expert on the costs and benefits of patient education efforts, especially financial, are an important source of expert power.

Positional power is always formal power, because it is invested in the person by an institution or organization. Persons with positional power have the ability to hire and fire, to authorize pay increases, and to set limits of acceptable behavior. Positional power is an obvious asset to the nurse who tries to initiate a patient education program. Nurses who have assumed the roles of care coordinator or case manager can learn to use their position and administrative mandates as a source of power (Marquis & Huston, 1998).

Personality, or charismatic, power is less effective than expert or positional power. All of us have known people with tremendous power because of a dynamism that sets them apart from others. Most people can name political or religious leaders with charismatic power. Likewise, most people know coworkers with power based on their personalities. We know a physician who began a successful in-house patient education program that was quickly adopted by the medical and nursing staff because of the power of his personality. Power by personality is more efficacious if it is combined with either expert or positional power. The support of a person with charismatic power can be a tremendous asset in beginning a patient education program.

Social power is the fourth and least effective type of power. Social power is the power that one has through social relationships and friendships. It is power given by a group to its

informal leader. The aspects of social power that make it least useful are its dependence on relationships, its lack of substance, and the underlying premise that something is owed in return for the granting of social power.

Social power, like expert power and charismatic power, can be formal or informal. Educators and nurse managers frequently use social power to get staff to accept changes. When launching a new patient teaching program, having a staff development session over lunch and sharing public acknowledgement with staff for their successful development efforts are helpful strategies that capitalize on social power. It is not unusual for chief nurse executives in large hospitals to use charismatic power to advocate for new programs; in fact, nurse executives are probably more productive if they can use these types of power in addition to the more formal kinds. A combination of power types is usually effective, but expert power is a necessity for anyone who wants to be recognized as an able leader for patient education.

Developing Power

Once the questions about who has the power have been answered and the type of power has been identified, many directions can be taken to gain support for patient education efforts. An obvious response is to develop expert power. Because this usually takes some time to develop, it may be desirable to gain knowledge from the one with expert power by spending time observing her modus operandi. This is also the time to gather as much formal training and education as possible, through reading books and journal articles and attending seminars and classes.

One nurse who was hired to develop and assume a job as coordinator for patient education in a community hospital spent the first 6 months in her new position identifying powerful figures among physicians, nurses, and other hospital personnel. She also improved her already formidable knowledge about patient education by attending conferences on patient education, by reading extensively, and by working closely with graduate students in health education to develop a needs assessment for the hospital. She researched innovative patient education models that had been shown to improve patient outcomes and decrease costs. After 6 months she solidified her power, which was previously positional, by displaying her knowledge of patient education needs in the hospital and by being recognized as an expert in her field. Positional power continued to undergird her authority, and expert power enhanced and strengthened her power in the hospital.

After assessment of the institutional power structure and establishment of a power base, change may be necessary.

Planned Change and Change-Agentry Skills

The nature and process of change is still not well understood, although many social scientists and some nursing leaders have developed theories and models that attempt to explain it (Bennis, Benne, & Chin, 1985; Watzlawick, Weakland, & Fisch, 1974; Lewin, 1951; Brooten, Hayman, & Naylor, 1978). Planned change entails organizing for change or applying scientific method and problem-solving skills: assessment, planning, implementation, and evaluation (Hall, 1985; Marquis & Huston, 1998). Examples of situations in which change-agentry skills (those skills the nurse uses to effect planned change) have been applied to the realm of patient education can illustrate the usefulness of these skills. As Hall states, these " . . . skills are those which can be employed to facilitate change in client systems and constitute the power armamentarium of the nursing practitioner as a change agent" (Hall, 1985).

Five skills listed below greatly enhance the professional image of nurses and help them to develop skills in these power-laden areas:

1. Coordinating
2. Collaborating
3. Consulting
4. Negotiating and bargaining
5. Confronting

We note two additional change-agentry skills—reframing and coercion—that are useful in diverse patient education settings.

Coordinating

Change agentry in patient education involves organizing and uniting various approaches and health care professionals in a way that ensures high-quality patient education is delivered. The nurse who uses this type of coordination as a change-agentry skill recognizes the contributions and capabilities of others involved in patient education and arranges patient education programs to meet the needs of varied client groups.

In a community hospital that hired an advanced practice nurse to establish a hospital-wide patient education program, the change-agentry skill of coordination was used in the following manner. In committee decision-making situations the coordinator repressed her tendency to want to control and, instead, facilitated the decision-making by *not* asserting her power or authority. She openly recognized the nurses and physicians on the patient education task force as the experts, and she assisted them in designing teaching protocols as part of the critical paths.

Coordination skills were also used to assist the patient education task force in setting goals. The goal was to create a product that would be strongly desired and then to make that product visible. By developing a product, the members of the task force enjoyed an enhanced image, and the entire task force was given increased credibility. Health care professionals were positively reinforced for patient education efforts and perceived payoffs from the patient education program were highlighted.

Collaborating

The process of working in a creative and egalitarian manner can further promote the welfare of the client in the patient education setting. Physicians, pharmacists, dietitians, and other health professionals respect the nurse who integrates such collaboration as a change-agentry skill, because he or she will share her expertise with others. Collaboration precludes the negative approaches of territoriality and ownership of patients.

In the community hospital example discussed above, collaboration was used creatively by the coordinator to set a tone of cooperation. She used validation as a strategy to prevent members of the task force from becoming entangled in the decision-making process. Validation consisted of documentation and carefully written minutes that were circulated before every meeting. By validating the process that was taking place, she could establish a spirit of mutual cooperation and appreciation of others' contributions.

Another way in which she used collaboration was through her obvious ability to work within the environment of the community hospital and to deal with the constraints imposed by the institution. Because she could work creatively with administrators and physicians, the nurse executive immeasurably improved her chances of successfully implementing a hospital-wide patient education program.

Consulting

> *I do a lot of one-on-one with staff nurses to help them prioritize patient education needs. A nurse might ask me to review her assessment and use me as a resource for a complicated patient. I help develop materials and programs to support the work of staff nurses.*

L.P. (Stallings, 1996)

The relationship between the nurse with proficiency in patient education (eg, the clinical nurse specialist) and the consultee who seeks his or her skills is reciprocal. The nurse shares expert knowledge to further the practice of sound patient education concepts. The nurse as

consultant has effective communication skills and uses them to assist the consultee in developing patient education resources and programs. Case managers and clinical specialists, by providing consultation for difficult patient situations, can empower staff nurses to teach and provide the precepting staff nurses need.

For example, the community hospital coordinator assumed her role as consultant by first clarifying her own understanding of her role. She realized that she occupied a staff position and not a line position; thus, there were limits on her authority and ability to discipline, hire and fire, or set policy. Instead, she had been employed for her considerable managerial and organizational skills and to provide the impetus for the establishment of a patient education program.

She avoided a common consultant mistake by refusing to actually practice patient education. She thus did not interject herself into the nurses' work setting. When a patient education coordinator uses consultation to effect change, it is inappropriate for her to assume the actual work of educating patients. Instead, she should teach the nursing staff the principles of teaching and learning theory and other relevant information.

Furthermore, this coordinator assumed the role of consultee herself when she sought help from other departments. In addition to increasing her visibility in the hospital, she managed to secure some valuable contacts for later use. For example, the coordinator consulted the medical records department to determine the most frequent diagnoses on admission. Her ability to move from the consultee to the consultant role provided beneficial role modeling for the nursing staff.

Negotiating and Bargaining

To promote and provide patient education, the nurse must negotiate agreements. The agreements usually involve the procurement or delivery of patient education to a needy client group. Negotiating is a positive process through which both parties derive satisfaction. In the patient education setting, bargaining may also occur between a nurse and a client with both parties negotiating for mutually satisfactory and achievable goals.

Bargaining is a splendid change-agentry skill that many of us rarely use. However, it must be accomplished in a setting in which rationality and calmness prevail. A patient education coordinator can avoid emotional debates; if someone exhibits obnoxious, strident behavior during meetings, it can be ignored and not held against the person in future meetings.

One coordinator bargained effectively when the goals of certain patient education programs were questioned. Instead of compromising goals, however, she agreed to changes in content and strategy. When bargaining is used as a change-agentry skill, the nurse must remember that negotiating a bargain is a give-and-take proposition and that some important ideas may have to be traded away.

A clinical nurse specialist who served as associate director of a diabetes teaching center negotiated to achieve her desired ends regarding establishment of outreach patient education centers for Chinese and Hispanic patients with diabetes. The medical director of the center was eager to have the center accredited by the American Diabetes Association, a long and tedious task that he was unwilling to do himself. The nurse informally bargained with the physician, using her willingness to oversee the accreditation process in exchange for the physician's willingness to approve the outreach programs.

Confronting

The various perceptions held by different people in a patient education setting must be clarified and compared. Confrontation involves a face-to-face encounter between the nurse and another health professional or the patient. Reserve the powerful change-agentry tool of confrontation for situations involving a lack of direct, open communication. Use confrontation only after other change-agentry skills have been exhausted.

When using confrontation as a change-agentry skill, be aware of the two levels of response it usually evokes: emotional and intellectual. Recognize and identify the emotional response but do not respond to it. The intellectual response allows room for reasoning. Do not use confrontation in an attempt to impose beliefs on another but to establish an environment that will encourage a new approach to the problem. For example, when a patient education coordinator realized that territoriality was becoming an issue, she turned the decision-making focus toward patient care and patients' rights.

When involved with confrontation, consider the amount of authority and support held by the person being confronted. If the person is not powerful, the optimal method of confrontation may be to override him or her. If he or she does possess support and authority, summon the committee members to attempt to change his or her mind. These group members must have equal influence and power for this method of confrontation to work. The term confrontation often has negative overtones. Attempt to remove the adversarial aspect of the term.

Reframing

When a situation is viewed in an entirely new light, old ideas and methods can be replaced with new approaches (Clark, 1977). This reframing is different from confronting in that the nurse reworks or restates the situation for the patient or client group. This frequently involves introducing an entirely different perspective into patient education. When old problems are broached in a different light, new avenues can be taken.

The patient or the institution may introduce this different perspective in patient education, or it may be the perspective of a particular committee member. An example of reframing occurred when we spoke to the medical staff of an outpatient center, presenting patient education as more than an attempt to gain compliance, but instead as a basic feature of the patient's right to know. One physician who had obviously pondered this idea said, "I see what you are saying; it's like informed consent."

Coercing

Legal authority can be used to gain an end that is not attainable in any other less forceful fashion. Coercion avoids emotional overtones, focusing instead on institutional and federal regulations. Coercion is better applied to recalcitrant groups of health professionals who are unwilling to institute patient education than it is to individual clients.

Coercion is usually a last-resort change-agentry tool; apply it only when all else has failed. When a patient education coordinator was stymied by one "blocker" physician, she used coercion by having an administrator exert power from above, after showing him that the blocker was obstructing the goals of the organization. This change-agentry skill makes many of us feel uncomfortable; it is not a skill we are taught as nursing students, or are encouraged to use in clinical practice. At times, however, it is the only effective way of achieving the desired goal.

The use of critical incidents, such as a high rate of diabetic readmissions or JCAHO probationary accreditation, can coerce reluctant people or institutions to affect change. When the staff of a community hospital was informed that they did not meet JCAHO criteria for acceptable patient education, they ceased arguing the merits of patient education and began planning better programs.

Other Strategies

Using open-ended questions to probe the attitudes of recalcitrant patient education task force members has led to greater understanding of some unspoken, underlying issues. When opposition is strong, retreating and compromising rather than continuing to wage war may be a good tactic. When using this strategy, however, it is unwise to go back to the be-

ginning of the process because all gains would thus be nullified.

Another strategy is to reinforce the base of support for change and make the base stronger. A change agent should constantly reinforce his or her position through the help of others. It is also important to look inward if things are not going well. Perhaps the change agent has provoked an undesirable response. Increasing credibility is another strategy to effect change. Showing is better than talking, and it is imperative that other health professionals believe the change agent is an expert in his or her area. High visibility in an institution does not guarantee credibility.

CLINICAL RELEVANCE: CASE STUDIES

A Case Management Model for Patients With HIV/AIDS

Case management is defined by the ANA as a system of health assessment, planning, delivery of care, coordination of care, and monitoring patients throughout the process to see that their needs are met (ANA, 1988). Nurse practitioners (NP) who work in primary care roles meet this definition of case managers of the patients in their care. HIV/AIDS care is very suitable for NP case management in the primary care setting (Kirton, Ferri, & Eleftherakis, 1999). The case management role of a primary care NP is not limited to this area, and many applications are currently used in practice (Bear, Brunell, & Covelli, 1997; Carlson, 1996; Johnson, Wise, & Jimmerson, 1995).

Since the advent of multidrug therapy, the treatment of people with HIV/AIDS has shifted from a focus of terminal illness to a long-term chronic illness. Caring for patients with HIV/AIDS is complex and these patients remain at risk for medical and psychosocial complications (Adinolfi, 1996; Kirton & Ferri, 1999). The excellent primary care and case management of this population by a nurse practitioner is illustrated by the following case.

A YOUNG MAN WITH HIV DISEASE

PRESENTATION AND PHYSICAL EXAMINATION

Chris is a 24-year-old male intravenous drug abuser with a three-year history of HIV disease. He is seen in a large university practice in San Francisco. During the initial encounter with the NP, a large amount of data is collected, including history of present illness, review of symptoms, and previous medical history, childhood illness, medication history, history of STDs, habits, dietary habits, travel history, and pets.

The physical examination consisted of laboratory studies and a complete physical examination, including a general assessment, oral exam, fundoscopic exam, lymph node assessment, skin, neurologic exam, cardiovascular exam, and gastrointestinal and genitourinary exam.

The NP uses this encounter to establish a therapeutic relationship with the patient. She listens to his concerns about his lifestyle and its impact on his illness. He has a history of male prostitution to obtain money for drugs, and he did not always use condoms. The NP and patient contract that the patient will cease any high-risk behaviors and only practice safe sex. In consultation with the consulting attending physician, the NP determines the degree of immune suppression and stages the disease for this patient.

Chris has HIV RNA levels above 5000 copies /ml of plasma and a CD4 count of less than 500 cells. This is within the guidelines for initiating antiviral therapy. The nurse practitioner consults with Chris and determines if he is ready to commit to an antiviral therapy, stressing the need for adherence. Initially the decision is made to hold off on treatment until Chris can stabilize his drug habit and housing issues.

Course

The NP sees Chris every 2 weeks. The NP and Chris agree that the priority is to place Chris into a drug rehabilitation program. The NP is familiar with resources in the community and helps Chris contact the admissions counselor.

In addition, Chris is referred to a social worker to locate a drug-free housing referral when he completes his detoxification program.

The NP schedule of health care maintenance activities included regular screening exam and lab studies to monitor his illness and complications. In addition, as the therapeutic relationship develops, the patient seeks additional information about therapies and medications. When his detoxification is complete, he makes an informed decision about therapy and begins a multiple drug therapy. Also once detoxed, the NP notices that Chris displays symptoms of depression and refers him to a mental health provider for counseling and group therapy.

With time, the NP refers Chris to a network of services available through the HIV community in the Bay Area. The NP meets regularly with other providers of care; she remains updated on intervention strategies and sources of services available in her area.

Case Commentary

Chris' case illustrates that patient education services are needed by patients with AIDS, especially during the period treatment decisions must be made. Now that the treatment armamentarium has been increased, a diagnosis of AIDS does not portend certain death, and patient education needs are similar to those for patients with all chronic illnesses. The gay community has successfully pushed the medical community to offer as many treatment options as possible and often informs health care providers of the treatment strategies. Thus, the nurse who

(case study continues on page 371)

attempts patient education with an informed person with AIDS should persevere in attempts to maintain the most up-to-date information about pharmacologic and nonpharmacologic interventions and be open to suggestions from patients.

Because many health care providers are unfamiliar with the lifeways of the gay community, the health care professional should admit this to the person with AIDS and maintain an open, caring, and professional relationship. As Scaffa and Davis (1990) point out, moral debates regarding sexual behavior and gay life choices have no place in the health care arena. If health care professionals cannot care for persons with AIDS in a nonjudgmental manner, then they should not work in this area of health care.

When nurses care for a gay man in the terminal stages of AIDS, they appreciate that this person may be faced not only with mortality but also with the need to tell his family of impending death and his lifestyle choices. The informed nurse can be exceptionally helpful to family members by giving them information, offering support, and allowing for privacy. The definition of family should be redefined to include the patient's partner and other gay friends who have become part of the family of the AIDS patient.

Intravenous drug abusers (IVDAs) are the fastest growing group of persons with AIDS in the United States. They may be of any gender, cultural, ethnic, or racial group. Sharing of syringes is responsible for a huge surge of cases in this population. The IVDAs are a challenging group with which to work. Because chemical dependency is often associated with denial, pharmacologic treatment may be more difficult to maintain. Patient education is difficult with this group until abstinence from alcohol and intravenous drugs has been achieved. Therefore, referral to Alcoholics Anonymous and Narcotics Anonymous support groups is essential. Self-destructive behavior is common and the health care provider should be alert to signs of impending suicide (Scaffa & Davis, 1990). The health care professional should be aware that this group of persons with AIDS is one of the most stigmatized groups in American society and is thus a vulnerable population. Patient education should always be accompanied by caring concern.

SUMMARY

This chapter addressed the innovation necessary to strengthen patient education as an integral component of case management systems. It is necessary to visibly incorporate patient teaching in the process of critical pathway design and implementation. Patient education should be realistic, based on length of stay as reflected by care maps; variances for patient teaching should be tracked with those for other interventions. Thus, patient education becomes part of total quality programs in the organization and outcomes can be evaluated. Positive outcomes (eg, safer discharges, cost savings) can provide needed support to justify staff time and resources for patient education programs. Patients and families should also be involved in planning care so that designs are patient centered.

Nurses in all roles can provide needed leadership for the patient education innovations that accompany case management. Staff nurses who know about critical paths, are skilled at teaching, and are enthusiastic about teamwork with other disciplines can help to make high-quality, low-cost care a reality. Nurses who are case managers, care coordinators, or patient education coordinators advocate for both the patient and the staff nurse not only through their clinical expertise, but also by developing consensus and gaining needed political support. Specifically, they advocate for two of the most needed resources to deliver quality patient education: allocating the time of RNs to teach and providing staff development to promote expertise in the practice of patient education for all professional staff.

STRATEGIES FOR CRITICAL ANALYSIS AND APPLICATION

1. Using Hanisch's model for cardiac rehabilitation teaching described in this chapter, discuss how a product-line patient education model could be developed for total hip replacement patients. Consider the various settings in which care is provided for the patient before, during, and after total hip replacement.
2. Using the above scenario, describe how the use of patient focus groups could help nurses identify learning priorities and redesign patient education for the inpatient period.
3. Describe how community-based nursing case management might improve patient education efforts for early discharge postpartum patients and their families.
4. Propose a strategy you could use to gain political support for an innovative new program you developed to replace an exiting program that is outdated because of decreased length of stay in your practice setting.

REFERENCES

(1998). Internet connections show promise in solving age-old patient education problems. *Patient Education Management, 5*(6), 69.

(1999). Type 2 diabetes runs in overweight families. *Diabetes Management, 2*(12), 138–140.

(1999a). Get physicians on your side. *Patient Education Management, 6*(1), 8.

(1999b). Make sure the right patient education measures are in your electronic records. *Patient Education Management, 6*(12), 133–134.

(1999c). A phone call a week cuts costs $8000 per patient. *Patient Education Management, 6*(12), 136–137.

Adinolfi, A. (1996). The role of the nurse in the care of patients with HIV infection. In Bartlett, J. (Ed), *Care and Management of Patients with HIV Infection*. Durham, NC: Clean Data, Inc. for Glaxo Wellcome.

American Nurses Association. (1980). *Nursing and social policy statement*. Kansas City, MO: Author.

American Nurses Association. (1988). *American Nurses Association Task Force on Case Management in Nursing: Nursing case management (Publication no. NS-32)* Kansas City, MO: Author.

American Nurses Association. (1994). ANA and SNAs testify on risks of decreasing skill mix. *American Nurse, 11*(11), 14.

Balik, B. (1998). The impact of managed care and integrated delivery systems on nursing education and practice. In O'Neil, E., and Coffman, J. (Eds.), *Strategies for the Future of Nursing*. San Francisco: Jossey-Bass.

Bartlett, E. (1986). Advocacy skill and strategies for patient education managers. *Patient Education and Counseling, 8*(4), 397–405.

Bear, M., Brunell, M., & Covelli, M., (1997). Using a nursing framework to establish a nurse-managed senior health clinic. *Journal of Community Health Nursing, 14*(4), 225–235.

Benner, P., Tanner, C., & Chesla, C. (1996). *Expertise in Nursing Practice: Caring, Clinical Judgement, and Ethics*. New York: Springer Publishing.

Bennis, W., Benne, K., & Chin, R. (1985). *The planning of change*. New York: Holt, Rinehart, and Winston.

Bower, K. (1988). Case management: Meeting the challenge of managed care: controlling costs, guaranteeing outcomes. *Definition, 3*(1), 1–3. Boston: The Center for Nursing Case Management, New England Medical Center Department of Nursing.

Brass-Mynderse, N. (1996). Disease management for CHF. *Journal of Cardiovascular Nursing 11*(1), 54–62.

Brooten, D., Hayman, L., & Naylor, M. (1978). *Leadership for change: A guide for the frustrated nurse*. Philadelphia: J. B. Lippincott.

Burr, W., Leigh, G., Day, R., & Constantine, J. (1979). Symbolic interactionism and the family. In W. Burr, R. Hill, F. Nye, & I. Reiss (Eds.), *Contemporary theories about the family* (Vol. II). New York: Free Press.

Cahill, J. (1995). Innovation and the role of the change agent. *Professional Nurse 11*(1), 57–58.

Carlson, K. (1996). Providing health care for children in foster care: A role for advanced practice nurses. *Pediatric Nursing, 22*(5), 418–422.

Clark, C. (1977). Reframing. *American Journal of Nursing, 77*(8), 840–841.

Collins, P., Sparger, K., Richardson, M., Schriver, T., & Bergenstock, D. (1999). Talking with physicians about pain. *American Journal of Nursing, 99*(10), 20.

Darby, M. (1999). Coordinating care in an integrated delivery system. *The Quality Letter, 11*(7), 1–15.

Freed, D. (1998). Please don't shoot me; I'm only the change agent. *Health Care Supervisor, 17*(1), 56–61.

Green, L. (1996). A better way to keep in touch with patients. *Medical Economics, 73*(20), 153–156.

Hall, J. (1985). Nursing as process. In J. Hall & B. Weaver (Eds.), *Distributive nursing practice: A systems approach to community health.* Philadelphia: J. B. Lippincott.

Hanisch, P. (1993). Informational needs and preferred time to receive information for phase II cardiac rehabilitation patients: What CE instructors need to know. *Journal of Continuing Education in Nursing, 24*(2), 82–89.

Health Care Benchmarks. (1997). *Written asthma plans cut hospitalizations in half, 4*(12), 180–181.

Hofmann, P. (1993). Critical path method: An important tool for coordinating clinical care. *Journal of Quality Improvement, 19*(7), 235–246.

Huggind, C., & Phillips, C. (1998). Using case management with clinical paths to improve patient outcomes. *Home Healthcare Nurse 16*(1), 15–20.

Jacobson, A. (1996). The psychological care of patients with insulin-dependent diabetes mellitus. *New England Journal of Medicine, 334*(19), 1249–1253.

Johnson, A., Wise, M., & Jimmerson, K. (1995). The nurse practitioner's role in a pediatric sleep clinic. *Journal of Pediatric Health Care, 9*(4), 162–166.

Joint Commission on the Accreditation of Healthcare Organizations. (1998). *Consolidated accreditation manual for hospitals.* Chicago: Author.

Kirton, C., Ferri, R., & Eleftherakis, V. (1999). Primary care and case management of persons with HIV/AIDS. *Nursing Clinics of North America, 34*(1), 71–92.

Kortbawi, P. (1993). An orientation plan for hospital-based case managers. *Journal of Continuing Education in Nursing, 12*(2), 69–73.

Kovner, C., Hendrikson, G., Knickman, J., & Finkler, S. (1993). Changing the delivery of nursing care: Implementation issues and quali-

tative findings. *Journal of Nursing Administration, 23*(11), 24–34.

Lachman, V. (1999). Breaking the quality barrier: critical thinking and conflict resolution. *Nursing Case Management 4*(6), 224–227.

Leininger, S. (1997). *Building Clinical Pathways.* Pittman, NJ: National Association of Orthopedic Nurses.

Lewin, K. (1951). *Field theory in social science.* New York: Harper & Row.

Mahn, V. (1993). Clinical nurse case management: A service line approach. *Nursing Management, 24*(9), 48–50.

Marrelli, T., & Hillard, L. (Eds.) (1996). *Home Care and Clinical Paths: Effective Care Planning Across the Continuum.* St. Louis: Mosby—Year Book, Inc.

Marquis, B., & Huston, C. (1998). *Management Decision Making for Nurses.* Philadelphia: Lippincott-Raven Publishers.

McEachern, J., Curley, C., & Neuhauser, D. (1995). Medical leadership in an era of managed care and continual improvement. *Health Care Management 2*(1), 19–32.

Menke, E. (1985). Conceptual basis for nursing intervention with human systems: Individuals. In J. Hall, & B. Weaver (Eds.), *Distributive nursing practice: A systems approach to community health.* Philadelphia: JB Lippincott.

New, K. (Ed.) (1998). *Making Patient Education Cross the Continuum of Care.* Atlanta: American Health Consultants.

Oermann, M., & Huber, D. (1999). Patient outcomes: a measure of nursing's value. *American Journal of Nursing, 99*(9), 40–47.

Orem, D. (1985). *Nursing: concepts of practice.* New York: McGraw-Hill.

Patterson, B., Thorne, S., & Dewis, M. (1998). Adapting to and managing diabetes. *Image—The Journal of Nursing Scholarship, 30*(1), 57–62.

Pollock, S. (1987). Adaptation to chronic illness: Analysis of nursing research. *Nursing Clinics of North America, 22*(3), 631–644.

Powell, S. (2000). *Case management: a practical guide to success in managed care.* Philadelphia: Lippincott, Williams, and Wilkins.

Redman, B., & Levine, D. (1987). Organizational resources in support of patient education programs: Relationship to reported delivery of instruction. *Patient Education and Counseling, 9*(3), 177–197.

Robbins, S. (1980). *The administrative process.* Englewood Cliffs, NJ: Prentice-Hall.

Roy, C. (1984). *Introduction to nursing: An adaptation model.* Englewood Cliffs, NJ: Prentice-Hall.

Scaffa, M., & Davis, D. (1990). Cultural considerations in the case of patients with AIDS. *Occupational Therapy and Health Care, 7*(1), 69–85.

Stallings, K. (1996). *Integrating patient education in your nursing practice.* [Video]. Reproduced with permission of GlaxoWellcome, Inc. (Produced by Horizon Video Productions, 4222 Emperor Boulevard, Durham, NC 27703).

Tahan, H. (1999). Clarifying case management: what is in a label? *Nursing Case Management, 4*(6), 268–277.

Tritsch, J. (1998). Application of King's theory of goal attainment and the Carondelet St. Mary's Case Management model. *Nursing Science Quarterly, 11*(2), 69–73.

Watzlawick, P., Weakland, J., & Fisch, R. (1974). *Change: Problem formation and problem resolution.* New York: W. W. Norton.

Wax, J. (1971). Power theory and institutional change. *Social Service Review, 45*(3), 284.

Wayman, C. (1999). Hospital-based nursing case management: Role clarification. *Nursing Case Management, 4*(5), 236–241.

Weaver, B. (1985). Distributive nursing practice. In B. Hall & B. Weaver (Eds.), *Distributive nursing practice: A systems approach to community health.* Philadelphia: J. B. Lippincott.

Weekes, D., & Savedra, M. (1988). Adolescent cancer: Coping with treatment-related pain, a pilot study. *Journal of Pediatric Nursing, 3*(5), 318–328.

Wright, D., & Arthur, H. (1996). An analysis of the impact of a management system on patients waiting for cardiac surgery. *Canadian Journal of Cardiovascular Nursing, 7*(1), 5–9.

Wu, R. (1973). *Behavior and illness.* Englewood Cliffs, NJ: Prentice-Hall.

Zander, K. (1988). Nursing case management: Strategic management of cost and quality outcomes. *Journal of Nursing Administration, 18*(5), 23–30.

Zander, K. (1991). Care maps: The core of cost/quality care. *The New Definition, 6*(3). Boston: The Center for Nursing Case Management.

Zander, K. (1992). Critical pathways. In M. Melum & M. Sinioris (Eds.), *Total quality management.* Chicago: AHA.

Zander, K. (1995). A look to the future. In Zander, K. (Ed.), *Managing Outcomes Through Collaborative Care.* Chicago: AHA.

Zander, K. (1997). Use of variance from clinical paths: coming of age. *Clinical Performance and Quality Health Care, 5*(1), 20.

Zander, K. (1998). Nursing case management: strategic management of cost and quality outcomes. *Journal of Nursing Administration, 18*(5), 23–30.

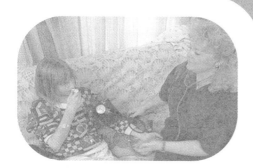

Community–Based Patient Education Programs

Marilyn P. Verhey

LEARNING OBJECTIVES

After reading this chapter, the nurse or student nurse should be able to:

1. Describe the purpose of a community needs assessment.

2. Develop a plan for a community-based health education program.

3. Identify settings for community-based health education programs.

4. Implement and evaluate a community-based health education program.

INTRODUCTION

Educating communities or groups of people is more difficult than educating one person or one family. The boundaries of communities are not always clearly defined. Rissel and Bracht (1999) identify two general categories of communities: *geographical communities* and *communities of interest*. Geographical communities include neighborhoods, towns, and cities. Communities of interest consist of aggregates of people who are linked through a common interest or characteristics (eg, breast cancer survivors, individuals committed to preventing domestic violence, or families of the chronically mentally ill). When a needs assessment indicates that community-based education is desirable, the implementation process must proceed in a careful and organized fashion. Evaluation methods must be included in the program design, and the economic realities of the program must be considered.

This chapter describes concepts relevant to tailoring patient education programs to meet the needs of community-based patients. It presents two examples of community-based programs: a health promotion and education program for adolescents in a school-based health center, and a peer advisor program for older patients who are recovering at home after a myocardial infarction.

COMMUNITY-BASED HEALTH EDUCATION PROGRAMS

Community Needs Assessment

Clients are assessed in the context of family, socioeconomic, educational, and cultural influences. Likewise, the community must be assessed in relation to many interfacing systems. A community health education program cannot be created as if the community existed in a vacuum. Social, economic, organizational, and environmental influences must be considered (Spradley & Allender, 1996). Each community is unique. For example, a community-based sexually transmitted disease (STD) education pro-

gram for teenagers in Los Angeles may differ considerably from a program planned for a small Appalachian community in West Virginia.

Just as a needs assessment is required for an individual patient, an assessment of the community's needs must be performed. Any type of health education or health promotion program should be requested by the community. Hospitals may use community programs to promote goodwill, market hospital network services, or promote their image as invested in health promotion. As capitation becomes the preferred method for insurance companies to contract with providers, preventive programs may both attract customers and maximize profitability by decreasing the need for illness care. Again, it is essential that the community recognize and express a need for services: planning and implementing community-based patient education programs requires significant time and financial expenditure, and the community as a whole, directly or indirectly, will probably pay for all or part of the program.

Community needs can be assessed in various ways. Approaching the medical personnel who deliver community health care is an effective method of gathering data pertaining to health education needs; the public health department is an obvious place to collect these data. Next, formal and informal community leaders should be polled about their perceptions of health education needs. Patient advisory groups, focus groups, or surveys can be used. Congruence between the needs as identified by health care and other professionals and the needs as identified by lay community members must then be determined. Community health education programs often fail if the program is perceived by health care professionals as needed but the population perceives neither the same need nor desire for the program. Chapter 7 presents a model and a tool for conducting a community needs assessment, and Table 14-1 summarizes the methods for learning about the community.

A comprehensive community assessment provides information about a community's strengths and its health problems and needs. After assessing the community's perceptions

TABLE 14.1 Methods for Community Needs Assessment

METHOD	DESCRIPTION
Literature review	Learn about community and social demographics as well as lifestyles, health beliefs, and health behaviors of the community. Types of literature include nursing and health care references, health intervention articles about the health problem, and behavioral and social science literature. Other sources include local newspapers and magazines, census data and maps, and government reports.
Observations	Observations can occur at community gathering places, businesses, worksites, and clinics. Explain who you are and why you are there.
Informal conversations	Information conversations can be a valuable way for nurses to discover what goes on in the community and other issues that might be relevant to the delivery of educational programs. Talk with a representative variety of individuals. Developing trust takes time. Listen carefully and take notes after you have left the interaction.
Written surveys	Surveys can be conducted of community members, community organization representatives and local professionals. Written surveys can be read to respondents if this is more appropriate and/or timely.
In-depth interviews	In-depth interviews of key community members are a rich source of community assessment data. Structured interview questions, prepared in advance, will ensure that the time is used wisely and the information you need is obtained.
Focus groups	Focus groups are a widely used method of gathering community information. A trained moderator guides a group of community members through a series of questions designed to gather in-depth information.

Adapted from AMC Cancer Research Center (1994). Beyond the Brochure: Alternative Approaches to Effective Health Communication. Atlanta: U.S. Centers for Disease Control and Prevention.

of its strengths and needs, a list of educational priorities should be developed. This list should include the community strengths and resources that can contribute to the educational process. To be successful, community-based education must involve community members in the needs assessment and in determining the priorities of the educational program.

Planning and Implementation

Most of the approaches for planning and implementing patient education services that are described in this text are also applicable to community settings, and this information should be used by the nurse in planning community-based educational interventions. Breckon, Harvey, and Lancaster (1998), in writing specifically about community-based education, have identified seven principles for planning (Table 14-2).

Financing is crucial when planning for a community-based education program. A community is willing to pay for the service when

it wishes to participate in health education. When considering a group such as school children, however, financing is usually provided by foundation grants or federal or state governments. Obviously, the state of the national economy is important to the funding of these programs. During recessions, federal funding is limited for programs that the government views as unessential. In the past decade, managed care has taken firm hold in the health care delivery system. Increased emphasis on disease management in managed care plans presents new opportunities for patient education. Because healthier clients use fewer health resources, health promotion programs will be supported by managed care plans if programs demonstrate cost effectiveness or cost saving.

Case Study: Program Planning in a Rural Community

Laura is a nurse who works in the health department of a rural county in Pennsylvania

TABLE 14-2. Principles of Planning for Community-Based Educational Programs

PRINCIPLE	DESCRIPTION
Principle 1: Plan the Process	The planning process itself takes careful thought and preparation. Consider community needs, strengths, and possible resistances. Establish timelines.
Principle 2: Plan with People	The involvement of community members is essential. Consider using a planning committee.
Principle 3: Plan with Data	The data obtained from a careful and comprehensive community needs assessment should provide a sound foundation for planning.
Principle 4: Plan for Permanence	Planning for community-based education takes time and resources. Plan for programs to occur on an ongoing basis to make the most of valuable planning time.
Principle 5: Plan for Priorities	Use your time to plan programs to meet the highest priority needs. Maintain a list of priorities that is reviewed and revised periodically. Continue to assess community needs and opportunities and incorporate this information into the planning process.
Principle 6: Plan for Measurable Outcomes in Acceptable Formats	Developing measurable objectives is a vital part of the planning process. Use Healthy People 2010 as a guide for community-based program planning.
Principle 7: Plan for Evaluation	Develop the way in which you will evaluate the outcomes of your educational program as part of the planning process. Also, evaluate the successes and areas for improvement of your planning processes.

Source: Breckon, Harvey & Lancaster, 1998.

Adapted from Breckon, D. J., Harvey, J. R., & Lancaster, R. B. (1998). *Community health education: Settings, role, and skills for the 21st century.* 4th ed. Gaithersburg, MD: Aspen.

that needs community-based case management and client education services to promote the growth and development of low-income children and families in the geographical area served by the department. The director of the health department has asked Laura to plan a program to meet this need. Laura uses the seven principles of planning for community-based educational programs from Table 14-2 to develop a comprehensive plan for the program.

Plan the Process

Laura develops a written document to use in the planning process. She talks with her colleagues to identify the specific needs of low-income children and families in the area. She lists the strengths of the community, the potential resistance to a new program of services, and the factors that may enhance the success of the program. Laura thinks about whom should be involved (eg, both members of the community and health care personnel) and the data needed to move forward with the planning process. Finally, she lists the steps and activities of the planning process and de-

velops a written timetable for each phase of the project.

Plan With People

By talking with her colleagues, Laura identifies two community agencies in the area that serve low-income families and children and decides that these agencies should be involved in planning the new program. In addition, two churches and one temple deliver services (eg, support and advocacy) to low-income families and children, and there is a child-care center located in the county's largest town. An ambulatory care clinic run by the county hospital and staffed by pediatricians and pediatric nurse practitioners provides most primary care to the potential clients of the new program. Laura asks one representative of each of these organizations to serve on a planning committee for the new program.

Plan With Data

Laura meets with the health department's assistant administrator to obtain data and reports that pertain to the needs that the program is intended to address. She discovers that a comprehensive needs assessment was conducted more than 1 year ago. She updates this with recent vital statistics and asks her planning committee members to supplement her data with reports they may have. She also researches the literature to gather information on similar programs, their interventions, and the evaluation of their services.

Plan for Permanence

Laura meets with the director of the health department to determine the department's long-range commitment to the program once it is developed. The director assures her that the department is prepared to fund the program for at least 3 years.

Plan for Priorities

Based on a careful review of all data sources and reports and discussions held during multiple meetings of the planning group, priorities for program development are determined. The planning committee decides to focus on developing programs for families with children from the prenatal stage to 3 years of age. Within this overall priority, more specific priorities for program development are delineated, and the committee agrees to review and revise the list periodically as the program planning process proceeds.

Plan for Measurable Outcomes in Acceptable Formats

Laura consults *Healthy People 2010* to ensure that the program addresses the objectives related to maternal, infant, and child health and those objectives related to access to quality health services (U.S. Office of Disease Prevention and Health Promotion, 2000). She uses the *Healthy People* objectives as a foundation for writing a set of program-specific objectives that cover both the processes of care and services that the program will provide and the expected client-centered outcomes for the

families and children served by the program. These objectives are reviewed, modified, and approved by the planning committee.

Plan for Evaluation

Laura builds an evaluation plan into her program proposal. She specifies what data will be collected, who will collect it, and how the data will be used to determine if the program objectives developed during Step 6 have been met.

After the completion of the seven steps of planning for the community-based educational program, Laura revises and adds to the document she developed in step one. She submits a comprehensive written program proposal to the health department director for her review and approval.

Models for Community-Based Health Education Programming

The use of a model for community-based health education programming provides direction to the process and helps organize the various phases of the project. Many models for the development of community-based health education programs have been developed. The PRECEDE-PROCEED model for health promotion planning (Green & Kreuter, 1999) is a well-known model. Other models include the PATCH model (Centers for Disease Control and Prevention, 1995), the ten-step planning model (Timmreck, 1995), and the five-stage model of organizing for health promotion (Bracht, Kingsbury & Rissel, 1999). A brief summary and resources for further information for these four models are presented in Table 14-3.

Types of Community Settings

Patient education can occur in many types of community settings. Breckon, Harvey, and Lancaster (1998) have identified several categories of community settings. In addition, grassroots community-based organizations provide an important venue for client education. These settings are briefly described and examples of

TABLE 14-3. Health Education and Promotion Models

MODEL	DESCRIPTION	RESOURCE FOR FURTHER INFORMATION
PRECEDE-PROCEED Model for Health Promotion	This model is comprised of two phases: 1) A diagnostic or needs assessment phase called PRECEDE (**P**redisposing, **R**einforcing, and **E**nabling **C**onstructs in **E**ducational/ environmental **D**iagnosis and **E**valuation, and 2) a developmental stage of health promotion planning that includes the implementation and evaluation processes (**P**olicy, **R**egulatory, and **O**rganizational **C**onstructs in **E**ducational and **E**nvironmental **D**evelopment). The two phases work simultaneously and provide a multi-dimensional assessment process that guides the policy, implementation and evaluation components of the model.	Green, L. W., & Kreuter, M. W. (1999). *Health promotion planning: An educational and environmental approach* (3rd ed.). Mountain View, CA: Mayfield Publishing Co.
PATCH (**P**lanned **A**pproach **to** **C**ommunity **H**ealth)	The PATCH process was developed by the Centers for Disease Control and Prevention for use by communities as they plan, conduct and evaluate health promotion and disease prevention programs. A hallmark of the PATCH process is the active participation of many community groups and leaders. The five stages of the process are 1) mobilizing the community, 2) collecting and organizing data, 3) choosing health priorities, 4) developing a comprehensive intervention strategy, and 5) evaluating the process.	Centers for Disease Control and Prevention. National Center for Chronic Disease Prevention and Health Promotion. (1995). *PATCH: Planned Approach to Community Health.* Atlanta: CDC.
Ten-Step Planning Model	The ten-step planning model provides a step-by-step approach to program planning, development and evaluation. The ten steps are 1) development of mission statement, 2) assessment and evaluation of organization, inventory of resources and review of regulations and policy, 3) writing of goals and objectives for needs assessment, 4) conduct of needs assessment, 5) determination of priorities, 6) writing of goals and objectives for project, 7) development of step-by-step activities and procedures, 8) development of timeline charts, 9) implementation of the project, and 10) evaluation and feedback.	Timmreck, T. C. (1995). *Planning, program development, and evaluation: A Handbook for health promotion, aging, and health services.* Sudbury, MA: Jones & Bartlett.
Five-Stage Model of Organizing for Health Promotion	This model has as its foundation the developer's own community work, general principals of social and community change, elements of organizational development and strategic planning, and community empowerment theory. The five stages, each of which have several interrelated steps and activities, are 1) community analysis, 2) community intervention design and initiation, 3) implementation, 4) program maintenance and consolidation, and 5) dissemination and reassessment.	Bracht, N., Kingsbury, L., & Rissel, C. (1999). A five-stage community organization model for health promotion: Empowerment and partnership strategies. In Bracht, N., (Ed.) *Health promotion at the community level,* 2d ed. (pp. 83–104). Thousand Oaks, CA: Sage.

client education programs representing several of the settings are provided.

Health Departments and Other Tax-Supported Agencies

Public health nurses who work in local health departments engage in client education during visits to client's homes. These nurses also organize and provide health education programs for health promotion, disease prevention, and disease management.

Traditional and Emerging Voluntary Health Agencies

Examples of these agencies include the American Cancer Society, the American Diabetes Association, and the National Stroke Association. At the local level, volunteer boards and committees may perform many of the agency's functions. Nurses who provide educational services in this community arena must develop expertise recruiting, training, supervising, and rewarding volunteer workers (Breckon, Harvey, & Lancaster, 1998).

Medical Care Settings

Medical care settings include primary care clinics, health care provider's offices, health maintenance organizations, and urgent care and same-day surgery centers. As the reorganization of the health care system continues and inpatient stays become both less frequent and of shorter duration, these settings emerge as key sites for the provision of patient education services.

For example, The Great Brook Valley Health Center in Worcester, Massachusetts, part of a community health center-owned Health Maintenance Organization, developed and implemented a six-session educational program for asthma management (Gallivan, Lundberg, Fiedelholtz, Andringa, Stableford, & Visser, 1998). The managed care health education program was designed to meet the needs of its Hispanic, often monolingual clients. A nurse conducted individualized teaching focusing on

specific content areas, with printed support materials in Spanish. Group education was offered as a supplement to the individual educational process and case management by the nurse was an adjunct to the overall educational program. The program has expanded to include outreach in other community settings, including health fairs and the homes of Worcester residents.

Worksites and Employee Assistance Settings

Nurses working in business and industry sites provide education on occupational health and safety, employee wellness, disease prevention, and disease management. Employee assistance programs provide services (often educational) to help prevent or solve problems that might interfere with an employee's job performance. The employee assistance program of the University of Texas at Houston (1999) provides special educational programs on drugs in the workplace, stress management, parenting skills, team building, AIDS awareness, sexual harassment, the Americans with Disabilities Act, and corporate wellness programs. Another model of worksite health education is that of Advocate Health Care, an organization of health care professionals that serves the health needs of individuals, families, and communities in northern Illinois. Advocate Health Care (1999) provides various educational services at local worksites, including health fairs, smoking cessation and weight loss programs, and a lecture series on health-related topics.

School Settings

During the past decade, programs that provide comprehensive health services in schools have grown substantially. For many children and adolescents, this growth in services has increased their access to health services. A major role of these programs is to educate students about healthy lifestyles, disease prevention, and the management of health problems.

For example, the *Healthy Schools, Healthy Communities* program (Martin, Gaston, Heppel, Horrigan, & Stinson, 1998) established new school-based health centers to serve some of the most disadvantaged, at-risk children and youth. The Edison School-based Health Center in Kalamazoo, Michigan, provides health education to fifth- and sixth-grade students in the areas of physical fitness, violence prevention, HIV prevention, and improving self-esteem. Sex education and nutrition education are targeted topics at the Nashville, Tennessee's East Middle School Health Center.

Many school-based educational programs focus on childhood asthma. One example is the *A+ Asthma Club* program for Black children in Baltimore and Washington, D.C. (Schneider, Richard, Huss, Huss, Thompson, Butz, Eggleston, Kolodner, Rand, & Malveaux, 1997). In six educational sessions during school hours and three booster sessions, children learned about their condition and how to manage it. Culturally and developmentally appropriate teaching strategies were used in program development and implementation.

Faith Community Settings

Churches, temples, and other faith community settings are often effective sites for health-related educational programs. A parish nurse employed by a Catholic Church in Colorado Springs, Colorado (Interfaith Health Program, 1999) is an example of a patient education practice model in the faith community. To provide health education, the parish nurse partners with community health agencies for workshops and disease prevention events. Some recent classes have covered topics such as CPR, babysitting, preschool health, cancer prevention, and menopause. The parish nurse also provides health counseling to individuals and families regarding special health needs. The Carter Center in Atlanta, Georgia, provides national leadership building collaborations between faith structures and health agencies in the government and private sector through its Interfaith Health Program *(www. ihpnet.org).*

Black churches have traditionally gone beyond attending to the spiritual needs of their members, and have also addressed needs, such as health education. Freeman-McGuire (1997)

conducted a program of hypertension education for Black seniors in San Francisco Bay Area churches. Registered nurses taught a series of three classes on understanding hypertension, the role of stress in hypertension, and managing hypertension. In addition, three telephone calls were made to follow-up on the seniors at the completion of the classes. An evaluation of the program found that the seniors had increased knowledge about hypertension, had decreased their dietary sodium intake, and had a decrease in systolic blood pressure.

In another program, the North Carolina Division of Adult Health Promotion and Black churches teamed up to fight cancer in ten counties of the state. They targeted a goal of improving diet as one way to decrease the risk of cancer in rural North Carolina's Black adult population and were awarded a grant from the National Cancer Institute. Five churches of various sizes and denominations were recruited from each county to participate in the dietary behavior change project entitled "Black Churches United for Better Health." Blacks are underserved by the traditional health care system; thus, health promotion messages may not reach them. The training of lay health advisors who have a tradition of being natural helpers, are sensitive to cultural norms, and are based at churches where people turn for everyday support and guidance had the greatest potential to affect health status (Cowan, 1994).

Other Community-Based Organizations

In a community-based organization, a group of individuals have organized for a common purpose. The purpose is identified by the community and the potential solutions are based on the values, traditions, and culture of the community. Leadership and decision-making are controlled by the community members. Any given community may have many community-based organizations with differing views on how to identify and approach a community problem. Examples of community-based organizations include adult learning centers, local health and human services councils, organizations for the homeless, and family service centers. Partnerships with community-based organizations can provide an important avenue for the delivery of health promotion and disease prevention educational programs.

For example, a nutrition education program was implemented within adult basic education reading classes at the Hamilton Terrace Learning Center, and welfare-to-work community site in Shreveport, Louisiana (Murphy, Davis, Mayeaux, Sentell, Arnold, & Rebouche, 1996). Principles of adult learning and guidelines for teaching individuals with low literacy skills were incorporated into the curriculum planning. Focus groups were held with potential learners to provide further information about learning activities that would be meaningful. Program staff incorporated many hands-on activities into the 8-hour, 8-day curriculum and student workbooks, using low-literacy principles, reinforced each teaching session. An evaluation conducted at the conclusion of the program showed that the program participants had a greater knowledge of nutrition concepts.

Evaluating Community-Based Education Programs

Many of the principles of evaluating individual patient educational efforts can be applied to the evaluation of community-based programs. An important concept in delivery of community-based educational services is the continuing connection with the community during all phases of the evaluation process. Box 14-1 presents a set of questions to evaluate community participation. An important consideration in evaluating community-based educational programs is the extent to which they can be sustained within the community after the initial planning and implementation efforts have been completed. The potential for sustainability should be addressed in the planning phase of educational program delivery, and the evaluation plan should measure the program's progress toward self-sufficiency. Developing program sustainability is part of the

---

BOX 14-1. Questions to Evaluate Community Participation

1. Is there open and frequent communication between educational program staff and community group members?
2. Have community group members participated in the community needs assessment process?
3. Did the community group members participate in the setting of educational priorities?
4. Have the community group members agreed upon the measurable objectives for the educational program(s)?
5. Do community group members support the educational interventions?
6. Are evaluation results shared with participants and community group members?

---

process of creating community capacity (ie, working with communities to influence the community's ability to identify, mobilize, and address social and health problems).

A detailed presentation of these concepts is beyond the scope of this chapter. For a fuller discussion of the dimensions of community capacity, refer to the resources in the Suggested Reading list at the end of the chapter.

CLINICAL RELEVANCE: TWO COMMUNITY-BASED HEALTH EDUCATION PROJECTS

Both of the following two community health projects could be implemented in any community. A program of educational services delivered by a school-based health center is discussed; a peer advisor program for unpartnered elders recovering at home in the community after a myocardial infarction is also discussed.

Mission High School Health Center[1]

The Mission High School Health Center (MHSHC) is a school-based nursing center that provides health care services to 1,200 students (considered to be among the city's most at-risk youth) in a San Francisco high school. A diverse ethnic distribution at the high school exists (more than 20 languages are spoken among the students). About one-third of the student population is Hispanic, one-third is Asian, approximately one-sixth is black, and the remainder are from other ethnic groups. More than 50% of the students have no access to health care services.

The Health Center operates under the aegis of the San Francisco State University (SFSU) School of Nursing and in collaboration with other university departments, community and government agencies, the University of California at San Francisco, and the San Francisco Unified School District. The clinic is staffed by a nurse director, two nurse practitioners, a registered nurse, a licensed social worker, and a health intake coordinator. A physician provides medical consultation and 24-hour backup. Two SFSU School of Nursing faculty members serve as the project director and the consultant for educational services, quality management, and program evaluation.

The services of MHSHC are organized according to four care delivery objectives:

1. To increase access to health services for students
2. To provide primary health care services
3. To case manage at-risk students
4. To provide a comprehensive health promotion and education program (the objective that pertains to this chapter)

---

[1]The Mission High School Health Center recently entered a collaboration with another community-based health center and relocated its services. The combined entity is called Valencia Pediatric, Adolescent, and Family Health Services and is a collaborative project between UCSF and SFSU Schools of Nursing.

Specific components of the health promotion and education program include the development of a learning resource center, the provision of organized classes at the Center and in the classroom, and individual staff contacts with students during the delivery of medical and mental health services. The Teen Advisory Board, established to provide a formal liaison between MHSHC staff and high school students, is also an important venue for health promotion and education.

Learning Resource Center

The Learning Resource Center is a collection of print and video health education materials for use by both MHSHC staff and high school students. The development of the Learning Resource Center began with an analysis of existing client health records to determine potential health promotion and health problem educational needs. In addition, a needs assessment of students was conducted. Commercial print and video materials were located and evaluated for developmental and cultural appropriateness. For topics of which commercially prepared materials were unavailable, MHSHC staff and students developed pamphlets, flipcharts, and other resources. Examples of the educational materials located in the Learning Resource Center are the Nutrition Education Resource and the Tobacco Education Resource Binders. Both binders contain a comprehensive collection of educational brochures, pamphlets, fact sheets, articles, posters, stickers and other items for both students and staff. Many materials are bilingual and culturally sensitive.

Classes in the Center and the Classroom

Various group educational and health promotion classes were organized and presented in the MHSHC community room. The use of group instruction and the incorporation of peers as educators is an effective strategy in the health education of adolescents. Examples of programs include:

- **Girls Group.** Facilitated by a high school teacher and a MHSHC nurse, the content covers many issues identified by the young women (eg, sexuality, self-esteem, body image). Field trips, discussions, and outside resources are methods used to address the interests identified by the girls at the beginning of the program.
- **Male Responsibility Group.** This group was formed to increase the awareness of roles and responsibilities with issues such as safe sex, relationships, parenting, conflict resolution, and anger management.
- **Latina Group.** This group was formed to help young women deal with issues of domestic violence. Several women in the community, who have experience in the juvenile justice system, conduct this program in Spanish with 13 young women. The participants learn strategies to recognize domestic violence situations, interventions to use in potentially violent situations, and resources in the community that provide help. The young women participate in self-defense courses, an outdoor challenge program, and peer education training workshops.
- **Freshman Drug Education.** This weekly class covers drug education on marijuana, alcohol, tobacco, and inhalants. The activities were designed to increase decision-making skills, explore possible consequences of drug use, and practice ways of dealing with peer pressure.

MHSHC nurses are invited into various high school classes to provide health education sessions. Examples include classes on health careers, safer sex, tobacco education, nutrition education, adolescent physical and emotional development, and CPR training.

Education During the Delivery of Other Health Services

Each student visit to MHSHC, whether for a physical examination or for intervention with an acute medical problem, is viewed as a teaching opportunity. Often, it is the informa-tion given to the student at a time of identified need that contributes most to the client's health education and growth. When a student comes to MHSHC for the first time, an assessment of educational needs is conducted through the Psychosocial and Medical History. In addition to an assessment of students' medical history, students are asked about their support system, alcohol and drug use, and sexual history. Learning needs are identified, and educational protocols are implemented as indicated. With each subsequent visit to MHSHC, learning needs are reassessed and addressed. The MHSHC Patient Encounter Form (Fig. 14-1) is completed by the provider at the conclusion of every visit, and includes specific sections for the documentation of health risk factors and education.

Teen Advisory Board

The Teen Advisory Board (TAB) was developed to provide a formal linkage between the high school youth and the staff of MHSHC. The Board allows the youth to have a voice in the development of new programs and services offered by MHSHC. In addition, the Board unites motivated youth who can be taught about MHSHC and its services; in this way, they can serve as a cadre of peer educators. Interested students are interviewed using the questions listed in Box 14-2 and eight youth are chosen to represent various ethnic groups and ages.

TAB members are active participants in conducting an educational needs assessment of their peers using a printed questionnaire developed during TAB meetings. Other TAB meetings are devoted to educational sessions on topics, such as reproductive anatomy, sexually transmitted diseases, relationships, and self esteem. All of the sessions incorporate many hands-on activities and lively group discussions. At the conclusion of the academic year, TAB members are incorporated into the staff of the high school's Peer Resource Center. Each fall, the process begins anew. Evaluations by TAB members are positive and several pursued health careers upon graduation.

MHSHC Patient Encounter Form

ID:

Name:

DOB:

School:

Date of Encounter:

Insurance Info

MediCal: No
Kaiser: No
Other Ins:

IZ Records ☐   OpenCase ☐

Self Consent:
Guard Consent:
Last Physical:
History:
Pysch/Soc:
Condom Ed:

Illness			☐ New ☐ Established ☐ Sensitive Services ☐ CHDP			
New Patient	**Established**	**Consultations**	**Psychosocial**	**Other Contact**	**Appt. Type**	
☐ Minor (10 m)	☐ Nurse Visit (5 m)	☐ Focused	☐ Assessment	☐ C.B.O.	☐ Scheduled ☐ Called down for F/U	☐ Crisis: Walk In
☐ Low Complex (20 m)	☐ Minor (10 m)	☐ Expanded	☐ Crisis	☐ Clinic	☐ Drop In ☐ Crisis: Called Out	☐ Phone
☐ Mod Complex (30 m)	☐ Low Complex. (15 m)	☐ Detailed	☐ Group Therapy	☐ Oth Family		
☐ Comp; Mod Comp. (45 m)	☐ Mod Complex. (25 m)	☐ Comprehensive	☐ Individual Therapy	☐ Parent	**Referred By**	
☐ Comp; High Comp. (60 m)	☐ Comp; High Comp. (60 m)	☐ Complex (Sexual Abuse)	☐ Family Counseling	☐ Teacher	☐ Everett ☐ School Admin.	☐ Social Worker
			☐ Case Management	Other: _____	☐ MHSHC ☐ School Security	☐ Teacher
Complaint:			Time: _____		☐ Parent ☐ Self	Other: _____

Diagnosis

DX/ICD-9:		**On-site Labs**	**Outside Labs**		**Immunizations/Inj.**
DX/ICD-9:		☐ 186: HCG Urine	☐ 180: CBC	☐ 190: HIV	173: Hep B Ser: _____
DX/ICD-9:		☐ 183: Hct	☐ 177: Chlamydia	☐ 175: Pap Smear	169: MMR Ser: _____
DX/ICD-9:		☐ 320: Strep A	☐ 181: Diff	☐ 174: Throat Culture	168 OPV Ser: _____
DX/ICD-9:		☐ 185: UA Dipstick/Micr	☐ 182: ESR	☐ 179: Urine Culture	171: TD Ser: _____
DX/DSM IV:	GAF:	☐ 188: Wet Prep	☐ 176: Gonorrhea Culture	☐ 178: VDRL	Oth: _____ Ser: _____
		☐ Oth:	☐ 333: Hep Panel	☐ Oth:	

Medications/Supplies

Qty	Unit		Qty	Unit		Qty	Unit	
____	____	216: Ace Bandage	____	____	196: Doxycyline	____	____	220: Throat Lozenge
____	____	204: Acetaminophen	____	____	197: Erythromycin	____	____	218: Tinactin
____	____	207: Albuteral MDI	____	____	209: Hydrocort. Cream	____	____	213: Tylenol
____	____	202: Amoxicillin	____	____	205: Ibuprofen	____	____	214: Vitamin C
____	____	191: Ampicillin	____	____	198: Metronidazole	____	____	Oth:
____	____	208: Analgesic Balm	____	____	217: Miconazole	____	____	Oth:
____	____	215: Antiacid	____	____	349: Multivitamin	____	____	Oth:
____	____	211: Antibiotic Oint.	____	____	201: Penicillin	____	____	Oth:
____	____	193: Benzoyl Peroxide	____	____	206: Pseudoephedrine			
____	____	194: Bicillin	____	____	348: Septra			
____	____	195: Ceftriaxone	____	____	219: Tetracycline			

Contraceptives

Qty	
____	314: Condoms
____	325: Depo
____	315: Diaphragm
____	316: Foam
____	317: Gel
____	318: Oral
____	319: Sponge
____	Oth: _____

Screenings/Other Procedures

☐ 313: Audiometry	☐ 339: Nebulized Rx
☐ 321: Blood Pressure	☐ 323: Pelvic
☐ 341: Burn Treatment	☐ 311: PPD
☐ 334: Condylomata	☐ 338: Rmve Foreign B
☐ 335: Debride. Skin Les.	☐ 340: Venipuncture >
☐ 336: Diaphragm Fitting	☐ 312: Vision Screen
☐ 337: Dressing Change	☐ Oth: _____
☐ 342: Ear Wash	☐ Oth: _____
☐ 324: Height/Weight	
☐ 344: I D	
☐ 345: Injection Antibiotic	
☐ 346: Injection Med	

Risk Factors

☐ 276: Abuse Neglect	☐ 278: Drugs	☐ 288: Peer Social Relation	☐ 298: Sexuality		
☐ 274: Abuse Physical	☐ 283: Family Relations	☐ 289: Peer Violence	☐ 300: Sleep		
☐ 275: Abuse Sexual	☐ 284: Family Violence	☐ 292: Pregnancy	☐ 304: Stress		
☐ 309: Abuse Verbal	☐ 285: Financial	☐ 291: Pregnancy Risk	☐ 297: Suicide		
☐ 303: AIDS	☐ 290: Gangs	☐ 293: School Performance	☐ 279: Tobacco		
☐ 277: Alcohol	☐ 302: HIV	☐ 301: S.T.D.s	☐ 328: Truancy		
☐ 305: Anxiety	☐ 286: Housing	☐ 294: Self Care	☐ 308: Vocational		
☐ 280: Crisis Boyfriend	☐ 330: Hygiene	☐ 295: Self Esteem	☐ 307: Oth: _____		
☐ 281: Crisis Girlfriend	☐ 306: Medical	☐ 296: Self Harm	☐ 307: Oth: _____		
☐ 282: Depression	☐ 287: Nutrition	☐ 299: Sexual Harassment			

Education

☐ 228: Alcohol	☐ 231: Nutrition	☐ 237: Oth: _____
☐ 227: Drugs	☐ 221: Pregnancy Counsel	☐ 237: Oth: _____
☐ 223: Family Planning	☐ 332: S.T.D.s	☐ 237: Oth: _____
☐ 232: Fitness	☐ 224: Safer Sex	
☐ 235: Harm Reduction	☐ 234: Safety	
☐ 229: Health Maint.	☐ 230: Self Exam	
☐ 331: Hygiene	☐ 226: Tobacco	
☐ 233: Medical Problem		
☐ 225: HIV		
☐ 236: Mental Health		

Follow Up

Location:	Date/Time:	Reason:	Resolved

Referral Categories

☐ Alcohol Tx	☐ Drug Tx	☐ FP	☐ lab	☐ Mental health (In)	☐ PHN	☐ Primary Care	☐ S.T.D.	☐ X-ray
☐ Dental	☐ Emergency	☐ Gyn	☐ Medical Specialty	☐ Mental health (Out)	☐ Prenatal	☐ Social Services	☐ Vision	☐ Oth:

REMINDER!! <<No insurance information has been entered for this patient>> REMINDER!! <<Patient's Self Consent Form>>
REMINDER!! <<Guardian Consent Form>>

Provider: _____   ☐ NP ☐ RN ☐ MD ☐ MSW ☐ Health Ed ☐ PHD Other _____   ☐ Student

Please write legibly   Primary provider Code:

FIGURE 14-1. MHSHC Patient Encounter Form.

BOX 14-2. Teen Advisory Board Interview Questions

1. Tell me a little bit about yourself, your interests, and any future plans that you have at this time in your life.
2. Why are you interested in being on the Teen Advisory Board for the Mission High School Advisory Board?
3. Do you have any experience or knowledge in the following areas that you believe would be helpful to the Teen Advisory Board?
   a) leadership
   b) club or organization involvement
   c) health care
   d) student government
   e) group projects
4. Are you comfortable talking about reproduction and contraception with your male and female peers?
5. Are you comfortable talking (presenting) in front of a group?
6. Can you contribute at least 8 hours to the Teen Advisory Board throughout this semester?
7. What do you want to learn from the experience of participating on the Teen Advisory Board?

Community Peer Advisor Program for Elders

An innovative, cost-effective program has been developed in the Cardiac Rehabilitation Program of a large New England teaching hospital. The program matches unpartnered older patients who have had a recent myocardial infarction (MI) to a peer advisor who has also sustained an MI in the past (Rankin & Carroll, 1995–1999). The program is targeted to elders without partners, because this population is at higher risk for morbidity and mortality than partnered elders. The intervention consists of 8 to 12 weekly phone calls by peer advisors to the unpartnered elders for the pur-

pose of providing information, problem solving, and social support.

The use of peer advisors has proven to be an effective educational intervention for risk reduction, health promotion, and for use in ill populations. Elders who have had an MI may offer a unique type of self-help to other elders who experience the same event. Access to another elder who serves as a confidante, a friend, and a trusted source of information provides a form of assistance not readily available to community-dwelling unpartnered elders. Talking with another age- and gender-matched peer who has similar health circumstances may be a more potent intervention than simply receiving social support and information from a nurse who does not offer an opportunity for reciprocation. Additionally, elders who serve as peer advisors may also experience improved quality of life and higher levels of perceived social support as a result of the benefits gained from giving social support.

Selection and Training of Peer Advisors

Potential peer advisors are identified by the director of the Cardiac Rehabilitation program, who is also an advanced practice nurse (APN). The peer advisors are required to be either active participants or graduates of a cardiac rehabilitation program. Criteria for selection include men and women who: are 65 years of age or older, are at least 12 months post-MI, can speak and read English, have a telephone, and are deemed by the program director to be willing to undergo training for the peer advisor role. Qualifications considered in the selection of peer advisors include successful completion of phase three or four of cardiac rehabilitation, the ability to be an empathic listener, use of adaptive psychosocial coping skills, and a willingness to participate in a training program.

The focus of Peer Advisor Training Program is to help peer advisors to develop empathic listening techniques, to learn how to role model successful recovery behaviors, and to develop techniques for building a helping relationship (Box 14-3). A review of coronary

---

BOX 14-3. Peer Advisor Training Program

The overall objectives of the Peer Advisor Training Program.

1. To reinforce previously learned content relative to cardiac disease and rehabilitation.
2. To provide an opportunity for peer advisors to share their own successful and difficult experiences in the rehabilitation process.
3. To provide an opportunity for peer advisors to recall strategies and persons who have helped them achieve successful outcomes in their rehabilitation.
4. To develop strategies that may be helpful as they guide fellow elders through the process of rehabilitation.
5. To discuss overall strategies that promote effective communication in a supportive relationship.
6. To learn strategies to help a peer sort out recovery issues.
7. To develop strategies to help a peer discern the seriousness of symptoms, and take accompanying actions when symptoms develop.

1. Listening to concerns and using strategies that had been successful for the peer advisors
2. Providing the advisors with additional techniques for handling difficulties that might arise (eg, how to respond with empathy during the death of a client's child)
3. Supplying updated information on the program
4. Providing an opportunity for the peer advisors to socialize with each other and with program staff

Support group activities have included holiday parties and luncheons. The second mechanism of support is ongoing, frequent contact between the APN and the peer advisors. The nurse has been called upon to give advice to peer advisors on various issues of the advising process, the advisors' own health, and various psychosocial issues related to their well-being.

Program Implementation

Peer advisors keep logs of their telephone calls to recovering elders; these telephone logs allow for retrieval of data regarding the various types of socially supportive and problem-solving interventions that they initiated. Logs reveal that at the beginning of the intervention and recovery period, telephone calls last longer; whereas toward the end of the intervention, phone calls are usually briefer.

Some advisors identify problematic symptoms in recovering elders and telephone the APN for advice. For example, one peer advisor called the APN because he was concerned about the recovering elder's nitrite usage. The APN solved the problem so that contacting the physician was unnecessary, thus saving the recovering elder time and money and alleviating that patient's anxiety. In another situation, a peer advisor relayed her concern to the APN about an elder's weakness and fatigue. The APN telephoned the daughter of the recovering elder who checked on her mother immediately. In all cases, appropriate follow-up is provided to the recovering elder, either

artery disease, its management, and methods of problem-solving situations involving potential health crises are included in these sessions. The 2 two-hour sessions are conducted by two APNs. Teaching methods include presentation of information, discussion, extensive use of role-play, and use of a study manual.

Ongoing Peer Advisor Support

Two mechanisms were put in place to support the peer advisors. One mechanism is the Peer Advisor Support Group. This group has the following goals:

through the intervention of the APN or through the advisor's suggestion to the participant that the physician be contacted.

Program Accomplishments

Many of the peer advisors find that being an advisor reinforces the healthy lifestyle changes they themselves had to make, deepening their understanding of themselves and contributing to a feeling of returning some of the care and support that they remember as an important part of their recovery. In addition to improving and reinforcing their own knowledge and skills about the subject matter, the elder peer advisors master important developmental tasks and add depth and fulfillment to their own lives.

This program provides a unique, community-based model for providing support, encouragement, and monitoring of recovering unpartnered elders in a cost-effective fashion. This type of program provides a linkage between nurses and other health care providers in the acute care setting and community-based nurses (eg, visiting nurses). The results of this program demonstrate that peer advisors can provide meaningful support and monitoring of other elders and provide a model for unpartnered elders experiencing other chronic illnesses.

SUMMARY

This chapter describes concepts relevant to developing educational programs to serve clients in community settings. Types of communities include health departments and other tax-supported agencies, traditional and emerging voluntary health agencies, medical care settings, worksites and employee assistance settings, school settings, faith community settings, and other community-based organizations.

The first step in developing community-based programs is to perform an assessment of the community's needs and strengths. The needs of communities can be determined in various ways, including interviews, patient advisory groups, focus groups, or surveys. After assessing the community's needs, a list of

educational priorities can be developed, which takes into consideration the community's strengths and resources. Planning and implementing community-based education involves paying special attention to the input of community members and coordination with other programs that serve the community. Developing the way in which the outcomes of the program will be evaluated is an essential part of the planning process. The extent to which a community-based program can be sustained within the community after the initial planning and implementation phases is a major goal of program evaluation. Two examples of community-based programs, a health promotion and education program for adolescents in a school-based health center, and a peer advisor program for elders recovering at home from a myocardial infarction, were presented to demonstrate the application of the principles of community-based health education.

STRATEGIES FOR CRITICAL ANALYSIS AND APPLICATION

1. Identify a need for health education in your community, which might be met by a community program.
2. How would you go about seeking more information about the health need and verifying a need for the program?
3. Describe how you might involve patients, family members, community leaders, and health care professionals to plan the program.
4. How would you evaluate the outcomes of your community-based program?
5. Develop a list of specific settings in your community in which patient/client education could occur.

REFERENCES

Advocate Health Care. (1999). Available: www.advocatehealth.com.
AMC Cancer Research Center. (1994). *Beyond the Brochure: Alternative Approaches to Effective*

Health Communication. Atlanta: U.S. Centers for Disease Control and Prevention.

Bracht, N., Kingsbury, L., & Rissel, C. (1999). A five-stage community organization model for health promotion: Empowerment and partnership strategies. In Bracht, N., (Ed.) *Health promotion at the community level* (2nd ed.). Thousand Oaks, CA: Sage.

Breckon, D. J., Harvey, J. R., & Lancaster, R. B. (1998). *Community health education: Settings, role, and skills for the 21st century* (4th ed.). Gaithersburg, MD: Aspen.

Centers for Disease Control and Prevention. National Center for Chronic Disease Prevention and Health Promotion. (1995). *PATCH: Planned Approach to Community Health.* Atlanta: Author.

Cowan, A. (1994). Division of Adult Health Promotion and Black churches team up to fight cancer. *Health Bulletin, 3*(7), 7–10.

Freeman-McGuire, M. (1997). Community-based hypertensive education for African American seniors: A replication study. *Journal of National Black Nurses Association, 9*(2), 57–68.

Gallivan, L. P., Lundberg, M. E., Fiedelholtz, J. B., Andringa, K., Stableford, S., & Visser, L. (1998). Promoting opportunities for community based health education in managed care. *Journal of Health Education, 29*(5), S28—S33.

Green, L. W., & Kreuter, M. W. (1999). *Health promotion planning: An educational and environmental approach* (3rd ed.). Mountain View, CA: Mayfield Publishing Co.

Interfaith Health Program. (1999). Available: www.ihpnet.org.

Martin, J., Gaston, M., Heppel, D., Horrigan, L., & Stinson, N. (1998). Health education in the Healthy Schools, Healthy Communities program. *Journal of Health Education, 29*(5), S23—S27.

Murphy, P. W., Davis, T. C., Mayeaux, E. J., Sentell, T., Arnold, C., & Rebouche, C. (1996). Teaching nutrition education in adult learning centers: Linking literacy, health care, and the community. *Journal of Community Health Nursing, 13*(3), 149–158.

Rankin, S. H., & Carroll, D. (1995–1999). *Improving health outcomes for unpartnered MI patients.* R15NR4255, National Institute of Nursing Research.

Rissel, C., & Bracht, N. (1999). Assessing community needs, resources and readiness: Building on strengths. In Bracht, N., (Ed.), *Health promotion at the community level* (2nd ed.). Thousand Oaks, CA: Sage.

Schneider, S. L., Richard, M., Huss, K., Huss, R. W., Thompson, L. S., Butz, A. M., Eggleston, P. A., Kolodner, K. B., Rand, C. S., & Malveaux, F. J. (1997). Moving health care education into the community. *Nursing Management, 28*(9), 40–43.

Spradley, B. W., & Allender, J. A. (1996). *Community health nursing: Concepts and practice* (4th ed.). Philadelphia: Lippincott.

Timmreck, T. C. (1995). *Planning, program development, and evaluation: A Handbook for health promotion, aging, and health services.* Sudbury, MA: Jones & Bartlett.

University of Texas at Houston (1999). Available: *www.uth.tmc.edu/schools/msi/eap.*

U.S. Office of Disease Prevention and Health Promotion. (2000). *Healthy People 2010: Understanding and improving health.* (Publication No. 017-001-00543-6). Washington, DC: U.S. Government Printing Office.

SUGGESTED READINGS FOR COMMUNITY CAPACITY

Creating capacity: A research agenda for public health education. (1995). Theme issue of *Health Education Quarterly, 22*(3).

Goodman, R. M., Speers, M. A., McLeroy, K., Fawcett, S., Kegler, M., Parker, E., Smith, S. R., Sterling, T. D., & Wallerstein, N. (1998). Identifying and defining the dimensions of community capacity to provide a basis for measurement. *Health Education & Behavior, 25*(3), 258–278.

Kang, R. (1995). Building community capacity for health promotion: A challenge for public health nurses. *Public Health Nursing, 12*(5), 312–318.

Shediac-Rizkallah, M. C., & Bone, L. R. (1998). Planning for the sustainability of community-based health programs: Conceptual frameworks and future directions for research, practice and policy. *Health Education Research, 13*(1), 87–108.

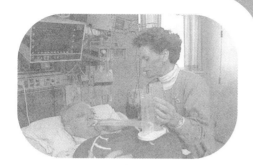

Research and
Patient Education

LEARNING OBJECTIVES

After reading this chapter, the nurse or student nurse should be able to:

1. List three challenges in patient education research.

2. Compare the progress of patient education research in diabetes mellitus, cancer, and heart disease.

3. Write two specific aims for a proposed study to test the efficacy of patient education for patients older than 65 years of age with type 2 diabetes.

INTRODUCTION

Nursing uses research as a basis for its science and its practice (Gortner, 1983; Kim, 1993; Monti & Tingen, 1999; Morse, 1996). Research—a tool of science—facilitates the development of a knowledge base for practice. Nursing research attempts to describe, explain, and predict outcomes of nursing interventions, and patient education is one of the most important of these interventions. This chapter describes the current state of research in patient education, examining primarily nursing research, but also appreciating the contributions made by other non-nursing health professionals.

The research covered in this chapter does not represent an exhaustive review of all research in patient education. Instead, we attempt to reflect the state-of-the-art in patient education research, so that research can be summarized and made useful for practitioners. Current trends in patient education research are highlighted, and implications for practice and future research directions are suggested. The chapter suggests methods of designing patient education research projects using concrete examples from our own research.

PATIENT EDUCATION RESEARCH: THE STATE-OF-THE-ART

Numerous factors have enhanced nursing research during the last two decades. The widespread growth of graduate programs in nursing, greater sophistication in research methods, and the technological availability of sophisticated statistical procedures have all greatly contributed to nursing research. Early research in patient education was usually pretest/post-test in design, and statistical procedures were generally univariate. Many reports of patient education programs were basically anecdotal in nature, with no outcome measures reported. Many of the earlier studies, particularly those by Lindeman and others in the 1970s (Lindeman & Stetzer, 1973; Lindeman & Van Aernam, 1971), were excellent studies and are still cited as models. However, later patient education research has demonstrated the importance of considering multiple independent variables and their impact on patient teaching outcomes.

Patient education, a primary cornerstone of health promotion and disease prevention, received a boost with the publication of two important documents: *Healthy People 2000 and 2010* (U.S. Department of Health and Human Services, 1990, 2000) and the *Guide to Clinical Preventive Services*. Patient education objectives are reflected in *Healthy People 2000 and 2010,* and techniques to effectively counsel and educate patients can be found in the *Guide to Clinical Preventive Services. Healthy People 2010* objectives were developed from a participatory process in which 467 objectives in 28 focus areas were developed to concentrate on contemporary public health and preventive medicine.

All of the focus areas explicitly address patient education or assume patient education as a means to achieve the desired outcomes. The two overarching goals of *Healthy People 2010* are: to increase the quality and years of healthy life and to eliminate health disparities (U.S. Department of Health and Human Services, 2000). Most of the focus areas require that they be conducted to determine achievement of the various goals. For example, focus area five deals with diabetes. The patient education portion states that diabetes patient education must be provided so that the economic burden can be decreased and the quality of life can be improved. Obviously, patient teaching oriented toward reduction of diabetes complications and better management of blood sugar levels will result in better quality of life for people with diabetes. Implications for the other areas of research are also clear using diabetes and other focus areas (eg, arthritis, kidney disease) as examples. As the objectives of *Healthy People 2010* are incorporated into preventive care and health promotion, research in the area of patient education should receive additional attention. Nursing has embraced *Healthy People 2000 and 2010* and has incorporated them into curricula, especially for advanced practice nurses.

An example of the use of *Healthy People 2010* objectives in research and practice is evident in a pediatric and family clinic owned, managed, and run as a faculty practice by the Department of Family Health Care Nursing at the University of San Francisco, California. In an effort to gauge the effectiveness of patient care at the faculty practice, *Healthy People 2010* objectives were examined in light of the achievement of such objectives within the San Francisco Bay area. When it was determined that San Francisco has lagged nationally in the achievement of focus areas related to mental health, sexually transmitted diseases, and immunizations, the clinic staff instituted a database that will provide concrete measures of the desired outcomes. These outcomes are predicated on effective patient education; therefore, the faculty who practice in this clinic will be measuring the effectiveness of their patient education interventions.

Challenges in Patient Education Research

Although patient education has become more formal since the first edition of this book in 1983, confusion still exists about the goals of patient education and which outcome measures are most appropriate to educational interventions (Oberst, 1989; Redman, 1997). Oberst (1989) notes that the most important outcomes in patient education research (and in practice) are knowledge, attitudes, and compliance.

Challenges in Measuring Educational Outcomes

Knowledge
In earlier attempts to determine the effectiveness of patient teaching, knowledge was often the only outcome measured. However, as a better understanding of behavioral change has emerged, research scientists realized that knowledge is not always linked with behavior change. Oberst states that even knowledge is not well evaluated because *norm-referenced measures* rather than *criterion-referenced measures* are usually used (Oberst, 1989). Norm-

referenced measures are used to determine cognitive performance as measured against a norm, such as the performance of others; criterion-referenced measures evaluate how the person performs in reference to certain predetermined criteria (Waltz, Strickland, & Lenz, 1993). A patient who demonstrates an understanding of the biochemical regulation involved in hypertension is not as important as the patient who demonstrates an understanding that hypertension is a chronic problem that requires constant, continuing medication and monitoring. Thus, a criterion-referenced test enables the health care provider to determine the patient's ability to manage his or her hypertension 100% of the time, whereas a norm-referenced test only indicates the patient's cognitive abilities in relationship to others, or perhaps to past scores on a knowledge test.

Attitudes
Attitude change is another outcome that can be problematic in terms of goals for patient education and measurement of the attainment of the goal (Oberst, 1989; Redman, 1997). It is more difficult to change an attitude toward a given health problem or belief than to change one's level of knowledge. For example, attitudes related to smoking cessation in adolescents are notoriously difficult to change, even with massive doses of health education, because 1) adolescents typically do not experience any noxious symptoms when they smoke, 2) they view themselves as essentially invulnerable, and 3) they find smoking pleasurable. On the other hand, adults resistant to exercise may change their attitudes once they discover that exercise promotes increased feelings of well-being and desired cardiovascular benefits. Therefore, measuring attitude change is complicated by issues related to the appropriate time of measurement (ie, after the new behavior has been inculcated) and the appropriateness of the attitude measure.

Compliance
Compliance to a treatment regimen is difficult to measure because of its multidimensional nature (Oberst, 1989). Oberst suggests that

compliance as an outcome has three levels: feasibility, adherence, and health status. Feasibility is the extent to which the patient has the needed information to act and the ability to master and apply the skills so that compliance can be achieved. For example, a problem achieving feasibility, such that appropriate outcomes can be achieved, is seen in the case of older women after myocardial infarction (MI) who are referred by their cardiologists for phase II and III cardiac rehabilitation programs. Although older women may have the knowledge regarding the importance of engaging in cardiac rehabilitation, they may neither have the financial resources nor the willingness to engage in behaviors that have not been part of their previous repertoire. If the nurse researcher were evaluating the program effectiveness of cardiac rehabilitation for women, she might note the lack of feasibility in terms of traditional cardiac rehabilitation to meet women's needs.

Adherence refers to the necessary behavior change that accompanies compliance. Behavior change is an elusive variable, because researchers cannot always assume that patient teaching is responsible for the behavior change. Additionally, because evaluation of behavior change usually hinges on the patient's self report, the data may be unreliable. Adherence is measured more easily in some disease processes, such as diabetes, because nearly all patients with type 1 and most patients with type 2 diabetes use home blood glucose monitoring devices. Many of these devices store the blood glucose levels with the date and time the reading is obtained. When the devices are downloaded into a computer, the researcher can obtain a 30-day history of blood glucose readings. The blood glucose monitor, therefore, not only allows the health care provider to obtain an indication of adherence to the medical regimen, but it also reveals whether the patient has monitored the blood glucose level as recommended. These devices are both useful data collection tools and an intervention that may induce desired behavior change.

Health status indicators are the third level of compliance that Oberst suggests should be considered in patient education research (Table 15-1). Again, diabetes is a good example of a disease with a rather straightforward health status indicator (ie, glycosylated hemoglobin blood tests). These blood tests give the health care provider an indicator of the degree to which the patient has engaged in behavior change to achieve euglycemia (appropriate blood sugar levels) during a 60-day to 90-day period. However, anyone who has worked extensively with clients who have diabetes, is aware that other variables influence blood sugar control and that some of the most com-

TABLE 15-1. Health Status Indicators Useful in Measuring Patient Outcomes

TYPE OF INDICATOR	WHAT INDICATOR MEASURES
Glycosylated hemoglobin	Measures metabolic control in patients with type 1 and 2 diabetes. Indicator gives an idea of control over the past 60–90 days.
Spot blood sugar	Measures current metabolic states; gives an up-to-date reading on how high or low blood glucose is during the past hour.
Blood pressure	Measures current state of arterial resistance which may be influenced by failure to take medications, or other causes.
Digital pedometer	Measures distance patient is walking, which may be a good proxy indicator of amount of exercise patient is obtaining.
Body weight	Measured in pounds or kilograms, this indicator measures the effectiveness, or lack of effectiveness, of dietary intervention. It may also measure fluid retention such as is found in congestive heart failure patients.
Pain	Indicators of pain include patients' verbal rating on a 0–10 scale with 0 referring to no pain and 10 referring to the worst pain ever. There are also "happy-sad face" drawings for children to rate pain.

pliant patients have the worst blood sugars, whereas some of the least compliant can have glycosylated hemoglobin readings within desired limits. Other disease processes may not have reliable indicators of health status. Therefore, patients who attend smoking cessation programs and who stop smoking may lead the program directors to believe that smoking cessation was a result of the patient education, when in fact it was caused by some other unrelated event.

Other Research Challenges

Other problems related to research methods have been identified (Holloway, Spivey, Zismer, & Withington, 1988; Oberst, 1989; Redman, 1997). For example, the teaching interventions themselves are usually incompletely described so that replication of both the intervention and the study are impossible. Because many patient education programs have developed outstanding curricula that could be used throughout the United States, reporting of patient teaching interventions must be carefully delineated. This reporting would provide greater support to the comparisons and meta-analyses that are frequently done to assess the efficacy of patient education.

Oberst (1989) points out that in some programs, no testable relationship exists between the program's objectives and the interventions. This problem is being solved as standards of practice are developed. The American Diabetes Association (ADA) developed standards of practice as guidance for educational programs that desire certification from ADA. The ADA requires that objectives be developed in 15 areas considered crucial to diabetes education. For ADA certification, the patient education program must demonstrate where and when achievement of the objectives is implemented and how the objectives are evaluated.

Other problems involve the failure to include a control, or comparison, group and to account for intervening or mediating variables (Holloway et al., 1988; Oberst, 1989). The nature of the teaching intervention for control groups is usually poorly described or simply referred to as "standard care." Thus, the reader of the research has a limited understanding as to what the experimental intervention is being compared.

Mediating variables include factors such as age, gender, socioeconomic status, and educational level. As Holloway and colleagues (1988) point out, variable factors also include personality and aptitude, which may interact in a manner that influences the effectiveness of the teaching intervention. Holloway's group notes that studies should have a sufficient sample size, so that a range of learner characteristics (eg, previous knowledge, personality factors, and attitudinal or predispositional attributes) can be measured. However, to search for such interactions mandates a large sample size and random selection.

Age, gender, socioeconomic status, and educational level are powerful mediating variables that should always be considered in research on patient education. As Chapter 4 points out, it is important to consider age, not only from the vantage point of maturation, but also from the viewpoint of contextual factors, such as historical and cohort effects that influence attitudes toward patient education. Gender effects intersect with age across the life span and these interactions require even larger sample sizes to determine their influence on patient educational outcomes. Socioeconomic status and education are also entwined and are frequently the most powerful predictors of patient educational outcomes (with higher education predictive of better outcomes).

In any patient education research, patient illness factors must be considered (Oberst, 1989). Most patient education occurs in the hospital setting; however, shortened hospital stays frequently mean that patients are no longer amenable to in-depth patient teaching while hospitalized because their physical condition mitigates against it. Surgical patients who still experience the effects of anesthesia and medical patients whose cardiac function has been impaired by an MI may be discharged to a long-term care facility or home before they are capable of understanding any but the most basic patient teaching. Therefore, the effects of the in-hospital patient teaching program are likely to be minimal and measurement of educational outcomes appears poor when the intervening variable, patient condition, is not considered.

Another important intervening variable is the characteristics of the patient educator (Oberst, 1989; Redman, 1997). If patient education research is supposed to test the efficacy of the intervention, then the people conducting the intervention should not vary. However, as all of us know, nurses and other health care providers vary in their ability to teach, their enthusiasm for teaching, and their commitment to patient education. If possible, differences between educators should be examined by group so that researchers can state with certainty that outcomes are a result of the entire program and not merely dependent on a particularly charismatic patient educator.

Characteristics of Patient Education Research

Carol Lindeman is a noted nurse researcher and educator who conducted some of the seminal research on patient education (Lindeman & Van Aernam, 1971; Lindeman & Stetzer, 1973). Her 1988 review of nursing research on patient education published in the *Annual Review of Nursing Research* is the last, systematic integrated review of nursing research in patient education. She examined five research variables that influence human learning (Lindeman, 1988):

1. Patient characteristics
2. Nurse characteristics
3. Nurse-patient interaction in teaching situations
4. Health- and disease-specific characteristics
5. Health care setting characteristics

Lindeman summarized the findings for each of the five variables that affect patient education outcomes. The following generalizations were made for those studies that were primarily examining patient characteristics. First,

psychological factors alone are not strong predictors of outcomes, but when used in interaction models with specific teaching strategies, psychological factors are predictive of patient education outcomes. Second, socioeconomic status and educational levels are positively related to patient education outcomes. A third generalization involved the timing of patient teaching. Lindeman's review indicated that the timing of teaching did not seem to be important.

 The fourth finding was related to family involvement. Research indicates that inclusion of the family enhances patient outcomes. Research by nurses and other health care providers increasingly documents the family stress caused by illness (Rankin & Monahan, 1991); however, it is not always easy to support the effectiveness of family education (Reeber, 1992). Some research conducted since Lindeman's review has substantiated the importance of including spouses and other family members in patient education (Gilden, Hendryx, Casia, & Singh, 1989), although there have been no systematic studies of the effects of family members participating in patient education in the period 1995 to 1999. Although most nurses pay lip service to the importance of including family members, research is unavailable to support the efficacy of such practices. ■

Only two studies focused on characteristics of the nurse as teacher, and, as Lindeman remarks, it is difficult to generalize from only two studies. One study cited by Lindeman, however, supported the authors' contention that higher levels of nursing education are related to better patient education outcomes.

The third and fourth variables in patient education research that Lindeman reviewed were health- and disease-specific patient populations and nurse-patient interaction in terms of instructional strategies developed for each. The greatest number of studies (n = 92) reviewed by Lindeman were in this group. The specific patient populations included in this review were maternal-child, surgical, cardiovascular, chronic illness, and psychiatric/mental health patients and patients undergoing diagnostic procedures. The first generalization involved the efficacy of patient teaching. Lindeman reports that although patients reflect knowledge and skill improvement after patient teaching, other more complex patient education outcomes, such as compliance, are affected by multiple independent variables in addition to exposure to patient education. A second generalization involved the effectiveness of various teaching strategies, and Lindeman states that most strategies are effective. She qualified this statement, however, by noting that it is impossible to determine if the teaching strategies themselves are effective or if findings are related instead to the nature of the research designs. Third, group teaching is reported to be as effective as individual teaching. Fourth, all patient groups showed some favorable outcomes as a result of patient teaching. More recent research supports most of Lindeman's statements. For example, Wilson (1997) found in a meta-analysis that both individual and group education can improve patient outcomes although some evidence exists that group teaching may be more effective in certain situations.

The fifth variable examined by Lindeman was the health care setting characteristics. Generalizations based on the nursing research reviewed indicated that the organizational structure of the health care setting was less important than the value attached to the delivery of patient education by staff and administration. Studies indicated that patients viewed education as important, and quality assurance programs are an effective vehicle for evaluating the effectiveness of patient education programs. Recently, attempts were made in an outpatient setting in New Mexico to determine if patient exposure to preventive measure materials (eg, on cholesterol screening, Pap smears, mammograms) would encourage them to ask their providers for such screening (Mead, Rhyne, Wiese, Lambert, & Skipper, 1995). When compared to a group of patients who had not been exposed to such materials, there was no difference in the number of patients who asked for screening; this led investigators to suggest that although these materials are inexpensive and readily available,

they may be ineffective in increasing patient screening (Mead et al, 1995).

Lindeman's review reflected nursing research on patient education published from 1965 through 1986, and, as mentioned earlier, there have been no published reviews by nurses on patient education since 1988. Although some of the 120 studies were conducted with scientific rigor, others were limited in their ability to be generalized by their small sample size, lack of randomization, and design and methodology problems. The following review of patient education research in major illnesses reveals problems; however, these problems are certainly not limited to nursing research.

The following section reviews research conducted by nurses and other health care professionals to determine what we presently know about patient education. Most of the research reviewed is based on meta-analyses or literature reviews and includes important work in the areas of diabetes, coronary heart disease, and cancer.

PATIENT EDUCATION RESEARCH IN DISEASE- AND CONDITION-SPECIFIC AREAS

Although the contribution nursing has made to patient education research is substantial, other disciplines and professions have participated in equally important ways. Important patient education research has been conducted for specific target populations by other health professionals. A review of patient education research follows. This review is in the area of three chronic illnesses: diabetes, cancer, and coronary heart disease. These illnesses are especially amenable to patient education and are among the greatest causes of morbidity and mortality in North America and Western Europe.

Diabetes

The efficacy of patient education in accomplishing desired outcomes in terms of diabetes management, metabolic control, and prevention of complications has been an area of controversy for some time. Although the evidence seems to support diabetes teaching and treatment programs (DTTP), the methods of best accomplishing the desired outcomes still require clarification (Albano, Jacquemet, & Assal, 1998; Assal, Muhlhauser, Pernet, Gfeller, Jorgens, & Berger, 1985; Brown, 1992; Brown, 1990; Delamater, Bubb, Davis, Smith, Schmidt, White, & Santiago, 1990; Muhlhauser, Overmann, Bender, Bott, Jorgens, Trautner, Siegrist, & Berger, 1998).

The emergence of laboratory tests [eg, glycosylated hemoglobin 1c (Hg1c)] and home blood glucose monitoring devices has led to more accurate evaluation of metabolic control. Brown's meta-analysis of diabetes research revealed that younger patients had better knowledge outcomes but that patients of all ages demonstrated improved glycosylated hemoglobin levels between 1 month and 6 months after the teaching intervention, but then declined to the 1-month level (Brown, 1992).

Muhlhauser and others documented long-term improvement in Hg1c values up to 22 months for patients with type I diabetes who attended DTTPs in West Germany, whereas Tildesley documented similar findings in Canada (Muhlhauser, Jorgens, Berger, Graninger, Grtler, Hornke, Kunz, Schernthaner, Scholz, & Voss, 1983; Tildesley, 1996). Assal and colleagues reported an incidence rate of 0.19 severe hypoglycemic reactions in 434 patients attending DTTPs (Assal et al., 1985). Muhlhauser and others compared this rate to 0.54 episodes per patient for the general diabetes population (Muhlhauser, Berger, Sonnenberg, Koch, Jorgens, Schernthaner, Scholz, & Padagogin, 1985). Abourizk's work demonstrated a similar improvement trajectory as measured by glycosylated hemoglobins to those found by Brown and Muhlhauser; however, sustained improvement was generally related to those subjects who had had diabetes for 2 years or less (1994). Abourizk surmises that improvement in metabolic control in people with diabetes who have been diagnosed more recently is probably related to increases in knowledge, whereas those with longer-term diabetes may improve metabolic control through knowledge reinforcement (Abourizk, O'Connor, Crabtree, & Schnatz, 1994).

Prevention of complications (eg, peripheral vascular problems, gangrene, amputations) has also been viewed as an important outcome of diabetes education for patients. Assal and associates found a decrease of 85% in below-knee amputations in a group of patients at the University Hospital of Geneva after specific foot care teaching (Assal et al., 1985). They asserted that the surgical savings are equivalent to the annual salaries of the entire staff of 12 at the Geneva Diabetes Treatment and Teaching Unit.

 The intrusiveness of diabetes into all aspects of individual and family life makes this disease especially conducive to patient education efforts.

Work by Gilden and colleagues (1989) suggests that older, married men with diabetes may be more amenable to diabetes education programs than younger men. For example, older men reported significantly higher quality of life and decreased stress than younger men after a teaching intervention.

Dunn (1986) also studied the importance of age in adjustment to diabetes by comparing a group of 300 subjects, ranging from young to middle-aged to elderly. The subjects were studied from the time of diagnosis up to 2 years after. He found that the youngest and oldest patients had more problems adjusting emotionally to the diagnosis of diabetes than did the middle-aged patients. Dunn surmised that middle-aged patients have so many family and career demands that the diagnosis had little emotional impact. Thus, findings regarding the influence of age and patient educational interventions on knowledge, metabolic, and quality of life outcomes appear to be contradictory although results of a more recent meta-analysis (Brown, 1992) suggest that age does influence knowledge outcomes (eg, older age is associated with lower levels of knowledge acquisition). ■

Patient perspectives on diabetes education have been assessed in research studies (Duchin & Brown, 1990; Wikblad, 1991; Hunt, Arar,

& Larme, 1998). Although it may seem self-evident that the patients should be polled about their specific needs, this practice has not been a part of most diabetes teaching programs. Therefore, the three studies cited are important examples of research that attempt to understand patient perceptions of their own learning needs. In general, patients with diabetes desire less pathophysiology and a greater emphasis on survival skills. They also report a need for individualized patient education based on their own disease trajectory and an understanding of their own personal attempts to control their diabetes when health care providers accuse them of being "out of control." The issue of control, including metabolic control, patient actions taken to manage diabetes, and provider attempts to exert control, is a fertile area of research for determining the most effective methods of helping patients with diabetes manage their diabetes.

Patient education in diabetes management has a long and distinguished history. Early studies conducted by Etzwiler (1967) looked at the knowledge young patients with diabetes and their parents had about diabetes and discovered that neither patients nor their parents had an adequate grasp of basic information about diabetes. Proper control was surmised to result from "well informed patients cooperating with interested and knowledgeable nurses, dietitians and physicians" (Etzwiler, 1967, p. 111). Patient education has become better regulated and precise with the entry of the American Association of Diabetes Educators (AADE), a professional group established in 1969 that certifies diabetes educators. AADE has also established a foundation that supports research in the area of diabetes and patient education. The ADA and the National Institute of Diabetes, Digestive, and Kidney Diseases (NIDDK) are two other organizations that underwrite research in diabetes and patient education.

Research in the area of diabetes patient education has demonstrated improved outcomes in terms of better metabolic control and decreased complications. The advent of glycosylated hemoglobins has given the diabetes health care provider a "gold standard" by which to judge the long-term effects of patient education, a tool that is not replicable in the study of other chronic illnesses. The importance of including the family in diabetes management classes and in focusing on psychosocial interventions needs greater attention by researchers (Padgett, Mumford, Hynes, & Carter, 1988).

Diabetes patient education research illustrates some provocative, although contradictory, findings related to age and the efficacy of diabetes patient education. Age is an important variable that should be included in studies of other chronic illnesses and patient education. Last, the use of new technologies in monitoring diabetes by telephone modem (Ahring, Ahring, Joyce, & Farid, 1992), computer assisted instruction (Glasgow, Toobert, & Hampson, 1996), and diabetes Web sites (McKay, Feil, Glasgow, & Brown, 1998) have proved useful in terms of decreased glycosylated hemoglobin values and enhancing knowledge acquisition. These new technologies should be monitored in the future as their promise for efficient and low cost education is immense.

Cancer

Patient education provided by nurses and directed toward cancer diagnosis, treatment, rehabilitation, and survival has helped change the way cancer is viewed (ie, cancer is considered a chronic rather than a terminal illness). Patient and health care provider partnerships have replaced the previous concept of the patient being the passive recipient of information from the physician (Adams, 1991). However, there are acute, unmet needs for knowledge during the diagnostic, treatment, rehabilitation, continuing care, and remission periods, and during recurrence or advanced disease (Adams, 1991; Coughlan, 1993; Corney, Everett, Howells, & Crowther, 1992; Palsson & Norberg, 1995).

Reviews by Rimer and Fawzy of research relating to patient education and cancer examined patient education approaches related to three categories [diagnosis, treatment, and rehabilitation and continuing care (Rimer, Keintz,

& Glassman, 1985)] or in terms of types of psychosocial interventions [eg, education, behavioral training, individual psychotherapy, and group interventions (Fawzy, Fawzy, Arndt, & Pasnau, 1995)]. Rimer's review is examined first.

During the diagnostic period, pertinent research studies (n = 9) revealed that patients wanted more information about all aspects of various treatment regimens and prognosis. Demographic characteristics (eg, age, educational background, socioeconomic status) were important predictors of the type of information desired. Agre and colleagues studied the amount of time nurses spend teaching cancer patients in the inpatient setting (Agre, Bookbinder, Cirrincione, & Keating, 1990). They documented that in one setting each cancer patient received 16.6 minutes of instruction each day, which they calculated as a significant amount of time. However, patients still do not believe they receive adequate information about diagnostic and treatment strategies despite the constant development of new approaches (Porter, 1998).

Research related to patient education and treatment of cancer (n = 13) indicated that information related to treatment diminished side effects and decreased oral infections. Additionally, several studies have demonstrated the efficacy of relaxation training, hypnosis, and guided imagery in reducing anticipatory nausea and vomiting related to chemotherapy. Studies related to compliance with treatment regimens have illustrated the usefulness of various educational approaches and professionals in improving compliance.

Patient education directed toward rehabilitation and continuing care (n = 3) has demonstrated to enhance coping strategies, improve relationships with health professionals, and increase self-concept and self esteem (Rimer et al., 1985). Generally, few studies of pain control with cancer patients are related to patient education or other aspects of continuing care.

Rimer and colleagues noted the following weaknesses in their review of various studies of patient education and cancer: lack of multiple impact measures, no health outcome measures,

inadequacy of process data documenting patient education, small sample size, unsatisfactory and inappropriate instruments, and inappropriate statistical tests (Rimer, Keintz, Glassman, 1985). The authors also point out that studies frequently tend to view multidimensional constructs, such as compliance, as unidimensional and tend to neglect the effects of patient education on health status or the costs of medical care.

The Fawzy review points out the importance of both educational and psychosocial approaches to achieving better quality of life and enhanced physical and psychological outcomes (1995). Their review suggests that a combination of treatment modalities, including health education, stress management and behavioral training, problem-solving and coping strategies, and group interventions, are most effective with patients who are newly diagnosed or in the early phases of treatment. A combination of strategies, rather than a single approach, is most likely to provide the necessary skills for living with cancer. They further propose, based on Spiegel's work (Spiegel, Bloom, & Yalom, 1981; Spiegel, Bloom, Kraemer, & Gottheil, 1989), that patients with advanced metastatic disease are likely to benefit from weekly group support that focuses on pain management, daily coping, and dealing with existential issues related to death.

A third review by Helgeson and Cohen (1996) finds overwhelming support for educational interventions, although the type of support most desired by cancer patients is emotional support. Their findings are mixed in terms of the efficacy of short-term peer discussion groups and they suggest that educational interventions directed at providing informational support appear to have an equal, if not greater, impact on adjustment than peer discussion. They suggest that one-on-one peer discussion might be more helpful than group discussion, because frequently, many differences exist in terms of prognosis, treatment, and diagnosis in peer discussion groups.

An important impetus in the education of patients with cancer is the recognition by the American Cancer Society (ACS) and the National Cancer Institute (NCI) that patient education should be an integral part of cancer care. The "I Can Cope" program, developed by two oncology nurses in Minnesota, was adopted nationally by the ACS and implemented in 1979 (Stevenson & Crosson, 1991). Concomitant with the adoption of the "I Can Cope" program was the federally sponsored NCI program, also implemented nationally in 1979, and entitled "Coping with Cancer." The two national cancer organizations have developed programs to benefit the public, although the NCI traditionally works through health care professionals (eg, the Oncology Nursing Society). The ACS focuses on the community, with 3000 ACS offices spread across the country (Stevenson & Crosson, 1991). Both the ACS and the NCI sponsor research related to cancer patient education for individuals and families.

The research related to patient education and cancer is not unlike that for heart disease and diabetes. For example, patients report they do not have adequate knowledge to make treatment decisions nor are they made aware of their trajectory of illness. As in the other two major chronic illnesses reviewed in this chapter, patient teaching research has gained during the past 20 years with the injection of doctorally prepared nurses competent in conducting research in the area of cancer and patient and family education.

Coronary Heart Disease

Coronary heart disease (CHD) causes more deaths than any other single disease for both men and women (Heart Facts, 1999). Shortened hospital stays for myocardial infarction (MI) make nurses and other health care providers question if patient teaching is even appropriate for the hospitalization period. Duryee's review (1992) and the meta-analysis of Mullen and colleagues (Mullen, Mains, & Velez, 1992) indicates that formal, structured education increases patients' knowledge and positively influences blood pressure, mortality, exercise, and diet.

Duryee's analysis concentrated on the inpatient phase of patient education after MI.

Although the national mean length of stay for the time she reviewed was 7 days to 11 days (currently, it is 4 days to 5 days for an uncomplicated MI), the authors speculate about whether the same knowledge outcomes would be achieved. Likewise, the authors question if patients can incorporate education that is supposed to result in lifestyle changes. In particular, teaching that attempts to effect behavioral changes is ineffective when provided on an inpatient basis (Waitkoff & Imburgia, 1990). Duryee's analysis indicates that most studies demonstrate lifestyle changes in areas of activity and smoking but less frequently in diet.

A third variable studied by Duryee that is influenced by shorter hospital stays is the most beneficial time for teaching in terms of anxiety level. Most of the studies she reviewed indicate that teaching during the stay in the coronary care unit is much less efficacious than teaching 7 days to 10 days after the cardiac event. Because most patients are discharged by this time, it seems that anxiety levels may be high enough during the contemporary hospitalization period that learning is not easily achievable. On the other hand, the coronary artery bypass graft patient (CABG) may incorporate information more easily and quickly. For example, Beggs and colleagues found in a study of collaborating institutions that overall patients were well prepared for discharge after CABG (Beggs, Willis, Maislen et al, 1998). These findings might be related to the fact that CABG patients are usually younger than MI patients and that teaching for these patients is more easily standardized.

Other helpful information from Duryee's and Mullen's systematic reviews involves the type of content and the type of educational strategy needed by CHD patients. Generally, staff and patients report that information on management of symptoms and reduction of risk factors is crucial; less crucial is material relating to pathophysiology of heart disease. Length of the patient education intervention was not found to be influential. Some studies indicated that use of audiovisual materials (eg, slide-tape presentations) were just as effective as live educators. A study of a patient-family pathway after CABG did not find any statistically significant differences in terms of length of stay, anxiety, and knowledge levels between those patients and families who experienced the pathway and the control group (Sagehorn, Russell, & Ganong, 1999).

Mullen and colleagues (1992) found that behavior-oriented interventions rather than didactic-oriented interventions were more successful in achieving the desired outcomes. The Mullen group noted that important educational principles were rarely applied. For example, attempts to educate patients to take recommended actions for symptoms or problems were uncommon. Reinforcement and feedback, important components of effective patient education, were also routinely neglected.

Because hospital stays are now so much shorter for acute cardiac events than in previous years, it may be more logical to institute patient education and lifestyle change programs on an outpatient basis. The nurse-managed smoking cessation program described by Taylor and colleagues (Taylor, Houston-Miller, Killen, & DeBusk, 1990) is an example of a useful model for inpatient and outpatient teaching. This program used written materials in the hospital that teach coping strategies for smoking cessation. Before hospital discharge, patients were oriented to audiotapes for progressive muscle relaxation and provided with written materials. After discharge, coronary care unit nurses with special training telephoned patients to provide instruction and support. Patients who were in the experimental group had significantly lower smoking rates 12 months after discharge from the hospital. This model demonstrates a low-cost, low-technology patient education intervention for lifestyle changes.

Taylor and colleagues have continued working with MI patients and have developed a multifactorial, risk-reduction program to reduce psychological distress. Their study of 585 men and women 70 years old or younger revealed no significant differences between the group that received the intervention during their recovery and the group that received standard care; psychological distress decreased significantly for both groups (Taylor, Miller, Smith, & DeBusk, 1997). The intervention worked well for subjects with low anxiety levels and also reduced anger in those subjects who had reported frequent episodes of anger (Taylor et al, 1997). These findings suggest that intervention should be tailored for different patient characteristics.

Carlsson and colleagues studied outcomes for MI patients referred to an intervention group that consisted of education regarding the effects of smoking cessation, dietary management, and regular physical activity (1997). The educational intervention was managed by a nurse; the control group was comprised of patients randomized to usual care provided by their primary care providers. Those subjects in the intervention group significantly improved their dietary management when compared to the controls and also improved in the area of smoking cessation, although the difference was not statistically significant. Exercise program results did not reflect a difference between the intervention and control patients. Carlsson and colleagues surmised that if the smoking cessation program had been initiated at the time of hospitalization and then had been followed by repeated counseling, the results might have been more favorable for the intervention group. Fifty percent of the smokers in the intervention group ceased smoking as compared to 29% of the smokers in the control group. This study is important to understanding the long-term effects of patient education, because the follow-up point was one year after hospitalization. Most studies do not follow subjects who participate in this type of intervention for one year, making this research an important contribution to the literature on MI and patient education research.

Patient education and research in the field of patient teaching and heart disease have been given impetus by two national organizations, the American Heart Association (AHA), a voluntary organization, and the National Heart, Lung, and Blood Institute. Like the ADA, most of the research funding within the AHA has been oriented toward physicians. However, this orientation has changed during the past 15 years through the strong nursing involvement in the AHA's Cardiovascular Nursing section.

The authors believe that patient education in heart disease has not been as well organized or as well studied by nurses as patient education in diabetes and cancer has. This may be because patient education in heart disease is less focused than in diabetes, owing to the diverse presentation and treatment of heart disease (eg, hypertension, coronary artery disease, congenital cardiac lesions); also, heart disease frequently has a longer period of chronicity than does cancer. Studies of patient education for preventive health behaviors important to heart disease have been strong in smoking cessation, nutrition, and weight control but weak in the areas of exercise and stress management (Simons-Morton, Calfas, Oldenburg, & Burton, 1998; Simons-Morton, Mullen, Mains, Tabak, & Green, 1992). Therefore, the authors recommend more nursing and other health professional research efforts in these areas.

Reviews of patient education directed toward cardiac patients reveal some of the same issues documented by research in diabetes patient education. Thus, it appears that the message, not the method, is important, and that the message should concentrate on survival skills needed to manage a chronic condition rather than the underlying pathophysiology. Programs oriented toward behavioral changes are more efficacious than those solely focused on knowledge acquisition. Shorter hospital stays mandate outpatient education, because memory and conceptualization abilities are influenced by changes in biochemical parameters.

Summary of Patient Education Research Findings

In summarizing findings from review articles, we note the emergence of pervasive themes across various diseases and as cited by health professionals in different fields. First, patient education is positively related to knowledge accrual and many beneficial psychosocial and physical health outcomes. Second, various teaching strategies, including one-on-one,

group, audiovisual, and psychoeducational strategies, have proved useful. The combination of strategies to reinforce learning is probably more effective than a single strategy. Third, to influence health outcomes and achieve maximal levels of adherence to medical regimen, patient education must be repetitive and reinforced at different time periods.

Fourth, demographic characteristics such as age, educational background, and socioeconomic status must be considered when patient education programs are designed because they have different impacts on patient education outcomes. Although psychological factors have been frequently studied as predictors of patient education outcomes, they are more important when considered in their interaction with various teaching strategies than when examined alone. A fifth finding involves social support as a strategy to enhance patient education. Whether social support is available as part of a group interaction technique or through inclusion of family members, the provision of social support probably interacts with the teaching intervention to increase the efficacy of patient education.

HEALTH OUTCOMES RESEARCH AND PATIENT EDUCATION

Health outcomes research is a body of research that covers quality of care to outcomes for patients. Generally, outcomes research serves as a guide to policy rather than as solely a guide to practice, although outcomes research obviously influences practice. The methodological perspective of outcomes research typically uses populations rather than individuals for samples and generally employs correlational designs that allow for statistical inferences. However, as Fig. 15-1 illustrates, it is possible to employ various levels of analysis to determine health outcomes.

In the past, quality of care has routinely been monitored in hospitals through outcomes such as mortality rates or infection rates. However, because of greater sophistication in sta-

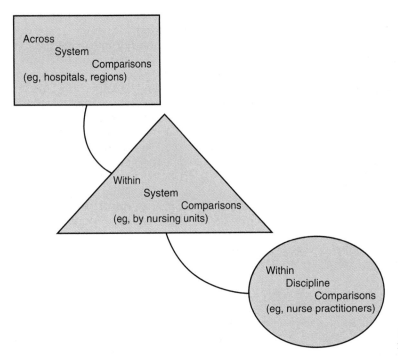

FIGURE 15-1. Levels of analysis for measuring quality of care.

tistical techniques and greater interest on the public's part, it has been found that quality of care and practice patterns vary from institution to institution, from provider to provider, and in different regions of the country (Brook, McGlynn, & Cleary, 1996). These variations are then reflected in the levels of analysis that must be considered when planning a study of quality of care.

Donabedian (1988) proposed that the quality of care can be evaluated on the basis of structure, process data, or outcomes data. *Structure* refers to organizational components, such as staffing patterns, collaborative practices, and characteristics of hospitals. *Process data* include the components of the encounter between the health care provider and the patient (ie, for nurses involved in patient education this includes knowledge levels of patients). *Outcomes data* refer to the patient's subsequent health status, such as an ability to perform self-care related to diabetes or improved mobility. To have nurse-sensitive patient outcomes, it is important to measure

outcomes that are amenable to nursing practice. Additionally, the outcomes should have reliable and valid measures. It is difficult to identify patient outcomes that are specific and sensitive to nursing intervention only (most outcomes are influenced by multiple care providers). Therefore, it is more logical to study the processes of care and, secondarily, to link processes to outcomes.

In terms of patient education and health outcomes research, the nurse is a key figure in bringing about positive health outcomes in areas such as functional status, behavioral changes, knowledge, family coping, and symptom control through the process of patient education. Research that could be conducted by the nurse to measure health outcomes includes a study designed to ascertain if all patients from three city hospitals in New York who received discharge teaching post-myocardial infarction had the same functional health outcomes at one year post-MI. Such a study would demand an across systems comparison of hospitals (see Figure 15-1).

DEVELOPING RESEARCH PROPOSALS TO STUDY THE EFFICACY OF PATIENT EDUCATION

As nursing research has increased, nurses continue to seek methods of evaluating the efficacy of their patient education efforts. We have been involved in the generation of research proposals and Sally H. Rankin has received funding from various sources, including the National Institute of Nursing Research, the NIDDK, and AHA.

Developing a research proposal is a precise and tedious process that involves following the grantor's guidelines and getting necessary materials together. The most difficult aspect of designing a research proposal is the conceptualization that must occur *before* writing the proposal. Answering the question *What do you want to know?* is the most difficult part of the proposal process. Once the investigators have determined what it is they want to know, research texts, methodologists, and statisticians can be consulted for aspects of design, sample specification, and data analysis.

The last section of this chapter outlines the different sections involved in producing a proposal that meets the guidelines of the various institutes of the National Institutes of Health (NIH), using the U.S. Department of Health and Human Services, Public Health Service (PHS) form 398. Examples are drawn from portions of an approved but unfunded proposal submitted by Dr. Rankin to the NIDDK. This proposal was chosen because the research involved patient education. The PHS format was chosen because it is one of the most rigorous and can be modified for submission to foundations or other funding sources. Form 398 is revised frequently, but the same basic elements of the application are consistent.

The same type of proposal format is used regardless if the research is qualitative or quantitative. In general, qualitative research seeks to generate hypotheses and deals with data that cannot be structured in a numbers format, whereas quantitative research includes data that can be structured in a numbers format or can be transposed into a numbers format (Brink & Wood, 1998). Whether research is qualitative or quantitative depends on the question being asked and the type of data available.

The longest and most important section of the proposal is the research plan. The proposal has nine sections (six of which are covered in this chapter):

1. Specific aims
2. Background and significance
3. Preliminary studies
4. Research design and methods
5. Human subjects
6. Vertebrate animals
7. Literature cited
8. Consortium/contractual arrangements
9. Consultants/collaborators

Items 7, 8, and 9 are well outlined in the PHS booklet and, in the case of vertebrate animals, do not apply to patient education research. These sections are found in almost all foundation and other agency proposal formats, although they may have different titles. Many private foundations ask the investigator to summarize in lay terms how the findings will benefit the population studied. We remind readers many different approaches to writing a research proposal exist and this discussion represents only one approach.

Specific Aims

The *specific aims* section of a proposal addresses the broad, long-term objectives of the proposed study. This section, which appears first, should be a concise and articulate attempt to grab the reader's interest. This section should be approximately one page; thus, the investigator must present a succinct, compelling argument for the study. Some investigators choose not to write their aims until they have developed the study in detail, so the aims reflect the study design and methods precisely. Specific aims should be translatable into research questions or hypotheses.

The specific aims that were derived for a

study to improve health outcomes for ethnic minorities with diabetes mellitus were twofold:

> The primary aim of the proposed study is: to conduct a randomized clinical trial to test the effectiveness of educational interventions (1 day versus 4 days) and family member support (family member present or absent) on selected outcome measures (metabolic control, knowledge levels, family support, quality of life, depression, and family function) at four data collection points (before intervention, and 3, 12, and 24 months after the intervention). A secondary aim describes the incidence of cardiovascular and renal complications in a sample of immigrated Chinese people with diabetes because the data are not now available.

The specific aims section also referred to a previous study funded by NIDDK that was preliminary to the randomized clinical trial and included operational definitions of important variables.

Background and Significance

The purpose of the *background and significance* section is to critically review the literature and document areas of existing knowledge that may be inadequate and specifically identify the gaps that the study is expected to fill. The background and significance section may include a theoretical model that will be tested in the study. Theoretical links to extant theories should be documented, so that the findings can later be interpreted within a theoretical framework. Literature that is reviewed should include recent work in the field and classic studies. Again, this section must be strongly stated and must demonstrate why the proposal is sufficiently unique and deserves funding.

The background and significance section in Dr. Rankin's proposal set the stage for continued study of Chinese immigrants with type II diabetes mellitus. Levanthal's self-regulation model was the theoretical framework used

(see Chapter 2). This section included the independent variables (the educational and family support interventions to enhance metabolic control) and the dependent variables (diabetes quality of life, depression, and glycosylated hemoglobin levels). The background and significance section concluded with the following statements:

> The importance of health education programs to teach self-care management skills to persons with diabetes has been highlighted by recent reports of the DCCT trial indicating that careful metabolic control in insulin dependent diabetes mellitus delays the onset of complications. Health education for people with chronic illnesses is also a national priority as described in the objectives of Healthy People 2000 (DHHS, 1990). It is a national goal to increase the proportion of people with chronic illnesses receiving formal patient education as part of illness management to 40%. Chinese Americans with NIDDM living in the San Francisco Bay Area are a rapidly growing minority population that has not been sufficiently studied. Although educational and psychosocial interventions can enhance not only short-term control of NIDDM but also quality of life for patients and their families (Padgett et al., 1988), failure to adequately address cultural factors in the designing, implementing, and testing of these interventions can reduce their effectiveness and perpetuate current disparities in health care for minorities.

The background and significance section of a proposal offers the investigator an opportunity to lay the groundwork for the study of an important phenomenon. Although the investigator may believe that her proposal offers a unique chance to study patient education, it should be recognized that many proposals to study the efficacy of patient education have been funded in the past; therefore, a proposal must be exceptional to garner funding.

Preliminary Studies

The *preliminary studies* section allows the investigator to report on his or her previous work in the same or similar areas. In this section, pilot work should be explained, so that the reviewers have an opportunity to review the investigator's expertise in the field. In nonfederal applications, this section may not be explicitly included. A summary of pilot work completed by the example study included the following statements:

This study allowed the Principle Investigator access to an important site for data collection from Chinese subjects with diabetes; critical contacts were made, and two data collection tools were translated into Chinese. This study also offered the opportunity to pilot a one-day course with the Chinese participants although there was no opportunity to compare a Chinese one-day to a four-day course during this study. Answers on the Diabetes Educational Profile (a questionnaire) indicated that diabetes mellitus was perceived as a stigmatizing illness over which this group had little control and about which they had little information. Other significant information related to the enthusiasm about doing self-blood glucose monitoring, which had not been in the repertoire of this group's behaviors before; with instruction in Chinese many of the subjects began self-blood-glucose-monitoring.

A second study, also of Chinese immigrants with type II diabetes mellitus, was also included in the preliminary studies section.

Research Design and Methods

The *research design and methods* section describes the design (eg, experimental versus quasiexperimental) and the procedures that will be used to achieve the specific aims of the study. This section also includes the methods by which data will be gathered, analyzed, and

interpreted. Any statistical procedures to be used in data analysis must be described in detail. A power analysis to determine sample size should also be included. If the methods are comprised solely of qualitative methods then, likewise, the procedures for analyzing qualitative data must be described. Some private foundations refer to this section simply as procedures; however, no matter how the section is titled, it should be sufficiently detailed to allow the reviewers to understand how the study will be carried out and how the data will be analyzed. With increasing sophistication on the part of reviewers and less funding available, the investigator must be comprehensive and articulate in describing the research design and methods. The following portion of the proposal describes the proposed design:

A three-factor, randomized clinical trial with a longitudinal, repeated measures design to test selected dependent variables is planned. The two between subjects factors are length of intervention (1 day versus 4 days) and family support (family present or absent) and the one within subjects factor is time (before intervention, 3, 12, and 24 months after intervention). Dependent variables are biobehavioral and cognition based: metabolic control measured by glycosylated hemoglobin tests, MDRTC diabetes knowledge levels, family support, and emotion based: psychosocial impact, quality of life, depression, and family function. Data are collected before the intervention begins, and at three, twelve, and twenty-four months after the intervention.

This section also included subsections on setting, recruitment strategies, sample criteria, sample size, descriptions of the teaching interventions, and descriptions of the various data collection instruments (questionnaires) and equipment (a piece of portable medical equipment that analyzed Hb1c), procedures and measurement, and data analysis. For example, the portion of the proposal that related to coding and missing data read:

> Data will be entered on a personal computer using the SPSS-9 for Windows statistical package. After data reduction to the appropriate subscales, analysis will proceed using SPSS-9. Two-tailed levels of significance will be set at .05. Missing data will be handled as follows: when no more than 20% of the items from a scale or subscale are missing, the mean of the scale or subscale will be substituted for that person's missing values; however, if more than 20% of the items are missing, the scale or subscale will be treated as missing for that person. Descriptive statistics will be computed on demographic and medical data including data pertaining to cardiovascular and renal complications. Additionally, the four groups will be compared on major covariates (eg, age, gender, education, income, and cardiovascular and renal complications) to determine that random assignment equally distributed the covariates.

The investigator should use precision and care for the research design and methods section. The authors recommend that a statistician be consulted to review this section of the proposal. Most institutions, whether hospitals or academic settings, have consulting statisticians available for this type of assistance.

Human Subjects

Human subjects is the last section in the PHS proposal format. Whether an agency requires this section in the formal proposal, the investigator must gain human subjects' clearance before commencing a study. In addition to describing the procedures that will be used with subjects or study participants, the principle investigator must also include the plans for the recruitment of subjects, the consent process, the nature of the information to be provided to prospective participants, and the method of documenting consent. Issues regarding con-

sent are covered in Chapter 6 of this book. The human subjects section of the proposal must include any potential risks to study participants and procedures for protecting subjects against potential risks. The purpose of obtaining human subjects' clearance through an institutional review board is to protect study participants to as great an extent as possible from any physical, psychological, social, legal, or other risks. This step of the grantsmanship process is of extreme importance and must never be neglected.

Concluding Remarks on Writing a Proposal

Conceptualizing, designing, and writing a research proposal is a creative endeavor that takes approximately 3 months to 6 months, depending on the resources needed. We have found that proposals that are reviewed by a group of one's peers before submission to the funding agency have a much better chance of receiving favorable reviews and funding. Colleague input may save valuable time and prevent having to rewrite proposals that are not favorably reviewed. Other means of learning the ropes of writing a proposal include mentorship by senior nurse scientists and proposal writing workshops. Many proposals are not funded during the first submission, but are patiently reworked and resubmitted for second or even third considerations. Although the process is time consuming, it is invaluable in terms of garnering funding and gaining clarity about one's own research directions.

SUMMARY

This chapter has reviewed the state-of-the-art of patient education research, reviewed research within three important chronic disease areas and the patient education research in each, and presented an approach to writing a research proposal using actual examples from a proposal. Research on patient education has become increasingly sophisticated, a fact that has helped the health care provider who needs to convince the skeptic of its efficacy. As the potential of patient education is increasingly appreciated, the research will continue to reflect the positive outcomes engendered by effective patient education.

STRATEGIES FOR CRITICAL ANALYSIS AND APPLICATION

1. If you had to convince the board of trustees in your local hospital to fund an office of patient education, which arguments based on research would you use?
2. You have been asked to design a teaching program for pediatric patients with asthma who have been prescribed inhaled bronchodilators. How would you measure the three levels of compliance—feasibility, adherence, and health status—outlined by Oberst?
3. What is the purpose of the background and significance section of a research proposal? What important points should be covered in this section if your proposal deals with prevention and detection of tuberculosis in the homeless community?

REFERENCES

Abourizk, N., O'Connor, P. J., Crabtree, B. F., & Schnatz, J. D. (1994). An outpatient model of integrated diabetes treatment and education: functional, metabolic, and knowledge outcomes. *Diabetes Educator, 20*(5), 416–421.

Adams, M. (1991). Information and education across the phases of cancer care. *Seminars in Oncology Nursing, 7*(1), 105–111.

Agre, P., Bookbinder, M., Cirrincione, C., & Keating, E. (1990). How much time do nurses spend teaching cancer patients. *Patient Education and Counseling, 16*(1), 29–38.

Ahring, K. K., Ahring, J. P., Joyce, C., & Farid, N. R. (1992). Telephone modern access improves diabetes control in those with insulin-requiring diabetes. *Diabetes Care, 15*(8), 971–975.

Albano, M. G., Jacquemet, S., & Assal, J. P. (1998). Patient education and diabetes research: A fail-ure! Going beyond the empirical approaches. *Acta Diabetologica, 35*(4), 207–214.

American Heart Association. (1999). *Heart Facts*. Dallas, TX: Author.

Assal, J. P., Muhlhauser, I., Pernet, A., Gfeller, R., Jorgens, V., & Berger, M. (1985). Patient education as the basis for diabetes care in clinical practice and research. *Diabetologia, 28*(8), 602–613.

Beggs, V. L., Willis, S. B., Maislen, E. L., Stokes, T. M., White, D., Stanford, M., Becker, A., Barber, S., Pawlow, P. C., & Downs, C. (1998). Patient education for discharge after coronary bypass surgery in the 1990s: Are patients adequately prepared? *Journal of Cardiovascular Nursing, 12*(4), 72–86.

Brink, P. J., & Wood, M. J. (1998). *Advanced design in nursing research* (2nd ed.). Newbury Park, CA: Sage.

Brook, D. H., McGlynn, E. A., & Cleary, P. D. (1996). Measuring quality of health care. *New England Journal of Medicine, 335*(13), 966–970.

Brown, S. A. (1990). Quality of reporting in diabetes patient education research: 1954–1986. *Research in Nursing and Health, 13*(1), 53–62.

Brown, S. A. (1992). Meta-analysis of diabetes patient education research: Variations in intervention effects across studies. *Research in Nursing and Health, 15*(6), 409–419.

Carlsson, R., Lindberg, G., Westin, L., & Israelsson, B. (1997). Influence of coronary nursing management follow up on lifestyle after acute myocardial infarction. *Heart, 77*(3), 256–259.

Corney, R., Everett, H., Howells, A., & Crowther, M. (1992). The care of patients undergoing surgery for gynaecological cancer: The need for information, emotional support and counseling. *Journal of Advanced Nursing, 17*(6), 667–671.

Coughlan, M. C. (1993). Knowledge of diagnosis, treatment and its side-effects in patients receiving chemotherapy for cancer. *European Journal of Cancer Care, 2*(2), 66–71.

Delamater, A. M., Bubb, J., Davis, S. G., Smith, J. A., Schmidt, L., White, N. H., & Santiago, J. V. (1990). Randomized prospective study of self-management training with newly diagnosed diabetic children. *Diabetes Care, 13*(7), 492–498.

Donabedian, A. (1988). The quality of care. How can it be assessed? *JAMA, 269*(12), 1743–1748.

Duchin, S. P., & Brown, S. A. (1990). Patients should participate in designing diabetes educational content. *Patient Education and Counseling, 16*(3), 255–267.

Dunn, S. (1986). Reactions to educational techniques: Coping strategies for diabetes and learning. *Diabetic Medicine, 3*(6), 419–429.

Duryee, R. (1992). The efficacy of inpatient education after myocardial infarction. *Heart and Lung, 21*(3), 217–227.

Etzwiler, D. D. (1967). Who's teaching the diabetic? *Diabetes, 16*(2), 111–117.

Fawzy, I., Fawzy, N. W., Arndt, L. A., & Pasnau, R. O. (1995). Cricial review of psychosocial interventions in cancer care. *Archives of General Psychiatry, 52*(2), 100–113.

Gilden, J. L., Hendryx, M., Casia, C., & Singh, S. P. (1989). The effectiveness of diabetes education programs for older patients and their spouses. *Journal of the American Geriatrics Society, 37*(11), 1023–1030.

Glasgow, R. E., Toobert, D. J., & Hampson, S. E. (1996). Effects of a brief office-based intervention to facilitate diabetes dietary self-management. *Diabetes Care, 19*(8), 835–842.

Gortner, S. R. (1983). The history and philosophy of nursing science and research. *Advances in Nursing Science, 5*(1), 1–8.

Helgeson, V. S., & Cohen, I. S. (1996). Social support and adjustment to cancer: Reconciling descriptive, correlational, and intervention research. *Health Psychology, 15*, 135–148.

Holloway, R. L., Spivey, R. N., Zismer, D. K., & Withington, A. N. (1988). Aptitude X treatment interactions: Implications for patient education research. *Health Education Quarterly, 15*(3), 241–257.

Hunt, L. M., Arar, N. H., & Larme, A. C. (1998). Contrasting patient and practitioner perspectives in type 2 diabetes management. *Western Journal of Nursing Research, 20*(6), 656–676.

Kim, H. S. (1993). Putting theory into practice: Problems and prospects. *Journal of Advanced Nursing, 18*(10), 1632–1639.

Lindeman, C. (1988). Patient education. *Annual Review of Nursing Research, 6*, 29–60.

Lindeman, C., & Stetzer, R. (1973). Effect of preoperative visits by operating room nurses. *Nursing Research, 22*(1), 4–16.

Lindeman, C., & Van Aernam, B. (1971). Nursing intervention with the presurgical patient—the effects of structured and unstructured preoperative teaching. *Nursing Research, 20*, 319–332.

Mead, V. P., Rhyne, R. L., Wiese, W. H., Lambert, L., & Skipper, B. (1995). Impact of environmental patient education on preventive medicine practices. *Journal of Family Practice, 40*, 363–369.

McKay, H. G., Feil, E. G., Glasgow, R. E., & Brown, J. E. (1998). Feasibility and use of an internet support service for diabetes self-management. *Diabetes Educator, 24*(2), 174–179.

Monti, E. J. & Tingen, M. S. (1999). Multiple paradigms of nursing science. *ANS. Advances in Nursing Science, 21*(4), 64–80.

Morse, J. M. (1996). Nursing scholarship: Sense and sensibility. *Nursing Inquiry, 3*(2), 74–82.

Muhlhauser, I., Jorgens, V., Berger, M., Graninger, W., Grtler, W., Hornke, L., Kunz, A., Schernthaner, G., Scholz, V., & Voss, H. E. (1983). Bicentric evaluation of a teaching and treatment programme for type I (insulin-dependent) diabetic patients: Improvement of metabolic control and other measures of diabetes care for up to 22 months. *Diabetologia, 25*(6), 470–476.

Mullen, P. D., Mains, D. A., & Velez, R. (1992). A meta-analysis of controlled trials of cardiac patient education. *Patient Education and Counseling, 19*(2), 143–162.

Oberst, M. T. (1989). Perspectives on research in patient teaching. *Nursing Clinics of North America, 24*(3), 621–628.

Padgett, D., Mumford, E., Hynes, M., & Carter, R. (1988). Meta-analysis of the effects of educational and psychosocial interventions on management of diabetes mellitus. *Journal of Clinical Epidemiology, 41*(10), 1007–1030.

Palsson, M. B., & Norberg, A. (1995). Breast cancer patients' experiences of nursing care with the focus on emotional support: The implementation of a nursing intervention. *Journal of Advanced Nursing, 21*(2), 277–285.

Porter, H. B. (1998). Effectiveness and efficiency of nurse-given cancer patient education. *Canadian Oncology Nursing Journal, 8*(4), 229–240.

Rankin, S. H., & Monahan, P. (1991). Great expectations: Perceived social support in couples experiencing cardiac surgery. *Family Relations, 40*(3), 297–302.

Redman, B. K. (1997). Patient education at 25 years; where we have been and where we are going. *Journal of Advanced Nursing, 18*(3), 725–730.

Reeber, B. J. (1992). Evaluating the effects of a family education intervention. *Rehabilitation Nursing, 17*(6), 332–336.

Rimer, B., Keintz, M. K., & Glassman, B. (1985). Cancer patient education: Reality and potential. *Preventive Medicine, 14*(6):801–818.

Sagehorn, K. K., Ruseell, C. L., & Ganong, L. H. (1999). Implementation of a patient-family pathway: Effects on patients and families. *Clinical Nurse Specialist, 13*(3), 119–122.

Simons-Morton, D. G., Calfas, K. J., Oldenburg, B., & Burton, N. W. (1998). Effects of interventions in health care settings on physical activity or cardiorespiratory fitness. *American Journal of Preventative Medicine, 15*(4), 413–430.

Simons-Morton, D. G., Mullen, P. D., Mains, D. A., Tabak, E. R., & Green, L. W. (1992). Characteristics of controlled studies of patient education and counseling for preventive health behaviors. *Patient Education and Counseling, 19*(8), 175–204.

Spiegel, D., Bloo, J. R., Kraemer, H., & Gottheil, E. (1989). Effect of psychosocial treatment on survival of patients with metastatic breast cancer. *Lancet, 2*(5), 888–891.

Spiegel, D., Bloom, J. R., & Yalom, I. (1981). Group support for patients with metastatic cancer. *Archives of General Psychiatry, 38*(2), 527–533.

Stevenson, E., & Crosson, K. (1991). Patient education: History, development, and current directions of the American Cancer Society and the National Cancer Institute. *Seminars in Oncology Nursing, 7*(3), 136–142.

Taylor, C. B., Miller, N. H., Smith, P. M., & DeBusk, R. F. (1997). The effect of a home-based, case-managed, multifactorial risk-reduction program on reducing psychological distress in patients with cardiovascular disease. *Cardiopulmonary Rehabilitation, 17*(3), 157–162.

Taylor, C. B., Houston-Miller, N., Killen, J. D., & DeBusk, R. F. (1990). Smoking cessation after acute myocardial infarction: Effects of a nurse-managed intervention. *Annals of Internal Medicine, 113*(2), 118–123.

Tildesley, H. D., Mair, K., Sharpe, J., & Piaseczny, M. (1996). Diabetes teaching-outcome analysis. *Patient Education and Counseling, 29*(1), 59–65.

Tolsma, D. D. (1993). Patient education objectives in Healthy People 2000: Policy and research issues. *Patient Education and Counseling, 22*(1), 7–14.

U.S. Department of Health and Human Services, Public Health Service. (1990). *Healthy people 2000: National health promotion and disease prevention objectives: Full report with commentary.* (DHHS Publication No. (PHS), 91–50212). Washington, D.C.: U.S. Government Printing Office.

Waitkoff, B., & Imburgia, D. (1990). Patient education and continuous involvement in a phase 1 cardiac rehabilitation program. *Journal of Nursing Quality Assurance, 5*(1), 38–48.

Waltz, C., Strickland, O., & Lenz, E. (1993). *Measurement in nursing research* (2nd ed.). Philadelphia: F. A. Davis.

Wikblad, K. R. (1991). Patient perspectives of diabetes care and education. *Journal of Advanced Nursing, 16,* 837–844.

Behavioral Change Strategies

Informing

Direct learning	Commonly uses a group setting such as the classroom and allows material to be shared and discussed by several individuals.
Audiovisual materials	Include written instructions, videos, tapes, structural models, computerized instruction, or even cartoons where the concepts being taught can be demonstrated.

Motivating

Self-instruction	A popular method but difficult to evaluate. An example of self-instruction is the use of "how to" books.
Bibliotherapy	A promising area of research using a combination of self-instruction and directed reading, evaluation, and group discussion. May involve inspirational story where crisis situation is resolved; reading about health risk information with follow-up counseling (Windsor et al., 1993).
Mass media	Uses persuasion and power of the written word in newspapers, radio, or TV. Influential in changing some behavior (Popham et al., 1993) but readers who experience cognitive dissonance may ignore the message or refute it (Chapman, Wong, & Smith, 1993). Mass media may also have a negative effect because of sensationalist themes of sex and violence and high power advertising.

Skill Building

Demonstration/return demonstration	Experiential method commonly used for teaching procedures, eg, how to prepare foods or engage in low-impact aerobics.
Simulation	A representation of a real-life situation to teach new behavioral responses. Practice sessions on responding to emergencies or conducting one's activities of daily living while blindfolded are examples.
Role play	A form of simulation whereby each participant assumes the characteristics of a player in a situation. Through role play, individuals can be taught in a nonthreatening atmosphere how to respond in an effective way (Weston & Cranton, 1986).

(table continued on page 414)

Skill Building

Inoculation	Also known as refusal skills training and assertiveness training are methods that prepare people for setbacks and challenges. Individuals role play potential stressful situations or exposure to real-life stress, and rehearse protective responses that will prevent backsliding (Barth, 1993). Assertiveness promotes the ability to say "no" in a comfortable and gracious way (such as upholding the decision to abstain from alcohol or refusing a high-calorie food) while respecting others' rights.
Activisim participation	Requires participation in activities such as letter writing or lobbying that create an unfavorable environment for the activity such as smoking. Also stimulates participants to resist or terminate the behavior (Edwards et al., 1992).

Modifying Attitudes and Behavior

Imagery	Creates a mental picture of a habit-free self by focusing on the competing behavior and visualizing the self without the habit. For example, individuals giving up smoking must imagine themselves as nonsmokers; seeing themselves with a cigarette in their hand or mouth must be incongruent with their picture of wholesomeness.
Cueing	A stimulus–response-based approach using human or computer-generated telephone calls, wall charts, or other types of messages to remind an individual to continue an activity. This intervention has been used to enhance medication compliance, immunizations, or appointments (Stehr-Green, Dini, Lindegren, & Patriarca, 1993).
Tailoring	Uses compromise as an interim step to change. Valuable when a suggested change is viewed as extremely difficult or impossible (eg, a stringent dietary restriction of salt or sugar).
Contracting	A verbal or written agreement toward one or more specific actions. Requires feedback to be effective.
Contingency contracting	An "if-then" approach that states a behavioral goal as well as the rewards for its achievement. Each step of change and reward are shared with a health care provider.
Graduated regimens	Implements the desired behavior changes in intermediate steps and goals. Acknowledges each level of success.
Self-monitoring	A method of self-tracking (eg, one's daily intake or weight) using a journal or diary. Frequently short-lived.
Self-confrontation	Consciously interrupts negative thinking. Person says "stop," claps hands. Works in conjunction with self-reinforcement.
Self-reinforcement	Acknowledges positive behavior and verbalizes it frequently out loud.
External reinforcement	Uses social support or continuity of care system to help maintain behavior change.
Self-generated aversive behavioral control	A method of urge control using a negative stimulus such as snapping an elastic band on the wrist or stimulating an acupressure point. Permits time to intervene between urge and acting. Is enhanced by urge replacement/response substitution with another behavioral strategy, such as taking a walk in lieu of smoking.

Other

Hypnosis	A method of behavior modification that requires the individual to be put into a receptive mental state where suggestion influences the behavior.
Acupuncture	Behavioral response believed to be a neurochemical reaction to endorphin production released by stimulating various superficial nerve endings.
Pharmacotherapy	Prescribed therapies often used with drug addictions, eg, nicotine patches or gum for tobacco addiction, Antabuse for alcoholism, and Methadone for heroin addiction.

Full reference info can be found in Chapter 7.

Index

Page numbers followed by a "t" indicate table, "b" indicates box, and "f" figure.